Midline Skull Base Surgery

Paolo Cappabianca • Luigi Maria Cavallo
Oreste de Divitiis • Felice Esposito
Editors

Midline Skull Base Surgery

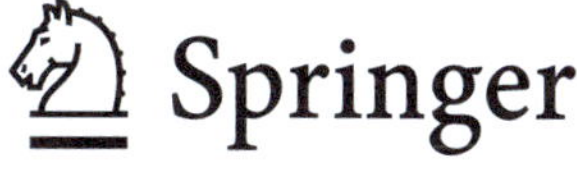

Editors
Paolo Cappabianca
Division of Neurosurgery
Department of Neurosciences
Reproductive and Odontostomatological Sciences
University of Naples "Federico II"
Naples
Italy

Oreste de Divitiis
Division of Neurosurgery
Department of Neurosciences
Reproductive and Odontostomatological Sciences
University of Naples "Federico II"
Naples
Italy

Luigi Maria Cavallo
Division of Neurosurgery
Department of Neurosciences
Reproductive and Odontostomatological Sciences
University of Naples "Federico II"
Naples
Italy

Felice Esposito
Division of Neurosurgery
Department of Neurosciences
University of Messina
Messina
Italy

ISBN 978-3-319-21532-7 ISBN 978-3-319-21533-4 (eBook)
DOI 10.1007/978-3-319-21533-4

Library of Congress Control Number: 2015956787

Springer Cham Heidelberg New York Dordrecht London

Printed on acid-free paper

Springer International Publishing AG Switzerland is part of Springer Science+Business Media (www.springer.com)

Preface

> Understand before you take any decision. Learn. Know.
> Then use the proper indications, the proper technique,
> the proper instruments.

Pier Paolo Pasolini, an Italian anti-conformist intellectual of great stature, stated that it is mandatory to revivify tradition in order to reinforce it, seldom antagonizing it with new ideas. This dictum perfectly suits the revolution that endoscopy has brought about within the fields of cerebral and ventricular neurosurgery during the past 30 years.

The endoscope is an instrument which, thanks to the intimate, close-up views that it affords, has contributed in expanding knowledge and in unlocking areas (e.g., the cavernous sinuses) and pathologies (e.g., craniopharyngiomas) in which progress was very much needed. This tremendous boost, however, did not mark the end for the preexisting techniques, approaches, and technologies; rather, endoscopy has aided the refinement of indications, improved the application of principles, helped in achieving paradigm shifts, and assisted in limiting nonscientifically based acclamation of results. Certainly, the use of the endoscope has not eliminated the use of the microscope in neurosurgery. The microscope remains a valuable instrument of visualization, but the endoscope has become an alternative or a complementary instrument that has generated real competition. Similar to cataract surgery within the field of ophthalmic surgery, endoscopy has emerged from a subspecialty within a vast subject area to have a dramatic impact. The initial innovation was the consequence of a shared effort among a small number of people, but it was soon greeted enthusiastically by experts in various subspecialties, lending them new life.

Personally, I had the good fortune and the privilege of being a topic editor on endoscopy for two issues of *Neurosurgical Focus* (the online publication of the Journal of Neurosurgery Publishing Group), a supplement of *Neurosurgery* (in *Surgery of the Human Cerebrum, part II*), and two supplements of *World Neurosurgery* (official journal of the WFNS). For these opportunities, I would especially like to thank John Jane Sr, editor of the *Journal of Neurosurgery* for more than 20 years, and Micheal L.J. Apuzzo, ex-editor in chief of *Neurosurgery* and founder of *World Neurosurgery*, whose superb attitude and devotion to the synthesis of science and humanism has helped to bring about the exponential spread of the neurosurgical message among the entire community. The flourishing of endoscopy within neurosurgery and its position within the international scientific literature also could not have been achieved without the painstaking work and study under the guidance of great teachers, above all Ed Laws, and constant cultural exchanges.

Moving the focus from the endoscope to the inspiration for this book, having thoroughly investigated the indications, techniques, and results of endoscopy with an enthusiasm akin to that of beginners, we felt a need to analyze our "journey" and to compare our experiences and conclusions with the thoughts and views of the neurosurgical community. With this in mind, we have brought together renowned experts in their respective fields and surgeons who have been trained in our school or with whom professional exchanges have been mutually beneficial, enabling both parties to develop further.

It is also worth recalling here to which extent our lives have been impacted by computers in recent decades. Computers have had huge effects on our knowledge, work, operating rooms, instrumentation, studies, and projects. All of us, to different degrees, have taken advantage of this revolutionary and tumultuous process, in which computer technology and other innovative ideas have merged to create the massive flow that has so sped up our lives.

Neurosurgery is alive and active; progress continues to be made in techniques, technology, and research. We are moving forward, striving for tomorrow. Among the present and the upcoming generation, I see those born to be surgeons and those able to take a guiding role or formulate new ideas; indeed, occasionally I detect these attributes within a single person.

Last but not least, all of us, editors and authors, feel indebted to Springer for the support provided by their special editorial staff during the production of this textbook in a period of extraordinary changes.

Naples, Italy Paolo Cappabianca
Luigi M. Cavallo
Oreste de Divitiis
Messina, Italy Felice Esposito

Contents

Part I Pituitary Adenomas

1 **Introduction** 3
Paolo Cappabianca, Marialaura Del Basso De Caro, and Alessandro Villa

2 **Endoscopic Endonasal Transsphenoidal Approach** 11
Paolo Cappabianca, Luigi Maria Cavallo, Ferdinando Caranci, Michelangelo de Angelis, Vita Stagno, Davide Luglietto, Domenico Solari, and Manfred Tschabitscher

3 **Endoscopic Endonasal Ethmoid-Pterygoid Transsphenoidal Approach to the Cavernous Sinus** 35
Giorgio Frank and Ernesto Pasquini

4 **Radiotherapy and Radiosurgery** 49
Giuseppe Minniti and Claudia Scaringi

Part II Craniopharyngiomas

5 **Introduction** 61
Paolo Cappabianca, Marialaura del Basso de Caro, and Arturo Brunetti

6 **Endoscopic Endonasal Transsphenoidal Approach** 69
Luigi Maria Cavallo, Alberto Di Somma, Francesco Briganti, Domenico Solari, Federico Frio, Luigi Maffei, and Paolo Cappabianca

7 **Cystic Craniopharyngiomas: Endoscopic Endonasal Transsphenoidal Approach** 89
Neil L. Dorward, Antonio Biroli, and Michelangelo de Angelis

8 **Endoventricular Cystic Craniopharyngiomas** 99
Michelangelo Gangemi

9 **Draining Techniques for Cystic Craniopharyngiomas** 105
Alberto Delitala, Renato Spaziante, Gianluigi Zona, Andrea Brunori, Daniele Marruzzo, and Ilaria Melloni

10 Rathke's Cleft Cyst: Endoscopic Endonasal Transsphenoidal Approach 113
Felice Esposito

11 Frontotemporal Approach 121
Oreste de Divitiis, Crescenzo Capone, Teresa Somma, Andrea Elefante, Pierpaolo Di Lorenzo, Paolo Cappabianca, and Peter A. Winkler

12 Supraorbital Approach 137
Masahiro Tanji, Ibironke Ogunbameru, Garni Barkhoudarian, and Daniel F. Kelly

13 Transcallosal Approach 155
Filippo Flavio Angileri, Francesca Granata, and Francesco Tomasello

14 Radiotherapy and Radiosurgery 163
Giuseppe Minniti and Claudia Scaringi

Part III Arachnoid Cysts

15 Endoscopic Endonasal Transsphenoidal Approach 173
Felice Esposito

16 Endoscopic Treatment of Arachnoid Cysts 179
Giuseppe Cinalli, Pietro Spennato, Giuliana Di Martino, Giuseppe Mirone, and Daniele Cascone

17 Transcranial Approaches 201
Francesco Maiuri

Part IV Anterior Cranial Fossa Meningiomas

18 Introduction 211
Oreste de Divitiis, Carmela Chiaramonte, and Gianluigi Califano

19 The Expanded Endonasal Approach to Skull Base Meningiomas 215
Amin Kassam, Martin Corsten, and Richard Rovin

20 Mini-Pterional Approach to Anterior Cranial Fossa Meningiomas 223
M. Yashar S. Kalani, Nicolas O. Koechlin, Hazem J. Abuhusain, and Charles Teo

21 Subfrontal Approach 237
Giuseppe Catapano, Matteo de Notaris, Roberto Granata, Vincenzo Seneca, Giuseppe Di Nuzzo, Joaquim Enseñat, and Alberto Prats-Galino

22 Supraorbital Approach 253
Henry W.S. Schroeder

23 Radiotherapy and Radiosurgery 269
Alfredo Conti and Antonio Pontoriero

Part V Clival Chordomas

24 Introduction 283
Paolo Cappabianca, Marialaura del Basso de Caro, and Alessandra D'Amico

25 Endoscopic Endonasal Transsphenoidal Approach 289
Domenico Solari, Luigi Maria Cavallo, Enrico Tedeschi, Chiara Caggiano, Massimo Niola, Rosa Maria Gerardi, and Paolo Cappabianca

26 Skull Base Approaches to Clival Chordomas 301
Salvatore Chibbaro, Damien Bresson, Philippe Herman, and Sebastien Froelich

27 Endoscopic Endonasal Odontoidectomy 313
Salvatore Chibbaro and Stephan Gaillard

28 Radiotherapy, Radiosurgery, and Proton Beam 323
Giuseppe Minniti and Claudia Scaringi

Part VI Cranial Base Recontruction After Transcranial and Transnasal Skull Base Surgery

29 Cranial Base Reconstruction After Transcranial and Transnasal Skull Base Surgery for Median Lesions 333
Raewyn G. Campbell, Hafiz Patwa, Ing Ping Tang, Bradley A. Otto, Daniel M. Prevedello, and Ricardo L. Carrau

Index 363

List of Videos

Video 2.1 Endoscopic Endonasal Transsphenoidal Approach

Video 3.1 Endoscopic Endonasal Ethmoid-Pterygoid Transsphenoidal Approach to the Cavernous Sinus

Video 6.1 Endoscopic endonasal extended approach showing the removal of an infundibular craniopharyngioma

Video 7.1 Cystic Craniopharyngiomas: Endoscopic Endonasal Transsphenoidal Approach

Video 9.1 Draining Techniques for Cystic Craniopharyngiomas

Video 10.1 Rathke's Cleft Cyst: Endoscopic Endonasal Transsphenoidal Approach

Video 11.1 Frontotemporal Approach

Video 12.1 Supraorbital Approach

Video 13.1 Transcallosal Approach

Video 15.1 Endoscopic Endonasal Transsphenoidal Approach

Video 22.1 Endoscope-assisted microsurgical resection of a tuberculum sellae meningioma (Created by H.W. Schroeder © Henry Schroeder 2015)

Video 25.1 Endoscopic Endonasal Transsphenoidal Approach

Video 27.1 Endoscopic Endonasal Odontoidectomy

Video 29.1 Cranial Base Reconstruction After Transcranial and Transnasal Skull Base Surgery for Median Lesions

Video 29.2 Cranial Base Reconstruction After Transcranial and Transnasal Skull Base Surgery for Median Lesions

Electronic supplementary material is available in the online version of the related chapter on SpringerLink: http://link.springer.com/

Contributors

Hazem J. Abuhusain Centre for Minimally Invasive Neurosurgery, Prince of Wales Private Hospital, Randwick, NSW, Australia

Filippo Flavio Angileri Division of Neurosurgery, Department of Biomedical Sciences, Dentistry, and Morphological and Functional Imaging, University of Messina, Messina, Italy

Garni Barkhoudarian Brain Tumor Center & Pituitary Disorders Program, John Wayne Cancer Institute and Saint John's Health Center, Santa Monica, CA, USA

Antonio Biroli Victor Horsley Department of Neurosurgery, National Hospital, London, UK

Damien Bresson Department of Neurosurgery, Lariboisiere University Hospital, Paris, France

Francesco Briganti Department of Advanced Biomedical Sciences, Neuroradiology Unit, University of Naples "Federico II", Naples, Italy

Arturo Brunetti Neuroradiology Unit, Department of Advanced Biomedical Sciences, University of Naples "Federico II", Naples, Italy

Andrea Brunori Division of Neurosurgery, Department of Neurosciences "G.M. Lancisi", San Camillo-Forlanini Hospital, Rome, Italy

Chiara Caggiano Division of Neurosurgery, Department of Neurosciences, Reproductive and Odontostomatological Sciences, University of Naples "Federico II", Naples, Italy

Gianluigi Califano Division of Neurosurgery, Department of Neurosciences, Reproductive and Odontostomatological Sciences, University of Naples "Federico II", Naples, Italy

Raewyn G. Campbell Department of Otolaryngology – Head and Neck Surgery, Wexner Medical Center, The Ohio State University, Columbus, OH, USA

Crescenzo Capone Division of Neurosurgery, Department of Neurosciences, Reproductive and Odontostomatological Sciences, University of Naples "Federico II", Naples, Italy

Paolo Cappabianca Division of Neurosurgery, Department of Neurosciences, Reproductive and Odontostomatological Sciences, University of Naples "Federico II", Naples, Italy

Ferdinando Caranci Neuroradiology Unit, Department of Advanced Biomedical Sciences, Università degli Studi di Napoli "Federico II", Naples, Italy

Ricardo L. Carrau Department of Otolaryngology – Head and Neck Surgery, Wexner Medical Center, The Ohio State University, Columbus, OH, USA

Department of Neurological Surgery, Wexner Medical Center, The Ohio State University, Columbus, OH, USA

Giuseppe Catapano Department of Neuroscience, Neurosurgery Operative Unit, "G. Rummo" Hospital, Benevento, Italy

Luigi Maria Cavallo Division of Neurosurgery, Department of Neurosciences, Reproductive and Odontostomatological Sciences, University of Naples "Federico II", Naples, Italy

Carmela Chiaramonte Division of Neurosurgery, Department of Neurosciences, Reproductive and Odontostomatological Sciences, University of Naples "Federico II", Naples, Italy

Salvatore Chibbaro Department of Neurosurgery, Strasbourg University Hospital, Strasbourg, France

Giuseppe Cinalli Division of Neurosurgery, Santobono Children's Hospital, Naples, Italy

Alfredo Conti Division of Neurosurgery, Department of Biomedical Sciences, Dentistry, and Morphological and Functional Imaging, University of Messina, Messina, Italy

Alessandra D'Amico Neuroradiology Unit, Department of Advanced Biomedical Sciences, University of Naples "Federico II", Naples, Italy

Michelangelo de Angelis Division of Neurosurgery, Department of Neurosciences, Reproductive and Odontostomatological Sciences, University of Naples "Federico II", Naples, Italy

Oreste de Divitiis Division of Neurosurgery, Department of Neurosciences, Reproductive and Odontostomatological Sciences, University of Naples "Federico II", Naples, Italy

Marialaura Del Basso De Caro Anatomopathology Unit, Department of Advanced Biomedical Sciences, University of Naples "Federico II", Naples, Italy

Alberto Delitala Division of Neurosurgery, Department of Neurosciences "G.M. Lancisi", San Camillo-Forlanini Hospital, Rome, Italy

Matteo de Notaris Department of Neuroscience, Neurosurgery Operative Unit, "G. Rummo" Hospital, Benevento, Italy

Pierpaolo Di Lorenzo Division of Legal Medicine, Department of Advanced Biomedical Sciences, University of Naples "Federico II", Naples, Italy

Giuseppe Di Nuzzo Department of Neuroscience, Neurosurgery Operative Unit, "G. Rummo" Hospital, Benevento, Italy

Alberto Di Somma Division of Neurosurgery, Department of Neurosciences, Reproductive and Odontostomatological Sciences, University of Naples "Federico II", Naples, Italy

Neil L. Dorward Victor Horsley Department of Neurosurgery, National Hospital, London, UK

Andrea Elefante Neuroradiology Unit, Department of Advanced Biomedical Sciences, University of Naples "Federico II", Naples, Italy

Joaquim Enseñat Department of Neurosurgery, Faculty of Medicine, Hospital Clinic, University of Barcelona, Barcelona, Spain

Felice Esposito Division of Neurosurgery, Department of Biomedical Sciences, Dentistry, and Morphological and Functional Imaging, University of Messina, Messina, Italy

Giorgio Frank Department of Neurosurgery, Center of Surgery for Pituitary Tumors and Endoscopic Skull Base Surgery, IRCCS Institute of Neurosciences, Bellaria Hospital, Bologna, Italy

Federico Frio Division of Neurosurgery, Department of Neurosciences, Reproductive and Odontostomatological Sciences, University of Naples "Federico II", Naples, Italy

Sebastien Froelich Department of Neurosurgery, Lariboisiere University Hospital, Paris, France

Stephan Gaillard Department of Neurosurgery, Foch Hospital, Sursenes, France

Michelangelo Gangemi Division of Neurosurgery, Department of Neurosciences and Reproductive and Odontostomatological Sciences, University of Naples "Federico II", Naples, Italy

Rosa Maria Gerardi Division of Neurosurgery, Department of Neurosciences, Reproductive and Odontostomatological Sciences, University of Naples "Federico II", Naples, Italy

Francesca Granata Division of Neuroradiology, Department of Biomedical Sciences, Dentistry, and Morphological and Functional Imaging, University of Messina, Messina, Italy

Roberto Granata Division of Neurosurgery, Department of Neurosciences and Reproductive and Odontostomatological Sciences, University of Naples "Federico II", Naples, Italy

Philippe Herman ENT Department, Lariboisiere University Hospital, Paris, France

M. Yashar S. Kalani Division of Neurological Surgery, Barrow Neurological Institute, Phoenix, AZ, USA

Centre for Minimally Invasive Neurosurgery Prince of Wales Private Hospital, Randwick, NSW, Australia

Amin Kassam Department of Neurosurgery, Aurora Health Care, Milwaukee, WI, USA

Daniel F. Kelly Brain Tumor Center and Pituitary Disorders Program, John Wayne Cancer Institute and Saint John's Health Center, Santa Monica, CA, USA

Nicolas O. Koechlin Centre for Minimally Invasive Neurosurgery, Prince of Wales Private Hospital, Randwick, NSW, Australia

Neurosurgery Clinic Lucerne Cantonal Hospital, Lucerne, Switzerland

Davide Luglietto Division of Neurosurgery, Department of Neurosciences, Reproductive and Odontostomatological Sciences, University of Naples "Federico II", Naples, Italy

Luigi Maffei Division of Neurosurgery, Department of Neurosciences, Reproductive and Odontostomatological Sciences, University of Naples "Federico II", Naples, Italy

Francesco Maiuri Division of Neurosurgery, Department of Neurosciences, Reproductive and Odontostomatological Sciences, University of Naples "Federico II", Naples, Italy

Daniele Marruzzo Division of Neurosurgery, Department of Neurosciences "G.M. Lancisi", San Camillo-Forlanini Hospital, Rome, Italy

Ilaria Melloni Department of Neurosurgery, San Martino University Hospital, Genoa, Italy

Giuseppe Minniti Department of Radiation Oncology, Sant' Andrea Hospital, University Sapienza, Rome, Italy

Radiation Oncology Unit, Department of Radiation Oncology, Sant' Andrea Hospital, University Sapienza, Rome, Italy

Department of Neuroscience, Neuromed Institute, Pozzilli (IS), Italy

Massimo Niola Division of Legal Medicine, Department of Advanced Biomedical Sciences, University of Naples "Federico II", Naples, Italy

Ibironke Ogunbameru Brain Tumor Center and Pituitary Disorders Program, John Wayne Cancer Institute and Saint John's Health Center, Santa Monica, CA, USA

Bradley A. Otto Department of Otolaryngology – Head and Neck Surgery, Wexner Medical Center, The Ohio State University, Columbus, OH, USA

Department of Neurological Surgery, Wexner Medical Center, The Ohio State University, Columbus, OH, USA

Ernesto Pasquini Department of Otolaryngology, Polyclinic Hospital of Budrio, Bologne, Italy

Hafiz Patwa Department of Otolaryngology – Head and Neck Surgery, Wexner Medical Center, The Ohio State University, Columbus, OH, USA

Antonio Pontoriero Radiation Oncology Unit, Department of Biomedical Sciences, Dentistry, and Morphological and Functional Imaging, University of Messina, Messina, Italy

Alberto Prats-Galino Laboratory of Surgical Neuroanatomy (LSNA), Faculty of Medicine, University of Barcelona, Barcelona, Spain

Daniel M. Prevedello Department of Neurological Surgery, Wexner Medical Center, The Ohio State University, Columbus, OH, USA

Department of Otolaryngology – Head and Neck Surgery, Wexner Medical Center, The Ohio State University, Columbus, OH, USA

Claudia Scaringi Radiation Oncology Unit, Department of Radiation Oncology, Sant' Andrea Hospital, University Sapienza, Rome, Italy

Henry W.S. Schroeder Department of Neurosurgery, University of Medicine Greifswald, Greifswald, Germany

Vincenzo Seneca Department of Neuroscience, Neurosurgery Operative Unit, "G. Rummo" Hospital, Benevento, Italy

Domenico Solari Division of Neurosurgery, Department of Neurosciences, Reproductive and Odontostomatological Sciences, University of Naples "Federico II", Naples, Italy

Teresa Somma Division of Neurosurgery, Department of Neurosciences, Reproductive and Odontostomatological Sciences, University of Naples "Federico II", Naples, Italy

Renato Spaziante Department of Neurosurgery, University of Salerno, Salerno, Italy

Vita Stagno Neurosurgical Unit, Alder Hey Children's Hospital, Liverpool, Merseyside, UK

Ing Ping Tang Department of Otolaryngology – Head and Neck Surgery, Wexner Medical Center, The Ohio State University, Columbus, OH, USA

Department of Otorhinolaryngology – Head and Neck Surgery, Faculty of Medicine, University Malaysia Sarawak, Kota Samarahan, Sarawak, Malaysia

Masahiro Tanji Brain Tumor Center and Pituitary Disorders Program, John Wayne Cancer Institute and Saint John's Health Center, Santa Monica, CA, USA

Enrico Tedeschi Neuroradiology Unit, Department of Advanced Biomedical Sciences, University of Naples "Federico II", Naples, Italy

Charles Teo Centre for Minimally Invasive Neurosurgery, Prince of Wales Private Hospital, Randwick, NSW, Australia

Francesco Tomasello Division of Neurosurgery, Department of Biomedical Sciences, Dentistry, and Morphological and Functional Imaging, University of Messina, Messina, Italy

Manfred Tschabitscher Department of Systematic Anatomy, Centre for Anatomy and Cell Biology, Medical University of Vienna, Vienna, Austria

Alessandro Villa Division of Neurosurgery, Department of Neurosciences, Reproductive and Odontostomatological Sciences, University of Naples "Federico II", Naples, Italy

Peter A. Winkler Department of Neurosurgery, Christian Doppler Klinik, Paracelsus Medical University, Salzburg, Austria

Gianluigi Zona Department of Neurosurgery, San Martino University Hospital, Genoa, Italy

Part I

Pituitary Adenomas

Introduction

1

Paolo Cappabianca, Marialaura Del Basso De Caro, and Alessandro Villa

Pituitary surgery is a distinct subspecialty of neurosurgery in which specific knowledge and interest of pituitary pathophysiology go with precise awareness of basic neurosurgical techniques and associated skills. Nowadays the neurosurgeon has more than one option, including the medical, surgical, and radiotherapeutic ones, alone or in various combinations, in order to manage many of the different pituitary syndromes. The best outcomes for pituitary surgery are obtained in centers where the entire range of pituitary specialties is offered in an environment of effective teamwork. The postoperative management with a long-term patient follow-up in pituitary surgery, perhaps more than other areas of neurosurgery, makes the difference between a satisfactory result and a poor result. It is in such a context that pituitary surgery should be approached today, where the neurosurgeon dealing with techniques, indications, and results resembles a member of an orchestra who is playing a refined instrument. The neurosurgeon must have a keen perception, good instincts, steady hands, and the ability to perform a tailor-made operation for the individual patient and not mass.

Pituitary adenomas are benign tumors arising from adenohypophyseal cells and represent 10–15 % of all intracranial tumors (third most common histotype). They are the most frequent lesions of the sellar region (80 %) with a prevalence of 0.02–0.03 % (200 cases per million of people); about 10 % of population has a hidden adenoma: for this reason we often have a radiological finding of a pituitary tumors (incidentaloma) in asymptomatic patients. The average age at diagnosis is 30–50 years old in 65–70 % of cases and these lesions are more common in women with a ratio of 2:1. Pituitary adenomas are classified into *secreting* (75 %) and *nonfunctioning adenomas;* following functional criteria and according to the lesion volume, we have *microadenomas* (<10 mm in diameter) and *macroadenomas* (>10 mm in diameter). Macroadenomas grow inside the pituitary fossa and can invade surrounding areas producing mass effect on important neurovascular structures. Secreting adenomas are classified according with endocrinological syndromes caused by the increase of one or more hormones:

PRL-secreting adenomas or prolactinomas cause an amenorrhea-galactorrhea syndrome in child-bearing potential women, while in men they provoke impotence. The high increase of serum prolactin levels is directly responsible for

P. Cappabianca, MD (✉) • A. Villa, MD
Division of Neurosurgery,
Department of Neurosciences,
Reproductive and Odontostomatological Sciences,
Università degli Studi di Napoli "Federico II",
Naples, Italy
e-mail: paolo.cappabianca@unina.it

M. Del Basso De Caro, BS
Anatomopathology Unit,
Department of Advanced Biomedical Sciences,
University of Naples "Federico II",
Naples, Italy

P. Cappabianca et al. (eds.), *Midline Skull Base Surgery*, DOI 10.1007/978-3-319-21533-4_1

the clinical manifestations. Diagnosis of prolactinoma is confirmed when a radiological finding of sellar lesion goes with a high increase of prolactinemia: a prolactin serum level >150 mcg/L is suggestive of a prolactinoma. On the other hand, a slight elevation in prolactin levels (25–100 mcg/L) can be caused by a functional hyperprolactinemia or a iatrogenic one (reduction of the dopamine-depending inhibitor mechanisms caused by psychotropic drugs, dopamine antagonist, estrogens, or a direct compression on the pituitary stalk). In those cases with an ambiguous diagnosis, it is possible to use functional tests as the TRH or L-DOPA stimulating test; despite these exams are effective, in most cases basal levels of PRL and neuroradiological imaging are sufficient to make a diagnosis once all the other causes of functional or iatrogenic prolactinemia have been excluded [1, 2].

GH-secreting adenomas cause pituitary gigantism during the growth and acromegaly in adults. Acromegaly determines an enlargement of extremities and of somatic characteristics of the face (enlargement of frontal bones, nose, cheekbones, eyebrows, paranasal sinuses, vocal cords, mandible, tongue, lips, and dental diastase) and is associated to systemic complications (cardiovascular, respiratory, metabolic, neoplastic), causing a higher rate of mortality in nontreated patients. As GH secretion is variable during the day, its serum sampling is not a reliable parameter. The IGF-1 serum level is a useful tool when there is the suspect of acromegaly. Another test which can confirm the diagnosis is the lack of suppression of GH levels under serum values of 0.1 ng/ml after OGTT [3–7].

ACTH-secreting adenomas are responsible of Cushing's disease, whose clinical symptoms are caused by glucocorticoid hormones' hypersecretion. Weight gain and truncal obesity with supraclavicular and cervical fat depots ("buffalo hump"), rounded "moonlike" facies, thinned skin with purple striae and multiple ecchymoses, acne and hirsutism, and proximal muscle weakness caused by muscle atrophy are the most common clinical characteristics. Hypertension, osteopenia, menstrual irregularities, and neuropsychological disturbances (e.g., depression, irritability, sleep disturbance, cognitive defects, or even frank psychosis) further characterize patients with Cushing's disease. The diagnosis of Cushing's disease requires a series of first-line tests, namely, measurement of 24 h urinary free cortisol (UFC) secretion and the evaluation of cortisol serum levels. In patients with discordant test responses, second-line testing may be performed. The dexamethasone-suppressed CRH test and desmopressin stimulation appear the most useful examinations to confirm the pituitary origin of the hypercortisolism [8]. If dynamic testing or pituitary imaging has not yield conclusive etiologic evidence, bilateral inferior petrosal sinus sampling (BIPSS) can be performed. The presence of a center-periphery ACTH gradient higher than 3 confirms the central origin of the disease and the gradient between the two sides can indicate the lateralization of the lesion.

TSH and FSH-LH adenomas are rare lesions causing, respectively, hyperthyroidism or hypogonadism syndrome, with patients often clinically asymptomatic.

On the other hand, *nonfunctioning adenomas* do not cause any specific endocrinological syndrome; usually they create deficits due to their mass effect on the surrounding structures, such as optic chiasm or cranial nerves of the cavernous sinus, and with a direct compression on the adenohypophysis provoking hypopituitarism (GH defect and hypogonadism are the most frequent) [9, 10]. The most common problems are the visual deficits caused by the compression of the optic chiasm with a partial or complete bitemporal hemianopia. In 10–15 % of cases, the cavernous sinus is invaded causing palsies of oculomotor nerves or trigeminal neuralgia. Especially with giant adenomas, when temporal or frontal lobe is involved, the mass effect on the brain tissue can lead to specific clinical manifestations such as memory deficits, personality disturbance, and seizures, while an hypothalamic compression can alter electrolytic balance or circadian rhythm. When the ventricular system is implicated, an obstructive hydrocephalus can result.

The anatomo-pathologic examination of pituitary adenomas allows to classify these entities according to their cell coloration, electronic microscope characteristics, or immunohistochemical reactions that recognize hormones produced by adenomas cells, even if the hormonal serum levels are too low to be noticed or hormones are functionally nonactive. As a matter of fact, it has been demonstrated how nonfunctioning adenomas can produce complete glycoproteic hormones (FSH, LH, TSH) or their subunits (alpha subunit, beta-FSH, beta-LH, beta-TSH) [10–12].

A neuroradiological evaluation is a key point for the diagnosis of pituitary adenomas with magnetic resonance imaging as the first choice. Coronal and sagittal images before and after gadolinium (Gd-DTPA) allow to define morphological and volumetric characteristics of the lesion, as its correlation with surrounding structures (suprasellar cistern, optic nerves, medial wall of the cavernous sinus, and internal carotid artery). In case a microadenoma is suspected, it is possible to use thin-slice acquisitions (3 mm) with dynamic sequences. CT scan has a secondary role for the sellar pathology; it can be useful for the preoperative planning of the approach, showing more details of paranasal and nasal cavities with their anatomic variations [13–15].

Therapeutic options available for the treatment of adenomas include medical therapy, surgery, and radiotherapy, but none of them is alone adequate to gain a total control of the disease. So a multidisciplinary approach is requested to choose the best option for the patient.

The normalization of excess hormone secretion, the preservation or restoration of normal pituitary function, the elimination of mass effect with restoration of normal neurological function, the prevention of tumor recurrence, and a complete histologic diagnosis are the multiple goals that therapy for pituitary adenomas is targeted to achieve.

Pituitary apoplexy is a relatively rare condition presenting with sudden headache, abrupt visual loss, ophthalmoplegia, altered level of consciousness, and collapse from acute adrenal insufficiency. It is caused by a hemorrhage in the tumor or by its acute necrosis, with subsequent swelling and frequent spreading into the subarachnoid space, leading to other signs of meningeal irritation; the related acute and severe clinical syndrome demands glucocorticoid replacement and surgical decompression, usually transsphenoidal, if visual loss is severe and progressive [16–19]. If the patient has a mild form of apoplexy and is clinically stable, it is prudent to measure the serum prolactin because some patients with prolactinoma present in this fashion and can be treated successfully with medical therapy.

Progressive mass effect is one more indication for surgical treatment. The compression of surrounding neurovascular structures usually causing visual deficit (due to compression of the optic chiasm) or less frequently cranial nerve palsy (due to compression of cranial nerves inside the cavernous sinus) needs an immediate intervention.

Having a biological, endocrinological, and anatomopathological heterogeneity, *the treatment of pituitary adenomas must be decided according with the tumor categories.*

For nonfunctioning adenomas the main goal must be the relief from the mass effect and the recovery of the endocrine functions if altered. Being the medical treatment ineffective, the first choice is surgery [20–22] and the transsphenoidal approach is the most effective. Visual deficits or endocrine dysfunction is an indication for the surgical treatment, while in all other cases, a conservative treatment can be preferred especially for those lesions smaller than 10 mm.

The normalization of the prolactin levels and the restoration from the sexual and gonadic function are the objectives of the treatment for prolactin-secreting adenomas, associated to the control and the reduction of the lesion volume. The first therapeutic option is represented by dopamine-agonist drugs such as cabergoline that in a high percentage of patients is sufficient to obtain the reduction in volume of the lesion and the normalization of the prolactin values [20, 23, 24] The surgical treatment is limited to those cases that develop a resistance, intolerance, or CSF leak after medical treatment, in case of patients with voluminous adenomas with severe neurological deficit or pituitary apoplexy or for patient's choice [25, 26]. In case of failure of both the medical and the surgical treatment, radiotherapy can be a useful tool.

For GH adenomas the surgical treatment is the option of choice with a normalization of GH and IGF-1 achieved in 44–76 % of cases. In the last decade, the preoperative treatment with somatostatin analogues or GH receptor antagonists (Pegvisomant) has been proposed as an alternative or a complement to surgery. The use of dopamine agonists is reserved for those cases in which the GH secretion is associated to high levels of prolactin [27–30].

The objective of the treatment in Cushing's disease is the normalization of the ACTH and cortisol levels and the option of choice is the surgical treatment via a transsphenoidal approach.

Pre- and postoperative pharmacological treatment and different drugs have been attempted and new agents are under investigation.

Stereotactic radiotherapy is used to treat recurrent adenomas or residual tumor after surgery. In case of all these options are not successful for the disease control, adrenalectomy is the last choice to solve the hypercortisolism.

As for the other secreting adenomas, the treatment of TSH adenomas must be direct to the mass effect relief and the hypersecretion normalization.

Transsphenoidal approach is the first option; the postoperative treatment with dopamine agonists and radiotherapy is reserved for those patients with residual tumor or still elevated levels of TSH.

Pituitary surgery was developed and has advanced on the basis of repeated innovations and exchanges between Europe and the USA. Starting with the British experience of Horsley in 1889, who performed the first operation on a pituitary tumor [31, 32], followed by Paul, a general surgeon in 1893, with a temporal decompression in an acromegalic patient [33, 34], we arrive to 1907 when with the Viennese surgeon Schloffer we had the first transsphenoidal approach [35]. Based on anatomic studies of the Italian physician Giordano [36, 37], who had analyzed the Egyptian technique used to extract cerebral tissue transnasally in the mummification process by means of special hooked instruments, without disfiguring the face, Schloffer performed a lateral rhinotomy, reflecting the nose to the right, removing the turbinates, and opening the maxillary, ethmoid, and sphenoid sinuses, before reaching the sella. In the same year, von Eiselsberg [38], in Vienna, performed a similar, if even more extended, procedure. Since then the evolution of the transsphenoidal technique had numerous contributions by eminent figures in the history of neurosurgery, such as Kocher, Kanavel, Hirsch, Hajek, and Kilian [39–46], that posed the basis for the sublabial approach performed by Cushing first and Halstead later, respectively, in 1909 and in 1910 [47–50]. After this initial enthusiasm for the transsphenoidal approach, Cushing himself abandoned this procedure [40, 51, 52] for the transcranial approach proposed by Dandy [53] who, in 1918, presented his experience in about 20 cases operated on through an intracranial intradural approach to the chiasm. A similar way had been originally used by Heuer in 1914, who described a frontotemporal route to the pituitary along the sylvian fissure [54, 55]. The two main transcranial options, subfrontal and frontotemporal, are still used today, together with more recent skull base approaches. The late 1920s to the 1960s was a relatively dark period for transsphenoidal surgery; the only one who kept this technique alive was Dott, neurosurgeon of the Royal Infirmary at Edinburgh and Cushing's pupil [40, 56], who taught the method to Guiot, laying the groundwork for the modern transsphenoidal surgery, formally started with Hardy in the late 1960s and 1970s with the introduction of the microscope [57]. Since then, the transsphenoidal approach was largely used and developed thanks to the efforts of eminent neurosurgeons such as Laws in the USA and Fahlbush in Europe. A new milestone in the evolution of this technique was the introduction of the endoscope [58]. Used for the first time by Guiot in 1963 [59] as an adjunct to the microscope to expand the field of vision (endoscope-assisted microneurosurgery), it had then been abandoned for years because it still was technically insufficient. The endoscope has come into regular use as a stand-alone visualizing and operating tool (pure endoscopic transsphenoidal surgery), thanks primarily to the work of Jho and Carrau in Pittsburgh, USA [60, 61], and of the group of Naples, Italy [62, 63]; these groups standardized an endonasal anterior sphenoidotomy approach to the sella, without the use of the operating microscope or of a transsphenoidal retractor. In the recent year the evolution of the endoscopic endonasal transsphenoidal approach allowed to remove giant and invasive adenomas by this procedure. The extended approach to the suprasellar region [64–66] as well as to the cavernous sinus [67, 68] has been recorded from several groups around the world.

Intraoperative magnetic resonance imaging (MRI), robotics, and miniaturization, as well as the rapidly emerging new insights from the biomolecular frontiers, are elements expected to change the world of pituitary surgery in the next years.

Bibliography

1. Naidich MJ, Russell EJ (1999) Current approaches to imaging of the sellar region and pituitary. Endocrinol Metab Clin North Am 28:45–79, vi
2. Casanueva FF, Molitch ME, Schlechte JA, Abs R, Bonert V, Bronstein MD, Brue T, Cappabianca P, Colao A, Fahlbusch R, Fideleff H, Hadani M, Kelly P, Kleinberg D, Laws E, Marek J, Scanlon M, Sobrinho LG, Wass JA, Giustina A (2006) Guidelines of the Pituitary Society for the diagnosis and management of prolactinomas. Clin Endocrinol (Oxf) 65:265–273
3. Giustina A, Casanueva FF, Cavagnini F, Chanson P, Clemmons D, Frohman LA, Gaillard R, Ho K, Jaquet P, Kleinberg DL, Lamberts SW, Lombardi G, Sheppard M, Strasburger CJ, Vance ML, Wass JA, Melmed S (2003) Diagnosis and treatment of acromegaly complications. J Endocrinol Invest 26: 1242–1247
4. Giustina A, Melmed S (2003) Acromegaly consensus: the next steps. J Clin Endocrinol Metab 88:1913–1914
5. Melmed S, Vance ML, Barkan AL, Bengtsson BA, Kleinberg D, Klibanski A, Trainer PJ (2002) Current status and future opportunities for controlling acromegaly. Pituitary 5:185–196
6. Scacchi M, Cavagnini F (2006) Acromegaly. Pituitary 9:297–303
7. Trainer PJ (2002) Editorial: acromegaly – consensus, what consensus? J Clin Endocrinol Metab 87:3534–3536
8. De Martin M, Giraldi FP, Cavagnini F (2006) Cushing's disease. Pituitary 9:279–287
9. Jaffe CA (2006) Clinically non-functioning pituitary adenoma. Pituitary 9:317–321
10. Katznelson L, Klibanski A (1996) Endocrine-inactive, FSH, LH and a-subunit adenomas: clinical findings and endocrinology. In: Landolt AM, Vance ML, Reilly PL (eds) Pituitary adenomas. Churchill Livingstone, New York, pp 127–138
11. Buurman H, Saeger W (2006) Subclinical adenomas in postmortem pituitaries: classification and correlations to clinical data. Eur J Endocrinol 154:753–758
12. Harris PE (1998) Biochemical markers for clinically non-functioning pituitary tumours. Clin Endocrinol (Oxf) 49:163–164
13. Chong VF, Fan YF, Lau D, Sethi DS (1998) Functional endoscopic sinus surgery (FESS): what radiologists need to know. Clin Radiol 53:650–658
14. Mason JD, Jones NS, Hughes RJ, Holland IM (1998) A systematic approach to the interpretation of computed tomography scans prior to endoscopic sinus surgery. J Laryngol Otol 112:986–990
15. Hardy J, Somma M (1979) Acromegaly. Surgical treatment by transsphenoidal microsurgical removal of the pituitary adenoma. In: Collins WF, Tindall GT (eds) Clinical management of pituitary disorders. Raven Press, New York, pp 209–217
16. Bills D, Meyer F, Laws ER Jr et al (1993) A retrospective analysis of pituitary apoplexy. Neurosurgery 33:602–609
17. Ebersold MJ, Laws ER Jr, Scheithauer BW et al (1983) Pituitary apoplexy treated by transsphenoidal surgery: a clinicopathological and immunocytochemical study. J Neurosurg 58:315–320
18. Laws ER Jr, Trautmann JC, Hollenhorst RW Jr (1977) Transsphenoidal decompression of the optic nerve and chiasm: visual results in 62 patients. J Neurosurg 46:717–722
19. Laws ER Jr (1997) Surgical management of pituitary apoplexy. In: Welch K, Caplan L, Reis D (eds) Primer on cerebrovascular diseases. Academic, New York, pp 508–510
20. Bevan JS, Webster J, Burke CW, Scanlon MF (1992) Dopamine agonists and pituitary tumor shrinkage. Endocr Rev 13:220–240
21. Lohmann T, Trantakis C, Biesold M, Prothmann S, Guenzel S, Schober R, Paschke R (2001) Minor tumour shrinkage in nonfunctioning pituitary adenomas by long-term treatment with the dopamine agonist cabergoline. Pituitary 4:173–178
22. Shomali ME, Katznelson L (1999) Medical therapy for gonadotroph and thyrotroph tumors. Endocrinol Metab Clin North Am 28:223–240, viii
23. Colao A, Di Sarno A, Cappabianca P, Di Somma C, Pivonello R, Lombardi G (2003) Withdrawal of long-term cabergoline therapy for tumoral and nontumoral hyperprolactinemia. N Engl J Med 349:2023–2033
24. Molitch ME, Elton RL, Blackwell RE, Caldwell B, Chang RJ, Jaffe R, Joplin G, Robbins RJ, Tyson J, Thorner MO (1985) Bromocriptine as primary therapy for prolactin-secreting macroadenomas: results of a prospective multicenter study. J Clin Endocrinol Metab 60:698–705
25. Molitch ME (2003) Dopamine resistance of prolactinomas. Pituitary 6:19–27
26. Semple PL, Webb MK, de Villiers JC, Laws ER Jr (2005) Pituitary apoplexy. Neurosurgery 56:65–72, discussion 72–63
27. Giusti M, Ciccarelli E, Dallabonzana D, Delitala G, Faglia G, Liuzzi A, Gussoni G, Giordano Disem G

(1997) Clinical results of long-term slow-release lanreotide treatment of acromegaly. Eur J Clin Invest 27:277–284
28. Giustina A, Barkan A, Casanueva FF, Cavagnini F, Frohman L, Ho K, Veldhuis J, Wass J, Von Werder K, Melmed S (2000) Criteria for cure of acromegaly: a consensus statement. J Clin Endocrinol Metab 85:526–529
29. Jaffe CA, Barkan AL (1992) Treatment of acromegaly with dopamine agonists. Endocrinol Metab Clin North Am 21:713–735
30. Schmitt H, Buchfelder M, Radespiel-Troger M, Fahlbusch R (2000) Difficult intubation in acromegalic patients: incidence and predictability. Anesthesiology 93:110–114
31. Fahlbusch R, Buchfelder M, Nomikos P (2002) Pituitary surgery. In: Melmed S (ed) The pituitary. Blackwell, Malden, pp 405–417
32. Horsley V (1906) Address in surgery on the technic of operation on the central nervous system. Br Med J 2:411–423
33. Caton R, Paul FT (1893) Notes on a case of acromegaly treated by operation. Br Med J 2:1421–1423
34. Jane JA Jr, Thapar K, Laws ER Jr (2002) A history of pituitary surgery. Oper Techn Neurosurg 5:200–209
35. Schloffer H (1907) Erfolgreiche Operationen eines Hypophysentumors auf Nasalem Wege. Wien Clin Wochenschr 20:621–624
36. Artico M, Pastore FS, Fraioli B et al (1998) The contribution of Davide Giordano (1864–1954) to pituitary surgery: the transglabellar-nasal approach. Neurosurgery 42:909–912
37. Giordano D (1911) Compendio di Chirurgia Operativa Italiana. UTET, Torino, pp 100–103
38. von Eiselsberg A, von Frankl-Hochwart L (1907) Uber die operative Behandlung der Tumoren der Hypophysisge- gend. Neurol Centralblatt 26:994–1001
39. Kocher T (1909) Ein Fall von Hypophysis-Tumor mit Operativer Heilung. Dtsch Zeitschrift Chir 100:13–37
40. Lanzino G, Laws ER Jr (2001) Pioneers in the development of transsphenoidal surgery: Theodor Kocher, Oskar Hirsch, and Norman Dott. J Neurosurg 95:1097–1103
41. Kanavel AB (1909) The removal of tumors of the pituitary body by an infranasal route: a proposed operation with a description of the technique. JAMA 53:1704–1707
42. Kanavel AB, Grinker J (1910) Removal of tumors of the pituitary body with a suggestion as to a two-step route, and a report of a case with a malignant tumor operated upon with primary recovery. Surg Gynecol Obstet 10:414–418
43. Hirsch O (1911) Uber Methoden der Behandlung von Hypophysistumoren auf endonasalem Wege. Arch Laryngol Rhinol 24:129–177
44. Hajek M (1904) Zur Diagnose und intranasalen chirurgischen Behandlung der Eiterungen der Keilbeinhöhle und des hinteren Siebbeinlabyrinthes. Arch Laryngol Rhinol 16:105–143
45. Kilian G (1904) Die submuköse Fensterresektion der Nasen- scheidewand. Arch Laryngol Rhinol 16: 362–387
46. Hamlin H (1981) Oskar Hirsch. Surg Neurol 16: 391–393
47. Halstead AE (1910) The operative treatment of tumors of the hypophysis. Surg Gynecol Obstet 10:494
48. Halstead AE (1910) Remarks on the operative treatment of tumors of the hypophysis: with the report of two cases operated on by an oronasal method. Trans Am Surg Assoc 28:73–93
49. Cushing H (1909) Partial hypophysectomy for acromegaly: with remarks on the functions on the hypophysis. Ann Surg 30:1002–1017
50. Cushing H (1914) Surgical experiences with pituitary disorders. JAMA 63:1515–1525
51. Cushing H (1932) Intracranial tumors: notes upon a series of two thousand verified cases with surgical-mortality percentages pertaining thereto. Charles C Thomas, Springfield, pp 69–79
52. Rosegay H (1981) Cushing's legacy to transsphenoidal surgery. J Neurosurg 54:448–454
53. Dandy WE (1934) The brain. In: Lewis D (ed) Practice of surgery. WF Prior, Hagerstown, pp 556–605
54. Heuer GJ (1920) Surgical experiences with an intracranial approach to chiasmal lesions. Arch Surg 1:368–381
55. Heuer GJ (1931) The surgical approach and the treatment of tumors and other lesions about the optic chiasm. Surg Gynecol Obstet 53:489–518
56. Liu JK, Das K, Weiss MH et al (2001) The history and evolution of transsphenoidal surgery. J Neurosurg 95:1083–1096
57. Hardy J (1969) Transsphenoidal microsurgery of the normal and pathological pituitary. Clin Neurosurg 16:185–217
58. Cappabianca P, de Divitiis O, Maiuri F (2003) Evolution of transsphenoidal surgery. In: de Divitiis E, Cappabianca P (eds) Endoscopic endonasal transsphenoidal surgery. Springer, New York, pp 1–7
59. Guiot G, Rougerie J, Fourestier M et al (1963) Explorations endoscopiques intracraniennes. Presse Med 71:1225–1228
60. Carrau R, Jho HD, Ko Y (1996) Transnasal-transsphenoidal endoscopic surgery of the pituitary gland. Laryngoscope 106:914–918
61. Jho HD, Carrau RL, Ko Y (1996) Endoscopic pituitary surgery. In: Wilkins H, Rengachary S (eds) Neurosurgical operative atlas. American Association of Neurological Surgeons, Park Ridge, pp 1–12
62. Cappabianca P, Alfieri A, de Divitiis E (1998) Endoscopic endonasal transsphenoidal approach to the sella: towards functional endoscopic pituitary surgery (FEPS). Minim Invasive Neurosurg 41: 66–73
63. de Divitiis E, Cappabianca P, Cavallo LM (2003) Endoscopic endonasal transsphenoidal approach to the sellar region. In: de Divitiis E, Cappabianca P (eds) Endoscopic endonasal T transsphenoidal surgery. Springer, New York, pp 91–130

64. Di Maio S, Cavallo LM, Esposito F, Stagno V, Corriero OV, Cappabianca P (2011) Extended endoscopic endonasal approach for selected pituitary adenomas: early experience. J Neurosurg 114(2):345–353. doi:10.3171/2010.9.JNS10262, Epub 2010 Nov 5
65. Komotar RJ, Starke RM, Raper DM, Anand VK, Schwartz TH (2012) Endoscopic endonasal compared with microscopic transsphenoidal and open transcranial resection of giant pituitary adenomas. Pituitary 15(2):150–159
66. Juraschka K, Khan OH, Godoy BL, Monsalves E, Kilian A, Krischek B, Ghare A, Vescan A, Gentili F, Zadeh G (2014) Endoscopic endonasal transsphenoidal approach to large and giant pituitary adenomas: institutional experience and predictors of extent of resection. J Neurosurg 2
67. Frank G, Pasquini E (2006) Endoscopic endonasal cavernous sinus surgery, with special reference to pituitary adenomas. Front Horm Res 34: 64–82
68. Woodworth GF, Patel KS, Shin B, Burkhardt JK, Tsiouris AJ, McCoul ED, Anand VK, Schwartz TH (2014) Surgical outcomes using a medial-to-lateral endonasal endoscopic approach to pituitary adenomas invading the cavernous sinus. J Neurosurg 120(5):1086–1094

2 Endoscopic Endonasal Transsphenoidal Approach

Paolo Cappabianca, Luigi Maria Cavallo, Ferdinando Caranci, Michelangelo de Angelis, Vita Stagno, Davide Luglietto, Domenico Solari, and Manfred Tschabitscher

2.1 Indications

The standard endoscopic endonasal transsphenoidal approach to the sella is suitable for the removal of pituitary tumors, both microadenomas and macroadenomas, and the indications are the same as those for conventional microscopic pituitary surgery [4, 13, 39].

Surgery for pituitary tumors has the goals of resection of tumor mass, normalization of hormonal hypersecretion, preservation or restoration of normal pituitary function, prevention of recurrence, and tissue sampling for diagnosis and research studies. The progressive visual loss from mass effect is a common indication for surgery as well as pituitary apoplexy, a condition caused by hemorrhage or necrosis into an existing pituitary tumor, characterized by sudden visual loss associated with headache, cranial nerves palsies, and sometimes acute adrenal insufficiency [6, 47, 57].

In case of nonfunctioning macroadenomas, owing that no medical treatment is clearly effective, the first therapeutic option is surgery being the transsphenoidal approach as the most effective [6]. Indeed, mass effect with visual defects or endocrine dysfunction (partial or total hypopituitarism) is an indication for surgical treatment; a conservative treatment can be preferred for those lesions smaller than 10 mm that do not alter any neurologic or endocrine condition [27].

Concerning secreting adenomas, transsphenoidal surgery has been advocated as the primary treatment for growth hormone-secreting lesions; however, it is worth reminding that preoperative treatment with somatostatin analogues is useful to improve the clinical conditions of the patient and can be adopted as an alternative in those cases with extremely increased surgical risk [8, 23, 25, 26].

Electronic supplementary material The online version of this chapter (doi:10.1007/978-3-319-21533-4_2) contains supplementary material, which is available to authorized users.

P. Cappabianca, MD (✉) • L.M. Cavallo, MD, PhD
M. de Angelis, MD • D. Luglietto, MS
D. Solari, MD, PhD
Division of Neurosurgery,
Department of Neurosciences,
Reproductive and Odontostomatological Sciences,
Università degli Studi di Napoli "Federico II",
Naples, Italy
e-mail: paolo.cappabianca@unina.it

F. Caranci, MD
Neuroradiology Unit, Department of Advanced Biomedical Sciences, Università degli Studi di Napoli "Federico II", Naples, Italy

V. Stagno, MD
Neurosurgical Unit, Alder Hey Children's Hospital, Liverpool, Merseyside, UK

M. Tschabitscher, MD
Department of Systematic Anatomy, Centre for Anatomy and Cell Biology, Medical University of Vienna, Vienna, Austria

P. Cappabianca et al. (eds.), *Midline Skull Base Surgery*, DOI 10.1007/978-3-319-21533-4_2

As well, the transsphenoidal surgical treatment is the first choice for the removal of radiologically evident ACTH pituitary adenomas causing Cushing's disease.

On the other hand, prolactinomas usually shrink with dopamine-agonist therapy [24]; however, in case of resistance or medical treatment-related complications, or in case patients don't tolerate or refuse it, surgical removal should be performed [14, 22, 35].

The use of the endoscopic transsphenoidal approach offers extra advantages in case of recurrent and/or residual tumors that are already treated with a transsphenoidal operation. The wide anatomical view of the surgical field provided by the endoscope helps to overcome disorientation related to eventual distorted anatomy, nasal synechiae, septum perforations, sphenoidal mucoceles, and intrasellar scars. Indeed, the direct and closeup control given along the entire procedure has reduced the risk of injury of intra- and parasellar structures [3, 20]. Furthermore, the endoscopic technique is preferred by patients having already been treated by means of the transsphenoidal microsurgical approach, thanks to the lesser postoperative nasal and breathing discomfort.

Recently, the endoscopic endonasal approach has permitted also the removal of giant adenomas, defined as lesions 4 cm or greater in maximum diameter with prevalent intracranial extension. In these cases the so-called "extended" variation of the approach with a wider bone opening over the planum sphenoidale provides a direct view of the suprasellar extension of the tumor along with a safer tumor removal [10, 30, 40, 45].

The introduction of the "extended" endoscopic endonasal approach (EEEA) has widened the indications of this technique to different pituitary adenomas such as dumbbell-shaped adenomas and pure suprasellar, recurrent, and/or fibrous lesions [7, 30]. A standard approach can be turn into an extended one when a relatively large suprasellar remnant of the lesion fails to descend and therefore cannot be removed. In such cases the use of the EEEA allows complete tumor removal, thus reducing the risk of swelling of the tumor remnant. In case of patients who have undergone a prior craniotomy, the EEEA offers a virgin surgical route, which allows the management of aspects of the lesion that could have not been accessed in the first transcranial operation. The EEEA indeed provides a double surgical corridor, intracapsular and extracapsular [30], making it complementary to craniotomy in some difficult-to-treat pituitary adenomas or representing an alternative to it [40, 45].

It has to be reminded that pituitary adenomas originate within the sella turcica so that, notwithstanding they could reach huge dimensions, the transsphenoidal route—with its standard or extended variations—represents the most direct and natural corridor to access this area. Conversely, when the tumor shows a significant intracranial extension that results out of the visibility and maneuverability of the endoscopic endonasal route, the transcranial approach still represents the most effective and viable surgical option [10].

We should conceive an "extended approach" also in its infrasellar variation, which thanks to the technique with a wider removal of nasal structures allows the surgeon to obtain an easier removal of those giant adenomas with a prevalent esocranial extension, such as adenomas invading the whole sphenoid sinus cavity, eroding the clival bone, or extending in the pterygopalatine fossa or into the nasal cavities [10].

Despite the surgeon must always attempt a "maximum-allowed" surgical outcome, it is very important to keep in mind that a wide variety of different options—medical, surgical, and radiotherapy—are now effective treatment in terms of long-term results. His/ her mind should be forged to relate the goal of surgery to the patient's needs, selecting the best option for the actual condition of the patient among all the options available, surgical or otherwise [10].

2.2 Anatomy of the Approach

The endoscopic endonasal approach represents a direct and minimally traumatic route for the removal of sellar and suprasellar lesions. Between the vestibule of the nasal cavities and the sellar floor, there are no major anatomical structures to be removed—aside from anterior wall of the sphenoid sinus—so that sella can be exposed just inserting an endoscope into the nostril and piercing the natural sphenoid ostium. As a matter of facts, the exposure does not allow a surgical procedure that requires a proper corridor to fit the instruments and handle them safely [17, 58].

Once the endoscope is inserted into the nasal cavity, the first two landmarks that are identified are the nasal septum and the lateral wall of nasal cavity that is lined out by three nasal turbinates: the inferior is the most anterior and it is recognizable as soon as the endoscope enters the nasal vestibule. Sliding further deeply, between the tail of the inferior turbinate and the nasal septum, it is possible to visualize the choana; this latter represents the most important landmark during this step, allowing the definition of the limit between the nasopharynx and the anterior wall of the sphenoid sinus. The middle and the superior turbinates are molded off the ethmoid bone; the first one can be seen angling the endoscope about 30° upward from the floor of the nasal cavities. The head of the middle turbinate can be less or more pneumatized. Its tail usually lies at the level of the sphenopalatine foramen through which the sphenopalatine artery enters into the nasal cavity. Thereafter, it divides in two branches, the nasopalatine artery medially and the posterior nasal artery, laterally. Though, the tail of the middle turbinate represents an important landmark for the control of eventual arterial bleeding during the anterior sphenoidotomy.

Posteriorly, superiorly, and medially to the middle turbinate, it is possible to identify the superior turbinate.

Above the choana, the sphenoethmoid recess forms the posterior wall of the nasal cavity: in its upper portion the sphenoid ostium can be identified, variable for shape, dimension, and location being sometimes covered by the tail of the superior turbinate. It represents the natural communication between the nasal cavity and the sphenoid sinus. Accordingly, during the surgical procedure, it is not mandatory to identify the sphenoid ostium, which definitely should not be considered as a main landmark of the approach (Fig. 2.1).

Hence, at the level of the sphenoethmoid recess, the nasal septum is detached from the prow of the anterior wall of the sphenoid bone; this latter is opened circumferentially and thus far the endoscope enters into the sphenoid cavity, often divided by one or more septa. The degree of pneumatization of the sphenoid bone is an important factor for the identification of the bony protuberances and depressions inside it. Depending on the degree of its pneumatization, a series of protuberances and depressions molded on its posterior and lateral walls can be identified. The sellar floor is at the center, the sphenoid planum is above, and the clival indentation is below; lateral to the sellar floor, the bony prominences of the intracavernous carotid artery and the optic nerve can be observed. Between them, the lateral optocarotid recess lies; it is molded by the pneumatization of the optic strut of the anterior clinoid process. The intracranial aspect of the upper border of the lateral optocarotid recess is covered by a thickening of the dura and periosteum that forms the distal dural ring, which separates the optic nerve from the clinoidal segment of the internal carotid artery (ICA). The inferior border of the lateral optocarotid recess also presents a thickening of the dura and periosteum, which forms the proximal dural ring, which separates the intra-cavernous portion of carotid artery from the clinoidal segment. The lateral aspect of tuberculum sellae represents the point where the bony prominences of the carotid artery and the optic nerve join medially (medial optocarotid recess). This recess is less evident than the lateral one; rather it represents the lateral limit to be opened to unlock the suprasellar area (Fig. 2.2).

The sella turcica is limited superiorly by the diaphragma sellae, a fold of dura with a central opening through which is pierced by the pituitary stalk and its blood supply. The diaphragma sellae separates the anterior lobe of the pituitary gland from the optic chiasm and the suprasellar cistern. The intercavernous sinus (anterior and posterior) lies in the anterior and posterior borders of the diaphragma sellae. Additional small venous sinuses in the base of the pituitary fossa drain into the intercavernous sinuses [53].

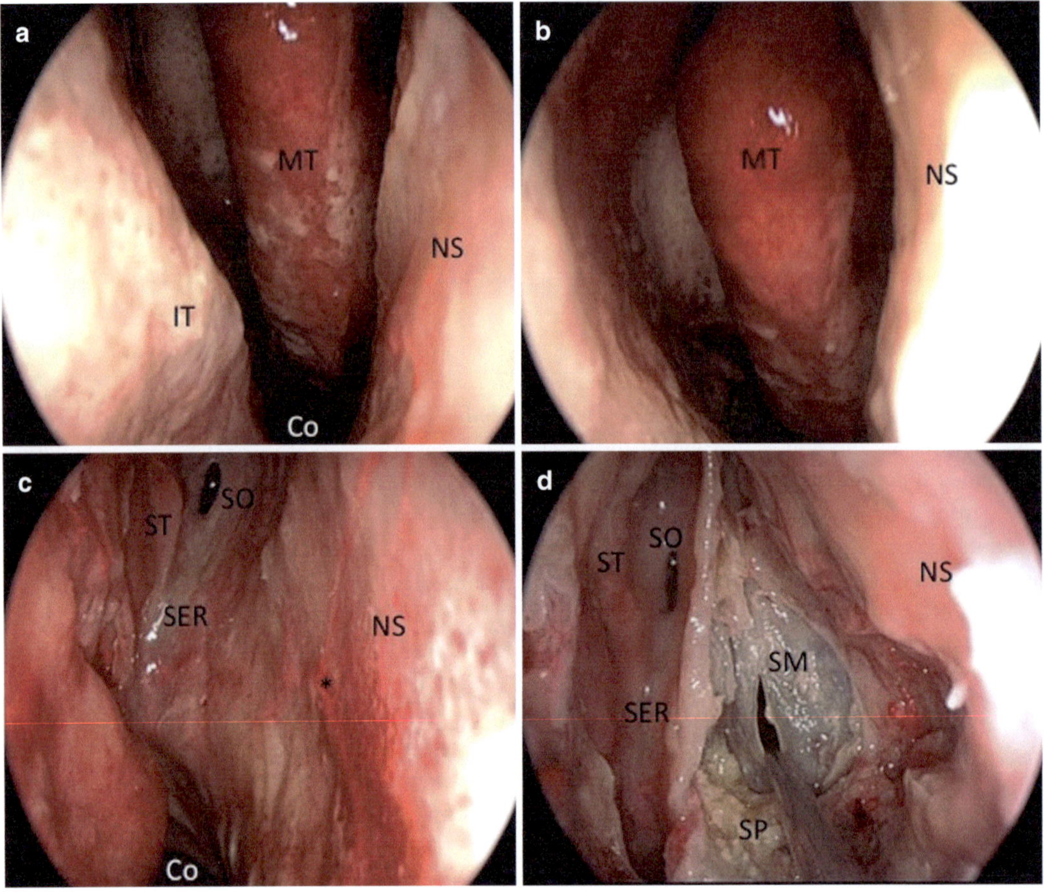

Fig. 2.1 Anatomical images of endoscopic exploration of the right nostril and identification of the nasal landmarks. (**a**) The inferior portion of the right nostril. (**b**) The middle turbinate. (**c**) The sphenoethmoid recess. (**d**) The sphenoid sinus mucosa after the opening of its anterior wall. *IT* inferior turbinate, *MT* middle turbinate, *SER* sphenoethmoid recess, *NS* nasal septum, *Co* choana, *SO* sphenoid ostium, *ST* superior turbinate, *SP* sphenoid prow, *SM* sphenoid mucosa, * branches of the nasopalatine artery

If the surgeon wants to explore the cavernous sinus, the bone that covers the intracavernous carotid artery (carotid protuberance) must be removed in order for both the medial and lateral compartments of the cavernous sinus to be exposed [15]. The space between the ICA and the pituitary gland varies depending on the anatomy of both structures. The medial wall may consist of tenacious connective tissue or may be fenestrated, incomplete, or inexistent, offering little or no anatomical resistance against tumor invasion. Surgical access to the medial and posterior wall of the cavernous sinus is possible by elevating or retracting the pituitary gland medially and by retracting the C4 (intracavernous segment) or C4–C5 bend of the ICA, laterally [21, 56]. The carotid artery itself is located in the major portion of the cavernous sinus so that the entire cavernous sinus will be disclosed only when the carotid artery is mobilized medially. Upon opening of the medial wall, the posterior and upper parts of the cavernous sinus are entered. The inferior hypophyseal artery is identified inferolaterally to the pituitary gland, arising from the meningohypophyseal trunk together with the dorsal meningeal and tentorial artery. Anteriorly to it, the inferolateral trunk, with its collaterals to the cavernous sinus cranial nerves, is detected, branching off the lateral aspect of the ICA; its origin can be seen by medial dislocation of the

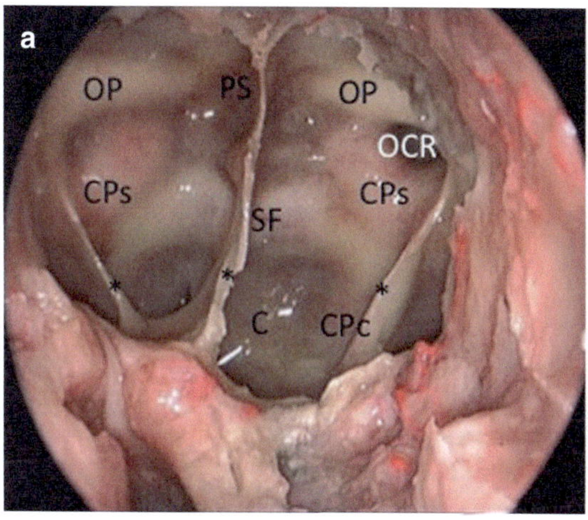

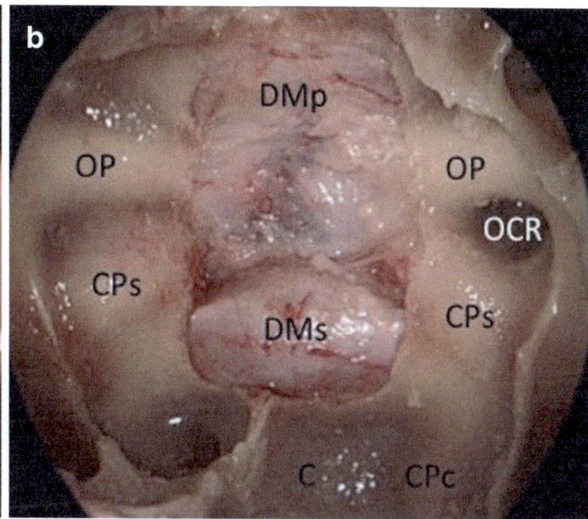

Fig. 2.2 Exposure of the sphenoid sinus after opening of its anterior wall and identification of the anatomical landmark. (**a**) Panoramic endoscopic view of the sphenoid sinus. (**b**) Bone removal of the sellar floor, the tuberculum sellae, and the posterior portion of the planum sphenoidale. *C* clivus, *SF* sellar floor, *PS* planum sphenoidale, *CPs* bony protuberance covering the parasellar tract of the intracavernous internal carotid artery, *CPc* bony protuberance covering the paraclival tract of the intracavernous internal carotid artery, *OP* bony protuberance covering the optic nerve, *OCR* opticocarotid recess, * sphenoid septum remnant. *DMp* dura mater of the planum sphenoidale, *DMs* sellar dura mater

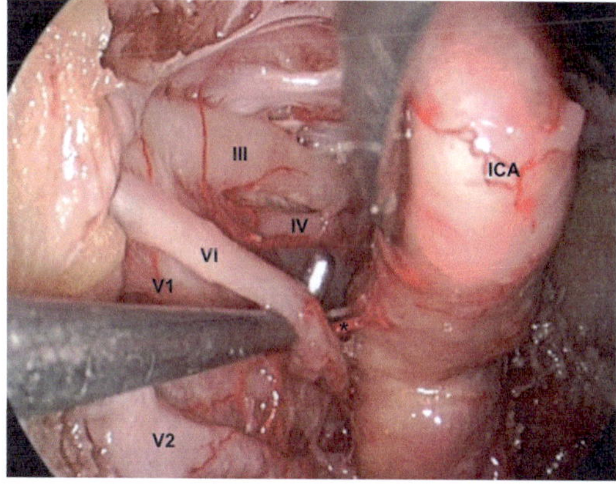

Fig. 2.3 Exploration of the cavernous sinus and medialization of the internal carotid artery. *ICA* internal carotid artery, *III* third oculomotor nerve, *IV* trochlear nerve, *VI* abducens nerve, *V1* ophthalmic branch of trigeminal nerve, *V2* maxillary branch of the trigeminal nerve, * inferolateral trunk (artery of the inferior cavernous sinus)

intracavernous segment of the ICA. Inferior hypophyseal artery divides into a medial and a lateral branch, which anastomose with the corresponding vessels of the opposite side, forming an arterial ring around the hypophysis [16, 28, 54] (Figs. 2.3, 2.4, and 2.5). The inferolateral trunk supplies all the cavernous sinus nerves, with the exception of the proximal segment of the VI cranial nerve, which receives blood from the tentorial artery. The oculomotor and trochlear nerves can be visualized from the sella through the C-shaped portion of the intracavernous sinus ICA. The oculomotor nerve enters the cavernous sinus under the posterior clinoid and then runs along the middle of the C-shaped ICA to enter into the cavernous sinus apex. At the apex, it runs along the inferior margin of the optic strut triangle until it reaches the superior orbital fissure. The trochlear nerve runs parallel and just inferior to the oculomotor nerve. When the ICA is displaced medially, the oculomotor nerve, the trochlear nerve, and the proximal and distal dural ring can be seen. The ophthalmic division of the trigeminal nerve runs obliquely in a rostral and anterior direction toward the cavernous sinus apex reaching the oculomotor and trochlear nerves at the superior orbital fissure. The abducens nerve passes through Dorello's canal approximately 5–10 mm inferior to the sellar floor at the medial aspect of the ICA and a few millimeters below the sellar floor at the lateral aspect of the ICA. The abducens nerve heads toward the orbital apex running inferiorly to the medial aspect of the ophthalmic branch of the trigeminal nerve [21, 31, 33, 34, 43] (Fig. 2.3).

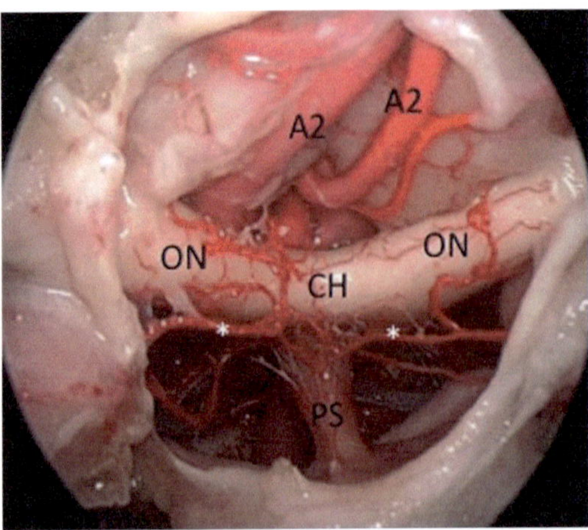

Fig. 2.4 Endoscopic endonasal view of the neurovascular structures localized above the pituitary gland. *CH* chiasm, *PS* pituitary stalk, *ON* optic nerve, *A2*, post communicating anterior cerebral artery, * superior hypophyseal artery (sha)

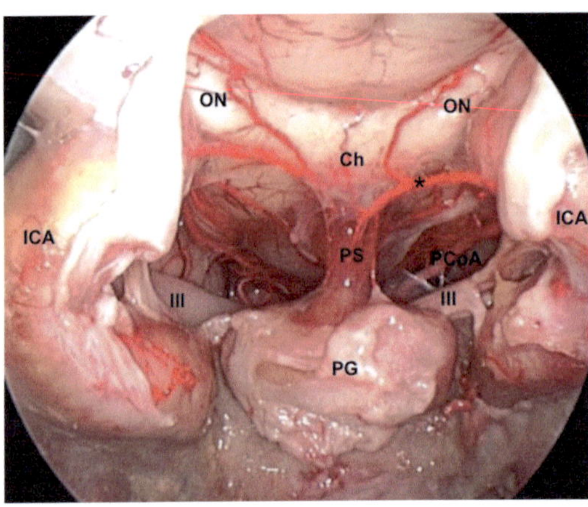

Fig. 2.5 Endoscopic endonasal view of the pituitary gland and surrounding neurovascular structures. *CH* chiasm, *PS* pituitary stalk, *Pg* pituitary gland, *ON* optic nerve, *PCoA* posterior communicating artery, *III* third cranial nerve, * superior hypophyseal artery

The exposure of the suprasellar region requires a more anterior trajectory: the posterior ethmoid cells and the anterior wall of the sphenoid sinus have to be widely removed. Above the sella, the angle formed by the convergence of the sphenoid planum with the sellar floor corresponds to the tuberculum sellae. This structure named after the classic Latin word "tuber," which etymologically means "small swelling, pimple, protuberance," appears to fit such a description when observed from above via a transcranial route, but it does not as seen from below through an endoscopic endonasal corridor. As a matter of fact, through direct visualization via an endoscopic endonasal approach, it has recently renamed "suprasellar notch" (SSN), that means "angular or V-shaped cut indentation" [29]. Indeed, in the majority of cases, the inferior point of view coincides with a sort of indentation between the superior aspect of the sella turcica and the declining part of the planum sphenoidale. Moving anteriorly, we can recognize the sphenoid planum, laterally delimited by the protuberances of the optic nerves. At this point, the bone of the suprasellar notch and the planum sphenoidale can be removed 1.5–2 cm in a posteroanterior direction and laterally up to the optic protuberances. The sellar and suprasellar dura are then opened to permit the exploration of the neurovascular structures localized above the diaphragma sellae. In the suprachiasmatic region, the chiasmatic and the lamina terminalis cisterns with relative contents are accessible. The anterior margin of the chiasm and the medial portion of the optic nerves, the anterior cerebral arteries, the anterior communicating artery, and the recurrent Heubner arteries, together with the gyri recti of the frontal lobes, can be identified. In the subchiasmatic space, the pituitary stalk is at the center of the field below the chiasm, with the superior hypophyseal artery and its perforating branches, supplying the inferior surface of the chiasm and the optic nerves. The superior aspect of the pituitary gland and the dorsum sellae are also visible. The superior hypophyseal arteries supply the optic chiasm, the floor of the hypothalamus, and the median eminence.

2.3 Neuroimaging

Magnetic resonance imaging (MRI) has replaced other techniques for the morphological study of the sellar region, because of the elevated tissue contrast and multiplanar capability. A complete MR protocol should include, at least, T1- and T2-weighted images and T1-weighted post-contrast (gadolinium) images, in the three orthogonal planes at max 3 mm sections. Complementary

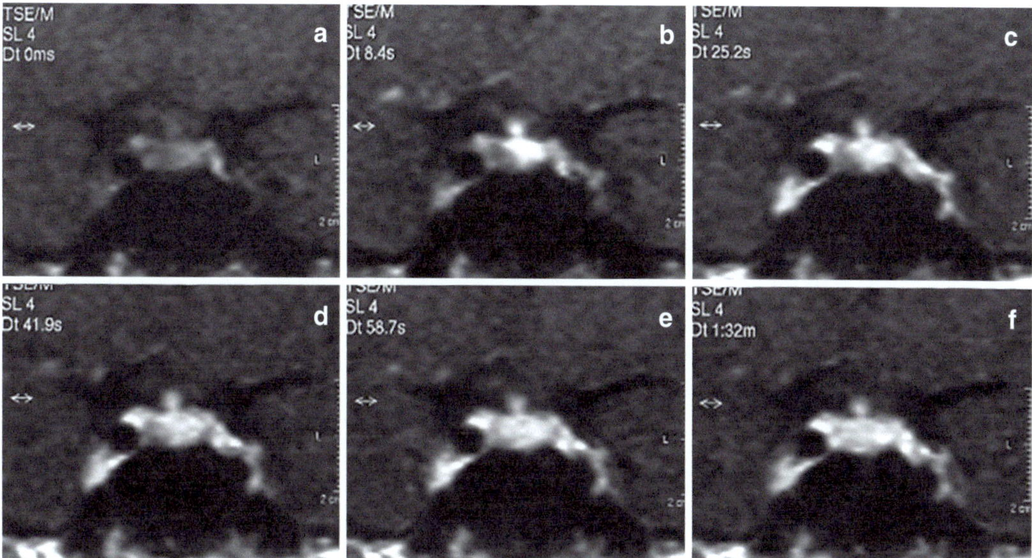

Fig. 2.6 Microadenoma. (**a–f**) Coronal T1-weighted dynamic images during contrast medium injection. Presence of a small hypointense area within the right lateral part of the gland, better demonstrated during the early phases of the dynamic scan (**b–d**), not identifiable in the delayed acquisition (**f**)

sequences, i.e., MR angiography, are also useful, especially upon the suspicion of a possible vascular nature of sellar lesion. Computed tomography (CT) should be used only in selected cases, to provide further details whether calcified components of the lesion are present, to achieve an accurate definition of the bony boundaries at presurgical planning of the approach, mainly sphenoid sinus septations. At the presurgical planning, CT remains the diagnostic imaging study of choice in patients who are unable to undergo an MR study. The purposes of the neuroradiologic study of pituitary adenomas are: to identify the lesion,; to define the spatial relationships of the lesion (presurgical planning), to monitor the medical treatment, and to clear the entity of the lesion (postsurgical follow-up) [2].

Pituitary microadenomas comprise lesions measuring 10 mm or less. They are the most common intrasellar neoplasms. The neuroradiologic diagnosis of microadenomas is drawn on the presence of indirect and direct findings. The indirect findings that should lead to diagnosis of microadenoma are: the lateral dislocation of the pituitary stalk and the alteration of the pituitary gland (upward convexity) or of the sellar floor (depression, slope, angulation). The stalk is usually found dislocated controlaterally off the tumor, but there have been reports describing homolateral stalk dislocation; as well it can be absent in contrast to tumor presence. The direct findings reveal proper MRI features of pituitary macroadenomas; they can be identified as rounded or ovular, sometimes flattened intrasellar lesions, and hypointense on T1-weighted images compared to the unaffected anterior pituitary gland (Fig. 2.6). Microadenomas can also exhibit hyperintensity on the T1-weighted images, due to the hemorrhage of a part or of whole lesion. At the T2-weighted images, pituitary microadenomas present a variety of aspects, according to the line of endocrine activity. T2 hyperintensity could be found in 80 % of prolactin-secreting microadenomas, while iso- or hypointensity is disclosed in ca 70 % of growth hormone-secreting microadenomas. The use of intravenous contrast medium injection becomes mandatory to further refine the diagnosis; upon half-dose gadolinium (0.05 mmol/kg) injection, most of microadenomas enhance less rapidly than the normal pituitary gland, appearing as hypointense areas. Late scans, 30–40 min after the injection, can sometimes show a late enhancement of the adenoma. Sometimes, in patients harboring a small lesion—particularly in case of Cushing disease—difficult to detect, specific dynamic techniques are performed to rule out diagnosis. This technique consists of repeated scans of the gland immediately upon intravenous injection of contrast medium, so that the progressive enhancement of the stalk and then of the gland is observed. The early phases of the acquisition demonstrate lesions that are not identifiable on conventional contrast-enhanced studies. In presence of clinical signs and symptoms of a functioning adenoma, with no lesion detected at the MRI, the inferior petrosal sinuses could be run to evaluate the hormonal output of the pituitary gland. This is most commonly performed in patients with Cushing's syndrome, because the corticotropin-secreting tumors may be extremely small and difficult to visualize [52].

On the other side, pituitary macroadenomas are bigger intrasellar masses, usually extending out of the sella. The aim of the neuroradiologic study is to clarify the origin side of the lesion (pituitary or not), its consistency (firm, cystic, necrotic, or hemorrhagic), and its relationships with anatomical surrounding structures. From these data an accurate differential diagnosis can be reached [11]. MRI typically demonstrates a mass arising from the pituitary fossa, completely filling the sella, which appears remodeled and enlarged. The normal pituitary tissue is compressed: after contrast medium injection, the normal gland appears as a strongly enhancing tissue, representing the pseudocapsula of the adenoma, usually posteriorly and/or on one side, between the tumor and the cavernous sinus. The posterior lobe and pituitary stalk appear more hyperintense as compressed and or displaced.

Pituitary macroadenomas may appear as homogeneous, soft-tissue masses, with variable signal intensity, often similar to gray matter. At the T2-weighted images, areas of inhomogeneous signal can be identified, because many macroadenomas harbor cystic, necrotic, or hemorrhagic components (Figs. 2.7 and 2.8). The adenoma may appear predominantly cystic, showing a typical hyperintense signal on the T1- and T2-weighted images (Fig. 2.9). Hemorrhage occurs in about 20 % of pituitary macroadenomas, revealed by spontaneous hypersignal intensity on the T1-weighted images. A fluid-fluid level can sometimes be seen within the hemorrhage, due to blood cell membranes remnants and hemoglobin residues. The clinical syndrome known as "pituitary apoplexy," representing hemorrhage into a pituitary adenoma, can be defected also on CT as hyperdense material in the pituitary fossa and possibly in the suprasellar cistern, within the lesion. MRI could differentiate various stages of the hemorrhage evolution. Small linear or curved spots, caused by hemosiderin deposits, can sometimes be found after intratumoral hemorrhage on the T2-weighted images. Concerning the consistency of the lesion, the T2-weighted scans are more helpful in providing relevant details: hyperintense lesions could be presumed as cystic, while hypointense ones as firmer. Additional data can be obtained by the diffusion-weighted imaging (DWI).

The use of contrast medium injection helps in defining the structure of the lesion, homogeneous or inhomogeneous, and the degree of its vascularization. After contrast medium, the tumor enhances moderately at early stage and retains this signal feature at later delayed scans.

The extension of the macroadenoma and its relationships with the surrounding structures constitute key-points of the neuroradiologic diagnosis. The tumor usually extends upward, to impinge and/or compress the optic chiasm, remaining subdiaphragmatic or breaching the diaphragma sellae with a typical "figure-eight" appearance, compressing the floor of third ventricle and sometimes the foramen of Monro. The adenoma can also extend downward, into the sphenoidal sinus, or laterally toward the cavernous sinus. Whether the cavernous sinus is compressed or invaded is of crucial importance for the neurosurgeon; this radiological diagnosis can be very difficult because the medial wall of the sinus is often thin and not directly visualized. The cavernous sinus invasion can be excluded in presence of normal pituitary tissue lying between the tumor and the sinus. In case of massive involvement of the cavernous sinus, complete encircling of the

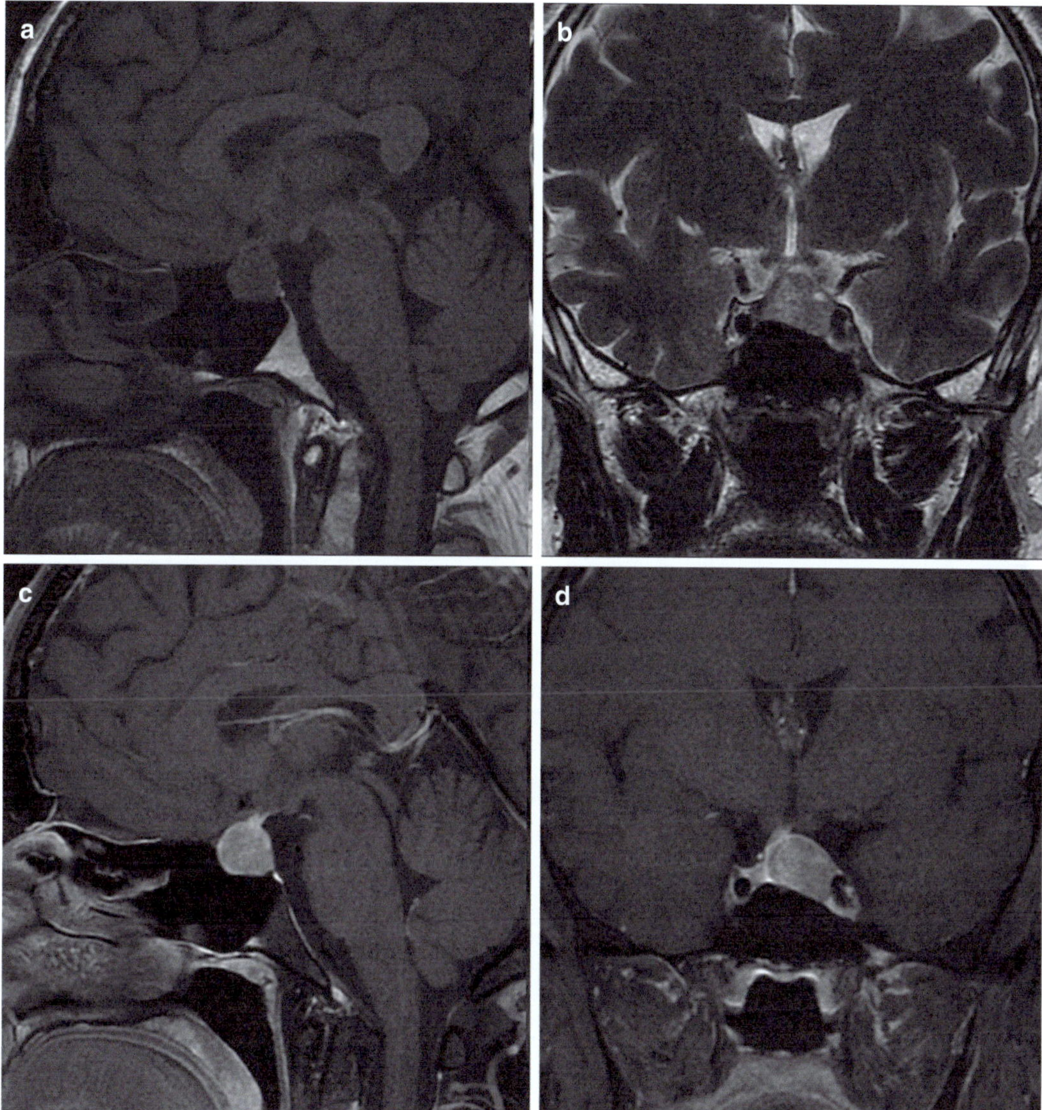

Fig. 2.7 Macroadenoma. (**a**) Sagittal T1-weighted image; (**b**) coronal T2-weighted image; (**c–d**) sagittal and coronal T1-weighted images after contrast medium injection. Presence of an intra- and suprasellar lesion, laterally displacing the axis and the left cavernous sinus

intra-cavernous internal carotid artery (ICA) tumor is visible and only tumor signal features are identified in this area. Prolactin or growth hormone-secreting adenomas are more often found to enter the cavernous sinus as compared to non-secreting tumors [44]. A grading system with a high predictive value for the identification of true cavernous sinus invasion has been proposed by Knosp et al., in 1993 [44] (Fig. 2.10).

The neuroradiology techniques play also an important role in evaluating the effects of the medical therapy for functioning adenomas [51].

In case of PRL-secreting adenomas, dopamine agonists can reduce the size of lesions since the 10th day of treatment and could last for several years. The shrinkage of macroadenomas caused by the medical treatment can determine the downward displacement of the optic tracts and

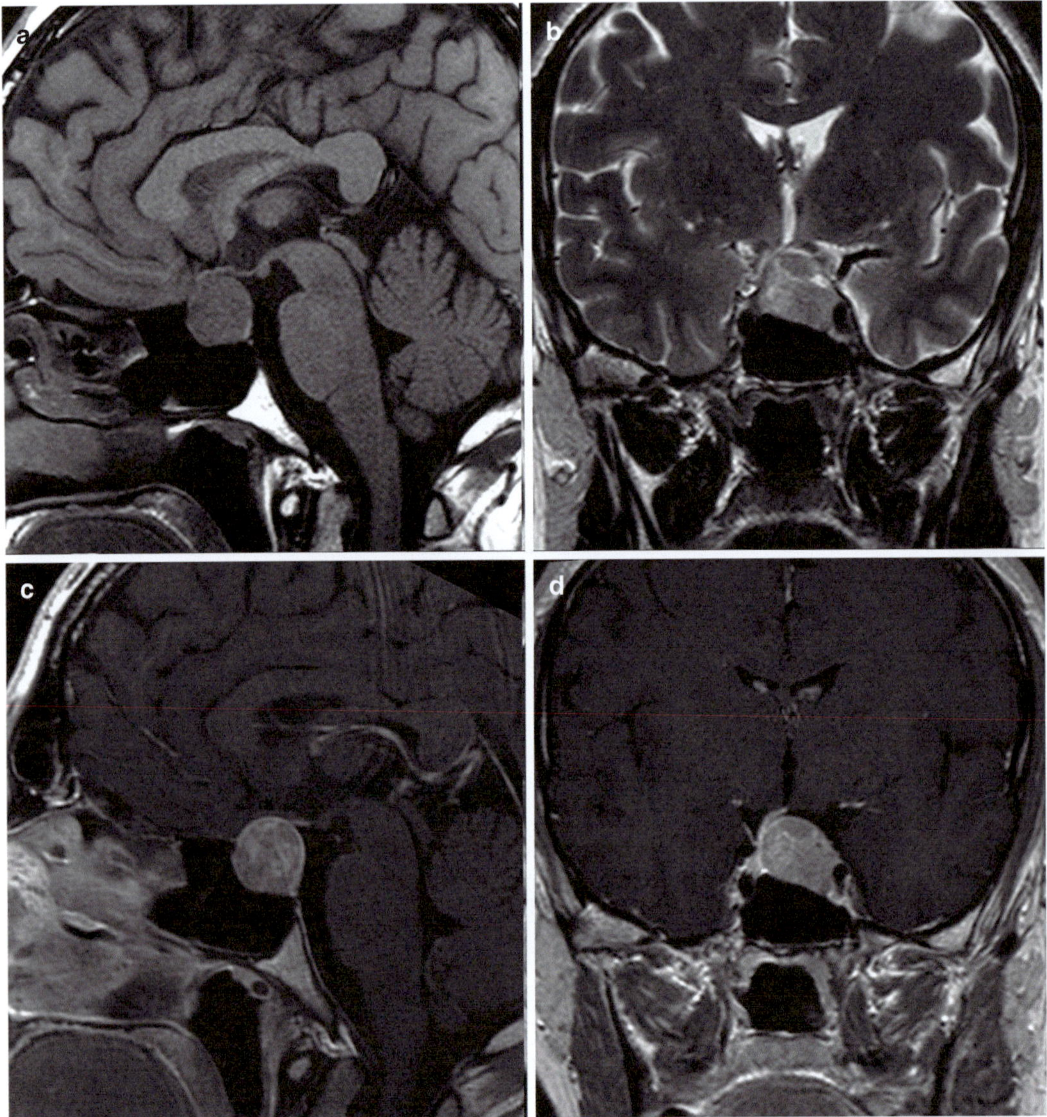

Fig. 2.8 Macroadenoma. (**a**) Sagittal T1-weighted image; (**b**) coronal T2-weighted image; (**c–d**) sagittal and coronal T1-weighted images after contrast medium injection. Presence of a large intra- and suprasellar lesion, clearly infiltrating the left cavernous sinus

chiasm although this usually doesn't produce symptoms. Within macroadenomas focal areas of necrosis or cysts, revealed by hypointense signal on T1-wieghted and hyperintense signal on T2-weighted images and an increasing T2 signal intensity, can occur. Hemorrhage within prolactinomas has also been observed.

It is worth reminding that, when an EEA is planned for the removal of pituitary adenoma, MRI and CT ease presurgical planning, giving details in regard to the bony boundaries of the approach, the anatomy of the nasal and paranasal sinuses, and eventual variations.

Thin-slice axial and coronal CT scans allow a detailed overview of major nasal cavities and bony structures, which are anatomical landmarks of the endoscopic route (nasal turbinates, uncinate processes, sphenoid ostium, etc.) and of the sinusal structures (symmetry and aeration of the sphenoid sinus and the relationships of the sphenoid septa with the sellar floor and carotid canal).

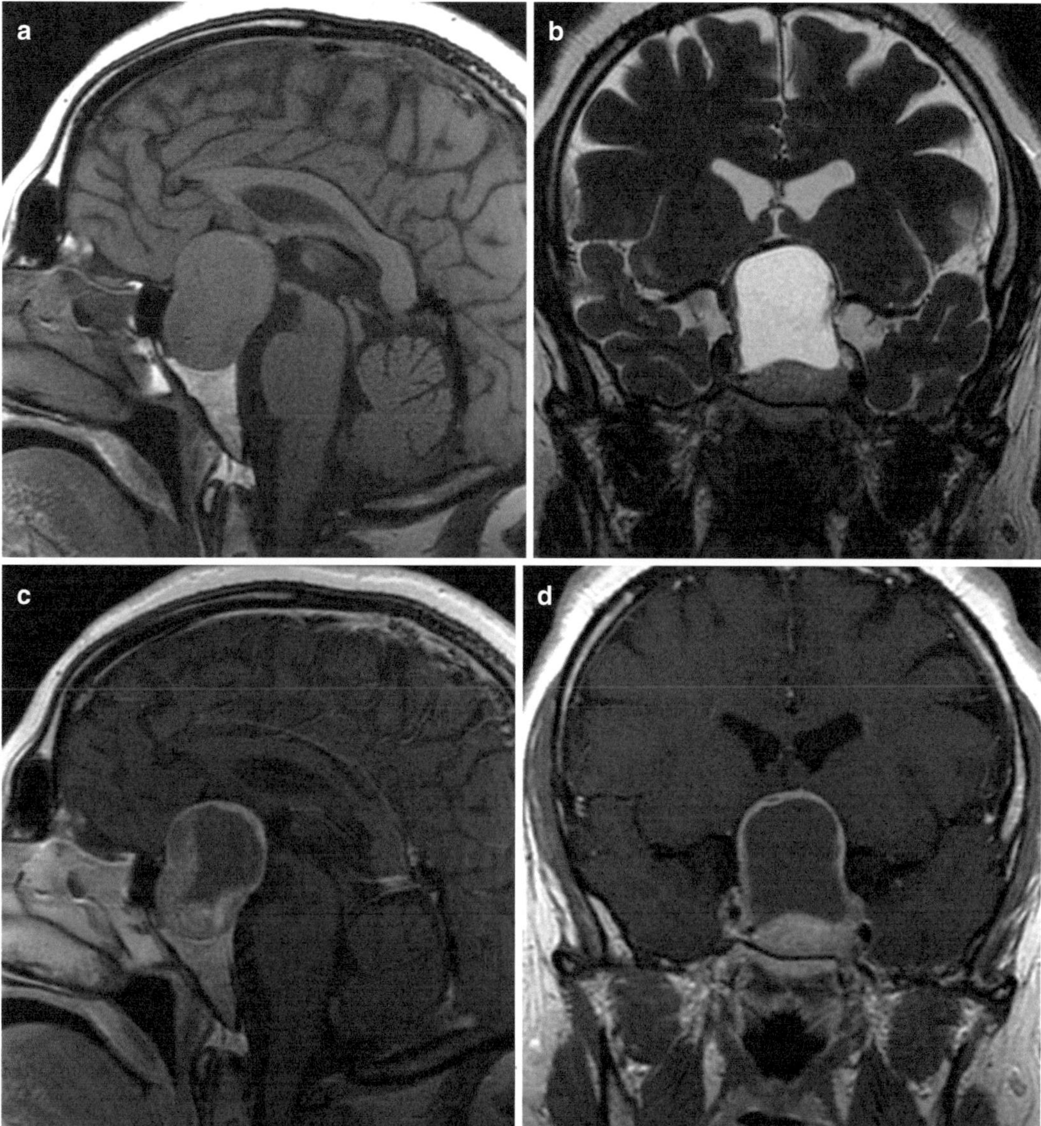

Fig. 2.9 Macroadenoma. (**a**) Sagittal T1-weighted image; (**b**) coronal T2-weighted image; (**c–d**) sagittal and coronal T1-weighted images after contrast medium injection. Presence of a very large intra- and suprasellar lesion with a prevalent, non-enhancing colliquative component

Finally, when MRI is adopted to diagnose any complication of surgery or to define eventual residual tumor or recurrence, the usual postoperative distortion of sellar anatomy should not be underestimated. Indeed, in the first 1 or 2 weeks following transsphenoidal resection, a sizeable "mass" may still be present; the surgical cavity is often filled with packing material (gelatin foam, autologous fat), soaked with blood and secretions, which slowly dissolves along following 2 or 3 months. The slow reduction of the "mass" in the surgical cavity, despite significant or complete removal of the tumor, reflects the reabsorption time of the reconstruction material or may represent peritumoral scars preserving the cavity from collapsing. Therefore, MRI examination should be required after 2 or 3 months after surgery (Fig. 2.11), after these changes have regressed. If fat or muscle grafts are used to reconstruct the sellar cavity, their reabsorption

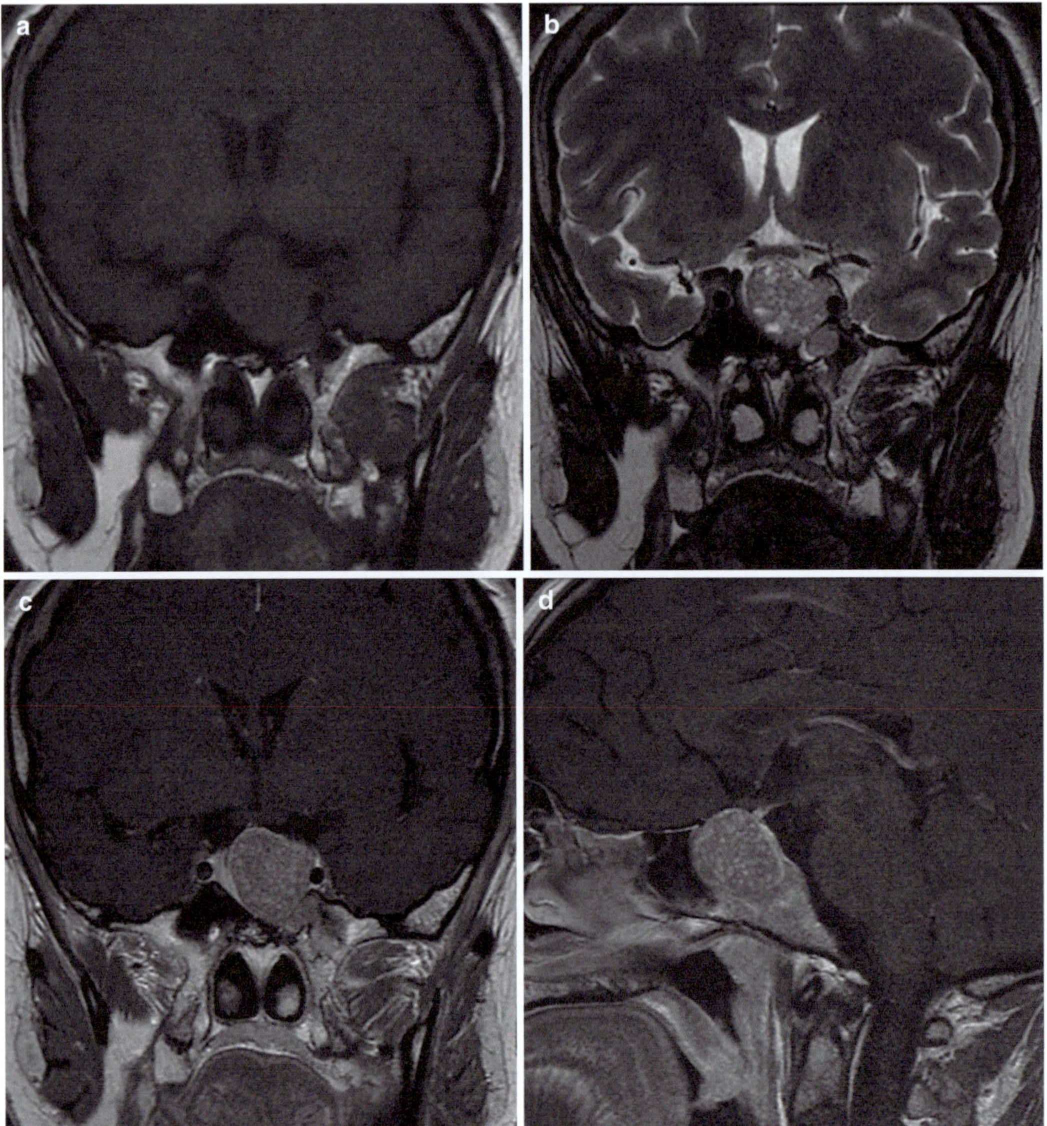

Fig. 2.10 Macroadenoma. (**a**) Coronal T1-weighted image; (**b**) coronal T2-weighted image; (**c–d**) coronal and sagittal T1-weighted images after contrast medium injection. Presence of a large intra- and suprasellar lesion, clearly infiltrating the left cavernous sinus and the sphenoid sinus

requires more time: that is, the fat may exhibit a hyperintense signal up to 2 or 3 years after surgery [55, 59].

2.4 Surgical Technique

Since the endoscopic transsphenoidal technique has been introduced during the 1990s, several variations of this procedure (endonasal, transnasal, single or binostril, with or without the use of the microscope, etc.) have been used worldwide for the removal of pituitary adenomas and of other variety of sellar lesions [3, 13, 32, 38, 48]. In this section we will describe the binostril procedure we currently adopt for the removal of the pituitary adenomas.

The patient is positioned supine with the trunk elevated 10° and the head turned 10° toward the surgeon seated in a horse-hole headrest.

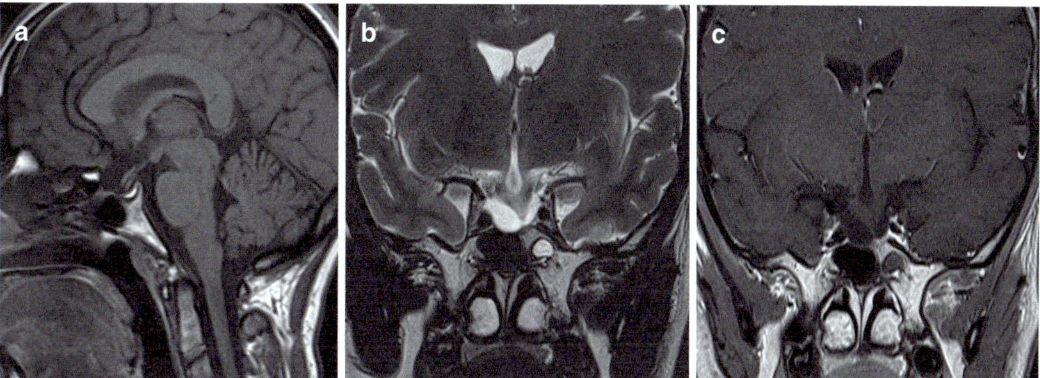

Fig. 2.11 Postoperative changes. (**a**) Sagittal T1 weighted image; (**b**) coronal T2-weighted image; (**c**) coronal T1-weighted image after contrast medium injection. The sellar cavity is completed filled by cerebrospinal fluid ("empty sella"), with downward retraction of the axis and the optic chiasm

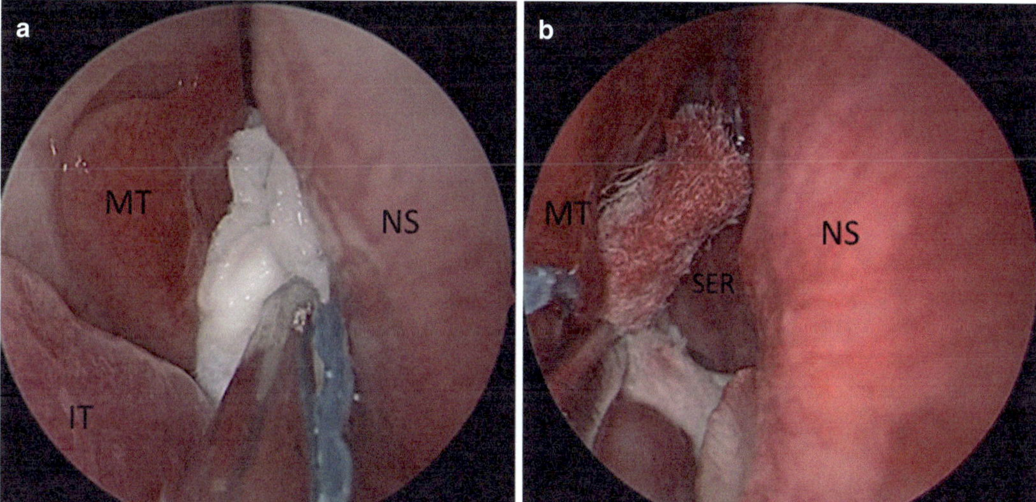

Fig. 2.12 Endoscopic endonasal intraoperative view through the right nostril (nasal phase of the approach). (**a**) Positioning of a cottonoid between the middle turbinate and the nasal septum. (**b**) Lateralization of the middle turbinate in order to reach the sphenoethmoid recess. *NS* nasal septum, *MT* middle turbinate, *SER* sphenoethmoid recess, *IT* inferior turbinate

Initially, cotton pledgets soaked in 3.5 % povidone iodine solution are placed along the floor of the nasal cavities and in the space between the nasal septum and the middle turbinates using a small Killian-type nasal speculum. Thereafter, with the same procedure described above, cotton pledgets soaked in a decongestant solution (2 ml of adrenaline, 5 ml of 20 % diluted lidocaine, and 4 ml of saline solution) are placed in order to reduce as much as possible blood tearing from the richly vascularized nasal mucosa. Though, they are left in place for ca. 10 min. Patient nose is prepped and draped and all the endoscopic equipment is set.

The endoscope is then introduced into the right nostril where it is possible to identify the inferior turbinate laterally and the nasal septum medially. The gently lateral dislocation of the middle turbinate protected with a cottonoid allows to widen the working space creating an adequate surgical corridor; sliding along the floor of the nasal cavity the choana and the sphenoethmoid recess can be identified (Fig. 2.12). A gentle monopolar coagulation of the mucosa of the sphenoethmoid recess

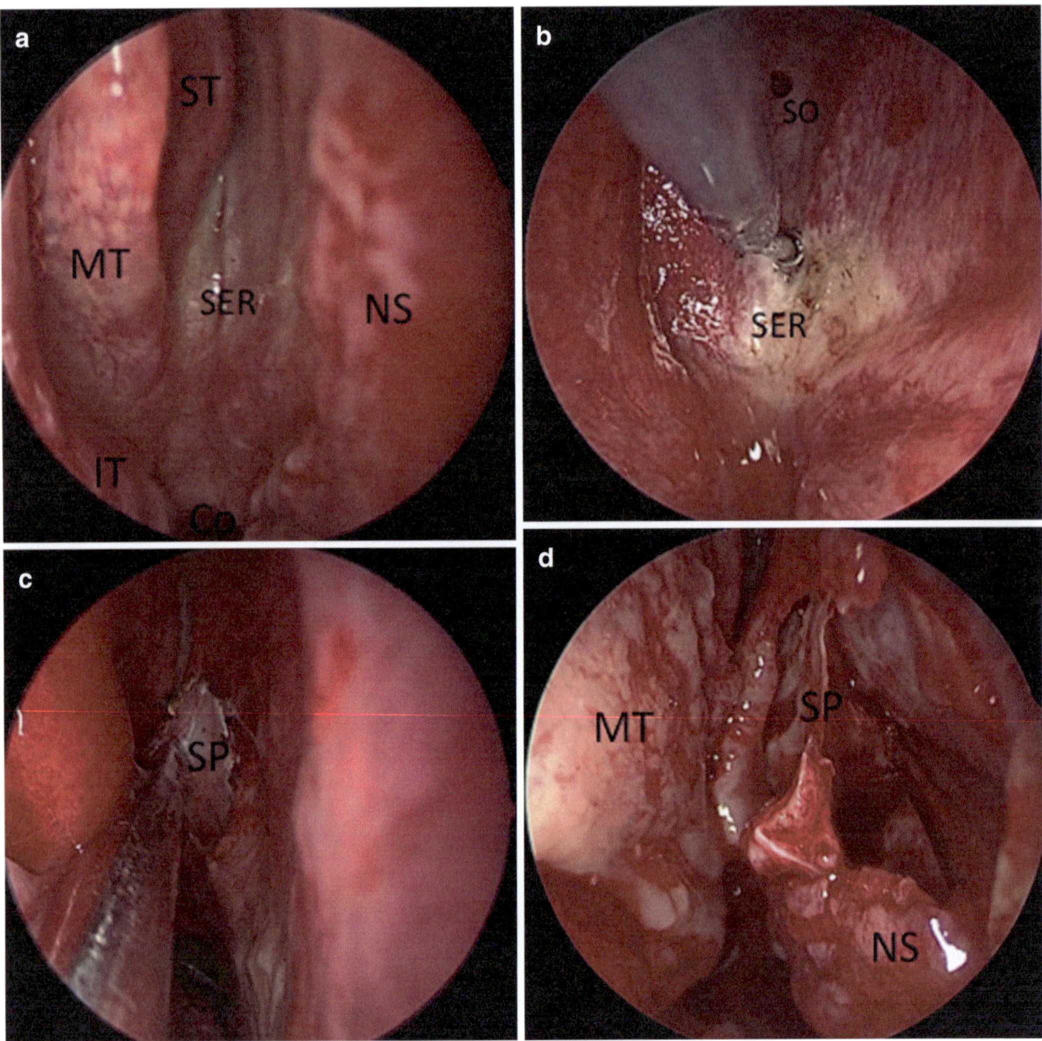

Fig. 2.13 (**a–b**) Coagulation of the sphenoethmoid recess. (**c–d**) Submucosal dissection performed in order to expose the sphenoid prow. *SP* sphenoid prow, *NS* nasal septum, *Co* choana, *MT* middle turbinate, *SO* sphenoid ostium, *ST* superior turbinate, *SER* spheno-ethmoid recess, *IT* inferior turbinate

prevents the bleeding of the septal branch of the sphenopalatine artery (Fig. 2.13). Thereafter, the nasal septum is detached from the sphenoid bone, thus allowing the exposition of the anterior wall of the sphenoid sinus; this latter is removed using a microdrill or bone punches paying particular attention in the inferolateral direction where sphenopalatine artery or its major branches lie. The wide opening of the anterior wall of the sphenoid sinus is a key point, to allow the proper maneuverability of the instruments inside the sphenoid sinus and later at the level of the sella (Fig. 2.14). An accurate check of eventual bleeding from the edges of the sphenoidotomy that could obscure the lens during the next steps has to be performed. The coagulation with bipolar forceps of the mucosa over the anterior wall of the sphenoid sinus could ensure preventing delayed bleedings.

The endoscope is then introduced in the other nostril and the mucosa of the sphenoethmoid recess is gently opened and removed after it is pushed laterally up to the roof of the nasal cavity. In this way the endoscope and another surgical instrument can be moved inside such nostril.

After the anterior sphenoidotomy has been enlarged, the removal of septa inside it permits to

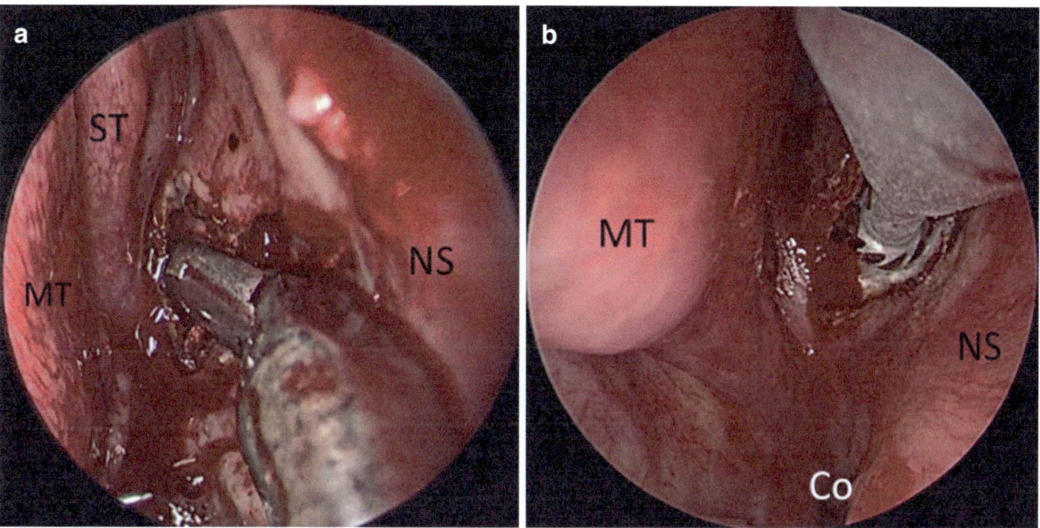

Fig. 2.14 Opening of the anterior wall of the sphenoid sinus. (**a–b**) Removal of the sphenoid prow. *ST* superior turbinate, *NS* nasal septum, *MT* middle turbinate, *Co* choana

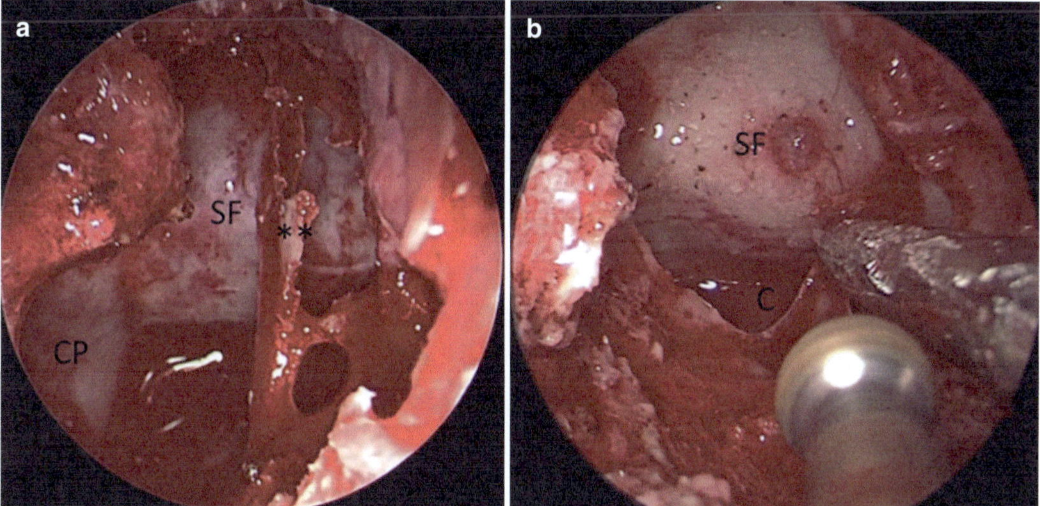

Fig. 2.15 (**a–b**) Enlargement of the anterior sphenoidotomy. *SF* sellar floor, *C* clivus, *CP* carotid protuberance, ** sphenoid septum

identify and to expose the posterior wall of the sphenoid sinus cavity with the sellar floor at the center, the planum sphenoidale above it, and the clival indentation below; lateral to the sellar floor, the bony prominences of the intracavernous carotid artery (ICA) and the optic nerve can be seen and between them is the optocarotid recess. In those cases where the identification of all these landmarks is not possible, or whether a presellar or conchal sphenoid sinus is present, the use of neuronavigation system can be useful, especially at the beginning of the learning curve in preventing misdirection (Fig. 2.15).

From this point on, the endoscope is hold by the second surgeon allowing the first operator to move two instruments through both nostrils.

According to the anatomical conditions of the sellar floor (intact, eroded, thinned), it can be

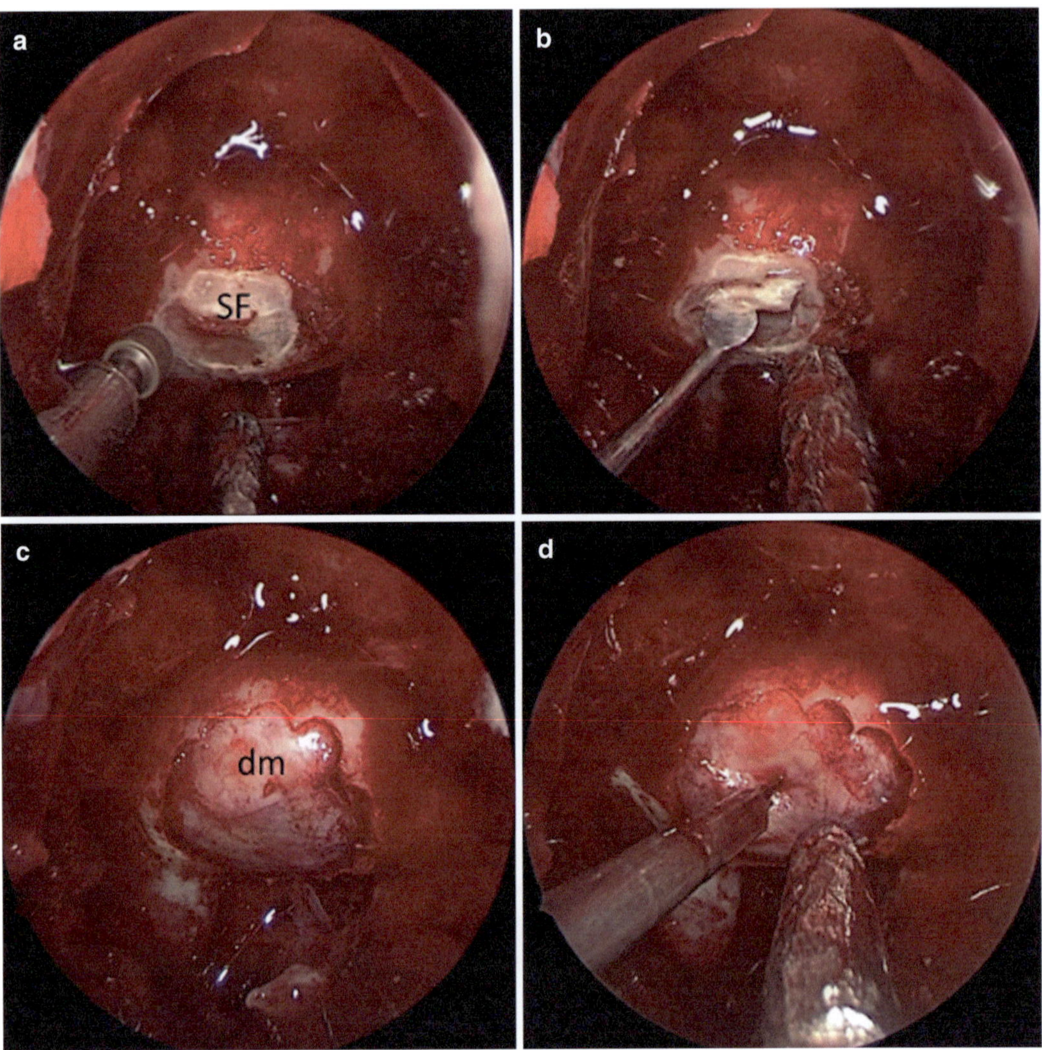

Fig. 2.16 (**a**) Drilling of the sellar floor, (**b**) enlarging the opening of the sellar floor, (**c–d**) incision of the dura mater using a scalpel with a telescopic blade. *SF* sellar floor, *dm* dura mater

opened in different ways and it is possible to extend the opening as required by the volume and the extension of the adenoma (Fig. 2.16). During this maneuver, care must be taken in avoiding injury of the underlying dura, which later can be incised in a linear, rectangular, or cruciate fashion. In patients with macroadenomas, inferior and superior cavernous sinuses are usually compressed making the dural incision almost bloodless; in case of microadenoma not so rarely, the inferior and/or superior intercavernous sinus has to be coagulated in order to perform an adequate dural opening.

The removal of macroadenomas must start from the inferior and lateral aspects of the lesion in order to avoid the premature delivery of the redundant diaphragm into the sella that could reduce the chance of a radical tumor removal.

After intracapsular debulking of the adenoma, its pseudocapsule can be dissected from the suprasellar cistern; it should be reminded that as the macroadenoma grows, it often stretches the residual pituitary so that it appears as a thin layer of tissue surrounding the adenoma. Nevertheless, the removal of this tissue could cause postoperative hypopituitarism (Figs. 2.17 and 2.18).

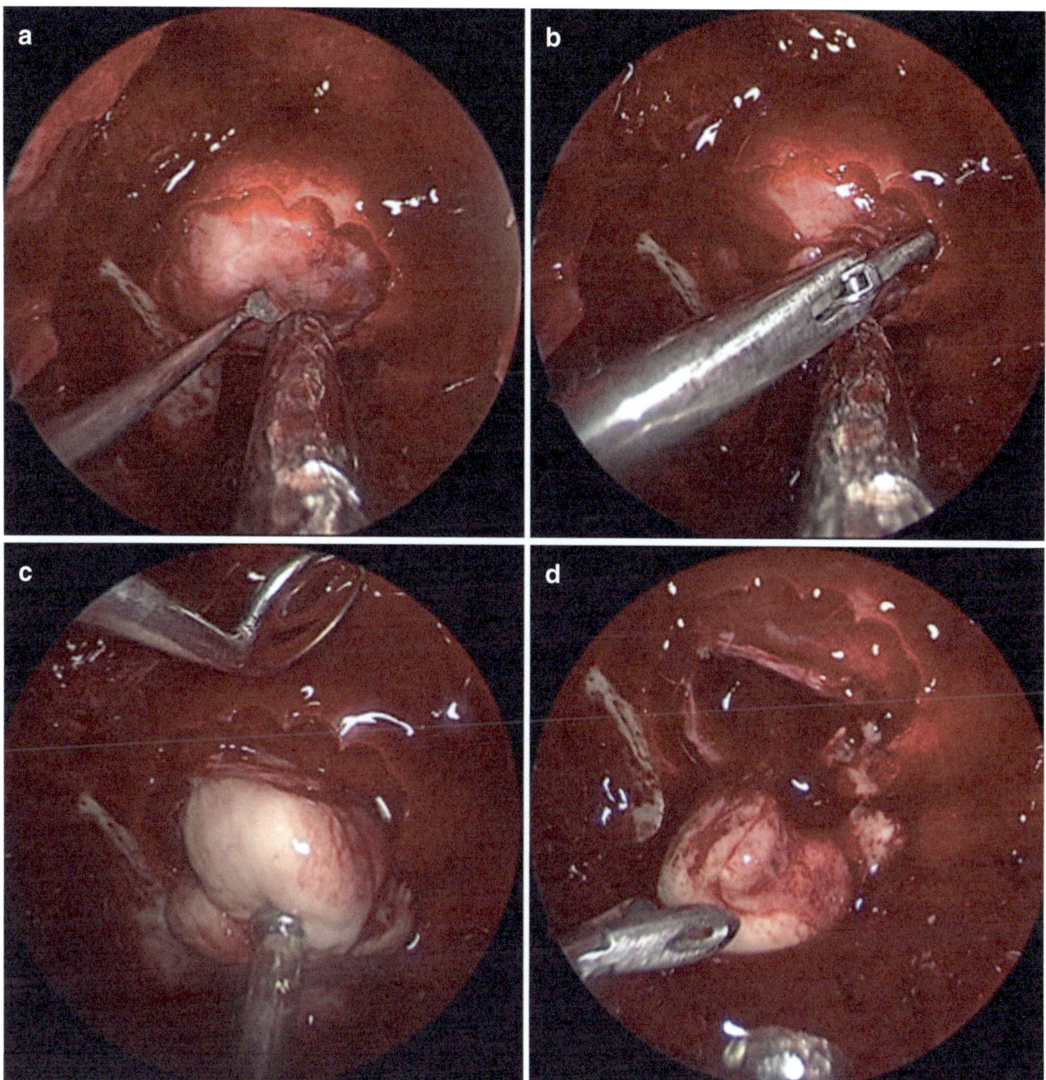

Fig. 2.17 (**a–b**) Opening of the sellar dura. (**c–d**) Extracapsular dissection and removal of the adenoma

Once the adenoma has been removed, if the descent of the suprasellar portion of the lesion is not obtained, a Valsalva maneuver can be useful (Fig. 2.19). In order to check if residual tumor is still present, the use of closeup intrasellar exploration with a 0° or angled endoscopes (30 or 45°) allows to visualize all the blind angles inside the sella. Recently, the so-called diving technique [50] that consists in the continuous irrigation into the residual cavity through the irrigation sheath of the endoscope allowing the surgeon to enter the death space filled with saline solution gives the opportunity to explore it and to eventually remove micro-residual of the lesion.

For lesions extending through the medial wall of the cavernous sinus, the removal can be performed using a curved suction cannula gently following the space within venous channels created by the lesion itself.

After tumor removal, reconstruction is properly achieved addressing the following principles: (1) protection of the suprasellar cistern; (2) filling of the "dead space," i.e., the residual sellar cavity; and (3) closure of the osteodural sellar

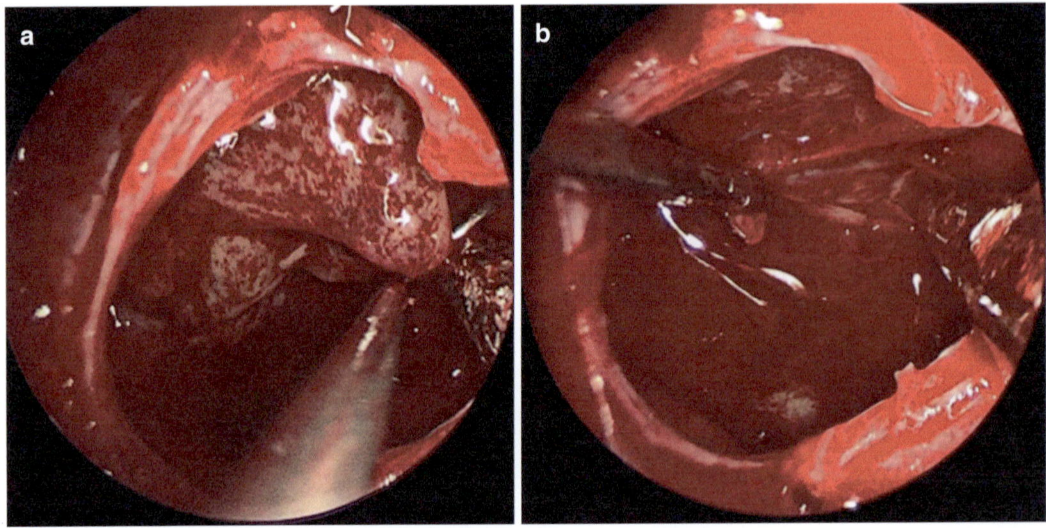

Fig. 2.18 (**a–b**) Dissection and removal of the tumor adherent to the suprasellar cistern

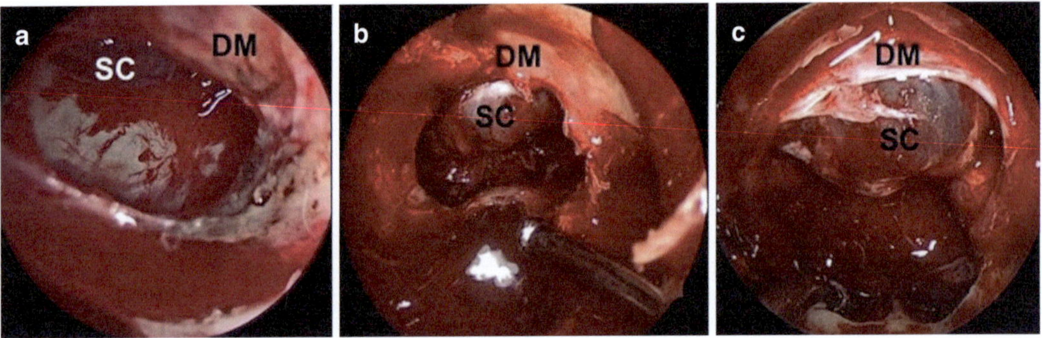

Fig. 2.19 (**a–c**) Different grade of descent of the suprasellar cistern after the removal of intra- and suprasellar macroadenomas in three different cases. *DM* dura mater, *SC* suprasellar cistern

defect. When no intraoperative CSF leak has occurred, it is possible to perform the reconstruction just protecting the suprasellar cistern with collagen sponge and fibrin glue to fill the eventual dead space. In case of intraoperative CSF leak, various techniques could be adopted to achieve an effective reconstruction depending mainly upon the size of the osteodural defect and of the "dead space" inside the sella. Besides the protection of the suprasellar cistern, a fat graft or pieces of collagen sponge can be positioned into the sellar cavity minding to avoid overpacking avoiding compression of the optic system. Different layers of dural substitute are positioned later in the intradural and above all extradural spaces to complete the sellar closure. It must be underlined that a good reconstruction starts from the sellar sealing. Therefore, generally it is important to preserve a good extradural plane in which the dural substitute foils should be wedged during the reconstruction. The extradural reconstruction of the sellar floor is considered the most effective in preventing postop CSF leak. Rarely, a nasoseptal pedicled flap is adopted for the reconstruction of the sella after standard endoscopic pituitary surgery or lumbar drainage is used [9, 12, 46] (Fig. 2.20).

At the end of the procedure, hemostasis along the basis of the anterior sphenoidotomy is performed and eventual bone residuals or blood

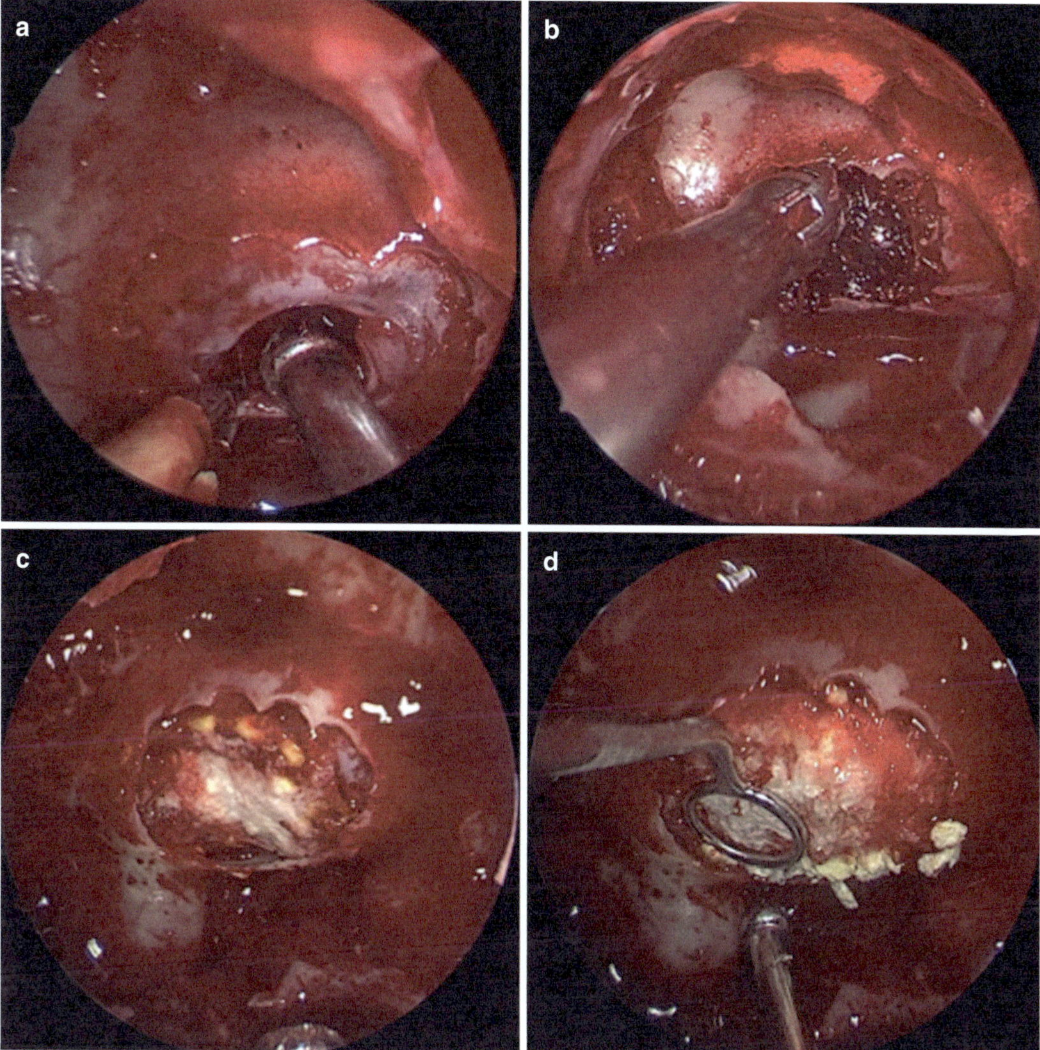

Fig. 2.20 Reconstruction of the sellar defect. (**a**) Coagulation of the inferior intercavernous sinus. (**b**) Hemostatic agent is placed to fill the sellar cavity. (**c–d**) Pieces of collagen sponge soaked with thrombin are positioned in the extradural space

clots are removed from the choanae and the rhinopharynx. Then, moving the endoscope backward, the middle turbinates are repositioned medially. Usually no nasal packing is required.

2.4.1 Extended Approaches

The exposure of the suprasellar area through an extended approach becomes necessary for those macroadenomas directly and extensively invading this area, breaching the diaphragma sellae.

A wider opening of the upper portion of the anterior wall of the sphenoid sinus is required and it can be obtained by removing the superior and/or the supreme turbinates and the opening of the posterior ethmoid cells, mostly in the nasal cavity where the endoscope will be introduced and hold by the assistant. This will allow reducing conflict between the endoscope and the surgical instruments that has to be moved along a more anterior trajectory and reach a deeper surgical target.

Once the sphenoid cavity is exposed and all the landmarks already described are recognized, the removal of the suprasellar notch and of the posterior planum sphenoidale is realized. The opening can be extended in a posteroanterior direction up to 1.5–2 cm, never beyond the anterior wall of the sphenoid sinus. Laterally, the boundaries of bone removal are represented by the protuberances of the optic nerves that, at the level of the suprasellar notch, are distant ca. 14 mm (ranging from 9 to 24 mm); therefore, the opening of the planum will have the shape of a trapezium with the smaller base posteriorly. In such cases, the superior intercavernous sinus is often obliterated as compressed by the lesion. Dura mater opening starts from the midline and diverging in a Y-shaped cut over the planum to permit the exploration of the neurovascular structures localized above the diaphragma sellae. The adenoma removal starts from the inferior and the lateral aspects as for standard pituitary adenomas. The suprasellar part of the lesion is then debulked and its capsule, dissected from the surrounding neurovascular structures, using microscissors and sharp dissection from arachnoid, as in conventional microsurgical technique. The extended approach gives the advantage of a double surgical corridor for the management of the suprasellar portion of the lesion: the first, intracapsular, allows the debulking of the adenomas, and the second, extracapsular, permits the dissection of the capsule from the surrounding neurovascular structures. This is of utmost importance, especially in case of giant adenomas with prevalent intracranial extension, to achieve safe management of the lesion, thus preventing the possibility of intralesional hemorrhage of residual tumor that often results in severe complications, seldom to death [10, 16, 30, 40, 45].

In case of adenomas extending into the cavernous sinus, it has to be highlighted that two different surgical corridors have been described to gain access to different areas of the cavernous sinus, in regard to the position of the intracavernous carotid artery (ICA); one permits access to the cavernous sinus through its medial wall, while the other one through its lateral wall. If the tumor itself enlarges the C-shaped parasellar segment of the intracavernous internal carotid artery, it could be easier to adopt a medial corridor and remove the lesion by mean of suctioning and curettage. The approach to the lateral compartment of the cavernous sinus is more rarely indicated, in those cases involving the entire cavernous sinus, i.e., Knosp grade 4 adenomas. Such tumors occupying mainly the lateral compartment of the cavernous sinus usually displace the ICA medially and push the cranial nerves laterally invading the lateral recess of the sphenoid sinus, which could be considered a "gate" to the cavernous sinus. The surgical approach requires the flattening of the pterygoid process and of the bone enclosed between the vidian canal and the foramen rotundum at the level of the anterior wall of the sphenoid sinus, in order to gain a wider exposure of the lateral recess of the sphenoid sinus. Delicate maneuvers of curettage and suction usually allow the removal of the lesion, in the same fashion as for the intrasellar portion [31, 33, 34].

When extending into nasal or paranasal cavities, giant adenomas have to be approached via a lower trajectory. The surgical approach has to be tailored to the extension of the lesion so that nasal and/or paranasal structures have to be widely removed to improve the width of the surgical field and the maneuverability of surgical instruments.

After removal of the lesion, the skull base defect must be repaired. In case of adenomas with a prevalent intra- or infrasellar extension, the reconstruction does not require peculiar strategies, namely, when the suprasellar cistern has not been violated (this latter has anyway to be protected). On the other hand, when the suprasellar cistern has been opened, i.e., after removal of giant adenomas with predominant intracranial extension, the reconstruction of the osteodural defect with multilayer technique is required; the same technique used for craniopharyngiomas or tuberculum sellae meningiomas has to be adopted. Recently we adopt the "sandwich technique" in the reconstruction of the skull base: the surgical cavity is filled with fat sutured to the inner foil of a three-layer assembly of fascia lata or dural substitute; the first two layers are positioned intradurally and the third one between the dura and the bone, wedged in the extradural space. A pedicled nasoseptal flap as described by Hadad and popularized by Kassam is used to support the reconstruction [18, 36, 37, 41, 42, 49].

Mucoperichondrium of the middle turbinate can be used as well in case of moderate intraop CSF leak and quite small skull base defect.

An inflated Foley balloon catheter, filled with 7–8 ml of saline solution, can be placed in the sphenoid sinus to support the reconstruction.

It is still controversial if the use of lumbar drainage is recommended.

2.4.2 Complications

Complications after endoscopic endonasal transsphenoidal surgery can be listed according to the anatomical region involved into the approach so that nasal, sphenoid sinus, sellar, suprasellar, and parasellar complications can be analyzed.

Nasal complications consist prevalently in the delayed bleeding from a branch of the sphenopalatine artery or in scars/crusting into the nostrils (usually after some extended approaches). In the first case, nasal packing or reoperation with coagulation of the sphenopalatine artery can be proposed, while the resolution of scars/crusting is usually achieved by irrigation of the nasal cavities with saline solution or in case of persistent ones with an endoscopic exploration of the nasal cavities and with aerosol therapy.

Concerning the sphenoid sinus complications, mucocele formation and sphenoidal sinusitis are described. In these cases the aerosol therapy can be advised. The reoperation must be considered only in symptomatic patients.

With regard to sella turcica complications, CSF leakage is the most common, even if its rate in the standard approaches is about 1 %. On the other hand, in the extended approaches, it reaches 4–5 %. When it occurs, a reoperation for a new reconstruction of the skull base is mandatory. In case of minimal discontinuous leak, it is possible to adopt the so-called awake sealant endoscopic endonasal technique [19].

There is a wide range of supra and parasellar complications depending of the anatomical, physiological, and biological features of the lesions treated. The most feared is the meningitis; this can be treated with targeted antibiotic therapy. Visual complication following optic chiasm or oculomotor nerves injuries can occur and usually could improve upon corticosteroid treatment. After an extended approach to the suprasellar region, massive pneumocephalus can be present; it usually requires bed rest and radiation therapy and CT scan have to be performed to evaluate the air reabsorption.

Although extremely rare, the injury of the internal carotid artery represents a serious intraoperative complication that can compromise surgery. Immediate sphenoid packing must be performed, so that angiography and the eventual stenting or embolization procedure could be run.

Finally, among the endocrinological complications, it should be reminded that posterior pituitary disfunction, as well as anterior pituitary defects, can occur thus leading to transient or permanent diabetes insipidus which can be managed with vasopressin administration [1, 5].

Bibliography

1. Berker M, Hazer DB, Yucel T, Gurlek A, Cila A, Aldur M, Onerci M (2012) Complications of endoscopic surgery of the pituitary adenomas: analysis of 570 patients and review of the literature. Pituitary 15(3):288–300. doi:10.1007/s11102-011-0368-2
2. Bonneville JF (2000) Pituitary adenomas: value of MR imaging. J Radiol 81(9):939–942
3. Cappabianca P, Alfieri A, Colao A, Cavallo LM, Fusco M, Peca C, Lombardi G, de Divitiis E (2000) Endoscopic endonasal transsphenoidal surgery in recurrent and residual pituitary adenomas: technical note. Minim Invasive Neurosurg 43(1):38–43. doi:10.1055/s-2000-8814
4. Cappabianca P, Alfieri A, de Divitiis E (1998) Endoscopic endonasal transsphenoidal approach to the sella: towards functional endoscopic pituitary surgery (FEPS). Minim Invasive Neurosurg 41(2):66–73. doi:10.1055/s-2008-1052019
5. Cappabianca P, Cavallo LM, Colao A, de Divitiis E (2002) Surgical complications associated with the endoscopic endonasal transsphenoidal approach for pituitary adenomas. J Neurosurg 97(2):293–298. doi:10.3171/jns.2002.97.2.0293
6. Cappabianca P, Cavallo LM, de Divitiis O, Solari D, Esposito F, Colao A (2008) Endoscopic pituitary surgery. Pituitary 11(4):385–390. doi:10.1007/s11102-008-0087-5
7. Cappabianca P, Cavallo LM, Esposito F, De Divitiis O, Messina A, De Divitiis E (2008) Extended

endoscopic endonasal approach to the midline skull base: the evolving role of transsphenoidal surgery. Adv Tech Stand Neurosurg 33:151–199
8. Cappabianca P, Cavallo LM, Esposito F, Romano I, Colao A, de Divitiis E (2003) Rationale of presurgical medical treatment with somatostatin analogs in acromegaly. J Endocrinol Invest 26(8 Suppl):55–58
9. Cappabianca P, Cavallo LM, Esposito F, Valente V, de Divitiis E (2002) Sellar repair in endoscopic endonasal transsphenoidal surgery: results of 170 cases. Neurosurgery 51(6):1365–1371; discussion 1371–1372
10. Cappabianca P, Cavallo LM, Solari D, de Divitiis O, Chiaramonte C, Esposito F (2014) Size does not matter. The intrigue of giant adenomas: a true surgical challenge. Acta Neurochir 156(12):2217–2220. doi:10.1007/s00701-014-2213-7
11. Cappabianca P, Cirillo S, Alfieri A, D'Amico A, Maiuri F, Mariniello G, Caranci F, de Divitiis E (1999) Pituitary macroadenoma and diaphragma sellae meningioma: differential diagnosis on MRI. Neuroradiology 41(1):22–26
12. Cappabianca P, Esposito F, Magro F, Cavallo LM, Solari D, Stella L, de Divitiis O (2010) Natura abhorret a vacuo – use of fibrin glue as a filler and sealant in neurosurgical "dead spaces". Technical note. Acta Neurochir 152(5):897–904. doi:10.1007/s00701-009-0580-2
13. Carrau RL, Jho HD, Ko Y (1996) Transnasal-transsphenoidal endoscopic surgery of the pituitary gland. Laryngoscope 106(7):914–918
14. Casanueva FF, Molitch ME, Schlechte JA, Abs R, Bonert V, Bronstein MD, Brue T, Cappabianca P, Colao A, Fahlbusch R, Fideleff H, Hadani M, Kelly P, Kleinberg D, Laws E, Marek J, Scanlon M, Sobrinho LG, Wass JA, Giustina A (2006) Guidelines of the Pituitary Society for the diagnosis and management of prolactinomas. Clin Endocrinol (Oxf) 65(2):265–273. doi:10.1111/j.1365-2265.2006.02562.x
15. Cavallo LM, Cappabianca P, Galzio R, Iaconetta G, de Divitiis E, Tschabitscher M (2005) Endoscopic transnasal approach to the cavernous sinus versus transcranial route: anatomic study. Neurosurgery 56(2 Suppl):379–389; discussion 379–389
16. Cavallo LM, de Divitiis O, Aydin S, Messina A, Esposito F, Iaconetta G, Talat K, Cappabianca P, Tschabitscher M (2008) Extended endoscopic endonasal transsphenoidal approach to the suprasellar area: anatomic considerations – part 1. Neurosurgery 62(6 Suppl 3):1202–1212. doi:10.1227/01.neu.0000333786.98596.33
17. Cavallo LM, Messina A, Cappabianca P, Esposito F, de Divitiis E, Gardner P, Tschabitscher M (2005) Endoscopic endonasal surgery of the midline skull base: anatomical study and clinical considerations. Neurosurg Focus 19(1):E2
18. Cavallo LM, Messina A, Esposito F, de Divitiis O, Dal Fabbro M, de Divitiis E, Cappabianca P (2007) Skull base reconstruction in the extended endoscopic transsphenoidal approach for suprasellar lesions. J Neurosurg 107(4):713–720
19. Cavallo LM, Solari D, Somma T, Savic D, Cappabianca P (2014) The awake endoscope-guided sealant technique with fibrin glue in the treatment of postoperative cerebrospinal fluid leak after extended transsphenoidal surgery: technical note. World Neurosurg 82(3–4):e479–e485. doi:10.1016/j.wneu.2013.01.017
20. Cavallo LM, Solari D, Tasiou A, Esposito F, de Angelis M, D'Enza AI, Cappabianca P (2013) Endoscopic endonasal transsphenoidal removal of recurrent and regrowing pituitary adenomas: experience on a 59-patient series. World Neurosurg 80(3–4):342–350. doi:10.1016/j.wneu.2012.10.008
21. Cebula H, Kurbanov A, Zimmer LA, Poczos P, Leach JL, De Battista JC, Froelich S, Theodosopoulos PV, Keller JT (2014) Endoscopic, endonasal variability in the anatomy of the internal carotid artery. World Neurosurg 82(6):e759–e764. doi:10.1016/j.wneu.2014.09.021
22. Colao A, Annunziato L, Lombardi G (1998) Treatment of prolactinomas. Ann Med 30(5):452–459
23. Colao A, Auriemma RS, Galdiero M, Lombardi G, Pivonello R (2009) Effects of initial therapy for five years with somatostatin analogs for acromegaly on growth hormone and insulin-like growth factor-I levels, tumor shrinkage, and cardiovascular disease: a prospective study. J Clin Endocrinol Metab 94(10):3746–3756. doi:10.1210/jc.2009-0941
24. Colao A, Di Sarno A, Cappabianca P, Di Somma C, Pivonello R, Lombardi G (2003) Withdrawal of long-term cabergoline therapy for tumoral and nontumoral hyperprolactinemia. N Engl J Med 349(21):2023–2033. doi:10.1056/NEJMoa022657
25. Colao A, Pivonello R, Cappabianca P, Vitale G, Lombardi G (2003) The treatment algorithm of acromegaly. J Endocrinol Invest 26(8 Suppl):39–45
26. Colao A, Pivonello R, Galderisi M, Cappabianca P, Auriemma RS, Galdiero M, Cavallo LM, Esposito F, Lombardi G (2008) Impact of treating acromegaly first with surgery or somatostatin analogs on cardiomyopathy. J Clin Endocrinol Metab 93(7):2639–2646. doi:10.1210/jc.2008-0299
27. Dallapiazza RF, Grober Y, Starke RM, Laws ER Jr, Jane JA Jr (2015) Long-term results of endonasal endoscopic transsphenoidal resection of nonfunctioning pituitary macroadenomas. Neurosurgery 76(1):42–53. doi:10.1227/NEU.0000000000000563
28. de Divitiis E, Cavallo LM, Esposito F, Stella L, Messina A (2008) Extended endoscopic transsphenoidal approach for tuberculum sellae meningiomas. Neurosurgery 62(6 Suppl 3):1192–1201. doi:10.1227/01.neu.0000333785.04435.2c
29. de Notaris M, Solari D, Cavallo LM, D'Enza AI, Ensenat J, Berenguer J, Ferrer E, Prats-Galino A, Cappabianca P (2012) The "suprasellar notch," or the tuberculum sellae as seen from below: definition, features, and clinical implications from an endoscopic

endonasal perspective. J Neurosurg 116(3):622–629. doi:10.3171/2011.11.JNS111162
30. Di Maio S, Cavallo LM, Esposito F, Stagno V, Corriero OV, Cappabianca P (2011) Extended endoscopic endonasal approach for selected pituitary adenomas: early experience. J Neurosurg 114(2):345–353. doi: 10.3171/2010.9.JNS10262
31. Doglietto F, Lauretti L, Frank G, Pasquini E, Fernandez E, Tschabitscher M, Maira G (2009) Microscopic and endoscopic extracranial approaches to the cavernous sinus: anatomic study. Neurosurgery 64(5 Suppl 2):413–421; discussion 421–422. doi:10.1227/01.NEU.0000338943.08985.73
32. Dusick JR, Esposito F, Mattozo CA, Chaloner C, McArthur DL, Kelly DF (2006) Endonasal transsphenoidal surgery: the patient's perspective-survey results from 259 patients. Surg Neurol 65(4):332–341; discussion 341–342. doi:10.1016/j.surneu.2005.12.010
33. Frank G, Pasquini E (2002) Endoscopic endonasal approaches to the cavernous sinus: surgical approaches. Neurosurgery 50(3):675
34. Frank G, Pasquini E (2006) Endoscopic endonasal cavernous sinus surgery, with special reference to pituitary adenomas. Front Horm Res 34:64–82. doi:10.1159/000091573
35. Gillam MP, Molitch ME, Lombardi G, Colao A (2006) Advances in the treatment of prolactinomas. Endocr Rev 27(5):485–534. doi:10.1210/er.2005-9998
36. Hadad G, Bassagasteguy L, Carrau RL, Mataza JC, Kassam A, Snyderman CH, Mintz A (2006) A novel reconstructive technique after endoscopic expanded endonasal approaches: vascular pedicle nasoseptal flap. Laryngoscope 116(10):1882–1886. doi:10.1097/01.mlg.0000234933.37779.e4
37. Harvey RJ, Nogueira JF, Schlosser RJ, Patel SJ, Vellutini E, Stamm AC (2009) Closure of large skull base defects after endoscopic transnasal craniotomy. Clinical article. J Neurosurg 111(2):371–379. doi:10.3171/2008.8.JNS08236
38. Jane JA Jr, Thapar K, Kaptain GJ, Maartens N, Laws ER Jr (2002) Pituitary surgery: transsphenoidal approach. Neurosurgery 51(2):435–442; discussion 442–444
39. Jho HD, Carrau RL (1997) Endoscopic endonasal transsphenoidal surgery: experience with 50 patients. J Neurosurg 87(1):44–51. doi:10.3171/jns.1997.87.1.0044
40. Juraschka K, Khan OH, Godoy BL, Monsalves E, Kilian A, Krischek B, Ghare A, Vescan A, Gentili F, Zadeh G (2014) Endoscopic endonasal transsphenoidal approach to large and giant pituitary adenomas: institutional experience and predictors of extent of resection. J Neurosurg 121(1):75–83. doi:10.3171/2014.3.JNS131679
41. Kassam A, Carrau RL, Snyderman CH, Gardner P, Mintz A (2005) Evolution of reconstructive techniques following endoscopic expanded endonasal approaches. Neurosurg Focus 19(1):E8
42. Kassam AB, Thomas A, Carrau RL, Snyderman CH, Vescan A, Prevedello D, Mintz A, Gardner P (2008) Endoscopic reconstruction of the cranial base using a pedicled nasoseptal flap. Neurosurgery 63(1 Suppl 1):ONS44–ONS52; discussion ONS52–ONS53. doi:10.1227/01.neu.0000335010.53122.75
43. Kawase T, van Loveren H, Keller JT, Tew JM (1996) Meningeal architecture of the cavernous sinus: clinical and surgical implications. Neurosurgery 39(3):527–534; discussion 534–536
44. Knosp E, Steiner E, Kitz K, Matula C (1993) Pituitary adenomas with invasion of the cavernous sinus space: a magnetic resonance imaging classification compared with surgical findings. Neurosurgery 33(4):610–617; discussion 617–618
45. Koutourousiou M, Gardner PA, Fernandez-Miranda JC, Paluzzi A, Wang EW, Snyderman CH (2013) Endoscopic endonasal surgery for giant pituitary adenomas: advantages and limitations. J Neurosurg 118(3):621–631. doi:10.3171/2012.11.JNS121190
46. Laws ER Jr, de Los Reyes K, Rincon-Torroella J (2013) Lumbar drains in transsphenoidal surgery. J Neurosurg 118(2):480–481. doi:10.3171/2012.8.JNS121702
47. Laws ER Jr, Thapar K (1999) Pituitary surgery. Endocrinol Metab Clin North Am 28(1):119–131
48. Laws ER, Kanter AS, Jane JA Jr, Dumont AS (2005) Extended transsphenoidal approach. J Neurosurg 102(5):825–827; discussion 827–828. doi:10.3171/jns.2005.102.5.0825
49. Liu JK, Schmidt RF, Choudhry OJ, Shukla PA, Eloy JA (2012) Surgical nuances for nasoseptal flap reconstruction of cranial base defects with high-flow cerebrospinal fluid leaks after endoscopic skull base surgery. Neurosurg Focus 32(6), E7. doi:10.3171/2012.5.FOCUS1255
50. Locatelli D, Canevari FR, Acchiardi I, Castelnuovo P (2010) The endoscopic diving technique in pituitary and cranial base surgery: technical note. Neurosurgery 66(2):E400–E401; discussion E401. doi:10.1227/01.NEU.0000363746.84763.A5
51. McGinn GJ, McClarty MB (1997) The posttherapeutic pituitary gland. Posttherapeutic neurodiagnostic imaging. Lippincott-Raven Publishers, New York
52. Pecori Giraldi F, Cavallo LM, Tortora F, Pivonello R, Colao A, Cappabianca P, Mantero F, Group obotAt-BCsS (2015) The role of inferior petrosal sinus sampling in ACTH-dependent Cushing's syndrome: review and joint opinion statement by members of the Italian Society for Endocrinology, Italian Society for Neurosurgery, and Italian Society for Neuroradiology. Neurosurg Focus 38(2), E5. doi:10.3171/2014.11.FOCUS14766
53. Rhoton AL Jr (2002) The sellar region. Neurosurgery 51(4 Suppl):S335–S374
54. Rhoton AL Jr (2002) The supratentorial arteries. Neurosurgery 51(4 Suppl):S53–S120
55. Rodriguez O, Mateos B, de la Pedraja R, Villoria R, Hernando JI, Pastor A, Pomposo I, Aurrecoechea J

(1996) Postoperative follow-up of pituitary adenomas after trans-sphenoidal resection: MRI and clinical correlation. Neuroradiology 38(8):747–754
56. Romano A, Zuccarello M, van Loveren HR, Keller JT (2001) Expanding the boundaries of the transsphenoidal approach: a microanatomic study. Clin Anat 14(1):1–9
57. Semple PL, Webb MK, de Villiers JC, Laws ER Jr (2005) Pituitary apoplexy. Neurosurgery 56(1): 65–72; discussion 72–73
58. Solari D, Chiaramonte C, Di Somma A, Dell'Aversana Orabona G, de Notaris M, Angileri FF, Cavallo LM, Montagnani S, Tschabitscher M, Cappabianca P (2014) Endoscopic anatomy of the skull base explored through the nose. World Neurosurg 82(6S):S164–S170. doi:10.1016/j.wneu.2014.08.005
59. Yoon PH, Kim DI, Jeon P, Lee SI, Lee SK, Kim SH (2001) Pituitary adenomas: early postoperative MR imaging after transsphenoidal resection. AJNR Am J Neuroradiol 22(6):1097–1104

3 Endoscopic Endonasal Ethmoid-Pterygoid Transsphenoidal Approach to the Cavernous Sinus

Giorgio Frank and Ernesto Pasquini

Since its introduction, the endoscopic endonasal approach has given a new horizon to the cavernous sinus (CS) surgery, permitting to extend the standard transsphenoidal approach toward the parasellar area and even to adopt a more lateral corridor transpterygoid approach, called ethmoid-pterygoid-sphenoidal (EPS), to face directly also the more lateral compartments of CS. Indeed, the endoscopic endonasal approach allows the surgeon to follow the extension of the tumor into the cavernous sinus though a direct, straightforward, and completely extracranial route. Thus, it permits to combine the high versatility and possibility to tailor the approach in each case of the endoscopic technique to the greater tolerability and safety given by the endonasal transsphenoidal route. Indeed, at the beginning of last decade, the main issue related to cavernous sinus surgery was still represented the high invasivity and elevated and sometimes unacceptable morbidity rate of the standard transcranial approaches [1–3]. These factors have had led from an initial phase of enthusiasm in the 1980s to a progressive abandoning of CS surgery in favor of the radiosurgery in the next decades [1–5]. The renewing of interest for the cavernous sinus surgery has started thanks to the works of Alfieri and Jho, who reconsidered the anatomy of the CS the endoscopic endonasal perspective [6, 7]. The effort of these authors, followed by many other papers, describing in deeper details this "upside-down" anatomy, allowed some surgical groups to adopt these anatomical corridors in living patients to obtain satisfactory results in terms of tumor removal and low rate of complications [8–10]. Schematically the CS can be divided in two regions: one medial and one lateral to internal carotid artery (ICA). As mentioned before, the former can be approached through a standard endoscopic endonasal approach, not needing lateral expansion of the corridor [11]. Conversely, the latter requires to EPS extended approach [11]. In this chapter, we will analyze the anatomical and surgical premised and the results of this approach that in these years has proved to be a replicable technique with similar results in different surgical series, and thus it represents a technique which can be learned, transmitted, and adopted with satisfaction by different generations of neurosurgeons. However, endoscopic endonasal approach is not a "magic bullet" for all cavernous sinus tumors. Its indications should be well considered, and even if it can

Electronic supplementary material The online version of this chapter (doi:10.1007/978-3-319-21533-4_3) contains supplementary material, which is available to authorized users.

G. Frank, MD (✉)
Department of Neurosurgery, Center of Surgery for Pituitary Tumors and Endoscopic Skull Base Surgery, IRCCS Istituto delle Scienze Neurologiche, Bellaria Hospital, Via Altura, 3, Bologna 40139, Italy
e-mail: giorgio.frank.46@gmail.com

E. Pasquini, MD, PhD
ENT Department, Azienda Unità Sanitaria Locale di Bologna, Via Benni, 44, Budrio (BO) 40054, Italy
e-mail: ernesto-pasquini@ausl.bo.it

P. Cappabianca et al. (eds.), *Midline Skull Base Surgery*, DOI 10.1007/978-3-319-21533-4_3

be the first choice for many tumors in the hands of a properly trained endoscopic endonasal surgeon in a well-equipped surgical center, it always is only one of the weapons that a skull base surgeon should have in his arsenal.

3.1 Indications

Many tumors with different biological features and paths of growth can involve the cavernous sinus; the knowledge of these aspects is of pivotal role to evaluate the indications to an endoscopic endonasal approach. Furthermore, the kind of invasion of the CS can greatly vary, from a limited involvement of just one compartment to the complete infiltration with ICA encasement, making the EPS rather than the standard approach more appropriate to achieve a satisfactory tumor removal. Insofar, starting from the consideration that different tumors involve differently the CS and thus they should be differently approached, we found that the two main parameters to be kept in consideration are the biological features in terms of tumor infiltration of vessels and nerves and its pattern of growth in particular in relationship with the dural layers (Fig. 3.1). Some tumors, for example, meningiomas, metastasis, or carcinomas, tend to infiltrate the walls of ICA and the CS nerves. Thus, for these cases, the endoscopic endonasal approach can bring to catastrophic consequences, such as ICA rupture or permanent CN palsies, because no dissection between the tumor and the surrounding structures is possible [9]. It is noteworthy that for these cases, and especially for meningiomas, the risk of massive intra- or postoperative bleeding is not only represented by the chance of ICA rupture but also by the risk of injuries to the enlarged, engorged, and hypertrophic vessels, deriving from the intracavernous ICA, such as the meningo-hypophyseal trunk and the inferolateral artery, which are the main tumor feeders [12]. That makes this surgery particularly hazardous, because it is quite complex to identify the course of these vessels even with neuronavigation or intraoperative Doppler; furthermore any injuries to these arteries can provoke postoperative CN permanent deficits [9, 12]. Basing on our experiences, thus we consider the endoscopic endonasal approach contraindicated for these cases. Indeed, some authors reported as exclusive indications of endoscopic endonasal approach for CS meningiomas or malignancies their osteodural decompression [13–15]. It consists in the drilling of the posterior wall of sphenoidal sinus in the sellar and parasellar area with opening of the dural layer, as reported by some authors, in order to reduce the compression of the tumor on the CNs with the limited palliative aim to the recovery of the ophthalmoplegia [13–15]. The second parameter on which we based the indication for the endoscopic endonasal approach is the relationship between the dural layer and the tumor. Some substantially extradural tumors, such as chondrosarcoma and to a lesser extent chordomas, can in their growth compress and displace the CS, without any invasion [16]. In these cases, the endonasal approach is effective and it appears as the more natural and appropriate one, because it allows to approach the tumor through an extradural route, with its the same adopted to the tumor to involve the CS region. The endonasal approach allows to reach the tumor in its direction of growth also in the case of pituitary adenomas (PTA). These tumors can trespass the medial wall, entering in the CS, from the sella [11]. Their invasion can be limited to one or more compartments or diffuse in all CS. When PTAs involve only the medial or posterosuperior compartments of CS, a midline transsphenoidal approach allows to reach the tumor, following the tumor through the medial wall of CS. Conversely, when the tumor involves the anteroinferior or lateral compartments, we considered the EPS the more appropriate approach. A third selection criterion is represented by the tumor consistency. When the tumor is soft, its resection is clearly favored; conversely a hard, fibrous consistency with hemorrhagic aspect greatly increases the surgical complexity, hampering the tumor resection with a greater risk of vessels or nerves damages during the surgical maneuvers. Unfortunately, this crucial feature of the tumor, which is associated to better outcome, is scarcely predictable before surgery and can be useful only in cases already

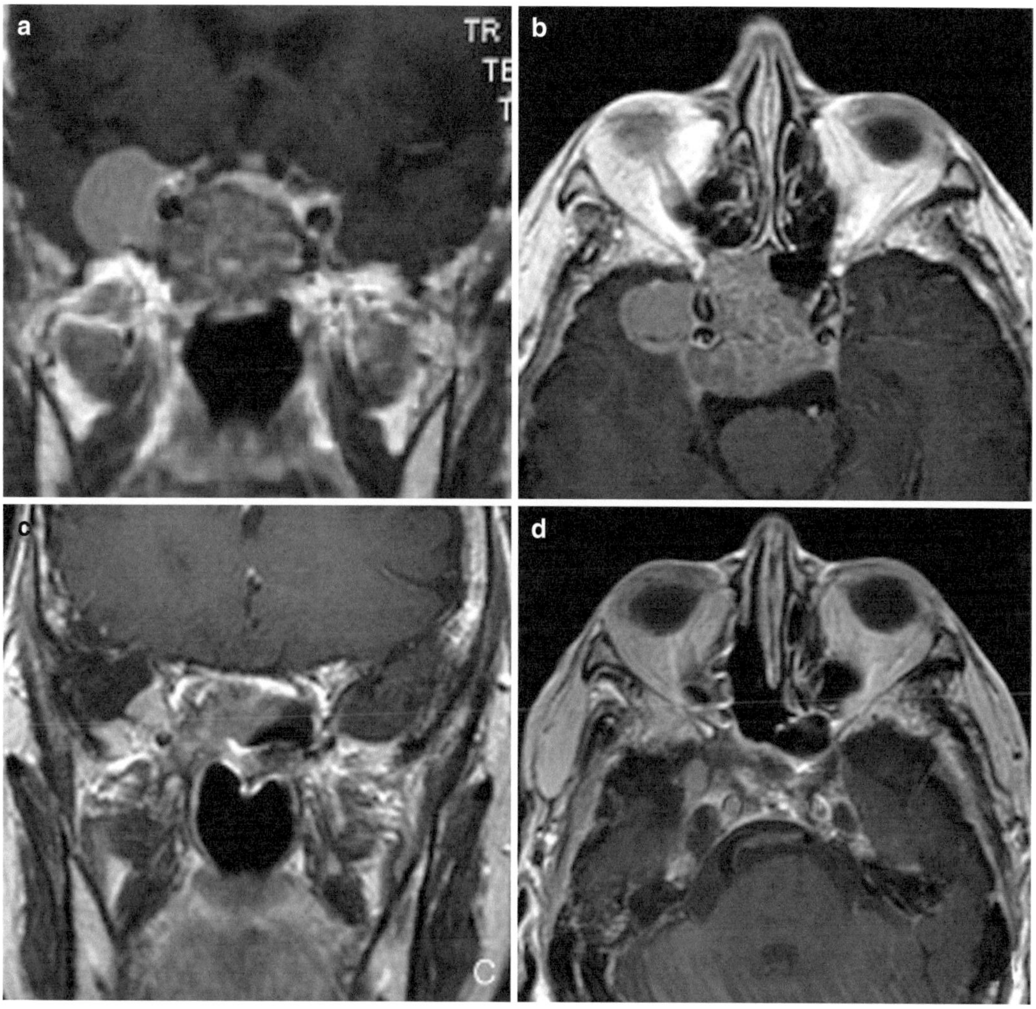

Fig. 3.1 MRI after gadolinium. Different tumors should be approached with different approaches, considering their different biological features and paths of growth. In (**a**, **b**) (coronal and axial views), the coexistence of a meningioma of lateral wall of right CS and of a clivus chordoma is appreciable, also involving the CS. The meningioma was treated first through a transcranial approach, while the chordomas was removed in the second stage through an EPS endoscopic endonasal approach. In (**c**, **d**) (coronal and axial views), the satisfactory surgical results with radical removal of both tumors are demonstrated

previously operated, of which, thus, the consistency is known. Hence, as long as a neuroradiological exam specific enough to assess the tumor consistency at the preoperative neuroimaging will not be validated, this selection criterion remains for the most only theoretical.

Following this criterion, in our experience from 1998 to December 2013, 435 patients with tumors involving the CS have been operated through an endoscopic endonasal approach. Their histology is reported in Table 3.1. PTAs represent the more common histotype, due to the higher incidence of this lesion compared to chordomas, chondrosarcomas, or rarer tumors such as schwannomas, epidermoid cysts, hemangiomas, or inflammatory diseases, such as a case of CS aspergillosis. However, even for PTA, the CS involvement represents a not extremely common condition: indeed, in the same time, 1170 PTAs have been operated; thus CS involvement is present in 32 %. Of these, an EPS was performed in 79 (7 % of the entire series) cases; thus the real

Table 3.1 The series of endoscopic endonasal surgeries for CS lesions from 1998 to 2013 at Center of Pituitary and Endoscopic Skull Base Surgery is presented

Pituitary adenomas	374	86 %
Chordomas/chondrosarcomas	49	11 %
Meningiomas	2	0.5 %
Neurinomas	3	0.75 %
Hemangioma	3	0.75 %
Epidermoid cyst	2	0.5 %
Inflammatory disease (Tolosa-Hunt S.)	2	0.5 %
Total	435	100 %

indication for this approach is very selected and reserved for tumors lateral to the ICA. On the contrary, for chordomas or chondrosarcomas, the involvement of CS is far more frequent, as in has been observed in 72 % of patients (49 out of 68). For these tumors, and especially for chondrosarcomas, which deriving from the spheno-petrous suture have a lateral to medial direction of CS involvement and thus are more frequently lateral to the ICA, EPS was adopted in 33 cases (48 %). Following the proper patient selection and tailoring the approach on the base of the tumor extension, we obtained a gross tumor removal in 66.3 %, a subtotal tumor removal (with remnant <20 %) in 28.1 %, and a partial tumor removal (with remnant >20 %) in 5.6 % cases of PTA. In the chordomas/chondrosarcomas series, the gross tumor removal was achieved in 51 % of cases, the subtotal tumor removal in 45 %, and partial tumor removal in 4 %. Postoperative definitive VI CN palsy occurred in 3 cases (6 %) after surgery for chordomas/chondrosarcomas, while in PTA series, two definitive (0.4 %) CN palsies were observed (in one case the VI CN and in one the III CN). One case of injury to ICA occurred on in a case of chordomas. Hemorrhage was controlled during surgery through gel foam and nasal packing and immediately after the vessels was closed via endovascular coiling. No neurological sequelae were observed.

3.2 Neuroradiology

Magnetic resonance imaging (MRI) is the gold standard to investigate CS involvement [17]. It is preferable to use high-field MRI, such as the 3 T, to obtain adequate images with the contrast enhancement and topographic resolution needed due to small dimension of the structures within it, their deep locations, and uneasy anatomical relationship especially when distorted by a tumoral mass [17]. The MRI study has 3 main goals. The first is to assess a radiological diagnosis, to identify the nature of the tumor. This is crucial in the patient selection phase to evaluate what surgical approach is preferable, in particular according to the selection criteria for the endoscopic endonasal approach. Even if only the histological confirmation can give the definite diagnosis, multiple neuroradiological signs can orientate the preoperative suspect, giving a working hypothesis, basing on which elaborate the treatment strategy. The recognizing of the origin of the tumor can strongly suggest the nature of the tumor. PTA derives from the pituitary gland, for macroadenomas is common to observe an enlarged sella, while only some small remnants of the gland are recognizable pushed in the periphery of the tumor for their evident enhancement after contrast [18]. Chordomas or chondrosarcomas take origin from the clivus or from the spheno-petrosal junction and are associated to erosion of these bony structures. Chondosarcoma are usually brightly hyperintense at T2WI, while chordomas have a more mixed pattern of hypo- and hyperintensity after gadolinium [19]. These tumors, PTA, chordomas, and condrosarcomas, can engulf or totally encase the ICA, but the vessels are of normal caliber, compared to the contralateral one, without any stenosis due to the tumor compression [19]. Conversely, this sign is commonly associated to meningiomas or malignancies which tend to infiltrate and finally to close the vessel. Malignant tumors, such as adenocarcinomas or nasal carcinoma, usually derive from the surrounding paranasal sinuses and occupy the nasal fossa and can present a dural tail as well as meningiomas. These have a uniform and diffuse contrast enhancement and can take origin from the CS, which completely filled by the tumor with a "bombé" or convex aspect [19]. Some exophytic portions can be observed in the sella or other surrounding regions. On the other hand, meningiomas can infiltrate the CS, taking origin in other places, such as the middle fossa, the sellar diaphragm, the anterior or posterior clinoid, or the pterygopalatine fossa. It is important to remark that also nontumoral lesions can involve the CS, and these lesser frequent lesions should be taken in consideration to avoid potentially disastrous event [20, 21]. This is particularly true for intracavernous ICA aneurysm. In these cases the flow sign from the lesion and the relationship with vessels are quite peculiar, but a confirmation through a MRA, CTA, or angiography is mandatory [21]. Finally, inflammatory disorders, such as infections or other idiopathic forms, must be considered for atypical lesions, sometimes enhancing and presenting a dural tail [20]. These patients can present a medical history of immunodepression, hematological disorders, or chemotherapeutic treatments, and they can have alterations in blood examinations. The second goal of the MRI is to determine the involvement of CS, showing where in its wall the tumor overwhelms the dural layer to enter into it; how the vasculo-nervous structures, mainly ICA and III, IV, V1, and VI CNs, are displaced; and what compartments of CS are occupied by the tumor. This evaluation is crucial for the surgical plan, to analyze which corridor can give the more wide and direct access to the tumor, avoiding to cross nervous and vascular structures. To be sufficiently accurate and precise in these determinations, the study should include multiple sequences such as thin (2–3 mm) coronal and sagittal T1W1 with and without contrast administration and thin T2WI multiplanar images. Basing on the information provided by these examinations, it is possible for PTAs to classify the tumor in 4° according to Knosp classification (Table 3.2) [22]. We analyzed in our series of 314 PTAs the reliability of Knosp grade to predict the effective CS invasion (Table 3.3). We found that especially for grade 1 and 2 this classification did not allow reliable conclusions, and in 68 % of cases, only a compression without a medial wall interruption was observed at surgical inspection (Fig. 3.2). Conversely, in 5 sporadic cases with no apparent CS invasion and preoperative imaging according to Knosp classification (Knosp 0), a limited invasion of the medial compartment of CS was

Table 3.2 The Knosp classification is presented

ICSI	
Knosp 0	PTA does not reach the medial aspect of the ICA
Knosp 1	Invasion extending to, but not past, the intercarotid line
Knosp 2	Invasion extending to, but not past, the lateral aspect of the ICA
Knosp 3	Invasion past the lateral aspect of the ICA but not completely filling the CS
Knosp 4	Completely filling the CS both medial and lateral to the ICA

Table 3.3 The comparison between Knosp grade and effective CS invasion at surgical inspection is provided

ICSI	0	1	2	3	4
Knosp 0	0	5	0	0	0
Knosp 1	87	8	2	0	0
Knosp 2	59	32	27	10	0
Knosp 3	19	17	38	20	8
Knosp 4	0	0	0	25	17
Total	165 (44.1 %)	62 (16.2 %)	67 (17.9 %)	55 (14.7 %)	25 (6.7 %)

ICSI 0 CS compression, *ICSI 1* invasion of medial compartment, *ICSI 2* invasion of medial and posterosuperior compartment, *ICSI 3* diffuse invasion including the anteroinferior compartment, *ICSI 4* complete invasion with involving of lateral compartment

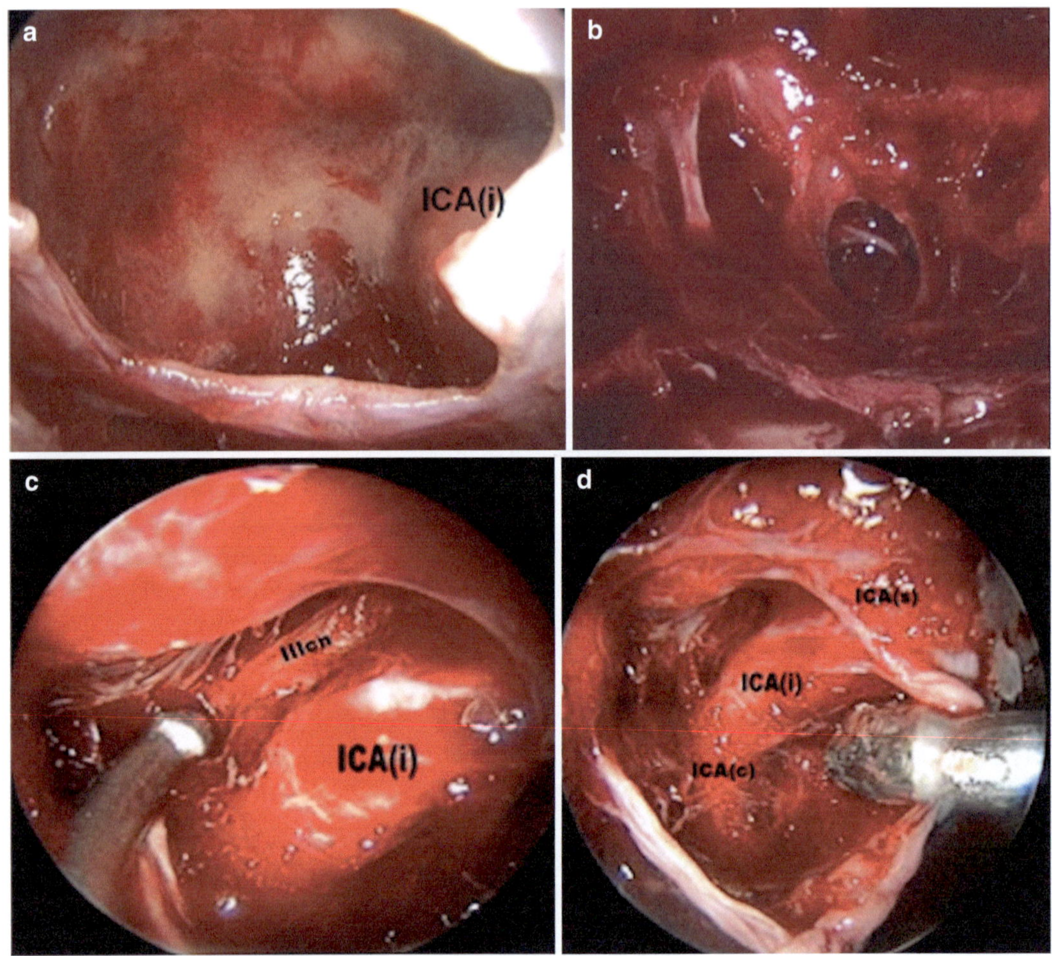

Fig. 3.2 Intraoperative images of PTA surgeries. (**a**) 0° endoscope. After tumor removal, at surgical inspection, the medial wall of Cavernous Sinus is intact and no invasion was observed. (**b**) 30° endoscope. A pit hole on the left medial wall was revealed after the tumor removal. The surgical inspection proved the focal invasion of medial compartment of CS. (**c**) 30° endoscope. The tumor was invading the medial and posterosuperior compartments of CS. Following the tumor invasion from a standard midline approach with a medial-to-lateral trajectory, it is possible to obtain a satisfactory tumor removal when this is mainly medial to ICA. (**d**) 0° endoscope. The anteroinferior and lateral compartments are exposed after tumor removal, performed through an EPS approach. The chance to extent the tumor removal lateral to ICA is shown

revealed. Also for chordomas or chondrosarcomas, the preoperative imaging can lead to inconsistent suspect of CS invasion, as showed in the Fig. 3.3. More innovative sequences, such as fast imaging employing steady-state acquisition (FIESTA) images, promise to assess with a higher accuracy than standard examination the tumor/CS relationship [23]. If the more wide and large experience will confirm these preliminary data, the role of these studies will become in the next years determining in the preoperative assessment of CS tumors. The distortion of the vasculo-nervous structures, and in particularly of the ICA, is crucial in the choice of the surgical approach. When the tumor pushes the artery anteriorly and laterally, mainly occupying the medial and posterosuperior compartments, a midline approach is more appropriate, permitting to approach the tumor from medial to lateral and reducing the chance of injury of the vessels. Conversely, if the ICA is pushed medially or is encased by the tumor, the EPS is preferred to work laterally to ICA with a direct orientation (Fig. 3.4). A few studies can be particularly help-

Fig. 3.3 (**a**, **c**) MRI after gadolinium and (**b**) intraoperative image 0° degrees endoscope. A chondrosarcoma is involving the left CS. The left ICA is completely encased by the tumor, but a hypointense linear sign, connecting the artery to the dura of middle fossa, is visible (*black arrow*). This sign represents the collapsed CS, which remains as dural envelope around the ICA. (**b**) When the tumor is completely removed, it is possible to observe that the ICA is covered by a dural envelope. Thus, the CS is not invaded by the tumor, but only compressed so far, it remains a virtual space around the ICA. (**c**) After tumor removal, the CS is decompressed, and it progressively re-expands to occupy its region

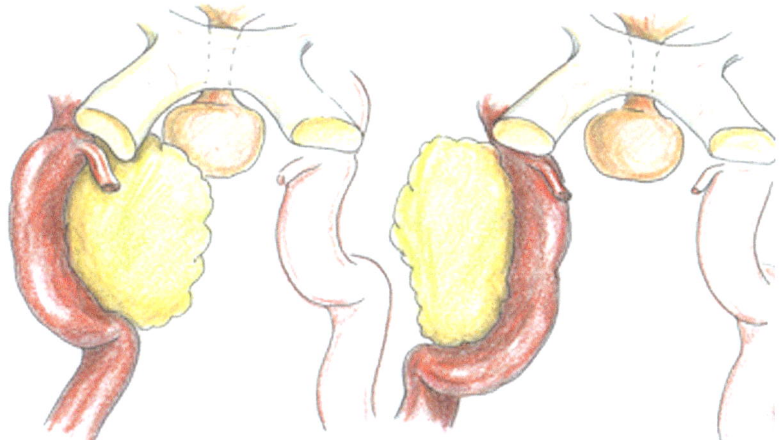

Fig. 3.4 Schematic drawing. In (**a**) the CS mass displaced the ICA laterally and posteriorly. This condition favors the approach of the tumor through a standard midline approach. In (**b**) the ICA is displaced medially; this requires an EPS approach to face directly the tumor, placed laterally to the artery

ful to evaluate the course of ICA, such as magnetic resonance angiography (MRA), and in particular sequences such as MRA+TOF with contrast, which shows in detail the relationship between tumor and ICA (Fig. 3.5). At present, it is not always evident to evaluate the course of the CNs, and in particular of the VI CN, which running free inside the CS is at major risk to be injured during the tumor removal. Some authors proposed diffusion tensor images (DTI) with tractography or 3D anisotropy contrast to identify with high precision the course of the CNs in the CS [24, 25]. Finally, the third goal of MRI consists in giving some information about the tumor consistency, to allow the surgeon to predict the outcome and assess its surgical strategy and even to plan preoperatively complementary treatments, such as radiosurgery, radiotherapy, or others. For lesions with a cystic component, the T2WI, marking the water content, can clearly identify this aspect, but to determine the consistency in solid tumors, these studies are lesser accurate [26]. Some authors propose to adopt the diffusion-weighted images (DWI), to predict the firmness of the tumors. Indeed, the apparent diffuse coefficient (ADC) is influenced by cellularity and extracellular fibrosis; thus a restricted diffusion is expression of a high reticulin content and thus a higher consistency of the tumor [27]. The efficacy of these analyses seems confirmed

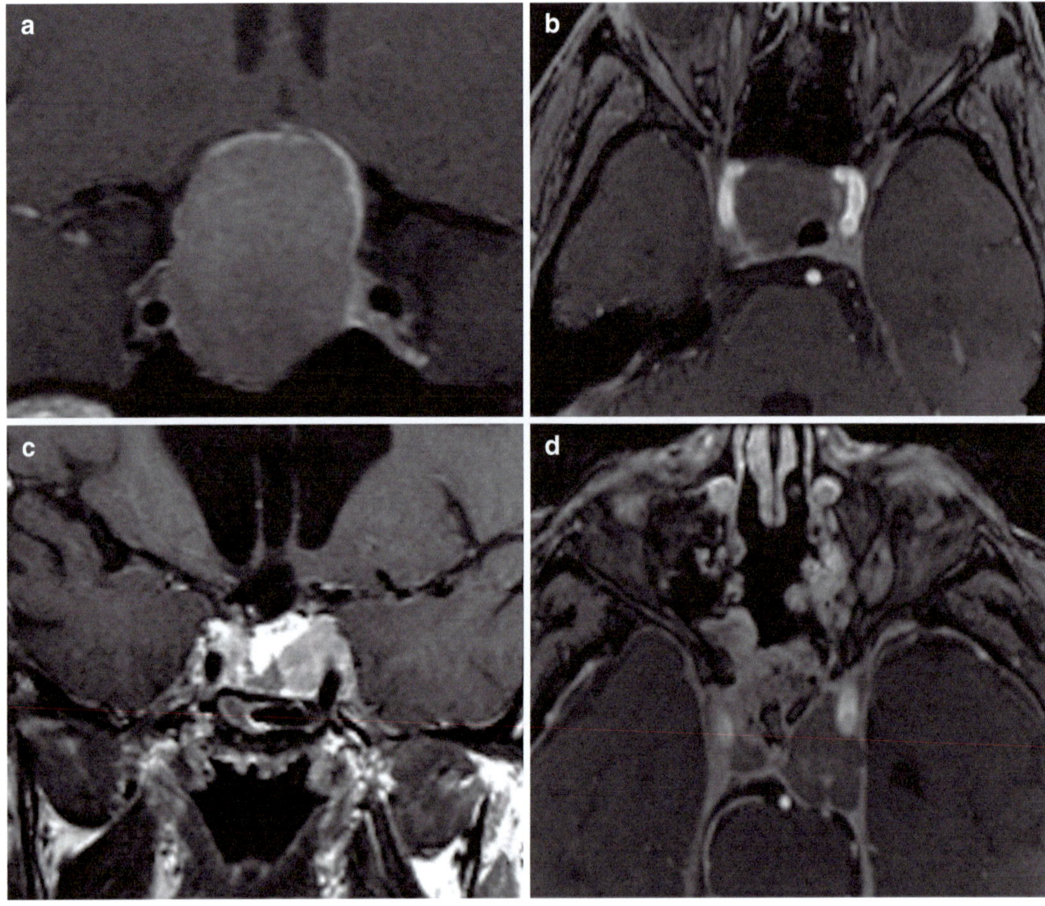

Fig. 3.5 (**a**, **c**) Coronal MRI T1WI after gadolinium. (**b**, **d**) Axial MRA+TOF after gadolinium. (**a**, **b**) An endo/suprasellar PTA with involvement of right CS is showed. Thanks to MRA+TOF sequences, the lateral displacement of right ICA appears more evident. (**c**, **d**) A recurrence in the left CS in a patient previously operated for a giant PTA is evident. The MRA+TOF shows how the tumor is displaced anteriorly and medially the ICA

by recent studies, and some authors proposed a threshold of ADC value of 1.1 to predict a more favorable tumor removal (Fig. 3.6) [27]. As we have seen, the MRI is more relevant preoperative study of neuroimaging, but also the CT scan and for some extent the angiography still have a role in the preoperative assessments. The CT scan is very helpful to precisely locate the bony landmarks of the approach, and thus a study of the nasal and paranasal anatomy is highly recommended before surgery especially for patients with anatomical variants, complete or partial lack of sphenoidal sinus pneumatization, pediatric cases, re-interventions, where the anatomy can be distorted by the previous approach, and in general for all cases in the early phases of the learning course of each single surgeon. The knowledge of the location of the bony landmarks in the patients can be essential to orientate the surgeon and avoid complications. This can be favored by the adoption of neuronavigation with the preoperative CT scan in the approaching phase of the surgery. The neuronavigation can obtain even a major role, if combined with CT angiography (CTA), which permits to locate the course of ICA, reducing the risk of injuring during the approach and the CS opening (Fig. 3.7). Finally, the angiography can provide information similar to those obtained by MRA, to analyze the course of ICA. Moreover, it is the mail examination that can provide information about the patency of anastomotic circuits by the contralateral ICA or basilar artery through the compression test (Fig. 3.8). This is important in case of

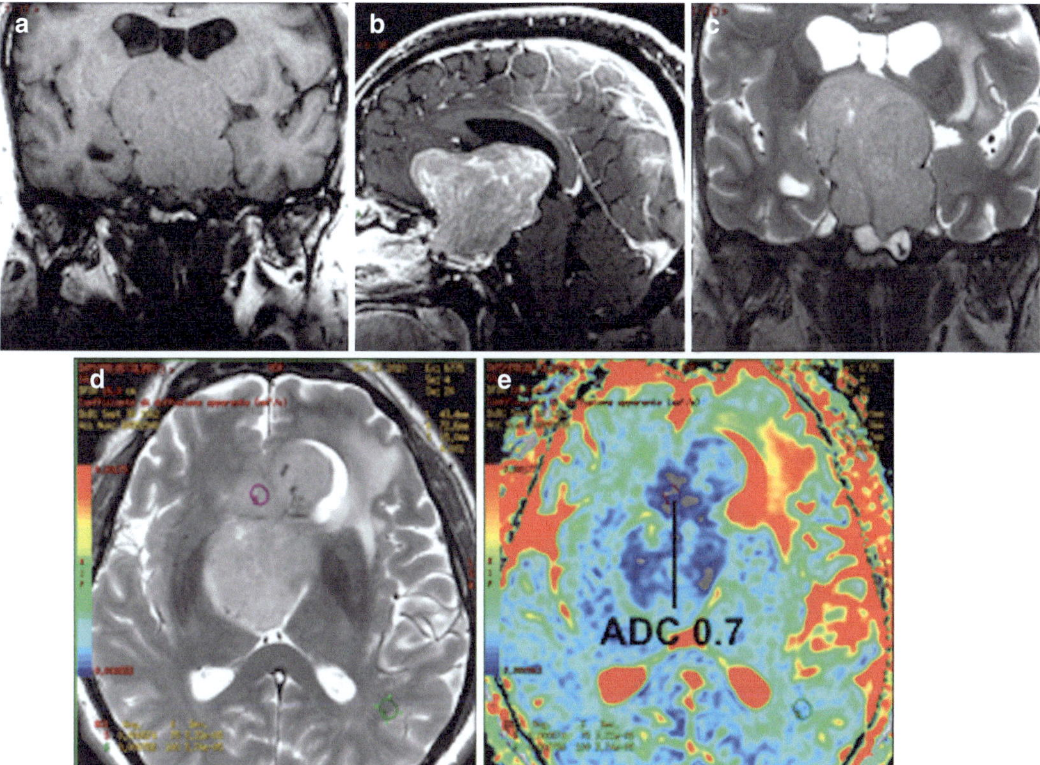

Fig. 3.6 MRI, (**a**) coronal T1W1, (**b**) sagittal T1WI after gadolinium, (**c**) T2WI, (**d**, **e**) DWI. A giant PTA with bilateral involvement of CS is showed. The tumor is hypointense at T1 and T2WI and enhances diffusely. The DWI shows a restricted diffusion, with a low ADC, which is consistent with a hard and fibrous tumor, as it was confirmed during surgery

ICA injury or pseudoaneurysm to plan a closure through coiling of the vessel and to determine the risk of neurological sequelae.

3.3 Anatomy of the Approach

The endoscopic endonasal approaches to CS require an advanced knowledge of skull base anatomy from an inverted point of view comparing to the classic neurosurgical perspective. Thus, we consider the knowledge of the anatomy of nasal and paransal sinuses and of skull base crucial as well as the experience in endoscopic endonasal surgery of the surgeon to avoid catastrophic complications. In the approach phase, the first target of the surgeon should be the identification of the sphenoidal ostium. The tail of superior turbinate points to this opening as an arrow, and it is the more useful landmark in the nasal stage. For a standard midline approach to CS, entering into this ostium and then its enlargement up to a complete sphenoidotomy are enough to identify the landmarks on posterior wall of sphenoidal sinus and to localize the sellar bulge and the ICA protuberances and the optic nerves. The quadrangular space comprised between the optic nerve superiorly, the sellar bulge medially, and a horizontal line inferiorly passing at the level of the vidian nerve or of the junction between petrosal and cavernous ICA represents the CS region (Fig. 3.9). This anatomical exposure allows to see laterally the course of ICA, but it is disadvantageous to work, because it imposed an angled trajectory to the surgeon. To expand laterally this approach, it is necessary to expose and partially remove the pterygoid plates. This maneuver requires to displace medially the middle turbinate and thus to observe the uncinate process and the bulla ethmoidalis

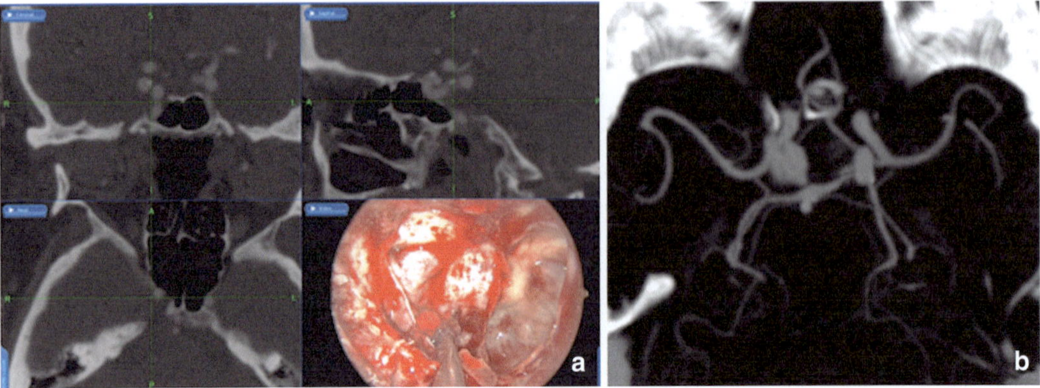

Fig. 3.7 CTA. (**a**) Neuronavigation with intraoperative image. The localization of the right ICA in the posterior wall of sphenoidal sinus in a clivus chordoma is showed. (**b**) CTA is helpful also in the differential diagnosis of CS tumors and aneurysm. An intracavernous aneurysm of right ICA, mimicking a parasellar mass, is demonstrated

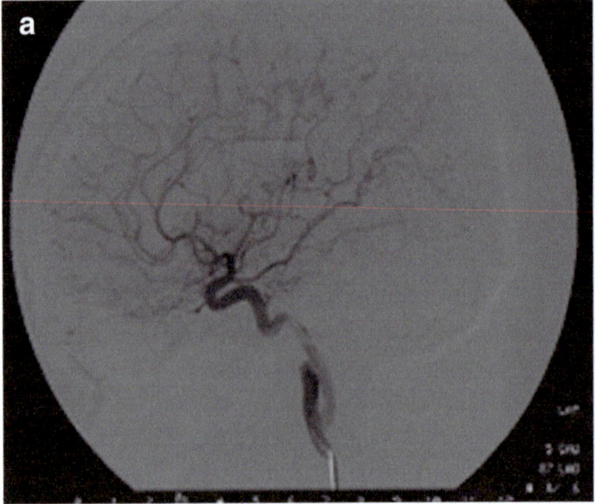

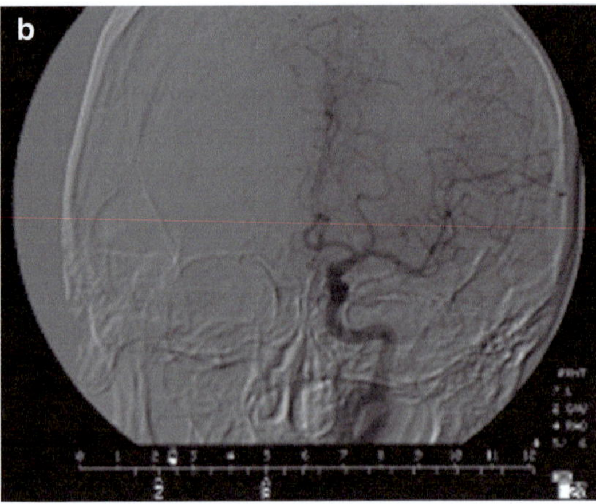

Fig. 3.8 Angiography in course of compression test. (**a**) Lateral view during left ICA. (**b**) Frontal view during right ICA injection and compression of the left. The injection demonstrates that left ICA is patent. During compression test, no injection of the left medial cerebral artery (MCA) is observed, concluding that no collateral circles are present to give adequate contralateral compensation

(Fig. 3.10 a,b). Removing these structures, the natural ostium of maxillary sinus is usually visible. The tail of middle turbinate allows to recognize the sphenopalatine foramen, which usually marked anteriorly by a bony ridge, called crista ethmoidalis. When this landmark is identified, it is possible to remove the vertical process of palatine bone, which lies posteriorly to maxillary sinus. After its removal, the medial and lateral pterygoid plates are exposed (Fig. 3.10c). The EPS approaches are concluded when the medial and superior aspects of these process are removed and the ethmoid is completely resected. That permits to identify from a more lateral perspective the same bony landmark on the posterior wall of sphenoidal sinus, previously illustrated (Fig. 3.10d). After dural skeletonization, the course of ICA with its anterior loop is clearly appreciable (Fig 3.10e). Opening the dura medial to ICA, the medial compartment of CS is accessed; in its inferior border, the anterior hypophyseal artery running toward the pituitary gland is present. It is derived from the meningo-hypophyseal trunk, which takes origin on the convexity of the supero-posterior surface of the posterior bend of the ICA (Fig. 3.11d). On the lateral wall surface

Fig. 3.9 Cadaveric endoscopic endonasal dissection. 0° endoscope. (**a**) The posterior wall of sphenoidal sinus is exposed. The main landmarks are recognizable, and they allow to localize the quadrangular projection of the CS region. (**b**) After bone removal and dural opening, the CS and its content are clearly showed

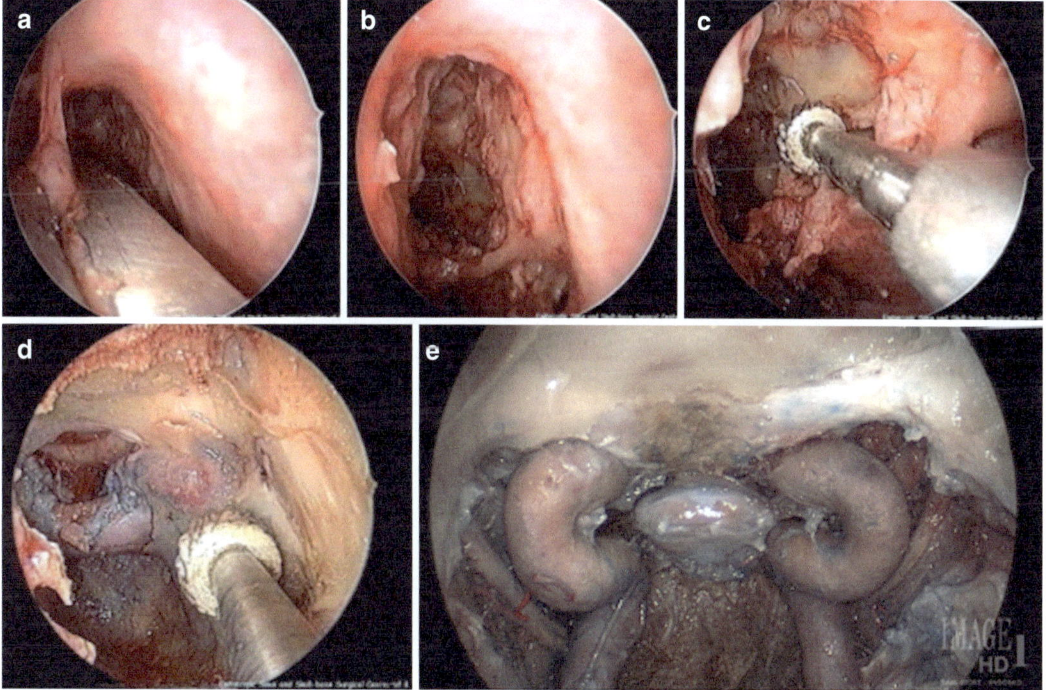

Fig. 3.10 Cadaveric endoscopic endonasal dissection. 0° endoscope. (**a**) The left middle turbinate resection is gently medialized and then resected. (**b**) That gives access to the ethmoid, which is removed. (**c**) The pterygoid plates are drilled in their medial and superior portion. (**d**) The posterior wall of sphenoidal sinus is exposed. (**e**) The dura of CS is opened and its structures are exposed

of the horizontal segment of ICA, in the lateral compartment, the inferolateral trunk is appreciable. This artery is a relevant landmark, because it covers the VI CN, where these nerves received the sympathetic fibers from the pericarotid plexus (Fig. 3.11b). More lateral, embedded in the lateral wall of CS, the III, IV, and V1 CNs are visible in their course toward the superior orbital fissure (Fig. 3.11c). In a small rate of case, the ophthalmic artery can take from the intravenous ICA, and thus particularly attention shout be taken on the superior portion of the lateral compartment.

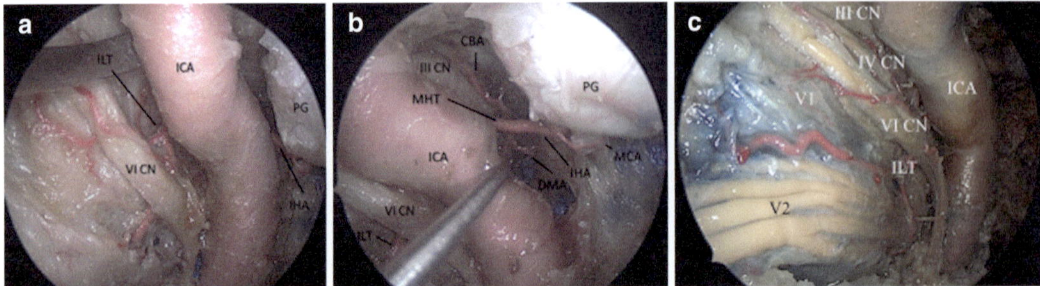

Fig. 3.11 Cadaveric endoscopic endonasal dissection. (**a**, **b**) 0° endoscope. (**c**) 30° endoscope. (**a**) The meningo-hypophyseal trunk deriving from the ICA in the medial compartment is exposed. (**b**) The inferolateral trunk and its relationship with the VI CN are evident. (**c**) The CN in the medial wall of CS and the VI CN, running free within it, are shown. *ICA* internal carotid artery, *PG* pituitary gland, *ILT* infero-lateral trunk, *CN* cranial nerve, *MHT* meningo-hypophyseal trunk, *CBA* Cassinari-Bernasconi Artery, *IHA* inferior hypophyseal artery, *DMA* Dorsal meningeal artery, *MCA* medial clivus artery

3.4 Technique

As we have seen, to approach tumors invading the CS, two main corridors can be adopted: the standard midline transsphenoidal (MTea) and the ethmoid-pterygoid-sphenoidal (EPS). The former consists in a wide anterior sphenoidotomy; we usually do not perform ethmoidectomy and middle turbinectomy, to expose the sellar bulge on the posterior wall of CS and identify the other anatomical landmarks, such as medial optic-carotid recess (Fig. 3.12a). After bone opening and dural incision at the level of sellar protuberance medial to the internal carotid artery (ICA), the tumor removal is performed with the microsurgical two-hand technique, dissecting the tumor from the surrounding dural structures and normal pituitary gland, with a progressive central debulking through suction or curettes, while the endoscope is fixed on a holder. The portion of the tumor invading the medial compartment is resected following the extension of the tumor and using the same opening in the medial wall of CS that the tumor created to invade the compartment (Fig 3.2b). In case of involvement of the postero-superior compartment of CS the resection through suction, curettes and dissectors is extended also to this portion passing through the intracavernous carotid loop. At the end of the tumor removal, venous bleeding was usually not noteworthy and can be generally well-controlled with hemostatic absorbable material. Afterward, the inspection of the surgical field through 30 and 45° angled endoscopes permitted the detection and removal of neoplastic residues (Fig. 3.2). The surgical defect can be closed using absorbable material, whereas in the case of a CSF leak, we usually repair using free graft with fat and/or mucoperiosteum taken from the middle turbinate. The EPS is the lateral extension of the MTea approaches, allowing to face frontally also the portion of the CS lateral to the ICA. EPS can be divided in three phases. The first stage is represented by the approach to the parasellar area. It requires an ethmoidal route through a middle turbinectomy and complete monolateral ethmoidectomy, followed by the sphenoidotomy. The medial portion of the posterior wall of the maxillary sinus is therefore resected to expose the posterior wall of the maxillary antrum and the vertical process of the palatine bone. After coagulation or clipping of pterygopalatine artery in the foramen, the vertical process is drilled out and the medial pterygoid process exposed. Its resection allows to reach the inferolateral portion of the cavernous sinus. In this stage the resection of the middle and superior turbinates is particular useful to gain a peripheral view of the entire sellar and parasellar region and improve the maneuverability of the surgical instruments in the region. The second stage is represented by the opening of the CS and by the tumor removal phase. With the auxilium of neuronavigation, the sellar and posterolateral wall of the sphenoid was removed to expose the external

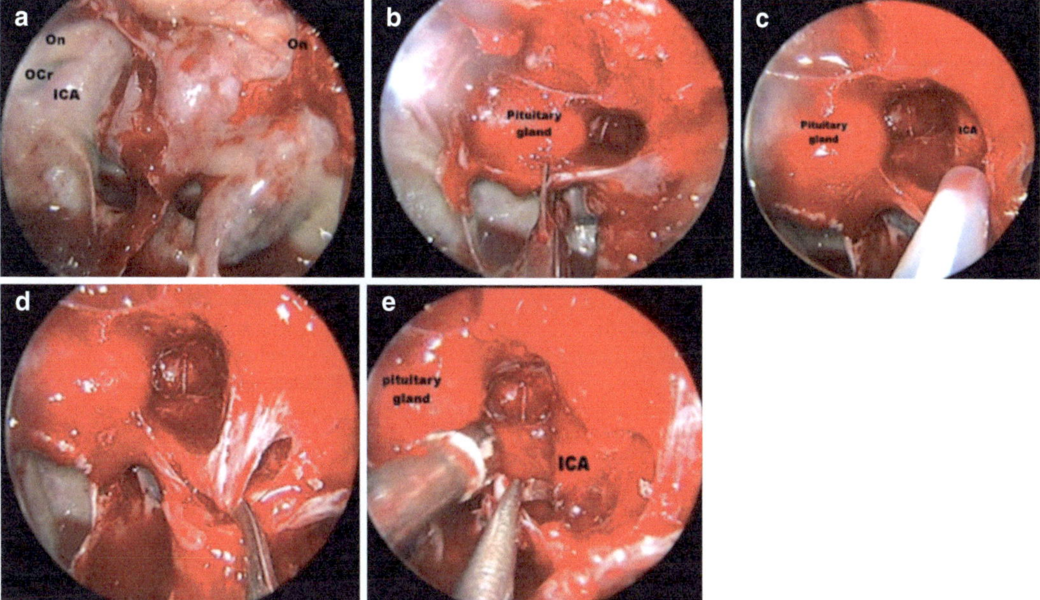

Fig. 3.12 Intraoperative images. 0° endoscope. (**a**) The posterior wall of cavernous sinus (*CS*) is exposed and the landmarks are visible. (**b**) The medial compartment is cleaned after the tumor is removed from this region. (**c**) With the intraoperative Doppler, the exact location of internal carotid artery (*ICA*) is recognized. (**d**) The dura is opened. (**e**) The ICA is visible and the tumor removal is completed. *ON* optic nerve, *OCr* optic-carotid recess, *ICA* Internal carotid artery

dural layer of the cavernous sinus. In this phase it is crucial to locate precisely the position of the ICA; this can be achieved with the combined use of neuronavigation and micro-Doppler. The dural opening can be performed medially to the ICA, to access to anteroinferior compartment of CS, or laterally to ICA to enter into the lateral compartment (Fig. 3.12 b). Using curettes, it was possible to mobilize the tumor fragments before their suction and/or removal. The last stage corresponds to the same of the previous approach: consisting in the final exploration and closure of the surgical defect. Bleeding from CS is usually not significant and well controlled with hemostatic absorbable material. After surgical field inspection through 30 and 45° angled endoscopes, the eventual CSF leak is repaired with multilayer free graft technique.

Acknowledgment Figures 3.2, 3.3, and 3.4 have been taken at the ALT-VISION at Wexner Medical Center, the Ohio State University, Columbus, Ohio, USA. We thank Dr. D. Prevedello, Dr. R. Carrau, and Dr. B. Otto, directors of the laboratory, for giving us the permission to use these pictures.

References

1. Dolenc VV (1997) Transcranial epidural approach to pituitary tumors extending beyond the sella. Neurosurgery 41(3):542–550
2. Eisenberg MB, Al-Mefty O, DeMonte F, Burson GT (1999) Benign nonmeningeal tumors of the cavernous sinus. Neurosurgery 44(5):949–954
3. Fahlbusch R, Buchfelder M (1988) Transsphenoidal surgery of parasellar pituitary adenomas. Acta Neurochir (Wien) 92(1–4):93–99
4. Kuo JS, Chen JC, Yu C, Zelman V, Giannotta SL, Petrovich Z, MacPherson D, Apuzzo ML (2004) Gamma knife radiosurgery for benign cavernous sinus tumors: quantitative analysis of treatment outcomes. Neurosurgery 54(6):1385–1393
5. Lee JP, Tsai MS, Chen YR (1993) Orbitozygomatic infratemporal approach to lateral skull base tumors. Acta Neurol Scand 87(5):403–409
6. Alfieri A, Jho HD (2001) Endoscopic endonasal cavernous sinus surgery: an anatomic study. Neurosurgery 48(4):827–836
7. Alfieri A, Jho HD (2001) Endoscopic endonasal approaches to the cavernous sinus: surgical approaches. Neurosurgery 49(2):354–360
8. de Divitiis E, Cappabianca P, Cavallo LM (2002) Endoscopic transsphenoidal approach: adaptability of the procedure to different sellar lesions. Neurosurgery 51(3):699–705

9. Cappabianca P, Cavallo LM, Esposito F, De Divitiis O, Messina A, De Divitiis E (2008) Extended endoscopic endonasal approach to the midline skull base: the evolving role of transsphenoidal surgery. Adv Tech Stand Neurosurg 33:151–159
10. Doglietto F, Lauretti L, Frank G, Pasquini E, Fernandez E, Tschabitscher M, Maira G (2009) Microscopic and endoscopic extracranial approaches to the cavernous sinus: anatomic study. Neurosurgery 64(5 Suppl 2):413–421
11. Frank G, Pasquini E (2006) Endoscopic endonasal cavernous sinus surgery, with special reference to pituitary adenomas. Front Horm Res 34:64–82
12. d'Avella E, Tschabitscher M, Santoro A, Delfini R (2008) Blood supply to the intracavernous cranial nerves: comparison of the endoscopic and microsurgical perspectives. Neurosurgery 62(5 Suppl 2):ONS305–ONS310
13. Walsh MT, Couldwell WT (2009) Management options for cavernous sinus meningiomas. J Neurooncol 92(3):307–316
14. Akutsu H, Kreutzer J, Fahlbusch R, Buchfelder M (2009) Transsphenoidal decompression of the sellar floor for cavernous sinus meningiomas: experience with 21 patients. Neurosurgery 65(1):54–62
15. Mendelson ZS, Patel AA, Eloy JA, Liu JK (2014) Endoscopic palliative decompression of the cavernous sinus in a rare case of a metastatic renal cell carcinoma to the clivus. Br J Neurosurg 9:1–2
16. Frank G, Sciarretta V, Calbucci F, Farneti G, Mazzatenta D, Pasquini E (2006) The endoscopic transnasal transsphenoidal approach for the treatment of cranial base chordomas and chondrosarcomas. Neurosurgery 59(1 Suppl 1):ONS50–ONS57
17. Linn J, Peters F, Lummel N, Schankin C, Rachinger W, Brueckmann H, Yousry I (2011) Detailed imaging of the normal anatomy and pathologic conditions of the cavernous region at 3 T using a contrast-enhanced MR angiography. Neuroradiology 53(12):947–954
18. Hess CP, Dillon WP (2012) Imaging the pituitary and parasellar region. Neurosurg Clin N Am 23(4):529–542
19. Patel SC, Silbergleit R, Talati SJ (1999) Sarcomas of the head and neck. Top Magn Reson Imaging 10(6):362–375
20. Mandrioli J, Frank G, Sola P, Leone ME, Guaraldi G, Guaraldi P, Collina G, Roncaroli F, Cortelli P (2004) Tolosa-Hunt syndrome due to actinomycosis of the cavernous sinus: the infectious hypothesis revisited. Headache 44(8):806–811
21. Locatelli M, Spagnoli D, Caroli M, Isalberti M, Branca V, Gaini SM, Lania A (2008) A potential catastrophic trap: an unusually presenting sellar lesion. Eur J Neurol 15(1):98–101
22. Knosp E, Steiner E, Kitz K, Matula C (1993) Pituitary adenomas with invasion of the cavernous sinus space: a magnetic resonance imaging classification compared with surgical findings. Neurosurgery 33(4):610–617
23. Amemiya S, Aoki S, Ohtomo K (2009) Cranial nerve assessment in cavernous sinus tumors with contrast-enhanced 3D fast-imaging employing steady-state acquisition MR imaging. Neuroradiology 51(7):467–470
24. Yamada K, Shiga K, Kizu O, Ito H, Akiyama K, Nakagawa M, Nishimura T (2006) Oculomotor nerve palsy evaluated by diffusion-tensor tractography. Neuroradiology 48(6):434–437
25. Yoneoka Y, Isogawa M, Terumitsu M, Matsuzawa H, Fujii Y (2010) Insidious extension of pituitary prolactinoma: two can't-miss findings depicted on a 3.0-T MR system. J Neuroimaging 20(3):267–271
26. Bahuleyan B, Raghuram L, Rajshekhar V, Chacko AG (2006) To assess the ability of MRI to predict consistency of pituitary macroadenomas. Br J Neurosurg 20(5):324–326
27. Boxerman JL, Rogg JM, Donahue JE, Machan JT, Goldman MA, Doberstein CE (2010) Original research. Preoperative MRI evaluation of pituitary macroadenoma: imaging features predictive of successful transsphenoidal surgery. Am J Roentgenol 195:720–728

4 Radiotherapy and Radiosurgery

Giuseppe Minniti and Claudia Scaringi

4.1 Introduction

External beam radiotherapy is an essential component of treatment of patients with benign skull base tumors. Radiotherapy is generally used in patients with residual or recurrent pituitary adenomas following surgery, with the aim of preventing tumor regrowth and normalizing elevated hormone levels. It is successful in achieving tumor control in up to 90–95 % of patients at 10 years, though excess hormone secretion may take some time to subside. However, despite the evidence that radiation reduces the rate of local recurrence and the low risk of toxicity when the treatment is delivered within the radiation tolerance limits of central nervous system, the role of postoperative radiation for these tumors is debated.

In the last three decades, advances in radiological imaging and the computer sciences and their application to radiotherapeutic planning and delivery have led to more accurate and focused treatment. Modern radiotherapy has evolved with the development of conformal and stereotactic techniques which allow higher doses of radiation to the tumor while limiting the amount of radiation to normal brain, with the hope of minimizing the long-term consequences of treatment while maintaining its effectiveness. The use of new techniques with potentially low toxicity has regained its place in the role of multimodal treatment approach for pituitary adenomas located at difficult accessible location.

4.2 Technical Advances in Radiotherapy

The aim of modern radiotherapy is to give maximum radiation dose to the tumor with least dose to normal brain. This is achieved by accurate localization of the tumor with computed tomography (CT) scan and magnetic resonance imaging (MRI), 3-dimensional (3D) computer treatment planning, precise immobilization, and radiation treatment delivery.

Patients are typically positioned on the couch in supine position and immobilized in a custom-made plastic mask with movement limited to 3–5 mm. For localization of pituitary adenomas, it is essential to use both CT and MRI

G. Minniti, MD (✉)
Radiation Oncology Unit, Department of Radiation Oncology, Sant' Andrea Hospital, University Sapienza, Via di Grottarossa 1035, Rome 00189, Italy

Department of Neuroscience, Neuromed Institute, Pozzilli (IS), Italy
e-mail: gminniti@ospedalesantandrea.it; giuseppeminniti@libero.it

C. Scaringi, MD
Radiation Oncology Unit, Department of Radiation Oncology, Sant' Andrea Hospital, University Sapienza, Via di Grottarossa 1035, Rome 00189, Italy

P. Cappabianca et al. (eds.), *Midline Skull Base Surgery*, DOI 10.1007/978-3-319-21533-4_4

imaging. Accurate delineation of visible tumor and possible residual disease should be based also on preoperative images and surgical notes. While the extent of the tumor and its relationship to critical structures are best seen with MRI, the co-registered CT scan provides the appropriate X-ray absorption characteristics necessary for accurate radiotherapy planning. A variable margin of 3–7 mm expanded in 3D beyond the gross tumor volume (GTV) to generate the planning target volume (PTV) is included in treatment planning to allow for patient movement and setup variation between treatments. During tumor delineation critical surrounding structures such as the optic apparatus or the brain stem are outlined. However, when doses of 45–50 Gy below tolerance limits of normal central nervous system (CNS) are used, the definition of the treatment or tumor volume should not be compromised by specific normal tissue avoidance.

3D treatment planning provides improved visualization of dose distribution within the target and the organs at risk of radiation toxicity, with the option of giving a more homogeneous target dose with a dose variation < 10 % and lower normal tissue dose to critical structures at risk of radiation toxicity. The CT image set is also used to reconstruct a plain film radiograph (digitally reconstructed radiograph – DRR) to confirm the treatment portal and arrangement for treatment quality assurance.

Localized irradiation is achieved by shaping the radiation beams to conform to the shape of the tumor, thus sparing more surrounding normal tissue. The technique of shaping radiation beams, described as conformal radiotherapy, is part of standard practice for all intracranial tumors and this is achieved with the use of a multileaf collimator (MLC). The leaves are automatically positioned to predefined shapes based on information transferred directly from the planning computer. Conventional external beam radiotherapy for skull base tumors uses 3–4 radiation beams. The total dose of 45–50 Gy for pituitary adenomas is achieved by daily doses of 1.8–2.0 Gy, with treatment lasting for 5–5.5 weeks.

MLC leaves can also be used to alter the intensity of radiation and this is described as intensity-modulated radiation therapy (IMRT). IMRT allows for better conformation of radiation to complex shape targets particularly with concave regions containing critical normal tissue and may improve sparing of normal brain tissue in selected patients with large residual tumors.

Stereotactic irradiation is a further refinement of conformal radiotherapy. Stereotactic irradiation can be given as single-fraction radiosurgery (SRS) using either multi-headed cobalt unit (Gamma Knife – GKSRS) or a linear accelerator (Linac SRS) or as fractionated stereotactic conformal radiotherapy (FSRT) delivered as fractionated treatment using a linear accelerator. The principal advances of stereotactic compared to conventional irradiation are improved immobilization using either fixed or relocatable frames. SRS is generally given with a patient immobilized in a fixed frame with an accuracy less than 1 mm. SRS is given as a single dose of 16–25 Gy generally with the preparation and treatment carried out in one day. FSRT is carried out using either a precision mask system or a relocatable frame which allows multiple treatments, with relocation accuracy in the region of 1–3 mm. Treatment delivery is improved with the use of multiple (usually 4–8) fixed shaped beams employing MLC with smaller leaves (mini or micro MLC).

Proton radiation has the appeal of superior conformality in dose distribution when compared to 3D-CRT and IMRT, therefore offering the potential for better sparing of normal tissue particularly beyond the principal target. The rationale for application in pituitary adenomas is the reduction of integral radiation dose to normal tissue, possibly limiting the long-term late effects of irradiation, and this could be especially important in pediatric tumors.

4.3 Clinical Outcome of Radiotherapy

Conventional external beam radiotherapy has traditionally been used following incomplete resection of pituitary adenomas and at the time of progression or recurrence of previously resected tumors. The aim of treatment is to achieve long-term local tumor control and normalization of hormone hypersecretion in patients with secreting pituitary adenomas.

Large series assessing the long-term effectiveness of radiation report an actuarial tumor growth control in the region of 80–90 % at 10 years and 75–90 % at 20 years [1–13]. The reported results are summarized in Table 4.1. Tumor control is similar for secreting and nonfunctioning pituitary adenomas regardless of the size of the residual tumor.

The reported tumor control is similar for doses ranging from 45 to 55 Gy at ≤ 2 Gy per fraction. The recommended dose for pituitary adenomas is generally 45–50 Gy at <2 Gy per fraction. There is no clear evidence that long-term control is influenced by timing of radiotherapy. Although some authors suggest that surgery followed by radiotherapy may provide the best therapeutic option for patients with residual tumor without major risks [14, 15], most of published series reported no difference in tumor growth control for patients who received immediate postoperative radiotherapy and those who received radiotherapy at the time of recurrence or progression [16]. In practice this means that deferring radiotherapy for patients with complete or near-complete resection seems to be a safe and reasonable approach. Tumor progression may be detected early with a close postoperative imaging follow-up and patients may be treated effectively with radiotherapy at time of tumor regrowth. Immediate postoperative RT as a potentially effective treatment modality can be reserved for patients with large and invasive pituitary adenomas after incomplete surgical removal. However, only prospective randomized trials can determine whether radiotherapy and its timing alter survival and quality of life in patients with subtotally resected pituitary adenomas.

In patients with secreting pituitary adenomas, the main goal of treatment is normalization of excess hormone production. Radiotherapy is effective in normalizing growth hormone (GH) and insulin-like growth factor I (IGF-1) levels in a consistent proportion of acromegalic patients, with a progressive rate of GH and IGF-1 declining. Most studies report the biochemical remission of disease in 30–50 % of acromegalic patients at 5–10 years and 75 % of patients at 15 years after treatment [9–12]. GH levels fall to around 50 % by 2 years with IGF-1 taking longer. Lower initial levels are associated with faster biochemical control of the disease.

Pituitary irradiation in patients with Cushing's disease in whom transsphenoidal surgery is unsuccessful achieves a biochemical remission of disease, measured as normalization of urinary and plasma cortisol concentration, in up to 80 % of patients at 5 years. After radiotherapy, the rate of reduction of urinary free cortisol is a 50 % drop in 6–12 months and the rate of decline of plasma cortisol is 50 % in 12 months [6, 13]. In a series of 42 patients with Cushing's disease treated with postoperative radiotherapy, the 10-year actuarial progression-free survivals were 93 % and 95 %. Biochemical remission of disease occurred in 80 % of patients with remission rates of 73, 78, and 83 % after 3.5 and 10 years [13]. Estrada et al. [6] reported a similar remission rate of 83 % in 30 patients with Cushing's disease after postoperative radiotherapy, with the majority of remissions that occurred within the first 2 years after the treatment.

Radiotherapy is less frequently used in the treatment of prolactinomas since medical treatment with dopamine agonists can achieve tumor shrinkage and normalize prolactin levels in more than 80 % of patients. It is employed in occasional patients who fail surgery and medical therapy with a reported hormone normalization rate of 30–50 % [17].

4.4 Toxicity

The risk of late normal CNS toxicity of external beam radiotherapy to doses <50 Gy at <2 Gy per fraction is low, with a reported incidence of optic neuropathy resulting in visual deficit of 1–3 % and risk of necrosis of normal brain structures of 0–2 % (Table 4.1). Hypopituitarism represents the most commonly reported late complication of radiotherapy, occurring in 30–60 % of irradiated patients 10 years after treatment, and the proportion is likely to increase with time. An increased

Table 4.1 Summary of results of published series on fractionated RT for pituitary adenomas

Authors	Type of irradiation	Type of adenoma	Patients (no)	Follow-up median (years)	Local control (%)	Late toxicity (%)	
						Visual	Hypopituitarism
Grigsby et al. (1989) [1]	CRT	NFA, SA	121	11.7	89.9 at 10 years	1.7	NA
McCollough et al. (1991) [2]	CRT	NFA, SA	105	7.8	95 at 10 years	NA	NA
Brada et al. (1993) [3]	CRT	NFA, SA	411	10.8	94 and 88 at 10 and 20 years	1.5	30 at 10 years
Tsang et al. (1994) [4]	CRT	NFA, SA	160	8.7	87 at 10 years	0	23
Zierhut et al. (1995) [5]	CRT	NFA, SA	138	6.5	95 at 5 years	1.5	27
Estrada et al. (1997) [17]	CRT	ACTH	30	3.5	73 at 2 years[a]	0	57
Breen et al. (1998) [7]	CRT	NFA	120	9	87.5 at 10 years	1	NA
Gittoes et al. (1998) [8]	CRT	NFA	126	7.5	93 at 10 and 15 years	NA	NA
Barrande et al. (2000) [9]	CRT	GH	128	11	53 at 10 years[a]	0	50 at 10 years
Biermasz et al. (2000) [10]	CRT	GH	36	10	60 at 10 years[a]	0	54 at 10 years
Epaminonda et al. (2001) [11]	CRT	GH	67	10	65 at 15 years[a]	0	NA
Minniti et al. (2005) [12]	CRT	GH	45	12	52 at 10 years[a]	0	45 at 10 years
Minniti et al. (2007) [13]	CRT	ACTH	40	9	78 and 84 at 5 and 10 years[a]	0	62 at 10 years
Milker-Zabel et al. (2001) [23]	FSRT	NFA, SA	68	38	93 at 5 years	7.5	5
Milker-Zabel et al. (2004) [24]	FSRT	GH	20	26	92[a]	0	3
Paek et al. (2005) [25]	FSRT	NFA	68	30	98 at 5 years	3	6
Colin et al. (2005) [26]	FSRT	NFA, SA	110	48	99 at 5 years	1.8	29 at 4 years
Minniti et al. (2006) [27]	FSRT	NFA, SA	92	32	98 at 5 years	1	22
Kong et al. (2007) [28]	FSRT	NFA, SA	64	36.7	97	0	27.3 at 5 years
Wilson et al. (2012) [30]	FSRT	NFA	67	60.1	93 at 5 years	1.5	7
Kim et al. (2013) [31]	FSRT	NFA, SA	76	80	97.1 at 7 years	0	48
Ronson et al. (2006) [62]	Protons	NFS,SA	47	>6 months	94	6	23

RT radiotherapy, *CRT* conformal radiotherapy, *NFA* nonfunctioning adenoma, *SA* secreting adenoma, *NA* not assessed, *ACTH* adrenocorticotropic hormone, *GH* growth hormone, *FSRT* fractionated stereotactic radiotherapy
[a]Biochemical remission of disease

incidence of cerebrovascular accidents and excess cerebrovascular mortality has been reported in patients with pituitary adenoma treated with conventional radiotherapy, although the risk has not been defined and the influence of radiation on its frequency is also not clear [18]. Radiation is associated with the development of a second, radiation-induced brain tumor. The reported frequency of development of gliomas and meningiomas following treatment of pituitary adenoma is 2 % at 20 years [19]. Although radiotherapy to large volumes of normal brain, particularly in children, is a recognized consequence of large-volume cranial irradiation [20, 21], there is little evidence that fractionated irradiation for pituitary adenomas may significantly alter cognitive function beyond the effect of other interventions and the tumor itself.

4.5 Fractionated Stereotactic Radiotherapy

The reported 5-year control for pituitary adenomas following FSRT is 85–100 % [22–30] (Table 4.1). In a series of 92 patients with either nonfunctioning or secreting pituitary adenomas treated with FSRT at a dose of 45 Gy delivered in 25 fractions at the Royal Marsden Hospital, the 5-year tumor control was 97 % and the 5-year survival 98 % [26]. Colin et al. [26] reported the clinical outcomes in 110 patients with pituitary adenomas who received FSRT at a mean dose of 50.4 Gy in 28 fractions. After a minimum follow-up of 48 months, the 5-year tumor control was 99 % and hormone hypersecretion normalization was 42 % out of 47 patients with a secreting tumor. Similar results have been reported by others using a dose of 45–54 Gy, with an overall median 5-year control of 95 % [27–30]. A reduction in size of the tumor after FSRT is reported in 15–45 % of patients. An improvement of visual deficits has been reported in up to 20–50 % of patients after FSRT.

Milker-Zabel et al. [23] reported normalization of elevated growth hormone level in 70 % of acromegalic patients at a median of 26 months. In another series of 34 acromegalic patients treated with FSRT, Roug et al. [29] reported the normalization of GH and IGF-1 levels in 30 % of patients at a median follow-up of 30 months, being 24 %, 38 %, and 64 % after 1, 3, and 5 years, respectively, similar to that seen following conventional radiotherapy. There is limited data on FSRT in patients with Cushing's disease or prolactinomas. In a small series of 12 patients, control of elevated cortisol concentration was reported in nine out of 12 patients (75 %) at a median time of 29 months [32].

Hypopituitarism is reported in 20–40 %% of patients at 5 years (Table 4.1). Even if FSRT may reduce radiation doses to the hypothalamus, theoretically reducing the incidence of hypopituitarism after the treatment, damage to the pituitary gland cannot be avoided when irradiating the pituitary fossa. So far, the incidence of hypopituitarism is likely to represent the major complication of radiation treatment even with the further optimization of techniques. Other late complications are rarely recorded; however, the relatively short follow-up requires caution in interpretation until more mature and reliable results are available both in terms of efficacy and late radiation-induced toxicity.

4.6 Stereotactic Radiosurgery

SRS is frequently used in patients with residual or recurrent pituitary adenomas. The reported 5-year tumor growth control with the use of SRS in patients with nonfunctioning pituitary adenomas is between 87 and 100 % (Table 4.2) [33–58]. In a large retrospective multicenter study of 512 patients with nonfunctioning pituitary adenomas treated with SRS, the reported actuarial tumor control was 95 and 85 % at 5 and 10 years [38], respectively, and similar results have been documented in few other large series using doses of 16–25 Gy [34–37].

SRS has been extensively used in patients with acromegaly after unsuccessfully surgery and/or resistant to medical therapy, with a reported normalization of serum GH concentration and IGF-1 in 30–50 % of patients at 5 years, and the biochemical remission of disease continues throughout the follow-up period (Table 4.2). Although initial reports suggested that the declining of serum GH concentration is faster after SRS compared with fractionated RT [59], recent reports show a hormone decline in the same region as following conventional treatment, depending from baseline GH/IGF-1 levels [41, 44, 46].

For patients with Cushing's disease treated with SRS using doses of 22–28 Gy, the biochemical remission of disease evaluated by normalization of 24-h urinary free cortisol and/or plasma cortisol concentration is reported in 40–70 % of patients and the time to hormonal response ranges from 6 months to 3 years [52–55] (Table 4.2). In

Table 4.2 Summary of recent published of SRS for pituitary adenomas

Authors	Patients (no)	Type of adenoma	Follow-up (months)	Tumor control (%)	Late toxicity (%)	
					Visual	Hypopituitarism
Losa et al. (2004) [33]	56	NFA	41	88 at 5 years	0	24
Mingione et al. (2006) [34]	100	NFA	45	92.2	0	25
Liscak et al. (2007) [35]	140	NFA	60	100	0	2
Park et al. (2011) [36]	125	NFA	62	94 at 5 years	0.8	24
Starke et al. (2012) [37]	140	NFA	50	97 at 5 years	12.8	30.3
Sheehan et al. (2013) [38]	512	NFA	36	95 at 5 years	6.6	21
Jezkova et al. (2006) [39]	96	GH	53.7	44 at 5 years	0	27.1
Voges et al. (2006) [40]	64	GH	54.3	14 and 33 at 3 and 5 years	1.4	13 and 18 at 3 and 5 years
Pollock et al. (2007) [41]	46	GH	63	11 and 60 at 2 and 5 years	0	33 at 5 years
Vik-Mo et al. (2007) [42]	53	GH	67	58 and 86 at 5 and 10 years	3.8	10 at 5 years
Jagannathan et al. (2008) [43]	95	GH	57	53	4	34
Losa et al. (2008) [44]	83	GH	69	52 and 85 at 5 and 10 years	0	10 at 10 years
Iwai et al. (2010) [45]	26	GH	84	17 and 47 at 5 and 10 years	0	8
Castinetti et al. (2009) [46]	43	GH	96	42,0	0	23
Sheehan et al. (2011) [47]	130	GH	31	53	2.4	24.4
Franzin et al. (2012) [48]	112	GH	71	58.3 at 5 years	0	14
Liu et al. (2012) [49]	40	GH	72	47.5	0	40
Wilson et al. (2013) [50]	86	GH	66	18.6	1.2	19.8
Devin et al. (2004) [51]	35	ACTH	35	49	0	40
Castinetti et al. (2007) [52]	40	ACTH	54	42.5	2.5	15
Jagannathan et al. (2007) [53]	90	ACTH	45	54	5.5	22
Sheehan et al. (2013) [54]	96	ACTH	48	70	5	36
Wilson et al. (2014) [55]	36	ACTH	66	25	0	13.9
Pan L et al. (2000) [56]	128	PRL	33	41	0	NA
Pouratian et al. (2006) [57]	28	PRL	55	26	7	28
Jezkova et al. (2009) [58]	35	PRL	75.5	37.1	NA	NA

SRS stereotactic radiosurgery, *NFA* nonfunctioning adenoma, *GH* growth hormone, *ACTH* adrenocorticotropic hormone, *PRL* prolactin, *NA* not assessed

a large retrospective series of 96 patients with Cushing's disease treated with GK SRS at the University of Virginia, Sheehan et al. [54] showed a tumor control and biochemical remission rate of 98 and 70 %, respectively, with a time to normalization of 16.6 months, and similar results have been reported by others [53–55].

SRS is usually reserved for prolactinomas resistant to medical therapy with dopamine agonists. In a series of 26 patients treated with GK SRS, Pouratian et al. [57] observed a tumor control and remission of the disease in 89 and 26 % of patients, respectively, with an average time to normalization of 24.5 months. In another large retrospective series of 112 patients with a prolactinoma treated with GK using a median dose of 31 Gy, Pan et al. [56] have reported hormonal normalization rate of 52 % at a median follow-up of 33 months.

The most commonly observed complication following SRS for secreting adenomas is hypopituitarism, with an incidence ranging between 10 and 40 % at 5 years (Table 4.2). Other complications, including cranial nerve deficits and optic neuropathy, are reported in 0–8 % of patients; however, for doses less than 10 Gy to the optic apparatus, the reported rate of radiation-induced optic neuropathy is < 2 %.

There is much debate about the relative efficacy of SRS and FSRT. Data from literature suggest no clear benefits in the efficacy and toxicity of SRS compared with FSRT for both nonfunctioning and secreting pituitary adenomas. In clinical practice, SRS is usually offered to patients with pituitary adenomas moderate in size away from the optic apparatus, whereas FSRT is preferred over SRS for lesions >2.5–3 cm in size and/or involving the anterior optic pathway.

More recently an image-guided robotic radiosurgery system (CyberKnife) has been employed for performing frameless SRS using either single-fraction or multi-fraction (2–5 fractions) SRS with promising results [60, 61]. Using doses of 21–25 Gy delivered in three to five sessions with CyberKnife, Iwata et al. [61] reported a local control rate of 98 % at 3 years in 100 patients with nonfunctioning pituitary adenoma with a low rate of hypopituitarism (4 %) and optic neuropathy (2 %). Similarly, Adler et al. [60] reported high rates of tumor control and preservation of visual function in a small group of patients with pituitary adenomas within 2 mm of the optic apparatus who received multi-fraction (2–5 fractions) SRS with CyberKnife.

4.7 Protons

Only a few series report on the use of protons for pituitary adenomas using either conventional fractionation [62] or SRS [63, 64]. In a series of 47 patients with either nonfunctioning or secreting pituitary adenoma treated with fractionated proton beam irradiation (54 cobalt-gray equivalent in 27 fractions), tumor control was observed in 93 % of patients with a minimum follow-up of 6 months. Complications included temporal lobe necrosis in 1 patient, new significant visual deficits in 3 patients, and new hypopituitarism in 11 patients. In a retrospective series of 33 patients with Cushing's disease at a median follow-up of 62 months, normalization of plasma and urinary free cortisol was achieved in 17 (52 %) patients, with a median time to remission of 18 months [64]. In another small series of 22 patients with GH-secreting pituitary adenomas who received proton SRS, normalization of GH/IGF-1 occurred in 50 % of patients, with a median time to complete response of 30.5 months [63]. The most frequent late toxicity was represented by the development of a new pituitary deficiency in up to 52 % of patients. Based on these preliminary experiences, the use of protons does not seem to offer clinical advantages when compared to photons.

References

1. Grigsby PW, Simpson JR, Emami BN et al (1989) Prognostic factors and results of surgery and postoperative irradiation in the management of pituitary adenomas. Int J Radiat Oncol Biol Phys 16: 1411–1417
2. McCollough WM, Marcus RB Jr, Rhoton AL Jr et al (1991) Long-term follow-up of radiotherapy for pituitary adenoma: the absence of late recurrence after greater than or equal to 4500 cGy. Int J Radiat Oncol Biol Phys 21:607–614
3. Brada M, Rajan B, Traish D et al (1993) The long-term efficacy of conservative surgery and radiotherapy in the control of pituitary adenomas. Clin Endocrinol (Oxf) 38:571–578
4. Tsang RW, Brierly JD, Panzarella T et al (1994) Radiation therapy for pituitary adenoma: treatment outcome and prognostic factors. Int J Radiat Oncol Biol Phys 30:557–565
5. Zierhut D, Flentje M, Adolph J et al (1995) External radiotherapy of pituitary adenomas. Int J Radiat Oncol Biol Phys 33:307–314
6. Rush S, Cooper PR (1997) Symptom resolution, tumor control, and side effects following postoperative radiotherapy for pituitary macroadenomas. Int J Radiat Oncol Biol Phys 37:1031–1034
7. Breen P, Flickinger JC, Kondziolka D et al (1998) Radiotherapy for nonfunctional pituitary adenoma: analysis of long-term tumour control. J Neurosurg 89:933–938
8. Gittoes NJ, Bates AS, Tse W et al (1998) Radiotherapy for non-function pituitary tumours. Clin Endocrinol (Oxf) 48:331–337
9. Barrande G, Pittino-Lungo M, Coste J et al (2000) Hormonal and metabolic effects of radiotherapy in acromegaly: long-term results in 128 patients followed in a single center. J Clin Endocrinol Metab 85:3779–3785
10. Biermasz NR, Dulken HV, Roelfsema F (2000) Postoperative radiotherapy in acromegaly is effective in reducing GH concentration to safe levels. Clin Endocrinol (Oxf) 53:321–327

11. Epaminonda P, Porretti S, Cappiello V et al (2001) Efficacy of radiotherapy in normalizing serum IGF-I, acid-labile subunit (ALS) and IGFBP-3 levels in acromegaly. Clin Endocrinol 55:183–189
12. Minniti G, Jaffrain-Rea ML, Osti M et al (2005) The long-term efficacy of conventional radiotherapy in patients with GH-secreting pituitary adenomas. Clin Endocrinol (Oxf) 62:210–216
13. Minniti G, Osti M, Jaffrain-Rea ML et al (2007) Long-term follow-up results of postoperative radiation therapy for Cushing's disease. J Neurooncol 84:79–84
14. Turner HE, Stratton IM, Byrne JV et al (1999) Audit of selected patients with nonfunctioning pituitary adenomas treated without irradiation – a follow-up study. Clin Endocrinol (Oxf) 51:281–284
15. Vlahovitch B, Reynaud C, Rhiati J et al (1988) Value of postoperative radiotherapy in various tumors of the pituitary gland. Presse Med 17:675–678
16. Minniti G, Gilbert DC, Brada M (2009) Modern techniques for pituitary radiotherapy. Rev Endocr Metab Disord 10:135–144
17. Estrada J, Boronat M, Mielgo M et al (1997) The long-term outcome of pituitary irradiation after unsuccessful transsphenoidal surgery in Cushing's disease. N Engl J Med 336:172–177
18. Tsagarakis S, Grossman A, Plowman PN et al (1991) Megavoltage pituitary irradiation in the management of prolactinomas: long-term follow-up. Clin Endocrinol (Oxf) 34:399–406
19. Laack NN, Brown PD (2004) Cognitive sequelae of brain radiation in adults. Semin Oncol 31:702–713
20. Taphoorn MJ, Klein M (2004) Cognitive deficits in adult patients with brain tumours. Lancet Neurol 3:159–168
21. Brada M, Asley S, Ford D et al (2002) Cerebrovascular mortality in patients with pituitary adenoma. Clin Endocrinol (Oxf) 57:713–717
22. Minniti G, Traish D, Ashley S et al (2005) Risk of second brain tumor after conservative surgery and radiotherapy for pituitary adenoma: update after an additional 10 years. J Clin Endocrinol Metab 90:800–804
23. Milker-Zabel S, Debus J, Thilmann C et al (2001) Fractionated stereotactically guided radiotherapy and radiosurgery in the treatment of functional and nonfunctional adenomas of the pituitary gland. Int J Radiat Oncol Biol Phys 50:1279–1286
24. Milker-Zabel S, Zabel A, Huber P et al (2004) Stereotactic conformal radiotherapy in patients with growth hormone-secreting pituitary adenoma. Int J Radiat Oncol Biol Phys 59:1088–1096
25. Paek SH, Downes MB, Bednarz G et al (2005) Integration of surgery with fractionated stereotactic radiotherapy for treatment of nonfunctioning pituitary macroadenomas. Int J Radiat Oncol Biol Phys 61:795–808
26. Colin P, Jovenin N, Delemer B et al (2005) Treatment of pituitary adenomas by fractionated stereotactic radiotherapy: a prospective study of 110 patients. Int J Radiat Oncol Biol Phys 62:333–341
27. Minniti G, Traish D, Ashley S et al (2006) Fractionated stereotactic conformal radiotherapy for secreting and nonsecreting pituitary adenomas. Clin Endocrinol (Oxf) 64:542–548
28. Kong DS, Lee JI, Lim do H et al (2007) The efficacy of fractionated radiotherapy and stereotactic radiosurgery for pituitary adenomas: long-term results of 125 consecutive patients treated in a single institution. Cancer 110:854–860
29. Roug S, Rasmussen AK, Juhler M et al (2010) Fractionated stereotactic radiotherapy in patients with acromegaly: an interim single-centre audit. Eur J Endocrinol 162:685–694
30. Wilson PJ, De-Loyde KJ, Williams JR et al (2012) A single centre's experience of stereotactic radiosurgery and radiotherapy for non functioning pituitary adenomas with the Linear Accelerator (Linac). J Clin Neurosci 19:370–374
31. Kim JO, Ma R, Akagami R et al (2013) Long-term outcomes of fractionated stereotactic radiation therapy for pituitary adenomas at the BC Cancer Agency. Int J Radiat Oncol Biol Phys 87:528–533
32. Colin P, Delemer B, Nakib I et al (2002) Unsuccessful surgery of Cushing's disease. Role and efficacy of fractionated stereotactic radiotherapy. Neurochirurgie 48:285–293
33. Losa M, Valle M, Mortini P et al (2004) Gamma knife surgery for treatment of residual nonfunctioning pituitary adenomas after surgical debulking. J Neurosurg 100:438–444
34. Mingione V, Yen CP, Vance ML et al (2006) Gamma surgery in the treatment of nonsecretory pituitary macroadenoma. J Neurosurg 104:876–883
35. Liscák R, Vladyka V, Marek J et al (2007) Gamma knife radiosurgery for endocrine-inactive pituitary adenomas. Acta Neurochir (Wien) 149:999–1006
36. Park KJ, Kano H, Parry PV et al (2011) Long-term outcomes after gamma knife stereotactic radiosurgery for nonfunctional pituitary adenomas. Neurosurgery 69:1188–1199
37. Starke RM, Williams BJ, Jane JA Jr et al (2012) Gamma Knife surgery for patients with nonfunctioning pituitary macroadenomas: predictors of tumor control, neurological deficits, and hypopituitarism. J Neurosurg 117:129–135
38. Sheehan JP, Starke RM, Mathieu D et al (2013) Gamma Knife radiosurgery for the management of nonfunctioning pituitary adenomas: a multicenter study. J Neurosurg 119:446–456
39. Jezková J, Marek J, Hána V et al (2006) Gamma knife radiosurgery for acromegaly – long-term experience. Clin Endocrinol (Oxf) 64:588–595
40. Voges J, Kocher M, Runge M et al (2006) Linear accelerator radiosurgery for pituitary macroadenomas: a 7-year follow-up study. Cancer 107:1355–1364
41. Pollock BE, Jacob JT, Brown PD et al (2007) Radiosurgery of growth hormone-producing pituitary

adenomas: factors associated with biochemical remission. J Neurosurg 106:833–838
42. Vik-Mo EO, Oksnes M, Pedersen PH et al (2007) Gamma knife stereotactic radiosurgery for acromegaly. Eur J Endocrinol 157:255–263
43. Jagannathan J, Sheehan JP, Pouratian N et al (2008) Gamma knife radiosurgery for acromegaly: outcomes after failed transsphenoidal surgery. Neurosurgery 62:1262–1270
44. Losa M, Gioia L, Picozzi P et al (2008) The role of stereotactic radiotherapy in patients with growth hormone-secreting pituitary adenoma. J Clin Endocrinol Metab 93:2546–2552
45. Iwai Y, Yamanaka K, Yoshimura M et al (2010) Gamma knife radiosurgery for growth hormone-producing adenomas. J Clin Neurosci 17:299–304
46. Castinetti F, Nagai M, Morange I et al (2009) Long-term results of stereotactic radiosurgery in secretory pituitary adenomas. J Clin Endocrinol Metab 94:3400–3407
47. Sheehan JP, Pouratian N, Steiner L et al (2011) Gamma knife surgery for pituitary adenomas: factors related to radiological and endocrine outcomes. J Neurosurg 114:303–309
48. Franzin A, Spatola G, Losa M et al (2012) Results of gamma knife radiosurgery in acromegaly. Int J Endocrinol 2012:342034
49. Liu X, Kano H, Kondziolka D et al (2012) Gamma knife radiosurgery for clinically persistent acromegaly. J Neurooncol 109:71–79
50. Wilson PJ, De-Loyde KJ, Williams JR et al (2013) Acromegaly: a single centre's experience of stereotactic radiosurgery and radiotherapy for growth hormone secreting pituitary tumours with the linear accelerator. J Clin Neurosci 20:1506–1513
51. Devin JK, Allen GS, Cmelak AJ et al (2004) The efficacy of linear accelerator radiosurgery in the management of patients with Cushing's disease. Stereotact Funct Neurosurg 82:254–262
52. Castinetti F, Nagai M, Dufour H et al (2007) Gamma knife radiosurgery is a successful adjunctive treatment in Cushing's disease. Eur J Endocrinol 156:91–98
53. Jagannathan J, Sheehan JP, Pouratian N et al (2007) Gamma knife surgery for Cushing's disease. J Neurosurg 106:980–987
54. Sheehan JP, Xu Z, Salvetti DJ et al (2013) Results of gamma knife surgery for Cushing's disease. J Neurosurg 119:1486–1492
55. Wilson PJ, Williams JR, Smee RI (2014) Cushing's disease: a single centre's experience using the linear accelerator (LINAC) for stereotactic radiosurgery and fractionated stereotactic radiotherapy. J Clin Neurosci 21:100–106
56. Pan L, Zhang N, Wang EM et al (2000) Gamma knife radiosurgery as a primary treatment for prolactinomas. J Neurosurg 93(Suppl 3):10–13
57. Pouratian N, Sheehan J, Jagannathan J et al (2006) Gamma knife radiosurgery for medically and surgically refractory prolactinomas. Neurosurgery 59: 255–266
58. Jezková J, Hána V, Krsek M et al (2009) Use of the Leksell gamma knife in the treatment of prolactinoma patients. Clin Endocrinol (Oxf) 70:732–741
59. Landolt AM, Haller D, Lomax N et al (2000) Octreotide may act as a radioprotective agent in acromegaly. J Clin Endocrinol Metab 85:1287–1289
60. Adler JR Jr, Gibbs IC, Puataweepong P et al (2008) Visual field preservation after multisession cyberknife radiosurgery for perioptic lesions. Neurosurgery 62(Suppl 2):733–743
61. Iwata H, Sato K, Tatewaki K et al (2011) Hypofractionated stereotactic radiotherapy with CyberKnife for nonfunctioning pituitary adenoma: high local control with low toxicity. Neuro Oncol 13:916–922
62. Ronson BB, Schulte RW, Han KP et al (2006) Fractionated proton beam irradiation of pituitary adenomas. Int J Radiat Oncol Biol Phys 64:425–434
63. Petit JH, Biller BM, Coen JJ et al (2007) Proton stereotactic radiosurgery in management of persistent acromegaly. Endocr Pract 13:726–734
64. Petit JH, Biller BM, Yock TI et al (2008) Proton stereotactic radiotherapy for persistent adrenocorticotropin-producing adenomas. J Clin Endocrinol Metab 93:393–399

Part II

Craniopharyngiomas

Introduction

5

Paolo Cappabianca, Marialaura Del Basso De Caro, and Arturo Brunetti

Craniopharyngiomas are rare epithelial tumors arising along the path of the craniopharyngeal duct, and as a consequence, they can be found from rhinopharynx to hypothalamus [6, 30, 31]. They develop in a deep-seated area of the brain, involving in many cases several vital structures, such as the hypothalamus, that are of paramount importance for vegetative, endocrine, and emotional functions as well as for maintaining body homeostasis. As a matter of fact, the functional impairment and anatomical distortion of the hypothalamus that may be caused by such kind of tumor have to be considered as critical factors influencing patient outcome.

However, apart from hypothalamic dysfunction, craniopharyngiomas may lead to the emergence of a large spectrum of symptoms and signs; usual clinical presentations include visual alteration, signs of chiasmatic and/or retrochiasmatic compression, and pituitary dysfunction, often presenting as panhypopituitarism [31].

Craniopharyngiomas account for only 2–5 % of the total amount of intracranial tumors. Generally, they tend to show a double-peak distribution model, i.e., during childhood (5–14 years) and in late adulthood, from 50 to 74 years [4]. A rather balanced distribution between sexes has been observed, with 55.6 % of lesions diagnosed in males and 44.1 % in females [46].

Historically, Friedrich Albert von Zenker firstly described a cystic suprasellar mass holding inside pieces of cholesterol crystals which was probably a craniopharyngioma [61]. Later, in 1904, Jakob Erdheim depicted the main histopathological aspects of such a kind of neoplasms [16], and, in agreement with the already obtained results presented by Mott and Barret [44], he endorsed that craniopharyngiomas develop from epithelial cells arising from a partially involuted hypophyseal-pharyngeal duct. On the other hand, from the clinical point of view, Rupert Boyce and Cecil Beadles were the pioneers to describe the case of a 35 year-old patient who became comatose and rapidly died because of a huge, ossified, and cystic lesion leading to brainstem, optic chiasm, and optic tract dysfunction; that mass was

P. Cappabianca, MD (✉)
Division of Neurosurgery, Department of Neurosciences, Reproductive and Odontostomatological Sciences, Università degli Studi di Napoli "Federico II", Naples, Italy
e-mail: paolo.cappabianca@unina.it

M. Del Basso De Caro, BS
Anatomopathology Unit, Department of Advanced Biomedical Sciences, University of Naples "Federico II", Naples, Italy

A. Brunetti, MD
Neuroradiology Unit, Department of Advanced Biomedical Sciences, Università degli Studi di Napoli "Federico II", Naples, Italy

P. Cappabianca et al. (eds.), *Midline Skull Base Surgery*, DOI 10.1007/978-3-319-21533-4_5

suspected to be a craniopharyngioma [3]. Hereinafter, Babinski [1] and Frohlich [21] reported analogue clinical features in patients with cystic pituitary masses but without any symptoms and/or signs of acromegaly, questionable to not be a pituitary adenoma but a cystic intrasellar craniopharyngioma.

Regarding the neuropathological outward, two subtypes of craniopharyngiomas have been described: adamantinomatous and papillary. The adamantinomatous form affects children (5–10 years) and adults (50–60 years), the papillary type almost only adults; in general, the adamantinomatous form is much more common than the papillary one (ratio: 9/1) [47, 60]. Regarding the main macroscopic characteristic, the adamantinomatous subtype shows adhesions to the nearby neurovascular structures as well as irregular interface, and its cystic components are usually filled with dark fluid, i.e., the so-called motor oil, containing cholesterol crystals; calcifications are present and described in the large majority of cases. Instead, the papillary form generally shows no adherence to the neighboring structures; cystic contents are often clear and no calcifications are found [11]. The two craniopharyngiomas histotypes have different immunohistochemical features leading to peculiar biological behavior. In particular, the adamantinomatous form shows positivity for CK7, CK8, and CK14 [35, 56, 59] and may contain mutations in CTNNB1 [37], encoding beta-catenin, a component of the adherents junction and mediator of Wnt signaling [27, 28, 53]. A mutated, degradation-resistant form of beta-catenin is implicated as the primary driver of oncogenesis in adamantinomatous craniopharyngioma and is usually present in the cellular nucleus [29]. Specifically, clusters of cells with nuclear beta-catenin form are principally represented in invasive tumors. This pattern is evocative of an implication of the beta-catenin signaling in the migratory behavior of these tumors; the cellular clusters with nuclear beta-catenin may coordinate the growth and infiltration of the tumor into the nearby vital tissues, thus explaining the increased aggressiveness of this adamantinomatous subtype versus the papillary one [6, 36].

Craniopharyngiomas originate from the midline skull base and, subsequently, they begin to insinuate into the nearby low-resistant structures, such as the arachnoid cisterns, the third ventricle, and the parasellar areas. However, as already said, differently from pituitary tumors, they often adhere to the neurovascular structures of the suprasellar space, such as perforating vessels coming from the anterior and posterior cerebral arteries and/or internal carotid arteries, the optic chiasm and optic pathways, and the hypothalamus. Despite of their histological classification as benign tumors, an aggressive and infiltrative behavior is often observed.

The peculiar location and significant size that such tumors may reach, together with the frequent implication of critical neurovascular structures as well as the presence of calcific components, can limit the degree of resection in many cases.

Moreover, craniopharyngiomas have a tendency to recur even after apparent total removal. Surgical removal of recurrent craniopharyngioma may be more difficult, principally due to scar tissue formation and new adhesions [8, 42]. The recurrent craniopharyngioma usually adheres intensively to the surrounding hypothalamic-hypophyseal areas, thus making the second surgery at a higher risk of fatal neural and vascular injury. According to major literature studies [8, 17, 57], the rate of recurrence ranges from 0 to 53 % in cases of total removal and from 30 to 100 % in cases of subtotal or partial removal.

Along many years, several authors defined classifications for craniopharyngiomas as related to the growth path and the surgical route used, all sharing the principle of subdividing craniopharyngiomas along the length of extension in the primary vertical axis, considering the optic chiasm, diaphragma sellae, third ventricle, and more recently to infundibulum.

Hoffman classified craniopharyngiomas with respect to the sella turcica, the optic chiasm, and the floor of the third ventricle into *prechiasmatic*, *retrochiasmatic*, *subchiasmatic*, and *intraventricular* craniopharyngiomas [26]. *Yasargil* divided them as follows: (a) *purely intrasellar–infradiaphragmatic*; (b) *intra- and suprasellar, infra- and supradiaphragmatic*; (c) *supradiaphragmatic parachiasmatic and extraventricular*; (d) *intra and extraventricular*; (e) *paraventricular*; and (f) *purely intraventricular* [60]. On the other hand, *Samii* et al. classified craniopharyngiomas into grades based on their vertical projections: *grade I* (intrasellar or infradiaphragmatic), *grade II* (cisternal with or without an intrasellar component), *grade III* (lower half of the third ventricle), *grade IV* (upper half of the third ventricle), and *grade V* (reaching the septum pellucidum or lateral ventricles) [51]. On another perspective, according to the relationships between the tumor, the arachnoid and the pia mater, *Ciric and Cozzens* classified craniopharyngiomas into different types, i.e., *intra-pial intraventricular*, *intra-pial intra-arachnoidal*, *extra-pial intra-arachnoidal* (invasive variant), *extra-pial extra-arachnoidal intrasellar*, *intra-arachnoidal suprasellar* (Dumbbell variant), and *intrasellar extra-arachnoidal* [9]. More recently, *Kassam* et al. proposed a further classification, principally linked with the use of the endoscopic and/or microscopic endonasal pathway, which is based on the relation of the craniopharyngioma with the infundibulum, accordingly, the authors described: *type 1, preinfundibular*; *type 2, transinfundibular*; *type 3, post- or retro-infundibular* (further subdivision is based on rostral or caudal extension, whether it is to the anterior third ventricular (infundibular recess, hypothalamic) and interpeduncular fossa); and *type 4, isolated third ventricular* [32]. When dealing with pediatric cases, classification criteria may be different, and, accordingly, Muller and coworkers proposed to classify craniopharyngiomas according to the degree of hypothalamic invasion, using the involvement of the mammillary bodies as a landmark of distinction between anterior and posterior hypothalamic implications [45].

Historically, regarding surgical resection of a craniopharyngioma, it has to be remained that the first surgical attempt was performed by A. E. Halstead [25], and, subsequently, Lewis [39], Cushing [12], and Schloffer [52] removed craniopharyngiomas using either transcranial or transnasal approach. However, craniopharyngiomas remain one of the most challenging intracranial tumors because of the everlasting controversy about the most appropriate surgical approach for each case. A major reason for this controversy is the enormous variability in the topographical location of the tumor, which can affect one to several compartments, from the sella turcica to the third ventricle, as well as its unpredictable degree of adherence [46]. As a consequence, many different possible transcranial approaches have been advocated for the management of such tumors (i.e., frontotemporal, subfrontal, supraorbital, transventricular). These pathways have been adopted and evolved through decades in the attempt of achieving better outcome with lower morbidity and mortality rates [9, 40, 50, 60]. Accordingly, variable modifications and combinations of these approaches have been used for resection of giant or extensive craniopharyngiomas, with the presumption that sufficient exposure of all parts of the tumor is essential for its safe and complete removal [23].

Surgical resection by means of the widely used frontotemporal approach provides the shortest path to the suprasellar space. This route has been accepted throughout the years as the standard technique for the surgical management of craniopharyngiomas, and its effectiveness has rendered it worldwide approved in the routinely neurosurgical practice [50, 60]. This safe and simple approach can be successfully used in craniopharyngiomas with a wide spectrum of extensions; it provides adequate access to the tumor and enables its complete removal with a reasonable morbidity and approach-related complication rate [23]. Many variations of this traditional approach have been used for lesions with hypothalamic extension. On the other hand, in the last decades, the evolution of surgical techniques has led to a progressive reduction of the invasiveness of any neurosurgical approaches, and, according to the keyhole concept, the supraorbital eyebrow route has been validated as an alternative to the conventional transcranial pathways. It allows bilateral and wide surgical exposition, offering the same possibilities with low approach-related morbidity, imputable to the minimal brain retraction obtained with this approach [19, 48].

On another perspective, besides transcranial approaches, transsphenoidal route has also been initially recommended for the craniopharyngiomas that are located within an enlarged sella without calcification and adhesion to parasellar structures. As a matter of fact, this route was introduced according to the indications defined by Guiot and Derome in the early 1960s [24], being proposed only for infradiaphragmatic lesions, with enlarged sella, that preferably already developed panhypopituitarism. Hereinafter, extended transsphenoidal approaches have been introduced for craniopharyngioma even with a significant suprasellar component. Weiss in 1987 [58] termed and originally described the extended transsphenoidal approach, intending a transsphenoidal approach with removal of additional bone along the tuberculum sellae and the posterior planum sphenoidale, between the optic canals, with subsequent opening of the dura mater above the diaphragma sellae. This novel pathway allows midline access and visibility to the suprasellar space from below, obviating brain retraction, and makes possible to manage transsphenoidally midline located suprasellar lesions, traditionally approached transcranially, namely, anterior cranial fossa meningiomas and craniopharyngiomas. First of all such procedures were done with the aid of the microscope [18, 33, 58]. Subsequently, endoscopy has contributed to the more contemporary knowledge and development of the possibilities of the transsphenoidal approach [5, 7, 13, 20, 22, 32, 34]. The wider and panoramic visualization given by the endoscope, and the rapid growth of neuroradiological diagnostic techniques together with the intraoperative neuronavigation systems, augmented the possibility of the transsphenoidal approach, thus allowing its extension toward different areas of the midline skull base. Accordingly, as craniopharyngiomas are often located at the midline, the endonasal pathway offers the advantage of accessing the tumor upon dural opening, without brain or optic nerve retraction and with a direct view through a straight surgical route, even if in a reverse modality as that obtained with the traditional transcranial approaches. Specifically, in recent years, the endoscopic endonasal approach has enabled to overcome many disadvantages of the microsurgical transsphenoidal route to the sella, permitting the management of different purely supra- and retrosellar cystic/solid craniopharyngiomas, regardless to the sellar size or the pituitary function.

Generally, craniopharyngiomas amenable to treat via an endonasal approach should possess key features, such as median midline location, absence of any solid parasellar component, and/or encasement of the main vascular structures. The transsphenoidal approach can avoid transcranial surgery with its inherent risks. However, especially when performing extended approaches, the possible risk of postoperative CSF leak and meningitis has to be highlighted. The validity of the endoscopic endonasal technique for the treatment of such featured craniopharyngiomas has been confirmed throughout recent surgical series, appeared in the pertinent literature [7, 13, 20, 34, 38].

At any rate, despite of the advancements in neurosurgical procedures, techniques, materials, and instrumentations, irregular margins, and tendency to adhere to the nearby vital neurovascular compartment, craniopharyngiomas resection continues to be a surgical challenge [43]. Relationships between the tumor and the surrounding nervous structures, in particular the third ventricle, optic pathways, the pituitary stalk, and major arteries and veins, may be predictive of a difficult surgical removal. Nowadays, the advantage of neuroimaging has led to a better knowledge of intricate relationship between craniopharyngiomas, hypothalamus, pituitary stalk, and optic apparatus, hence ensuring proper selection of surgical approaches.

As a matter of fact, historically, although patients with large craniopharyngiomas involving the third ventricle usually showed symptoms of hypothalamic derangement, such as increased weight gain, impaired sexual function, abnormal somnolence, unexplained high body temperature, inappropriate emotional responses, and/or defective memory, these disturbances were largely ignored or not linked to the anatomical involvement of the hypothalamus by the lesion [46]. Therefore, in the past years, initial surgical approaches for such kind of neoplasm were designed with the primary aim of radical tumor removal and relief of chiasm compression caused by the tumor [46], being unaware of preoperative and eventually postoperative hypothalamic-related symptoms.

As a consequence, proper treatment of every craniopharyngioma remains to be found, and even if total surgical resection has to be thought as the gold standard, several other options and techniques can be taken into account for the optimal general management of craniopharyngiomas. Cyst drainage [54, 55], wide marsupialization of the cysts into CSF spaces (cysto-ventriculo-cisternostomy) with neuroendoscopic technique [14], stereotactic aspiration with the instillation of bleomycin or interferon-alpha [2, 41], and endocavitary irradiation [15] have been proposed for the treatment of cystic components of craniopharyngiomas.

When approaching pediatric patients, given that total tumor excision at the first attempt, whenever possible, is the preferred strategy for these difficult neoplasms, it may be suggested to accept the risk of a subtotal surgical resection—above all when hypothalamus is involved—in order to allow adequate neuropsychic and motor development and reduce the risk of hypothalamic injuries [10, 49].

Owing these data, the management of craniopharyngioma patients requires interdisciplinary cooperation of different expertise of the cogent disciplines and should be reserved to specialized centers.

The attempt of total removal is the most suitable aim of the surgical treatment, with lower morbidity and mortality: nowadays, preservation of the quality of life and neurocognitive functioning as long-term survival maintenance are important aspects to be considered. In particular, apart from the pre- or postoperative neurological disorders, hypothalamic obesity can lead to a significant decline in the quality of life and should be taken into consideration in the follow-up of patients with craniopharyngiomas. These aspects concerning the general management of craniopharyngiomas can be thought as "modern treatment targets."

In conclusion, craniopharyngiomas remain one of the most challenging intracranial tumors requiring patience, flexibility, surgical insight, and diligent postoperative management [6]. In every case, treatment should be patient-tailored according to age, presenting symptoms, tumor characteristics, prior treatment, treatment tolerance, and comorbidities.

References

1. Babinski J (1900) Tumeur du corps pituitaire sans acromé´galie et avec arrê`t de dé´veloppement des organes genitaux. Revue neurologique, Paris
2. Backlund EO, Axelsson B, Bergstrand CG, Eriksson AL, Noren G, Ribbesjo E et al (1989) Treatment of craniopharyngiomas–the stereotactic approach in a ten to twenty-three years' perspective. I. Surgical, radiological and ophthalmological aspects. Acta Neurochir (Wien) 99:11–19
3. Boyce R, Beadles CF (1893) A further contribution to the study of the pathology of the hypophysis cerebri. J Pathol 1:359–383
4. Bunin GR, Surawicz TS, Witman PA, Preston-Martin S, Davis F, Bruner JM (1998) The descriptive epidemiology of craniopharyngioma. J Neurosurg 89:547–551
5. Cappabianca P, Cavallo LM, Esposito F, De Divitiis E (2008) Craniopharyngiomas. J Neurosurg 109:1–3
6. Cappabianca P, Cavallo LM, Solari D, Di Somma A, Del Basso De Caro ML (2015) Introduction and outcome. In: Evans JJ, Kenning TJ (eds) Craniopharyngiomas: a comprehensive guide to diagnosis, treatment, and outcome. Elsevier, Amsterdam, pp 137–153
7. Cavallo LM, Frank G, Cappabianca P, Solari D, Mazzatenta D, Villa A et al (2014) The endoscopic endonasal approach for the management of craniopharyngiomas: a series of 103 patients. J Neurosurg 121(1):100–113
8. Cavallo LM, Prevedello DM, Solari D, Gardner PA, Esposito F, Snyderman CH et al (2009) Extended endoscopic endonasal transsphenoidal approach for residual or recurrent craniopharyngiomas. J Neurosurg 111:578–589
9. Ciric IS, Cozzens JW (1980) Craniopharyngiomas: transsphenoidal method of approach – for the virtuoso only? Clin Neurosurg 27:169–187
10. Cohen M, Bartels U, Branson H, Kulkarni AV, Hamilton J (2013) Trends in treatment and outcomes of pediatric craniopharyngioma, 1975–2011. Neuro Oncol 15:767–774
11. Crotty TB, Scheithauer BW, Young WF Jr, Davis DH, Shaw EG, Miller GM et al (1995) Papillary craniopharyngioma: a clinicopathological study of 48 cases. J Neurosurg 83:206–214
12. Cushing H (1932) Intracranial tumors. Charles C Thomas, Baltimore

13. de Divitiis E, Cappabianca P, Cavallo LM, Esposito F, de Divitiis O, Messina A (2007) Extended endoscopic transsphenoidal approach for extrasellar craniopharyngiomas. Neurosurgery 61:219–227; discussion 228
14. Delitala A, Brunori A, Chiappetta F (2004) Purely neuroendoscopic transventricular management of cystic craniopharyngiomas. Childs Nerv Syst 20: 858–862
15. Derrey S, Blond S, Reyns N, Touzet G, Carpentier P, Gauthier H et al (2008) Management of cystic craniopharyngiomas with stereotactic endocavitary irradiation using colloidal 186Re: a retrospective study of 48 consecutive patients. Neurosurgery 63:1045–1052; discussion 1052–1043
16. Erdheim J (1904) Uber hypophysenganggeschwwuste und hirncholesteatome. Gerold, Wien
17. Fahlbusch R, Honegger J, Paulus W, Huk W, Buchfelder M (1999) Surgical treatment of craniopharyngiomas: experience with 168 patients. J Neurosurg 90:237–250
18. Fahlbusch R, Honneger J, Buchfelder M (2000) Transsphenoidal microsurgery for craniopharyngiomas. In: Schmidek HH (ed) Shmidek & sweet operative neurosurgical techniques. Indications, methods and results, vol 1. W. B. Saunders, Philadelphia, pp 503–511
19. Fatemi N, Dusick JR, de Paiva Neto MA, Malkasian D, Kelly DF (2009) Endonasal versus supraorbital keyhole removal of craniopharyngiomas and tuberculum sellae meningiomas. Neurosurgery 64:269–284; discussion 284–266
20. Frank G, Pasquini E, Doglietto F, Mazzatenta D, Sciaretta V, Farneti G et al (2006) The endoscopic extended transsphenoidal approach for craniopharyngiomas. Neurosurgery 59(suppl 1):ONS75–ONS83
21. Frohlich A (1901) Ein fall von tumor der hypophysis cerebri ohne akromegalie. Wien klin Rdsch
22. Gardner PA, Prevedello DM, Kassam AB, Snyderman CH, Carrau RL, Mintz AH (2008) The evolution of the endonasal approach for craniopharyngiomas. J Neurosurg 108:1043–1047
23. Gerganov V, Metwali H, Samii A, Fahlbusch R, Samii M (2014) Microsurgical resection of extensive craniopharyngiomas using a frontolateral approach: operative technique and outcome. J Neurosurg 120:559–570
24. Guiot G, Derome P (1972) Indications for transsphenoid approach in neurosurgery. 521 cases. Ann Med Interne (Paris) 123:703–712
25. Halstead AE (1910) Remarks on the operative treatment of 256 tumors of the hypophysis. Surg Gynecol Obstet 10:494–502
26. Hoffman HJ, De Silva M, Humphreys RP, Drake JM, Smith ML, Blaser SI (1992) Aggressive surgical management of craniopharyngiomas in children. J Neurosurg 76:47–52
27. Hofmann BM, Kreutzer J, Saeger W, Buchfelder M, Blumcke I, Fahlbusch R et al (2006) Nuclear beta-catenin accumulation as reliable marker for the differentiation between cystic craniopharyngiomas and rathke cleft cysts: a clinico-pathologic approach. Am J Surg Pathol 30:1595–1603
28. Holsken A, Kreutzer J, Hofmann BM, Hans V, Oppel F, Buchfelder M et al (2009) Target gene activation of the Wnt signaling pathway in nuclear beta-catenin accumulating cells of adamantinomatous craniopharyngiomas. Brain Pathol 19:357–364
29. Hussain I, Eloy JA, Carmel PW, Liu JK (2013) Molecular oncogenesis of craniopharyngioma: current and future strategies for the development of targeted therapies. J Neurosurg 119:106–112
30. Jane JA Jr, Laws ER (2006) Craniopharyngioma. Pituitary 9:323–326
31. Karavitaki N (2014) Management of craniopharyngiomas. J Endocrinol Invest 37(3):219–228
32. Kassam AB, Gardner PA, Snyderman CH, Carrau RL, Mintz AH, Prevedello DM (2008) Expanded endonasal approach, a fully endoscopic transnasal approach for the resection of midline suprasellar craniopharyngiomas: a new classification based on the infundibulum. J Neurosurg 108:715–728
33. Kitano M, Taneda M (2009) Extended transsphenoidal surgery for suprasellar craniopharyngiomas: infrachiasmatic radical resection combined with or without a suprachiasmatic trans-lamina terminalis approach. Surg Neurol 71(3):290–298
34. Koutourousiou M, Gardner PA, Fernandez-Miranda JC, Tyler-Kabara EC, Wang EW, Snyderman CH (2013) Endoscopic endonasal surgery for craniopharyngiomas: surgical outcome in 64 patients. J Neurosurg 119(5):1194–1207
35. Kurosaki M, Saeger W, Ludecke DK (2001) Immunohistochemical localisation of cytokeratins in craniopharyngioma. Acta Neurochir (Wien) 143:147–151
36. Larkin SJ, Ansorge O (2013) Pathology and pathogenesis of craniopharyngiomas. Pituitary 16:9–17
37. Larkin SJ, Preda V, Karavitaki N, Grossman A, Ansorge O (2014) BRAF V600E mutations are characteristic for papillary craniopharyngioma and may coexist with CTNNB1-mutated adamantinomatous craniopharyngioma. Acta Neuropathol 127:927–929
38. Leng LZ, Greenfield JP, Souweidane MM, Anand VK, Schwartz TH (2012) Endoscopic, endonasal resection of craniopharyngiomas: analysis of outcome including extent of resection, cerebrospinal fluid leak, return to preoperative productivity, and body mass index. Neurosurgery 70:110–123; discussion 123–114
39. Lewis D (1910) A contribution to the subject of tumors of the hypophysis. JAMA 55:1002–1008
40. Liu JK, Christiano LD, Gupta G, Carmel PW (2010) Surgical nuances for removal of retrochiasmatic craniopharyngiomas via the transbasal subfrontal translamina terminalis approach. Neurosurg Focus 28, E6
41. Liu W, Fang Y, Cai B, Xu J, You C, Zhang H (2012) Intracystic bleomycin for cystic craniopharyngiomas in children (abridged republication of cochrane systematic review). Neurosurgery 71:909–915

42. Minamida Y, Mikami T, Hashi K, Houkin K (2005) Surgical management of the recurrence and regrowth of craniopharyngiomas. J Neurosurg 103:224–232
43. Mortini P, Gagliardi F, Boari N, Losa M (2013) Surgical strategies and modern therapeutic options in the treatment of craniopharyngiomas. Crit Rev Oncol Hematol 88(3):514–529
44. Mott FW, Barret JO (1899) Three cases of tumor of the third ventricle. Arch Neurol 1:417–440
45. Muller HL, Gebhardt U, Teske C, Faldum A, Zwiener I, Warmuth-Metz M et al (2011) Post-operative hypothalamic lesions and obesity in childhood craniopharyngioma: results of the multinational prospective trial KRANIOPHARYNGEOM 2000 after 3-year follow-up. Eur J Endocrinol 165:17–24
46. Pascual JM, Prieto R, Castro-Dufourny I, Carrasco R, Strauss S, Barrios L (2014) Development of intracranial approaches for craniopharyngiomas: an analysis of the first 160 historical procedures. Neurosurg Focus 36, E13
47. Paulus W, Stockel C, Krauss J, Sorensen N, Roggendorf W (1997) Odontogenic classification of craniopharyngiomas: a clinicopathological study of 54 cases. Histopathology 30:172–176
48. Reisch R, Perneczky A (2005) Ten-year experience with the supraorbital subfrontal approach through an eyebrow skin incision. Neurosurgery 57:242–255
49. Sainte-Rose C, Puget S, Wray A, Zerah M, Grill J, Brauner R et al (2005) Craniopharyngioma: the pendulum of surgical management. Childs Nerv Syst 21:691–695
50. Samii M, Samii A (2000) Surgical management of craniopharyngiomas. In: Schmidek HH (ed) Schmidek & sweet operative neurosurgical techniques. Indications, methods and results, vol 1. W. B. Saunders, Philadelphia, pp 489–502
51. Samii M, Tatagiba M (1997) Surgical management of craniopharyngiomas: a review. Neurol Med Chir (Tokyo) 37:141–149
52. Schloffer H (1907) Erforgleiche operationen eines hypophysentumors auf nasalem wege. Wien Klin Wochenschr 20:621–624
53. Sekine S, Shibata T, Kokubu A, Morishita Y, Noguchi M, Nakanishi Y et al (2002) Craniopharyngiomas of adamantinomatous type harbor beta-catenin gene mutations. Am J Pathol 161:1997–2001
54. Spaziante R, de Divitiis E (1997) Drainage techniques for cystic craniopharyngiomas. Neurosurg Quart 7:183–208
55. Spaziante R, de Divitiis E, Irace C, Cappabianca P, Caputi F (1989) Management of primary or recurring grossly cystic craniopharyngiomas by means of draining systems. Topic review and 6 case reports. Acta Neurochir (Wien) 97:95–106
56. Tateyama H, Tada T, Okabe M, Takahashi E, Eimoto T (2001) Different keratin profiles in craniopharyngioma subtypes and ameloblastomas. Pathol Res Pract 197:735–742
57. Van Effenterre R, Boch AL (2002) Craniopharyngioma in adults and children: a study of 122 surgical cases. J Neurosurg 97:3–11
58. Weiss MH (1987) The transnasal transsphenoidal approach. In: Apuzzo MLJ (ed) Surgery of the third ventricle. Williams & Wilkins, Baltimore, pp 476–494
59. Xin W, Rubin MA, McKeever PE (2002) Differential expression of cytokeratins 8 and 20 distinguishes craniopharyngioma from rathke cleft cyst. Arch Pathol Lab Med 126:1174–1178
60. Yasargil MG, Curcic M, Kis M, Siegenthaler G, Teddy PJ, Roth P (1990) Total removal of craniopharyngiomas. Approaches and long-term results in 144 patients. J Neurosurg 73:3–11
61. Zenker FA (1857) Enorme Cystenbildung im Gehirn, vom Hirnanhang ausgehend. Arch Pathol Anat Physiol Klin Med 12:454–466

Endoscopic Endonasal Transsphenoidal Approach

6

Luigi Maria Cavallo, Alberto Di Somma, Francesco Briganti, Domenico Solari, Federico Frio, Luigi Maffei, and Paolo Cappabianca

6.1 Indications

There are several kinds of craniopharyngioma that can be managed via two variations of the endoscopic endonasal transsphenoidal procedure: the "standard" approach to the sellar region and the "extended" approach to the suprasellar area. These two variations have different indications.

The indications for the standard approach were postulated more than 50 years ago, in the early 1960s, when Guiot and Derome [1] identified the possibilities of transsphenoidal surgery for craniopharyngiomas retaining suitable for this approach infradiaphragmatic lesions, with enlarged sella that preferably already caused panhypopituitarism. Still today these guidelines are absolutely valid for both the microsurgical and endoscopic transsphenoidal approaches. The standard transsphenoidal route for infradiaphragmatic craniopharyngiomas provides the advantage of accessing the tumor immediately after dural opening, without entering the subarachnoid space.

Later on, during the 1980s, some authors expanded the classic indications of transsphenoidal microscopic approach, adopting this route for the management of craniopharyngiomas with extension above the diaphragma sellae, i.e., with an involvement of the subarachnoid space. Accordingly, in order to allow the proper handling of surgical instruments and the adequate exposure of the tumor, the refinement of bone and dural opening beyond the limits of the sella, i.e., over the tuberculum sellae and the posterior portion of the planum sphenoidale, was described. A new variation of the transsphenoidal pathway, i.e., the so-called "extended" transsphenoidal approach, was though defined [2].

During more recent years, there have been a worldwide diffusion and acceptance of the endoscope in transsphenoidal approaches. The panoramic and wider view offered by the endoscope increased the versatility of the transsphenoidal pathway, thus permitting the removal even of supradiaphragmatic lesions, including craniopharyngiomas [3–6]. The use of the endoscope through this route provides an access to the suprasellar supradiaphragmatic area, regardless of the sellar size (even a not enlarged sella).

Electronic supplementary material The online version of this chapter (doi:10.1007/978-3-319-21533-4_6) contains supplementary material, which is available to authorized users.

L.M. Cavallo, MD, PhD • A. Di Somma, MD
D. Solari, MD, PhD • F. Frio, MD • L. Maffei, MD
P. Cappabianca, MD (✉)
Division of Neurosurgery, Department of Neurosciences, Reproductive and Odontostomatological Sciences, Università degli Studi di Napoli "Federico II", Naples, Italy
e-mail: lcavallo@unina.it; d.solari.md@gmail.com; paolo.cappabianca@unina.it

F. Briganti, MD
Neuroradiology Unit, Department of Advanced Biomedical Sciences, Università degli Studi di Napoli "Federico II", Naples, Italy

P. Cappabianca et al. (eds.), *Midline Skull Base Surgery*, DOI 10.1007/978-3-319-21533-4_6

It was the group of Pittsburgh, initially Jho [7] and later Kassam and Carrau [8], that defined and popularized the use of the endoscope in the so-called "extended" endoscopic transsphenoidal approaches for the removal of suprasellar lesions.

The proposed indications for an extended endoscopic transsphenoidal approach are different from the standard one: the relationship of lesions with the diaphragma sellae is a key aspect for choosing either a standard or an extended transsphenoidal approach. However, craniopharyngiomas that can be considered amenable for an extended endoscopic endonasal approach should have particular features, such as midline position, without a solid parasellar component or encasement of the main neurovascular structures, small-to-medium size, with main pattern of growth along the stalk-infundibulum axis, as these can be identified running along the same path of the endoscopic endonasal route [9–13]. Nevertheless, other characteristics, above all the degree of tumor and capsule adhesion to critical neurovascular structures, could make this surgery difficult and risky. On the contrary, it is possible to assume that patients who have undergone earlier operations, radiation therapy, or both could harbor lesions presenting such troublesome features. However, if a previous open craniotomy has been used, the endoscopic endonasal approach may offer the benefit of a naive surgical route, thus providing a safer option for recurrence surgery.

Finally, it should be reminded that when endoscopic endonasal route is chosen, many different aspects in regard to the approach itself should be taken into account.

First of all, the sphenoid sinus pneumatization has to be considered. Differently from tuberculum sellae meningiomas, when dealing with a craniopharyngioma, the degree of pneumatization of the sphenoid sinus is not a limiting factor. Indeed, if the craniopharyngioma develops in the sub- and/or retrochiasmatic areas, it is not necessary to have a large sphenoid sinus to obtain a proper exposure of these regions.

Secondarily, the location of the pituitary stalk in relation to the craniopharyngioma should be highlighted: the correlation between the craniopharyngioma and the pituitary stalk is of utmost importance for properly planning the optimal surgical strategy. As a matter of fact, the surgical classification proposed by Kassam et al. [14] relates the craniopharyngioma to the infundibulum and therefore identifies type I, preinfundibular; type II, transinfundibular; type III, post- or retroinfundibular, further subdivided based on rostral or caudal extension; and type IV, isolated third ventricular (generally, not removable via endonasal route).

The size and location of the craniopharyngioma should be assessed in relation to the width of osteo-dural defect that is necessary to realize an adequate exposure of the lesion. In case of a very large predominantly cystic craniopharyngioma with components of the lesion getting into the retro and/or parasellar space, extending beyond the limit of the surgical maneuverability of the instruments, the endoscopic endonasal route should not be adopted. Moreover, a very narrow surgical corridor due to minimal distance between the supraclinoid tracts of the internal carotid arteries could represent a relative contraindication to the use of this route.

The endoscopic endonasal approach, with both its standard and extended variation, provides a shorter intradural corridor, a median closeup and symmetric view of suprasellar neurovascular structures, and, above all, a greater exposure of the subchiasmatic and retrochiasmatic areas, as well as of the stalk-infundibulum axis and the anterior part of the third ventricle, which definitely represents a crucial area in the growth path of craniopharyngiomas [15, 16].

Anyway it is important to underline that the endonasal approach is not the only route used to treat craniopharyngiomas. Many transcranial approaches have been and are successfully used to manage such kind of lesions [17–21].

6.2 Neuroradiology

Magnetic resonance imaging (MRi) is more commonly used to define the features of a craniopharyngioma. High-resolution sequences of the sellar region, pre- and post-contrast enhancement should be obtained in all cases, thus providing more details regarding the relationship of the tumor to the nearby neurovascular structures (Figs. 6.1, 6.2, and 6.3).

Adamantinous craniopharyngioma, the most common type, appears as a lobulated mass located within the suprasellar area or, less frequently, in the sellar, parasellar, and retrosellar regions; it could present cystic, calcic, and solid components.

Cysts can be found in 90 % of cases, commonly hypointense on the T1- and hyperintense on the T2-weighted (w) images; the typical hyperintense signal on the T1-w images and hypointense signal on the T2-w images, eliciting a "motor-oil" content, are mainly influenced by high protein concentrations and by the presence of blood degradation products; cholesterol and triglycerides concentrations have little effect on the signal. A fluid-fluid level can be present.

The cystic part usually shows a post-gad rim enhancement.

A calcified ring, not always complete, or calcified clusters can be found in 90 % of cases, better showed on CT images; x-rays of the skull is nowadays rarely performed, sometimes demonstrating the presence of calcifications and providing some information about the size and shape of the sella.

The identification of a cystic, partially calcified suprasellar mass, is suggestive for a craniopharyngioma.

The solid portion of the tumor appears isointense and/or hypointense on the T1-w images, almost always hyperintense on the T2-w images; it is characterized by a strong post-gad enhancement.

Hyperintense signal in the parenchyma adjacent to tumor may indicate gliosis, tumor invasion, or indirect injury due to cyst fluid leaking and/or edema from compression of optic chiasm/tracts. Obstructive hydrocephalus is a possible concomitant characteristic of large tumors.

Magnetic resonance angiography (MRA) images may better characterize vascular displacement and/or encasement, in particular when the anterior cerebral artery complex is involved.

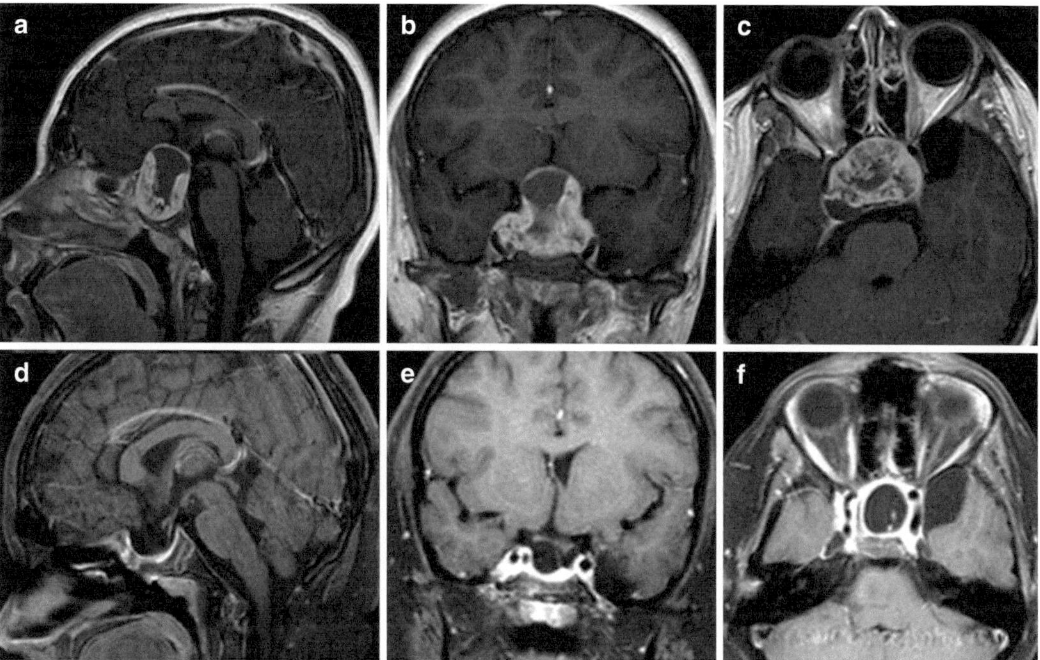

Fig. 6.1 (**a**) Sagittal, (**b**) coronal, and (**c**) axial preoperative MRi scans showing an intra- and suprasellar infradiaphragmatic craniopharyngioma, partially cystic, displacing upward the optic chiasm and the floor of the third ventricle. (**d**) Sagittal, (**e**) coronal, and (**f**) axial postoperative MRi scans showing complete tumor removal

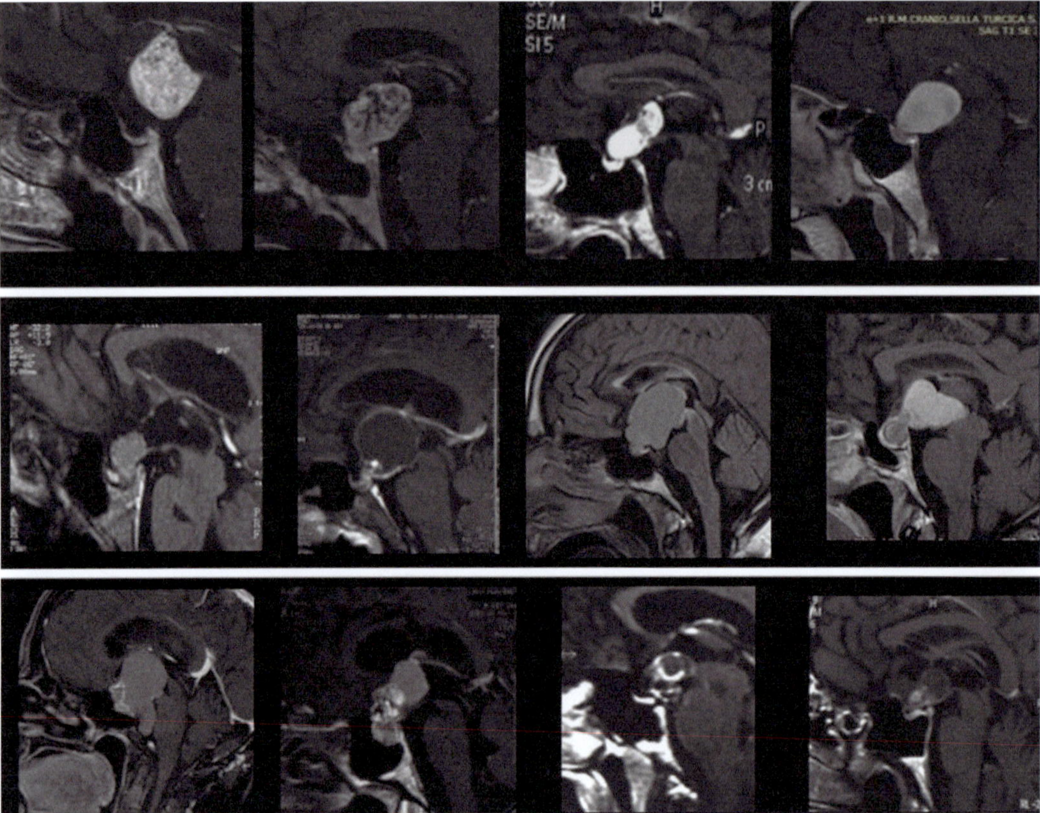

Fig. 6.2 Preoperative sagittal MRi scans showing different kinds of craniopharyngiomas involving the third ventricle

Squamopapillary craniopharyngioma appears as a rounded, solid, or both solid and cystic mass located in the third ventricle; it shows a hypointense signal on the T1-w images and hyperintense signal on the T2-w images and enhances strongly post-gad injection, although not homogeneously, because of the presence of necrotic areas.

However, it has to be reminded that there are no radiologic features that can absolutely discriminate among the subtypes of craniopharyngioma; lobulated shape, vessel encasement, and calcification have all been postulated to be indicative of the adamantinomatous subtype.

6.3 Anatomy of the Approach

The main structures related to the standard endoscopic endonasal approach have been already described in details in the homonymous section of the pituitary adenomas chapter (see Chap. 1). Although the anatomy of the nasal and paranasal cavities is the same, during surgical treatment of craniopharyngiomas, there are some relevant structures, which it is useful to focus on, especially in case of extended approaches.

First of all, whether a pedicled nasoseptal flap should be used, its anatomy has to be understood. The flap consists of the mucoperiosteum and mucoperichondrium of the nasal septum, and it is pedicled on the posterior septal artery, a branch of the sphenopalatine artery. The posterior septal artery arises from the sphenopalatine artery, branch of the internal maxillary artery, in the pterygopalatine fossa and bifurcates into a superior and inferior branch with the latter being the larger one. The branches of the posterior septal artery then form a dense network along the septum to supply the inferior two thirds of the septum and a large portion of the nasal floor.

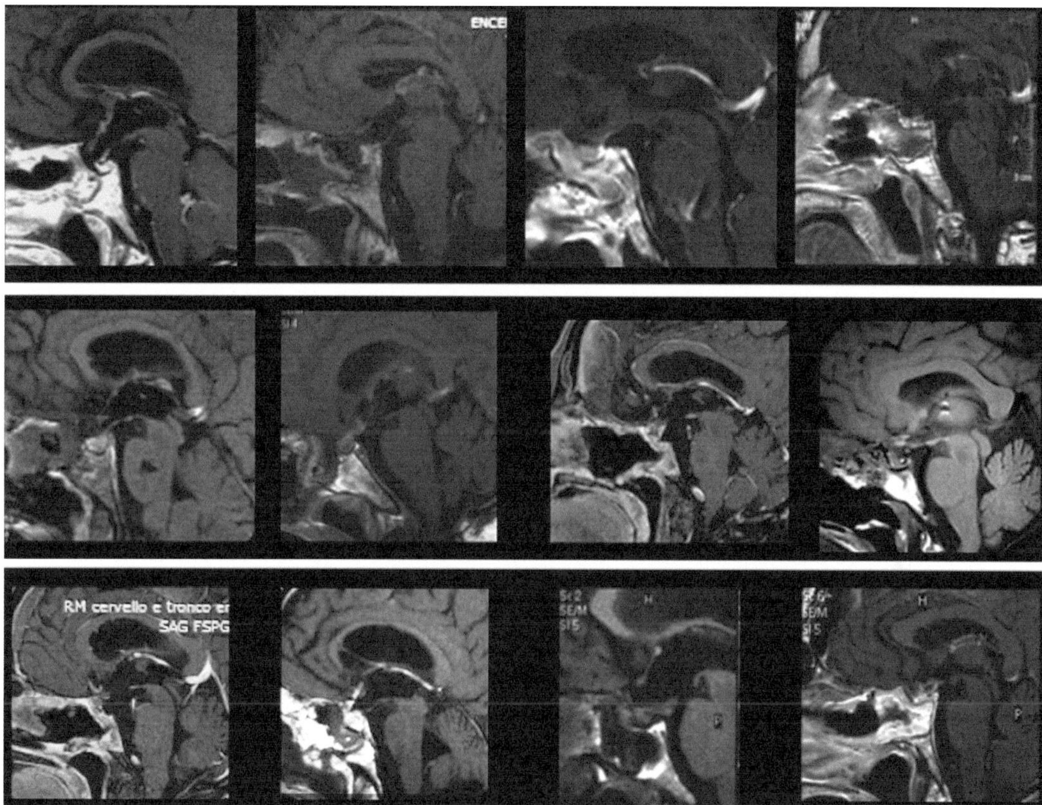

Fig. 6.3 Postoperative sagittal MRi scans of the cases shown in Fig. 6.2. The tumors have been removed via an extended endoscopic endonasal approach

As well, the configuration of the sphenoid sinus has to be addressed properly: the sphenoid sinus could present an extreme variability in terms of size and shape and, above all, degree of pneumatization. Accordingly, in the adulthood, the sphenoid sinus could be identified as follows: sellar (≅75 %), presellar (≅24 %), and conchal (≅1 %). The sellar type of sphenoid sinus is the most common; in this case the air cavity extends into the body of sphenoid below the sella and as far posteriorly as the clivus. On the other hand, in the presellar type of sphenoid sinus, the air cavity does not penetrate beyond a vertical plane parallel to the sellar floor, whereas in the conchal type, the area below the sella is a solid block of bone without an air cavity [22].

During the approach, after all the sphenoidal septa have been flattened down, the posterior and lateral walls of the sphenoid sinus are visible. The sellar floor is positioned at the center of the surgical field with the cavernous sinuses laterally to it and the planum sphenoidale above with the bony protuberances of the optic nerves laterally to it and the clival indentation below. The bony prominences of C4 and C5 segments of the internal carotid artery (ICA) [23] can be seen laterally to the sellar floor and, above them, the optic nerves prominences can be observed; between them the optocarotid recesses lie. The ICA prominences are more evident as more the sphenoid sinus is pneumatized; the molding can be different depending on the shape and course of the carotid arteries. It is useful to remind that the bone covering the artery at the level of the sphenoid sinus may be very thin, especially at bony lateral aspects of the tuberculum sellae. The lateral optocarotid recess (LOCR) lies in between the inferior aspect of the optic nerve and the lateral aspect of the carotid artery bone protuberances and corresponds to the optic strut; it varies in depth accordingly to its degree of pneumatization. On the other hand, the medial optocarotid recess (MOCR) can be identified at the medial confluence of the optic and carotid bone protuberances.

Immediately above the sellar floor, the angle formed by the convergence of the sphenoid planum with the sellar floor can be observed; this latter structure, recently named "suprasellar notch" [24], from an endoscopic standpoint resembles a "mirror image" of the tuberculum sellae. It is limited superiorly by a line joining the 2 lateral optocarotid recesses, inferiorly by a line crossing just above the superior margin of the sella, and laterally by the medial aspect of the parasellar tract of the carotid arteries.

Once the bone of the sella and of the planum sphenoidale has been removed, venous sinuses that interconnect the cavernous sinuses appear: the intercavernous connections are named on the basis of their relationship to the pituitary gland; the anterior, or superior, intercavernous sinus passes anterior to the hypophysis, while the posterior, or inferior, intercavernous sinus passes behind the gland. However, these intercavernous connections can run at any site along the anterior, inferior, or posterior surface of the gland, or eventually they may be absent. There is also a large intercavernous venous connection, i.e., the basilar sinus that passes posteriorly to the dorsum sellae and upper clivus and connects the inferior and posterior aspects of both cavernous sinuses.

The dura is opened and it is possible to explore the entire suprasellar region. It should be said that a brief intercarotid distance – measured at the level of the supraclinoid tracts – could narrow the width of the endonasal corridor. Though, when adopting an extended endoscopic endonasal approach, this feature should be carefully evaluated preoperatively.

As well, the anatomical variability of the optic chiasm as related to the anterior skull base and surrounding structures should be highlighted: several anatomical studies showed that about 80 % of the optic chiasms overlie the diaphragm sellae, so defined as normal positioning. The remaining 20 % was equally distributed between the prefixed variant – when sitting above the tuberculum sellae – and the postfixed variant – when lying over to the dorsum sellae.

From the endoscopic endonasal perspective, the suprasellar area can be divided into four areas by two ideal planes, one passing through the inferior surface of the chiasm and the mammillary bodies and another passing through the posterior margin of chiasm and the dorsum sellae; these two lines define four regions, i.e., the suprachiasmatic, the subchiasmatic, the retrosellar, and the ventricular (Fig. 6.4) [3].

In the *suprachiasmatic region*, the chiasmatic and lamina terminalis cisterns with relative contents are accessible. The anterior margin of the chiasm and the medial portion of the optic nerves, the anterior cerebral arteries, the anterior communicating artery, and the recurrent Heubner arteries, together with the gyri recti of the frontal lobes, are identified.

In the *subchiasmatic space*, the pituitary stalk is at the center of the view, below the chiasm, with the superior hypophyseal arteries and its perforating branches, supplying the inferior surface of the chiasm and the optic nerves. The superior aspect of the pituitary gland and the dorsum sellae are also visible. The superior hypophyseal arteries supply the optic chiasm, the floor of the hypothalamus, and the median eminence. On the other side, the inferior hypophyseal artery divides into a medial and a lateral branch, which anastomose with the corresponding vessels of the opposite side, forming an arterial ring around the hypophysis.

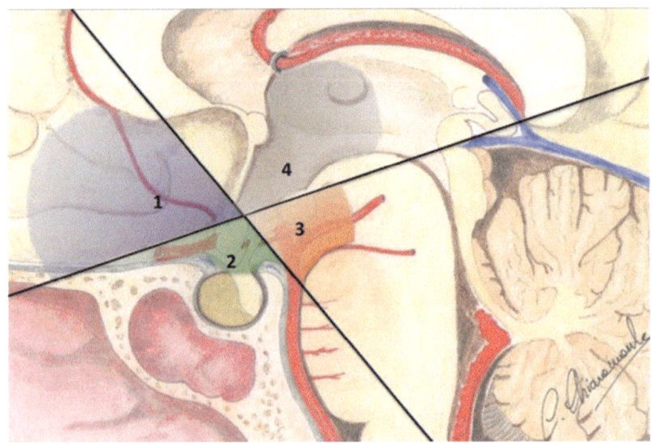

Fig. 6.4 Areas above the sella that can be explored via the extended endoscopic endonasal approach to the planum sphenoidale: *1* suprachiasmatic, *2* infrachiasmatic, *3* retrosellar, and *4* intraventricular

The *retrosellar area* can be explored passing with the endoscope between the pituitary stalk and the internal carotid artery, sliding above the dorsum sellae; it encloses the upper third of the basilar artery, the pons, the superior cerebellar arteries, the oculomotor nerves, the posterior cerebral arteries, and lastly the mammillary bodies and the floor of the third ventricle at the level of the tuber cinereum (Fig. 6.5).

Concerning the *third ventricle* area, it has to be highlighted that, as seen from the endonasal perspective, this cavity can be divided into four areas by means of two ideal planes, one passing through the optic chiasm and the interthalamic commissure and one passing through the posterior edge of the foramen of Monro and the interthalamic commissure. Accordingly, two anterior (infundibular and foraminal) and two posterior

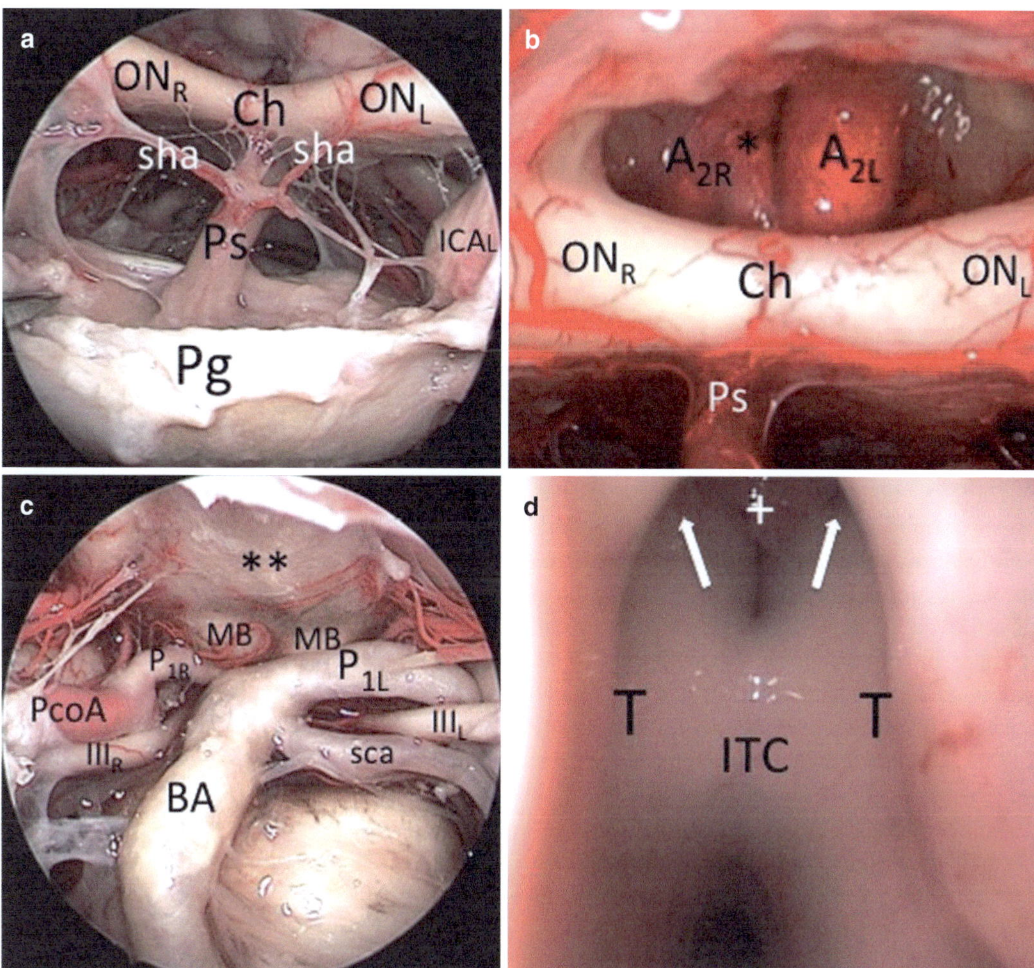

Fig. 6.5 Endoscopic endonasal anatomical view of the (**a**) infrachiasmatic, (**b**) suprachiasmatic, (**c**) retrosellar, and (**d**) intraventricular areas. *Pg* pituitary gland, *Ps* pituitary stalk, *PcoA* posterior communicating artery, *BA* basilar artery, *ICA* internal carotid artery, *ONL* left optic nerve, *ONR* right optic nerve, *Ch* chiasm, *A2L* post-communicating tract of the left anterior cerebral artery, *A2R* post-communicating tract of the right anterior cerebral artery, *IIIR* right oculomotor nerve, *IIIL* left oculomotor nerve, *P1R* pre-communicating tract of the right posterior cerebral artery, *P1L* pre-communicating tract of the left posterior cerebral artery, *sca* superior cerebellar artery, + choroid plexus, * fronto-polar artery, *ITC* interthalamic commissure, *MB* mammillary bodies, ** tuber cinereum, *white arrows* access to the foramina of Monro, *T* thalamus

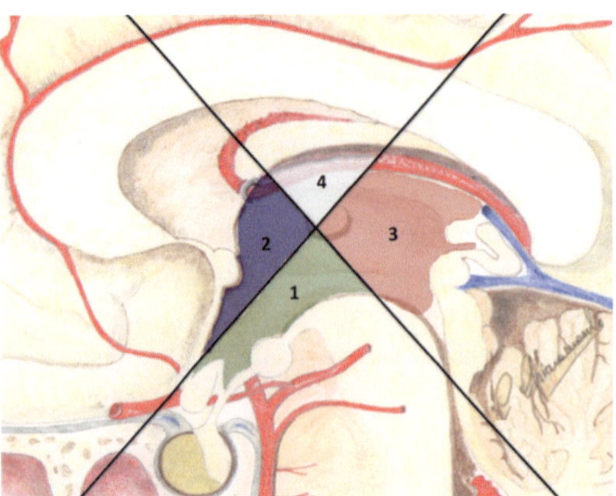

Fig. 6.6 Artistic drawing showing a sagittal view of the third ventricle. The third ventricle chamber has been divided into four areas by means of two ideal lines passing the first one between the optic chiasm and the interthalamic commissure and the second one between the posterior edge of the foramen of Monro and the interthalamic commissure. *1* anterior-inferior (infundibular) area, *2* anterior-superior (foraminal) area, *3* posterior-inferior (mesencephalic) area, *4* posterior-superior (tectal) area

(mesencephalic and tectal) areas can be defined (Fig. 6.6). Furthermore, two separate endoscopic endonasal corridors can be identified, namely, the suprachiasmatic and the subchiasmatic [25].

Through the suprachiasmatic pathway, the lamina terminalis cistern is entered above the optic chiasm. Once the lamina terminalis is opened, the *infundibular area* of the third ventricle can be accessed. As soon as the third ventricle chamber is entered, the endoscopic inspection with 0° endoscope permits to visualize the thalami laterally and the interthalamic commissure. The use of angled endoscopes permits a better view, especially of the foraminal area.

On the other hand, the subchiasmatic route allows the entry into the third ventricle cavity through its floor. In this case the third ventricle is accessed through the tuber cinereum, which is located on the floor of the third ventricle between the pituitary stalk and the mammillary bodies. It has to be stressed that, entering the third ventricle through the tuber cinereum, the extradural removal of the dorsum sellae and eventually of the posterior clinoids along with the anterior transposition of the pituitary gland are useful.

As the endoscope is advanced in an inferior-superior trajectory through the tuber cinereum inside the ventricular cavity, a wide panoramic view is obtained (not only its infundibular area): the thalami and the interthalamic commissure and the foramen of Monro are visualized anteriorly, while the bulging of mammillary bodies can be seen posteriorly.

Advancing further inside the ventricular chamber, a panoramic view of the *foraminal area* is obtained: the endoscopic endonasal exploration of the foraminal area permits to show the inner surface of the foramina of Monro, i.e., the aspect appearing at the third ventricle. As seen from this perspective, the body of the fornix is located on the middle of the field and it continues upward and laterally with its columns; on the other hand, the inferior-lateral surface of each foramen of Monro, as seen from below, is formed by the ipsilateral thalamus. The choroid plexus extends within each foramen of Monro, surrounding the body of the fornix like a collar before entering the lateral ventricle through the choroidal fissure. The anterior commissure is identified anteriorly to the foramen of Monro.

Finally, passing under the interthalamic commissure, the posterior portion of the third ventricle, i.e., the *mesencephalic area*, can be reached up to the pineal and suprapineal recesses, the posterior commissure, the habenular commissure, the habenular trigone, the stria medullaris, the tela choroidea, and the beginning of the cerebral aqueduct. The pineal gland and the internal cerebral veins lateral to the pineal gland can be seen as well (Fig. 6.7). The tectal area is generally not accessible through an endoscopic endonasal approach, neither via a suprachiasmatic or a subchiasmatic route.

6.4 Technique

As a general rule, it should be said that as position and orientation of the microscope could turn around the patient's head, the same concept should be adopted during the endoscopic endonasal procedure. The position of the endoscope and instruments inside the nasal cavities should be variable and versatile, according to the target surgical area. Whether the surgeon is right-handed or left-handed, the endoscope is inserted, respectively, into the right or left nostril, at the high or

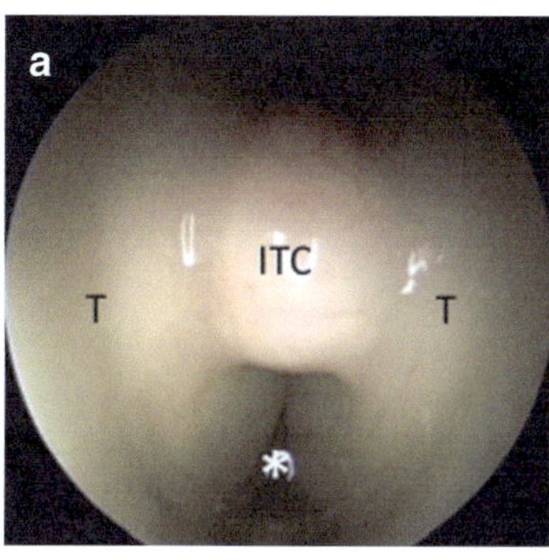

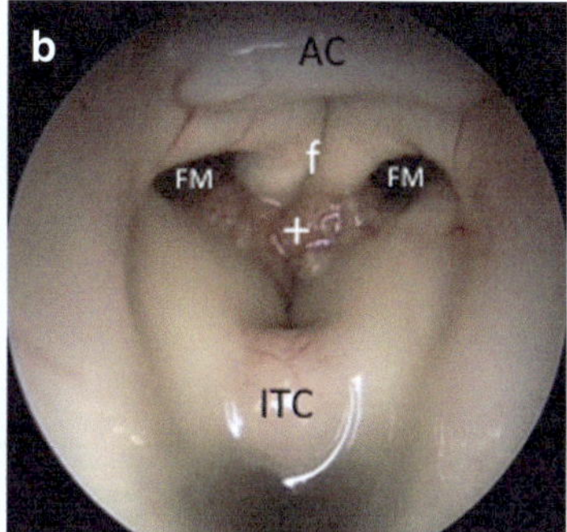

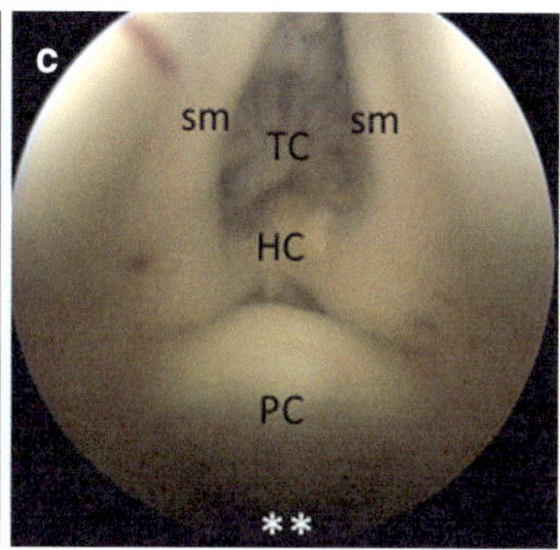

Fig. 6.7 Endoscopic endonasal anatomical view of the (**a**) infundibular, (**b**) foraminal, and (**c**) mesencephalic regions of the third ventricle. *T* thalamus, *ITC* interthalamic commissure, *FM* foramina of Monro, *f* fornix, *AC* anterior commissure, *TC* tela coroidea, *sm* striae medullaris, *HC* habenular commissure, *PC* posterior commissure, * mesencephalic region, ** aqueduct of Sylvius

low portion of the nasal cavity, with the aim of reaching the area of the surgical field that must be displayed. The first surgeon uses the nostril not occupied by the scope for his first instrument and the other for a second tool, while the second surgeon holds the scope in one nostril and another instrument in the contralateral nostril. This strategy attains to the strictly proper neurosurgical part of the operation, let's say from the sphenoid sinus on, where a microsurgical attitude with using an instrument for each surgeon's hand is mandatory. The same principle has to be applied to the surgical instruments; as a matter of fact, their position inside the nasal cavities should allow the most comfortable trajectory in order to reach each visible area of the surgical field, avoiding any conflict with the endoscope.

In case of infradiaphragmatic craniopharyngiomas, the surgical procedure is the same as described for pituitary adenomas (see Chap. 1). The endoscopic endonasal approach begins in the same way; in case of a craniopharyngioma, after the dura is opened, any cystic component of the lesion is aspirated, while the solid component has to be sharply dissected from the sellar walls and/or from the suprasellar cistern trying to not damage this structure to avoid intraoperative CSF leak (Figs. 6.8, 6.9, and 6.10). It has to be stressed that infradiaphragmatic craniopharyngiomas may be purely intrasellar or, more frequently, present a considerable suprasellar extension, pushing upward the diaphragma sellae. Those tumors can be approached via a standard endoscopic endonasal pathway as well. During the removal of infradiaphragmatic craniopharyngiomas, it is often possible to preserve the integrity of the suprasellar cistern: thus far, the sellar floor can remain open allowing the drainage of any eventual fluid part of the lesion inside the sphenoid sinus. The introduction of an X-shaped silastic catheter inside the sella grants the communication of the sella with the sphenoid sinus and/or the nasal cavities also after tissue healing (see Fig. 6.21) [26].

In case of supradiaphragmatic craniopharyngioma, an "extended" endoscopic endonasal approach has to be performed.

Lumbar drainage is placed at the beginning of the procedure. The patient is placed supine and the head is positioned in a slightly extended position in order to optimize the access to the anterior cranial base. The face is turned 5–10° toward the surgeons. The procedure starts, dealing with nasal steps as previously described for pituitary adenomas, with some modifications according to the principle of the extended endoscopic endonasal surgery [27, 28, 14]. Besides, the periumbilical area has to be prepped and draped in order to allow to harvest autologous fat for the reconstruction phase.

Cottonoids, soaked with diluted adrenaline and lidocaine, are inserted in both nostrils between the middle turbinate and the nasal septum and left in place for about 5 min; then, unilateral middle turbinectomy with removal of the posterior ethmoidal cells is performed in the same cavity where the nasoseptal flap will be raised. Moreover, the posterior aspect of the nasal septum is removed

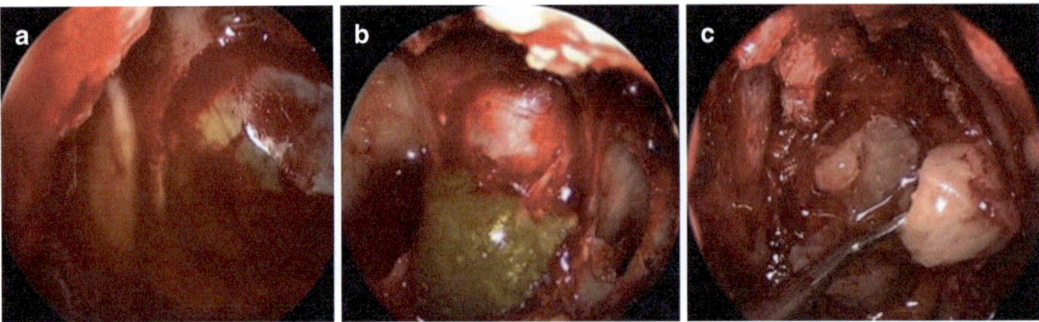

Fig. 6.8 Intraoperative picture showing a standard endoscopic endonasal approach for the removal of infradiaphragmatic craniopharyngiomas. Different consistencies of craniopharyngioma content. (**a**) Liquid; (**b**) motor-oil like; (**c**) solid

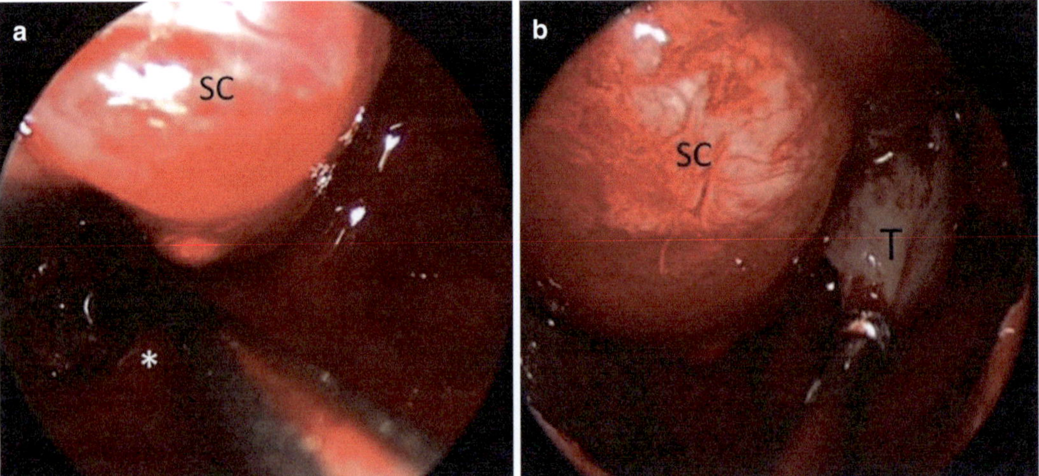

Fig. 6.9 Intraoperative endoscopic closeup intrasellar view during the removal of an infradiaphragmatic craniopharyngioma (**a**, **b**). *T* tumor, *SC* suprasellar cistern, * dorsum sellae

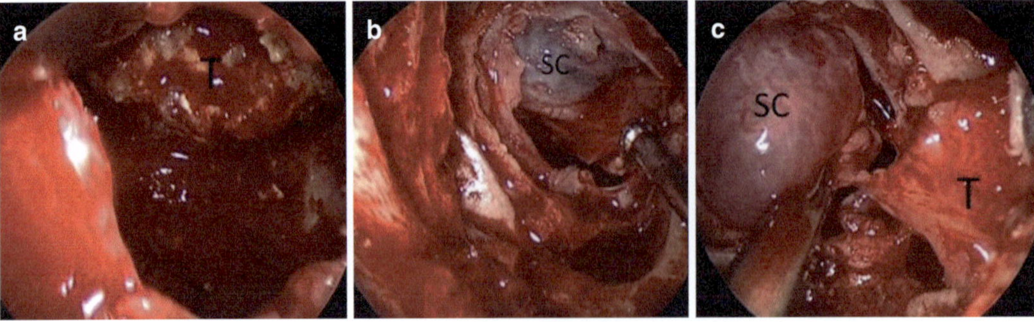

Fig. 6.10 Intraoperative endoscopic endonasal approach for the removal of infradiaphragmatic craniopharyngioma: (**a**–**c**) dissection of the solid component of an infradiaphragmatic craniopharyngioma from the suprasellar cistern. *T* tumor, *SC* suprasellar cistern

minding to not extend anteriorly to the head of the contralateral middle turbinate to reduce scars to a single nasal cavity and therefore limit the patient's postoperative breathing discomfort.

At the beginning of the surgical procedure, the nasoseptal flap is usually drawn – tailored according to size and shape of the defect – on the septum while raised and rotated on the osteo-dural defect at the end of the surgery. Two parallel incisions are performed following the sagittal plane of the septum, one over the maxillary crest and the other 1–2 cm below the most superior aspect of the septum (this preserves the olfactory epithelium) and joined anteriorly by a vertical cut. Elevation of the flap is realized at the end of the procedure, in order to reduce the nasal bleeding during surgery and eventually avoid the ischemia of the flap due to the twisting of its pedicle and, at the same time, increase the adhesive property of the same flap that is lifted from the septum and immediately placed on the osteo-dural defect. The nasoseptal flap is elevated with a Cottle dissector or similar instrument taking care of preserving the posterolateral neurovascular pedicle [29].

At this point, the nasal septum is detached from the anterior wall of the sphenoid sinus with the aid of a dissector or with a high-speed microdrill and the posterior edge of the nasal septum (1–2 cm) is resected with backbiting forceps. It is crucial to widely open the anterior wall of the sphenoid sinus in order to gain a proper working angle for the instruments. Subsequently, the contralateral middle turbinate is laterally displaced. All intrasinus septae are flattened down. The main anatomical landmark of the posterior wall of the sphenoid sinus must be recognized (Fig. 6.1). These include the optic nerves and intracavernous carotid artery (ICA) canals as well as lateral and medial opticocarotid recesses (MOCR and LOCR, respectively) and the clival recess.

A complete removal of the tuberculum sellae, i.e., the suprasellar notch [24] as seen from the endonasal perspective up to both medial optocarotid recesses, is mandatory to enter the suprasellar area and reach the third ventricle: the bone is thinned with the drill and then removed with a Kerrison rongeur. The extent of bone removal, in anteroposterior direction, is determined by the size and location of the tumor and can be measured intraoperatively using neuronavigation.

Before opening the dura, it can be useful to dissect the epidural space alongside the edge of the bone opening in order to allow a comfortable extradural reconstruction at the final stage of the surgery.

Prior than dural opening, micro-Doppler ultrasonography can be used to avoid injury to the ICA, especially when its proximal supraclinoid portion courses toward midline and the superior intercavernous sinus should be coagulated and closed (Fig. 6.11). The dura is initially incised horizontally few millimeters above and below the superior intercavernous sinus, with the aim of dissecting the two dural layers in which the sinus lies; thereafter, it is totally closed with bipolar coagulation and cut in its median portion. This technique avoids the use of hemoclips that conversely can narrow the dural opening, hindering the access to the suprasellar space.

The dural incision is though performed in a median position passing over the superior intercavernous sinus diverging superiorly in a "Y shape" toward both the optic prominences and downward as well in "Y shape" to the inferolateral corners of the pituitary gland. It is crucial to avoid coagulation and/or removal of the dural leaflets, as they can help supporting the reconstruction.

The removal of a craniopharyngioma via an endoscopic transsphenoidal approach suits the same goals and principles of the microsurgical transcranial routes: internal debulking of the solid part and/or cystic evacuation, followed by fine tumor dissection from the main surrounding neurovascular structures.

Hence, upon dural opening the craniopharyngioma will came into view covered by the arachnoidal layers of the suprasellar cistern (Figs. 6.12 and 6.13): the surgical removal proceeds in an anteroposterior direction taking extreme care while managing the lower part of the tumor, in

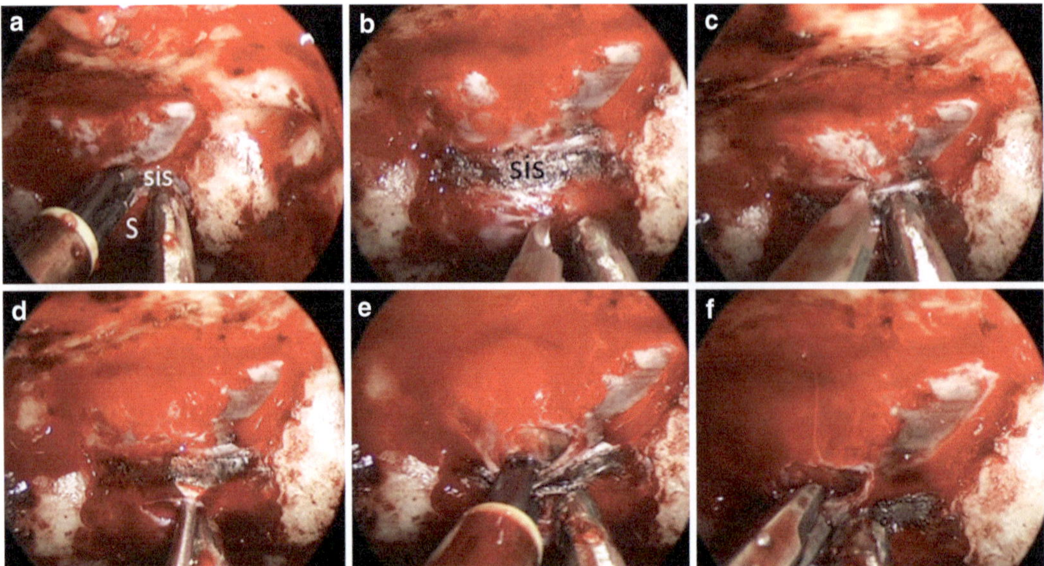

Fig. 6.11 Management of the superior intercavernous sinus during extended endoscopic endonasal approach to the planum sphenoidale. (**a**) The sinus is first coagulated and then the dura is cutted (**b**) below and (**c**) above it. (**d**) A dissector is inserted underneath the superior intercavernous sinus in order to detach it from the arachnoid and the pituitary gland. Then, (**e**) both layers of the dura mater containing the venous connection are coagulated and the sinus is (**f**) divided to allow safe entry inside the subarachnoid space. *sis* superior intercavernous sinus, *s* sella

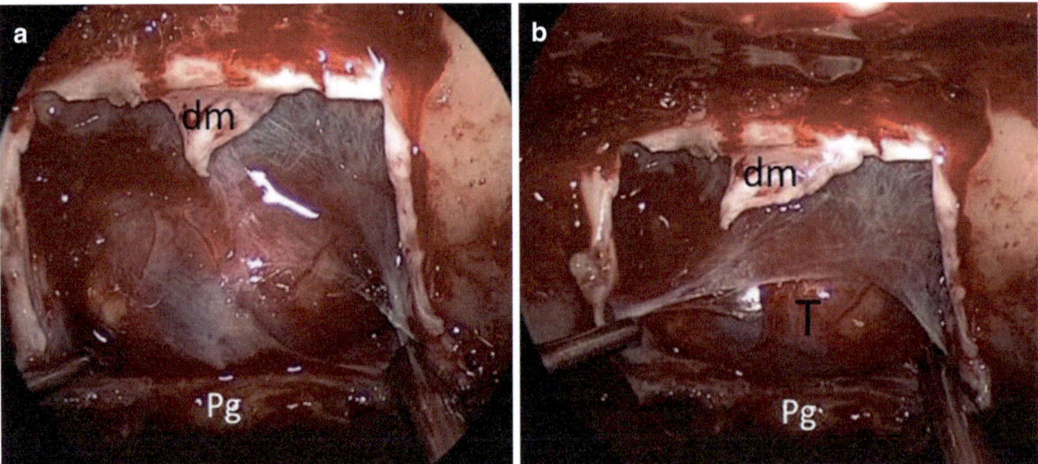

Fig. 6.12 Intraoperative endoscopic enondasal view. Once the dura has been opened, (**a**) the tumor is visualized. (**b**) Thin layer of arachnoid covers the tumor. *dm* dura mater, *T* tumor, *Pg* pituitary gland

close contact with to the pituitary gland and stalk, and, as well, dealing with the upper part, in a strict relationship with the optic chiasm and optic nerves. During the early intracapsular debulking of the craniopharyngioma, it is mandatory to identify and preserve the superior hypophyseal arteries as they greatly contribute to the blood supply of the optic chiasm (Fig. 6.14).

Proceeding with the removal of the posterior portion of the lesion, the relationships of

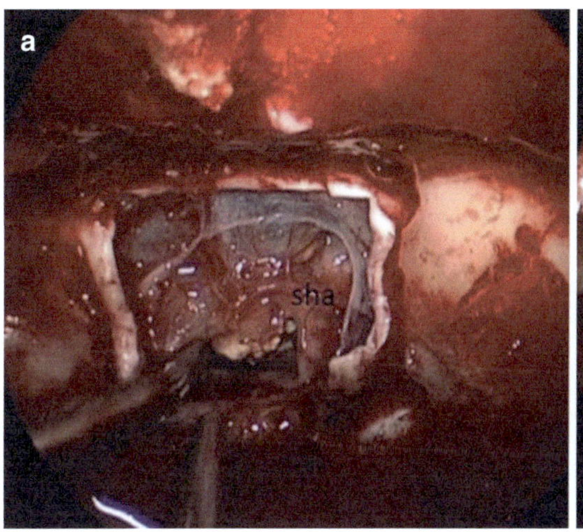

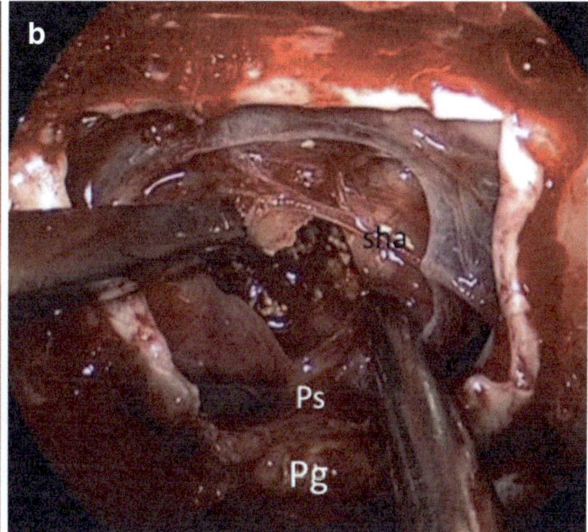

Fig. 6.13 Intraoperative endoscopic endonasal approach for the removal of an infundibular craniopharyngioma: (**a**) debulking of the solid part and (**b**) identification of the main anatomical landmarks. *sha* superior hypophyseal artery, *Pg* pituitary gland, *Ps* pituitary stalk

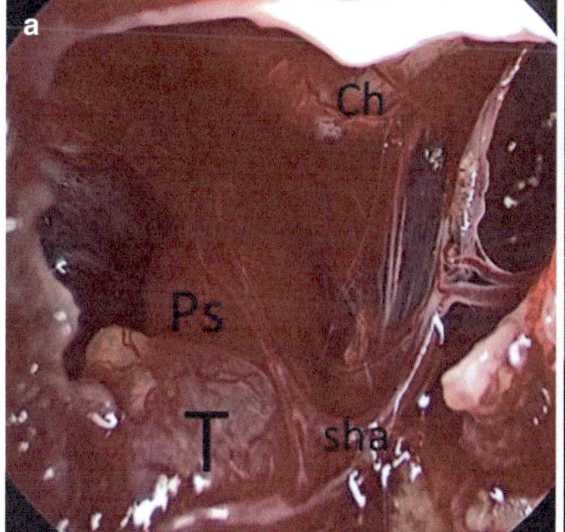

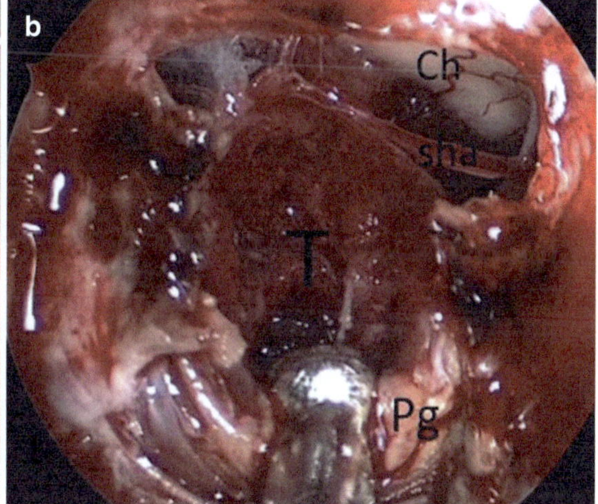

Fig. 6.14 Intraoperative endoscopic endonasal view: identification of the superior hypophyseal artery during the removal of (**a**) a preinfundibular and (**b**) infundibular craniopharyngioma. *T* tumor, *sha* superior hypophyseal artery, *Ps* pituitary stalk, *Pg* pituitary gland, *Ch* chiasm

the craniopharyngioma with the infundibulum and the floor of the third ventricle have to be ruled out (Figs. 6.15, 6.16, and 6.17): in these terms the endoscopic endonasal route for the management of craniopharyngiomas provides the advantages of a peculiar surgical trajectory that follows the origin and development of craniopharyngioma (Fig. 6.18). The endoscopic closeup view gives the opportunity to understand the amount of involvement of the main neurovascular structures along the axis stalk-infundibulum-third ventricle and their supplying vessels (Fig. 6.19).

Debulking of the craniopharyngioma can be effectively performed according to its consistency using mostly the ultrasonic aspirator; delicate "countertraction" can be very useful to identify the arachnoid cleavage plane that could allow sharp dissection from other neurovascular structures [30, 31].

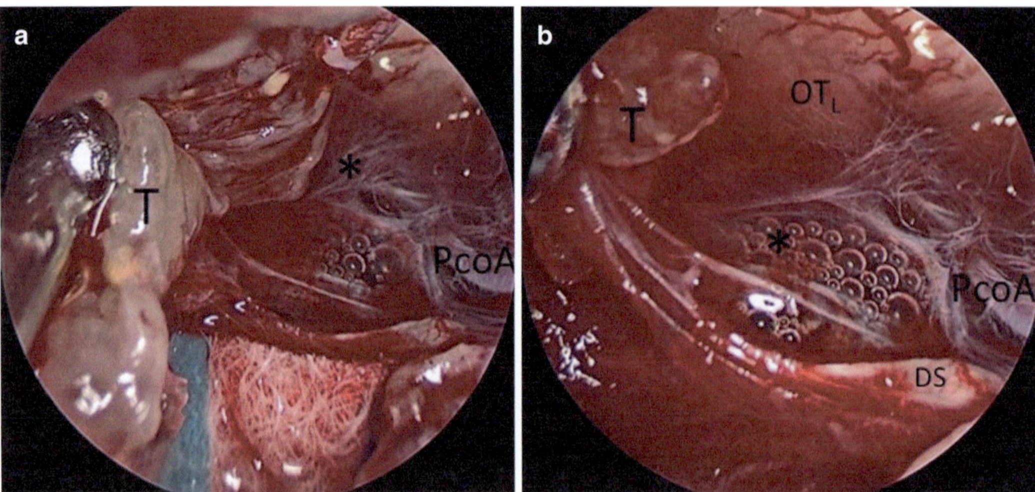

Fig. 6.15 Intraoperative endoscopic endonasal view (**a, b**) showing the Liliequist membrane during the removal of an infundibular craniopharyngioma. *T* tumor, *PcoA* posterior communicating artery, * Liliequist membrane, *MB* mammillary body, OT_L left optic tract

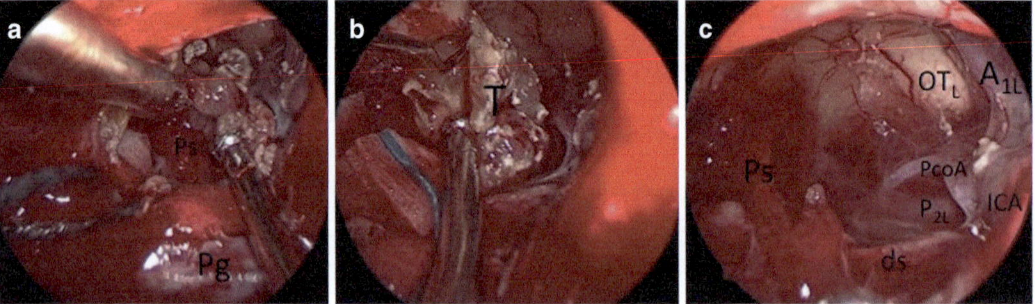

Fig. 6.16 Intraoperative endoscopic endonasal picture showing a preinfundibular craniopharyngioma (type I). (**a**) Identification of the tumor in front of the pituitary stalk. (**b**) Tumor dissection and removal from the main neuronal structure. (**c**) Exploration of the surgical field after total tumor removal. *T* tumor, *Pg* pituitary gland, P_{2L} post-communicating tráct of the left posterior cerebral artery, *PcoA* posterior communicating artery, *ICA* internal carotid artery, A_{1L} precommunicating tract of the left anterior cerebral artery, *OTL* left optic tract, *Ps* pituitary stalk, *ds* dorsum sellae

The endoscopic endonasal approach provides some advantages, i.e., a shorter intradural corridor, a median closeup view of suprasellar neurovascular structures, and, above all, a great exposure of sub- and retrochiasmatic areas, as well as of stalk-infundibulum axis, which definitely represents a crucial area in the craniopharyngiomas growth path. Indeed, a minimal displacement of the surrounding neurovascular structures is performed as compared to transcranial microsurgical approaches [9, 32].

6.4.1 Reconstruction Techniques

It has to be minded that the reconstruction technique is different among infradiaphragmatic craniopharyngiomas and those with supradiaphragmatic extension.

For infradiaphragmatic craniopharyngiomas, which require in most cases a standard endoscopic endonasal approach, the reconstruction phase of the surgical procedure, when no intraop CSF leak has occurred, aims

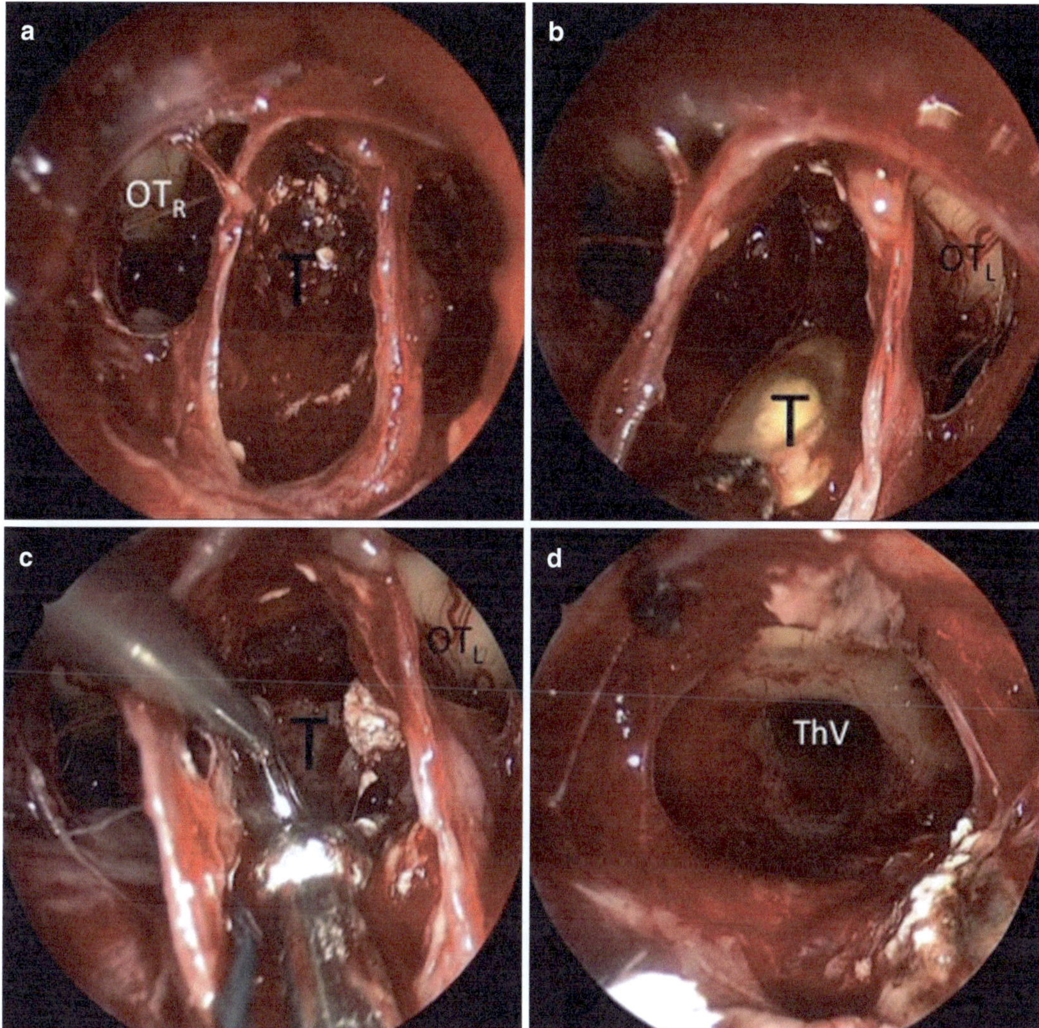

Fig. 6.17 Intraoperative endoscopic endonasal picture showing an infundibular craniopharyngioma (type II). (**a–c**) The infundibulum has been enlarged by the craniopharyngioma and through it the tumor is gradually removed. (**d**) At the end of the procedure, the infundibular part of the third ventricle cavity comes into view. *T* tumor, OT_R right optic tract, OT_L left optic tract, *ThV* third ventricle

to protect the suprasellar cistern, placing over it collagen sponge or dural substitute foils (Fig. 6.20), and to fill then the sellar dead space. In case of cystic craniopharyngiomas, after the emptying of the lesion, the insertion of an X-shaped silastic catheter into the residual cavity may be performed, in order to avoid cyst reformation and continuously drain fluid contents into the sphenoid sinus and/or nasal cavities during complementary postop radiotherapy and radiosurgery (Fig. 6.21).

On the other hand, for supradiaphragmatic craniopharyngioma, which requires an "extended" endoscopic endonasal approach, meticulous closure is mandatory for minimizing the risk of postoperative CSF leakage that may lead to potential fatal complications. A variety of reconstruction methods and materials are currently available and

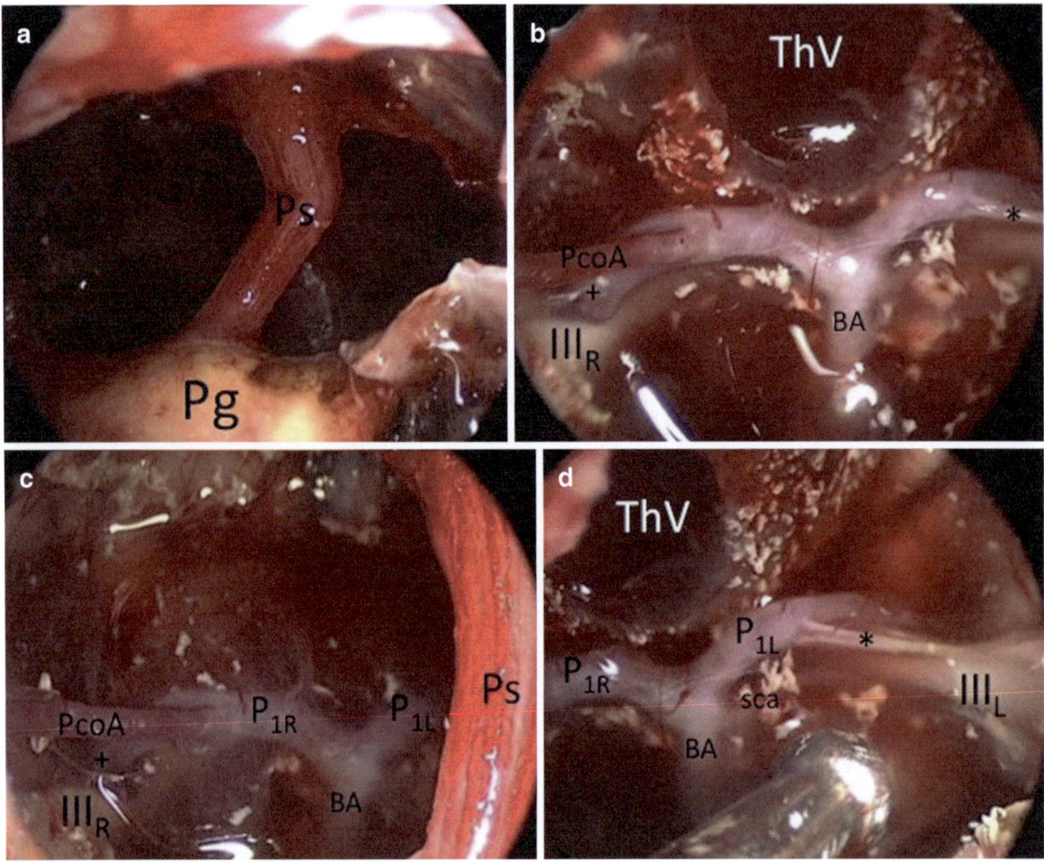

Fig. 6.18 Intraoperative endoscopic endonasal picture (**a**) showing retroinfundibular craniopharyngioma (type III). View of the retrosellar area after the removal of a retroinfundibular craniopharyngioma (**b–d**). *Pg* pituitary gland, *Ps* pituitary stalk, *ThV* third ventricle, *PcoA* posterior communicating artery, *BA* basilar artery, III_R right oculomotor nerve, III_L left oculomotor nerve, P_{1R} pre-communicating tract of the right posterior cerebral artery, $P1_L$ pre-communicating tract of the left posterior cerebral artery, *sca* superior cerebellar artery, + post-communicating tract of the right posterior cerebral artery, * hypoplastic left posterior communicating artery

used (Fig. 6.22). First of all, intradural closure with obliteration of the dead space, using autologous fat and fibrin glue, is performed. Then, we rather prefer to use the so-called sandwich technique: the surgical cavity is filled with fat graft sutured to three layers of fascia lata or dural substitute. The first two layers are positioned intradurally and the third one extradurally, wedged in between the dura and the bone. A pedicled nasoseptal flap is used to cover the skull base defect and the posterior wall of the sphenoid sinus (Fig. 6.23). An inflated Foley balloon catheter is placed, inside the sphenoid sinus to support the reconstruction [33].

Finally, bipolar hemostasis is performed over the lateral wall of the sphenoidotomy and irrigation of the nasal cavities is obtained. Lumbar drainage is usually left in place for 3–5 days.

6.4.2 Postoperative Management

Craniopharyngiomas treated via an endoscopic endonasal approach require an intensive and watchful postoperative care [34]. New-onset diabetes insipidus (DI) should be diagnosed promptly and treated with desmopressin (DDAVP).

The patient should rest in bed with the head raised at 30° in order to facilitate venous return and CSF flow toward the spine; besides, patients are asked to adopt postoperative habits in order

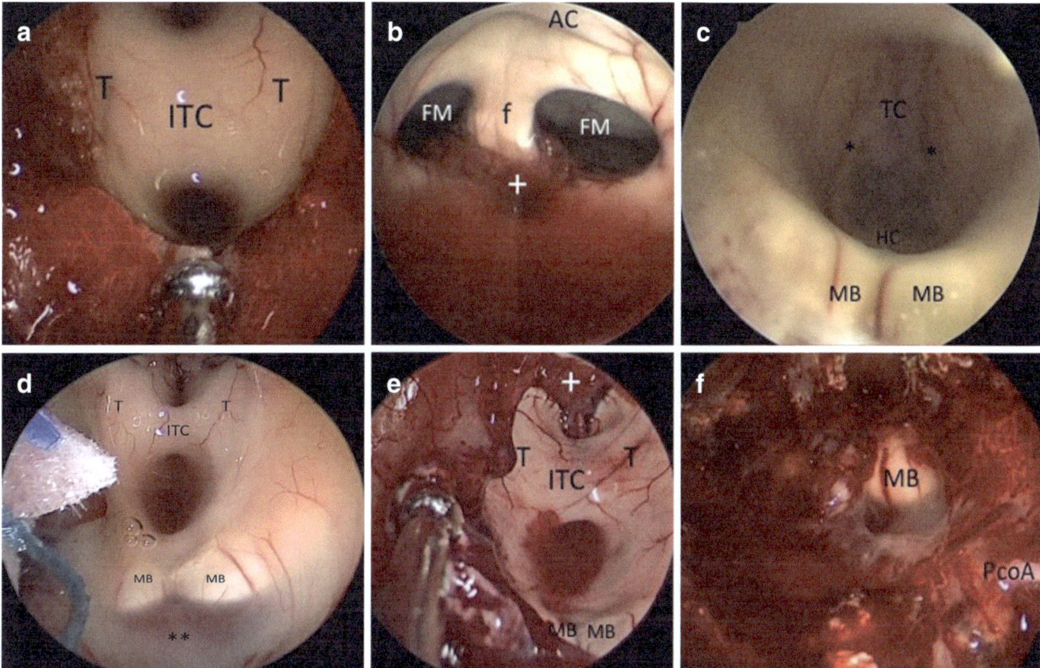

Fig. 6.19 Endoscopic views showing third ventricle cavity exploration during removal of craniopharyngiomas. (**a**) Infundibular area of the third ventricle cavity; (**b**) closeup view of the foraminal area of the third ventricle after the removal of a large intra and suprasellar craniopharyngioma in a patient with hydrocephalus. (**c**) Surgical view of the third ventricle mesencephalic area. At this level the third ventricle floor can present different degrees of pial invasion: (**d**) no involvement; (**e**) partial involvement; (**f**) diffuse involvement. *f* fornix, *FM* foramina of Monro, *PcoA* posterior communicating artery, + choroid plexus, *MB* mammillary bodies, * striae medullaris, *T* thalamus, *ITC* interthalamic commissure, *fThV* floor of the third ventricle, ** tuber cinereum

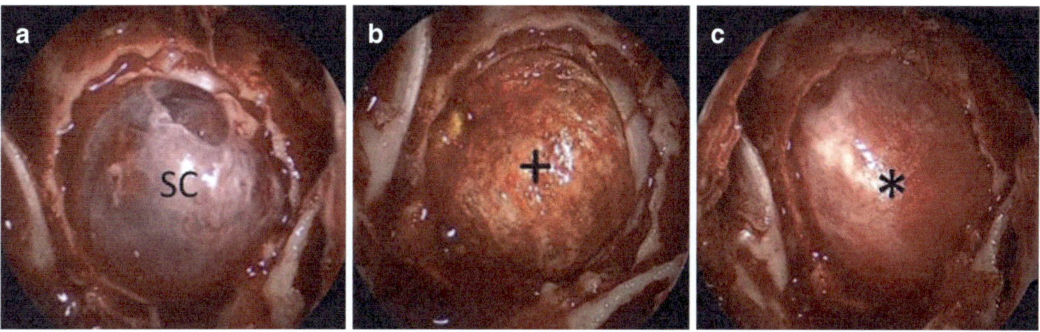

Fig. 6.20 Reconstruction technique used in case of infradiaphragmatic craniopharyngioma: (**a**) the suprasellar cistern has descent into the sellar cavity. Though, (**b**) it is protected with collagen sponge and (**c**) the floor is closed with dural substitute wedged in the extradural space. *SC* suprasellar cistern, + collagen sponge, * dura mater substitute

to prevent any ICP increase and the eventual displacement of skull base reconstruction. It is preferable to avoid the use of straws, to cough and/or sneeze with the mouth open, to assume as early as possible a stand-up position and start walking, to avoid bending over nor squatting, and to assume stool softeners.

Computed tomography (CT) scan is performed routinely at POD#1 in order to evaluate any neurosurgical complication and/or the amount of pneu-

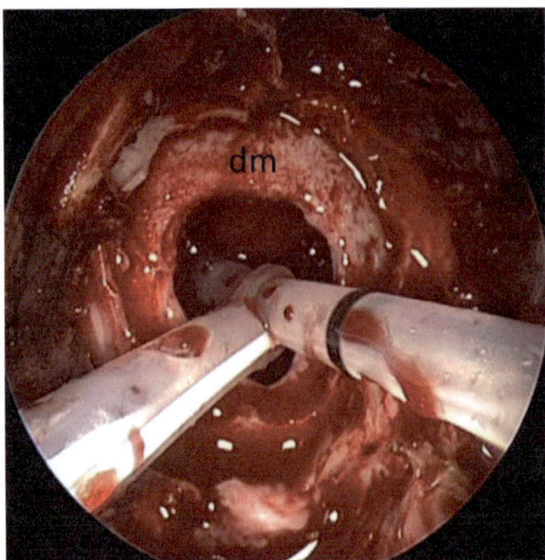

Fig. 6.21 Positioning of an X-shaped silastic catheter in case of cystic infradiaphragmatic craniopharyngioma. *dm* dura mater

mocephalus. According to a recent contribution [35], frontal and intraventricular pneumocephalus is not necessarily associated with a postoperative CSF leak; on the other hand, a "suspicious" pattern of air, namely, pneumocephalus in the convexity, interhemispheric fissure, and sella, parasellar, or perimesencephalic locations, may be significantly associated with a postoperative CSF leak occurrence and for such reason these patients require closer observation. An initial sign of not yet recognizable CSF leak may be a sudden fever onset in the early post-op period (fever sign).

It has to be highlighted that patients with minimal postoperative CSF leak can be managed without reoperation: repeated endoscope-guided fibrin glue injections – while they were awake in the outpatient operating room – can be performed if the CSF leak is minimal or moderate [36].

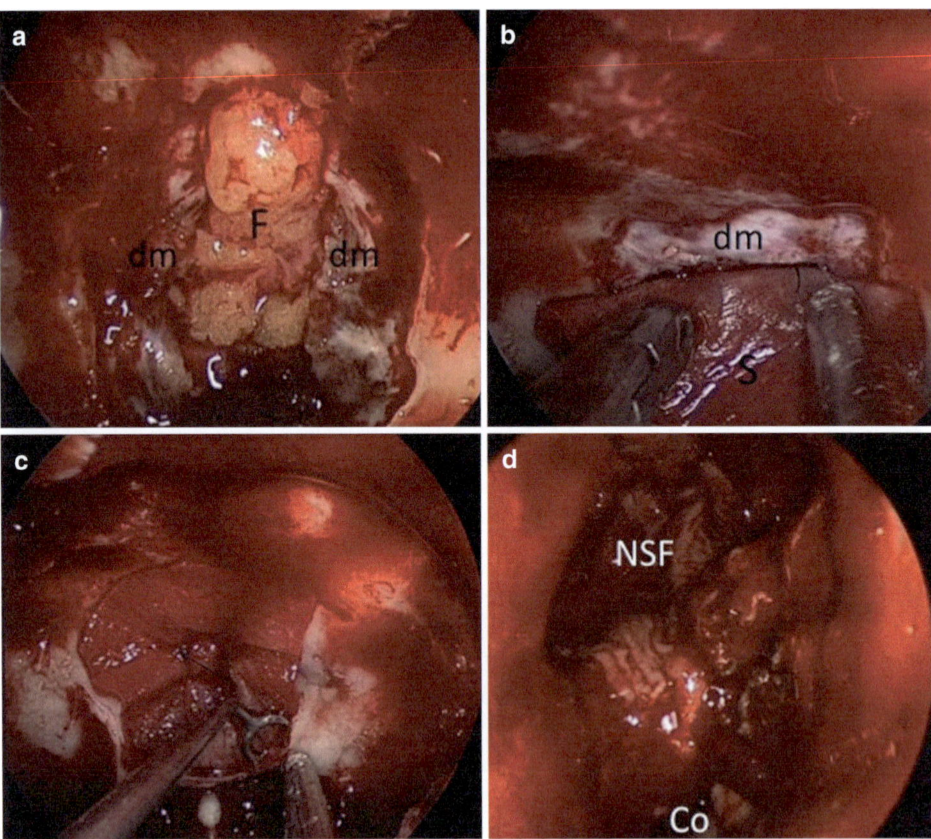

Fig. 6.22 Reconstruction technique used after endoscopic endonasal removal of a supradiaphragmatic craniopharyngioma. (**a**) Obliteration of the suprasellar dead space, using autologous fat. (**b**, **c**) Closure of the osteodural defect using the so-called sandwich technique. Finally, (**d**) the nasoseptal flap is reflected posteriorly over the skull base defect. *F* fat, *dm* dura mater, *S* "sandwich", *NSF* nasoseptal flap, *Co* choana

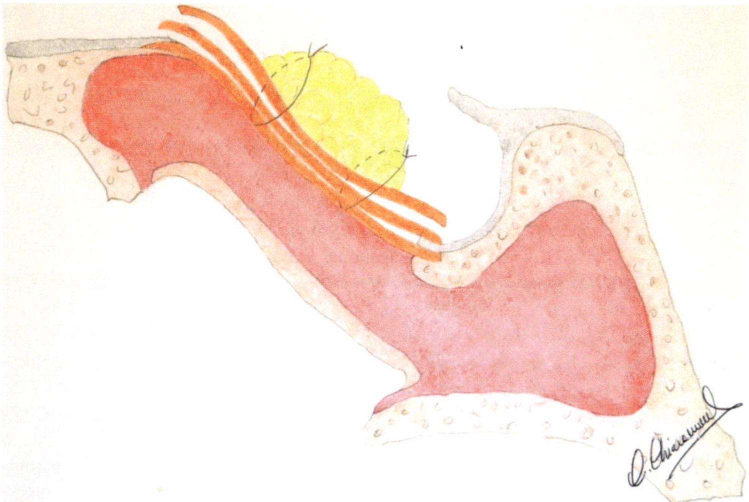

Fig. 6.23 Schematic drawing showing the reconstruction technique used after extended endoscopic endonasal approach to the suprasellar area

However, in case of severe CSF leak, displacement of the reconstruction materials, and/or evident communication of the sphenoid sinus with the intradural compartment, immediate transsphenoidal reoperation is needed.

Acknowledgment The editors wish to thank Doctor Carmela Chiaramonte for the original drawings prepared for this chapter.

References

1. Guiot G, Derome P (1972) Indications for transsphenoid approach in neurosurgery. 521 cases. Ann Med Interne (Paris) 123(8):703–712
2. Weiss MH (1987) The transnasal transsphenoidal approach. In: Apuzzo MLJ (ed) Surgery of the third ventricle. Williams & Wilkins, Baltimore, pp 476–494
3. Cavallo LM, de Divitiis O, Aydin S, Messina A, Esposito F, Iaconetta G, Talat K, Cappabianca P, Tschabitscher M (2008) Extended endoscopic endonasal transsphenoidal approach to the suprasellar area: anatomic considerations – part 1. Neurosurgery 62(6 Suppl 3):1202–1212. doi:10.1227/01.neu.0000333786.98596.33
4. Couldwell WT, Weiss MH, Rabb C, Liu JK, Apfelbaum RI, Fukushima T (2004) Variations on the standard transsphenoidal approach to the sellar region, with emphasis on the extended approaches and parasellar approaches: surgical experience in 105 cases. Neurosurgery 55(3):539–550
5. Dusick JR, Esposito F, Kelly DF, Cohan P, DeSalles A, Becker DP, Martin NA (2005) The extended direct endonasal transsphenoidal approach for nonadenomatous suprasellar tumors. J Neurosurg 102(5):832–841
6. de Divitiis E, Cappabianca P, Cavallo LM (2002) Endoscopic transsphenoidal approach: adaptability of the procedure to different sellar lesions. Neurosurgery 51(3):699–705; discussion 705–707
7. Jho HD (2001) The expanding role of endoscopy in skull-base surgery. Indications and instruments. Clin Neurosurg 48:287–305
8. Kassam A, Snyderman CH, Mintz A, Gardner P, Carrau RL (2005) Expanded endonasal approach: the rostrocaudal axis. Part I. Crista galli to the sella turcica. Neurosurg Focus 19(1):E3
9. Cavallo LM, Frank G, Cappabianca P, Solari D, Mazzatenta D, Villa A, Zoli M, D'Enza AI, Esposito F, Pasquini E (2014) The endoscopic endonasal approach for the management of craniopharyngiomas: a series of 103 patients. J Neurosurg 121(1):100–113. doi:10.3171/2014.3.JNS131521
10. Koutourousiou M, Gardner PA, Fernandez-Miranda JC, Tyler-Kabara EC, Wang EW, Snyderman CH (2013) Endoscopic endonasal surgery for craniopharyngiomas: surgical outcome in 64 patients. J Neurosurg 119(5):1194–1207. doi:10.3171/2013.6.JNS122259
11. Cappabianca P, Frank G, Pasquini E, de Divitiis O, Calbucci F (2003) Extended endoscopic endonasal transsphenoidal approaches to the suprasellar region, planum sphenoidale & clivus. In: de Divitiis E, Cappabianca P (eds) Endoscopic endonasal transsphenoidal surgery. Springer, Wien
12. Cappabianca P, Cavallo LM, Esposito F, de Divitiis O, Messina A, de Divitiis E (2008) Extended endoscopic endonasal approach to the midline skull base: the evolving role of transsphenoidal surgery. In: Pickard JD, Akalan N, Di Rocco C et al (eds) Advances and technical standards in neurosurgery. Springer, Wien/New York, pp 152–199
13. Jane JA Jr, Kiehna E, Payne SC, Early SV, Laws ER Jr (2010) Early outcomes of endoscopic transsphenoidal surgery for adult craniopharyngiomas. Neurosurg Focus 28(4):E9. doi:10.3171/2010.1.FOCUS09319

14. Kassam AB, Gardner PA, Snyderman CH, Carrau RL, Mintz AH, Prevedello DM (2008) Expanded endonasal approach, a fully endoscopic transnasal approach for the resection of midline suprasellar craniopharyngiomas: a new classification based on the infundibulum. J Neurosurg 108(4):715–728. doi:10.3171/JNS/2008/108/4/0715
15. Cavallo LM, Prevedello DM, Solari D, Gardner PA, Esposito F, Snyderman CH, Carrau RL, Kassam AB, Cappabianca P (2009) Extended endoscopic endonasal transsphenoidal approach for residual or recurrent craniopharyngiomas. J Neurosurg 111(3):578–589. doi:10.3171/2009.2.JNS081026
16. Cappabianca P, Cavallo LM (2012) The evolving role of the transsphenoidal route in the management of craniopharyngiomas. World Neurosurg 77(2):273–274
17. Samii M, Samii A (2000) Surgical management of craniopharyngiomas. In: Schmidek HH (ed) Schmidek & Sweet operative neurosurgical techniques, vol 1, Indications, methods and results. W. B. Saunders, Philadelphia, pp 489–502
18. Yasargil MG, Abdulrauf SI (2008) Surgery of intraventricular tumors. Neurosurgery 62(6 Suppl 3):1029–1040. doi:10.1227/01.neu.0000333768.12951.9a, 00006123-200806001-00010 [pii]; discussion 1040–1021
19. Yasargil MG, Curcic M, Kis M, Siegenthaler G, Teddy PJ, Roth P (1990) Total removal of craniopharyngiomas. Approaches and long-term results in 144 patients. J Neurosurg 73(1):3–11
20. Fatemi N, Dusick JR, de Paiva Neto MA, Malkasian D, Kelly DF (2009) Endonasal versus supraorbital keyhole removal of craniopharyngiomas and tuberculum sellae meningiomas. Neurosurgery 64(5 Suppl 2):269–284. doi:10.1227/01.NEU.0000327857.22221.53; discussion 284–266
21. Gerganov V, Metwali H, Samii A, Fahlbusch R, Samii M (2014) Microsurgical resection of extensive craniopharyngiomas using a frontolateral approach: operative technique and outcome. J Neurosurg 120(2):559–570. doi:10.3171/2013.9.JNS122133
22. Rhoton AL Jr (2002) The sellar region. Neurosurgery 51(4 Suppl):S335–S374
23. Bouthillier A, van Loveren HR, Keller JT (1996) Segments of the internal carotid artery: a new classification. Neurosurgery 38(3):425–432; discussion 432–423
24. de Notaris M, Solari D, Cavallo LM, D'Enza AI, Ensenat J, Berenguer J, Ferrer E, Prats-Galino A, Cappabianca P (2012) The "suprasellar notch," or the tuberculum sellae as seen from below: definition, features, and clinical implications from an endoscopic endonasal perspective. J Neurosurg 116(3):622–629. doi:10.3171/2011.11.JNS111162
25. Cavallo LM, Di Somma A, de Notaris M, Prats-Galino A, Aydin S, Catapano G, Solari D, de Divitiis O, Somma T, Cappabianca P (2015) Extended endoscopic endonasal approach to the third ventricle. Multimodal anatomical study with surgical implications. World Neurosurg. doi:10.1016/j.wneu.2015.03.007
26. Spaziante R, De Divitiis E, Irace C, Cappabianca P, Caputi F (1989) Management of primary or recurring grossly cystic craniopharyngiomas by means of draining systems. Topic review and 6 case reports. Acta Neurochir (Wien) 97(3–4):95–106
27. de Divitiis E, Cappabianca P, Cavallo LM, Esposito F, de Divitiis O, Messina A (2007) Extended endoscopic transsphenoidal approach for extrasellar craniopharyngiomas. Neurosurgery 61(5 Suppl 2):219–227. doi:10.1227/01.neu.0000303220.55393.73, 00006123-200711001-00006 [pii]; discussion 228
28. Frank G, Pasquini E, Doglietto F, Mazzatenta D, Sciaretta V, Farneti G, Calbucci F (2006) The endoscopic extended transsphenoidal approach for craniopharyngiomas. Neurosurgery 59(Suppl 1): ONS75–ONS83
29. Hadad G, Bassagasteguy L, Carrau RL, Mataza JC, Kassam A, Snyderman CH, Mintz A (2006) A novel reconstructive technique after endoscopic expanded endonasal approaches: vascular pedicle nasoseptal flap. Laryngoscope 116(10):1882–1886
30. Conger AR, Lucas J, Zada G, Schwartz TH, Cohen-Gadol AA (2014) Endoscopic extended transsphenoidal resection of craniopharyngiomas: nuances of neurosurgical technique. Neurosurg Focus 37(4):E10. doi:10.3171/2014.7.FOCUS14364
31. Kassam A, Snyderman CH, Mintz A, Gardner P, Carrau RL (2005) Expanded endonasal approach: the rostrocaudal axis. Part I. Crista galli to the sella turcica. Neurosurg Focus 19(1):E3:1–12
32. Cavallo LM, Solari D, Esposito F, Cappabianca P (2013) The endoscopic endonasal approach for the management of craniopharyngiomas involving the third ventricle. Neurosurg Rev 36(1):27–37. doi:10.1007/s10143-012-0403-4; discussion 38
33. Snyderman CH, Kassam AB, Carrau R, Mintz A (2007) Endoscopic reconstruction of cranial base defects following endonasal skull base surgery. Skull Base 17(1):73–78. doi:10.1055/s-2006-959337
34. Ditzel Filho LFS, Prevedello DM, Kerr EE, Jamshidi AO, Ottoy BA, Carrau RL (2015) Endonasal resection of craniopharyngiomas: post-operative management. In: Evans JJ, Kenning TJ (eds) Craniopharyngiomas: comprehensive diagnosis, treatment and outcome. Elsevier, Inc. USA, pp 271–280
35. Banu MA, Szentirmai O, Mascarenhas L, Salek AA, Anand VK, Schwartz TH (2014) Pneumocephalus patterns following endonasal endoscopic skull base surgery as predictors of postoperative CSF leaks. J Neurosurg 121(4):961–975. doi:10.3171/2014.5.JNS132028
36. Cavallo LM, Solari D, Somma T, Savic D, Cappabianca P (2014) The awake endoscope-guided sealant technique with fibrin glue in the treatment of postoperative cerebrospinal fluid leak after extended transsphenoidal surgery: technical note. World Neurosurg 82(3–4):e479–e485. doi:10.1016/j.wneu.2013.01.017

Cystic Craniopharyngiomas: Endoscopic Endonasal Transsphenoidal Approach

7

Neil L. Dorward, Antonio Biroli, and Michelangelo de Angelis

7.1 Introduction

Craniopharyngiomas (CPs) are uncommon, benign, extra-axial, epithelial neoplasms of the sellar and parasellar region. They represent 3–4 % of all intracranial neoplasms and occur without any sex predilection [2, 25, 35]. Among children CPs are the most common intracranial tumors of non-glial origin, accounting 6–13 % of all childhood brain tumors and representing more than 90 % of the tumors of the pituitary region in childhood [33, 36]. Clinical presentation may occur at any age but with a bimodal age distribution, with peaks at 5–14 years and 50–74 years [2]. The properties of secretion in squamous epithelium account for the fact that approximately 90 % of CPs have a cystic portion containing secreted fluid, cholesterol crystals, and epithelial cells. According to the different series, CPs are defined as purely or predominantly cystic in 46–64 % of cases [18, 20]. Despite their benign histological nature, CPs frequently display a locally aggressive behavior and cause damage to critical neural and vascular structures in the sellar and parasellar regions. This can cause endocrine, behavioral, and visual deficits. These tumors have a high propensity to recur after resection and, given their site, are associated with significant morbidity and mortality rates.

The pioneering neurosurgeons of the turn of the twentieth century considered the region of the hypothalamus and suprasellar space to be virtually inaccessible and attempts at transcranial removal of tumors in this region met with failure. Contemporary approaches were presaged by the recognition that they could be approached via a transsphenoidal approach and in 1909 Albert Halstead performed the first successful resection of a CP, via the transsphenoidal route. Despite this early success, the transsphenoidal approach was not widely adopted; rather various transcranial approaches were developed [13, 15, 18, 21]. The renaissance of transsphenoidal surgery for pituitary adenomas opened the way to resect sellar CPs via this route and smaller midline suprasellar CPs via the extended transsphenoidal method. The use of endoscopes has thrown open the door to using this approach for a far wider range of CPs, and in many centers this is now the preferred approach [3, 5, 15].

Historically the benign histology and high initial survival rates were seen as supporting complete resection as the method of choice. However, adhesion to the optic chiasm and hypothalamus limited

Electronic supplementary material The online version of this chapter (doi:10.1007/978-3-319-21533-4_7) contains supplementary material, which is available to authorized users.

N.L. Dorward, MD (✉) • A. Biroli, MD
Victor Horsley Department of Neurosurgery, National Hospital, London, UK
e-mail: neil.dorward@uclh.nhs.uk

M. de Angelis, MD
Division of Neurosurgery, Department of Neurosciences, Reproductive and Odontostomatological Sciences, Università degli Studi di Napoli Federico II, Naples, Italy

P. Cappabianca et al. (eds.), *Midline Skull Base Surgery*, DOI 10.1007/978-3-319-21533-4_7

true gross total resection (GTR) and morbidity was high [27, 33]. The modern surgical approach is more concerned with preserving total quality of life [34], and recent data suggests that selective subtotal resection (STR) followed by adjuvant therapies can provide similar rates of tumor control to GTR, without the endocrine and behavioral morbidity associated with aggressive resection [31, 33]. CPs are now viewed more as a chronic condition [10], and in this context, endoscopic transsphenoidal surgery has a clear role in achieving less invasive, safe, and accurate GTR/STR.

7.2 Pathology

CPs are epithelial neoplasms that develop from remnants of Rathke's pouch. These rests occur from the sella to the floor of the third ventricle. Two principal subtypes are described: adamantinomatous and papillary. The adamantinomatous CPs are more frequent and are the main form encountered in the pediatric population. These are mixed cystic and solid lesions. The papillary type is less frequent, more often seen in the adult population (14–50 % of CPs in adults, 2 % of CPs in children), and these tumors are mainly solid [10, 35]. The cysts of CPs contain turbid, yellow-brown, cholesterol-rich fluid containing phospholipids and keratin. The solid component consists of clusters of organized palisading columnar cells [25]. Desquamated cells form masses called "wet keratin." The papillary type does not calcify and usually is a well-circumscribed lesion. The genetic basis of CPs has not been fully elucidated, but aberrant patterns of β-catenin expression are seen [34].

7.3 Radiology

On MR imaging, the solid elements are usually iso- or hypointense on T1-weighted series, exhibit inhomogeneous high intensity on T2-weighted images, and heterogeneously enhance following gadolinium (Gd) administration. The cystic elements of adamantinomatous CPs typically display a high intensity on T1-weighted images, high or mixed intensity on T2-weighted images, and contrast enhancement of the cyst wall. Several topographic classifications have been described based on relationship to surrounding structures. These provide a guideline to the most appropriate surgical approach [17]. These however are modified via reference to individual high-definition imaging.

7.4 Presenting Symptoms

Given their site, CPs may present with a spectrum of clinical symptoms, mainly related to visual problems, endocrine dysfunction, headaches, and hypothalamic involvement. In a series of 309 patient, Shi et al. found a decrease in visual acuity or a visual field deficit in 133 patients, moderate to severe headache in 107 patients, diabetes insipidus (DI) in 27 patients, amenorrhea in 21 women, and growth retardation in 11 patients [29]. Children (<18 years old) are significantly less likely to present with visual symptoms than adults and tend to present with endocrine dysfunction [37]. Comparing transcranial with endoscopic series, presenting features were visual disturbance in 53 % and 75 %, headache in 52 % and 35 %, hypopituitarism in 28 % and 55 %, and DI in 12 % and 32 % [22].

7.5 Indications and Aims

Stalk or suprasellar CPs of a modest size and mainly midline can readily be approached by several routes, both transcranial and transsphenoidal. The choice is often dictated by the surgeon's experience as much as the anatomy. The transsphenoidal route has the advantage of avoiding brain retraction, better visualization, and no driving ban. Also, the transsphenoidal procedure can be performed regardless of the position of the chiasm. Tumor and capsule extending into the third ventricle present a formidable challenge to access transcranially, and major retraction is often required even with a wide Sylvian split and orbito-zygomatic disassembly. In contrast, the third ventricle is readily accessed via the extended transsphenoidal route, lying directly along the surgical pathway. Lateral extension into the temporal lobes and basal ganglia is difficult to resect via either route and will possibly require a combined approach. In some cases however transsphenoidal removal is feasible as deflation of the cysts relaxes the temporal compression bringing the capsule into view for dissection. Encasement of the suprasellar carotid or anterior cerebral arteries is very difficult to deal with safely via the endoscopic transsphenoidal approach, so in such a case the favored approach would either be purely transcranial or combined with transsphenoidal subtotal resection [9, 8, 22, 32].

7.6 Equipment

While it is feasible to operate with minimal endoscopic equipment that is available in most large hospitals (ENT endoscopes, FESS sets), having the full range of special equipment transforms the level of control the surgeon has, enables far greater dissection and delicacy of technique, and opens further possibilities, indications, and potential procedures.

Rigid Hopkins lens endoscopes with irrigation sheaths are used, most often the 0° of 4 mm diameter and 18 cm length. A small diameter 2.7 mm scope is useful for narrow nostrils and children, but the illumination is a little compromised. For lateral and superior viewing, an 18 cm scope of 30° angle is needed, and for extended transsphenoidal cases scopes of 30 cm length, both 0° and 30° are required. Currently 3-D endoscopes are in their infancy and are still either rather large or of inferior image quality. The irrigation system with pump provides a means of clearing the lens without removing the scope. There are several designs of holding arm available of equal merit, but most important are a low profile attachment and sufficient length to allow positioning away from the surgical access (Fig. 7.1).

A broad freer for initial nasal dissection does little mucosal damage and reduces nasal bleeding. Upcut and downcut punches are used to open the sphenoid, taking bites of mucosa with the bone and a 1 mm upcut to open the pituitary fossa. For complex intracranial endoscopic procedures, the full set of long dissecting instruments should be available. Image guidance is invaluable for the extended and intracranial cases. Given the number of metal instruments required for the procedure, accuracy is better maintained with infrared-based navigation rather than electromagnetic tracking. A long-tipped CUSA and a small disposable Doppler probe are also very useful.

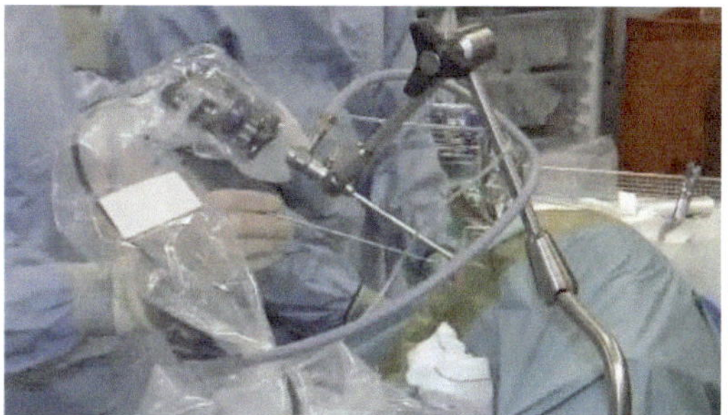

Fig. 7.1 The holding arm with endoscope. The arm is positioned arched out of the way from the surgical field, in order not to interfere with the surgeon's movement

2 ml of 10 % Cocaine HCL solution

2.2 ml of 1 % Sodium Bicarbonate solution

1 ml of 1:1000 Adrenaline solution (1 mg/ml)

Made up to 10 ml with 0.9 % NaCl

Fig. 7.2 Recipe for Moffat's solution

7.7 Surgical Technique

Here we will describe the surgical approach to suprasellar cystic CPs. Those occurring purely within the pituitary fossa are approached precisely as for adenomas and therefore require no further description [4, 6].

After induction of anesthesia, the patient is positioned with neck extended (nose-to-ceiling position) and the nasal mucosa sprayed with Moffat's solution (Fig. 7.2) [1]. A lumbar drain is inserted (as long as the ventricles are not

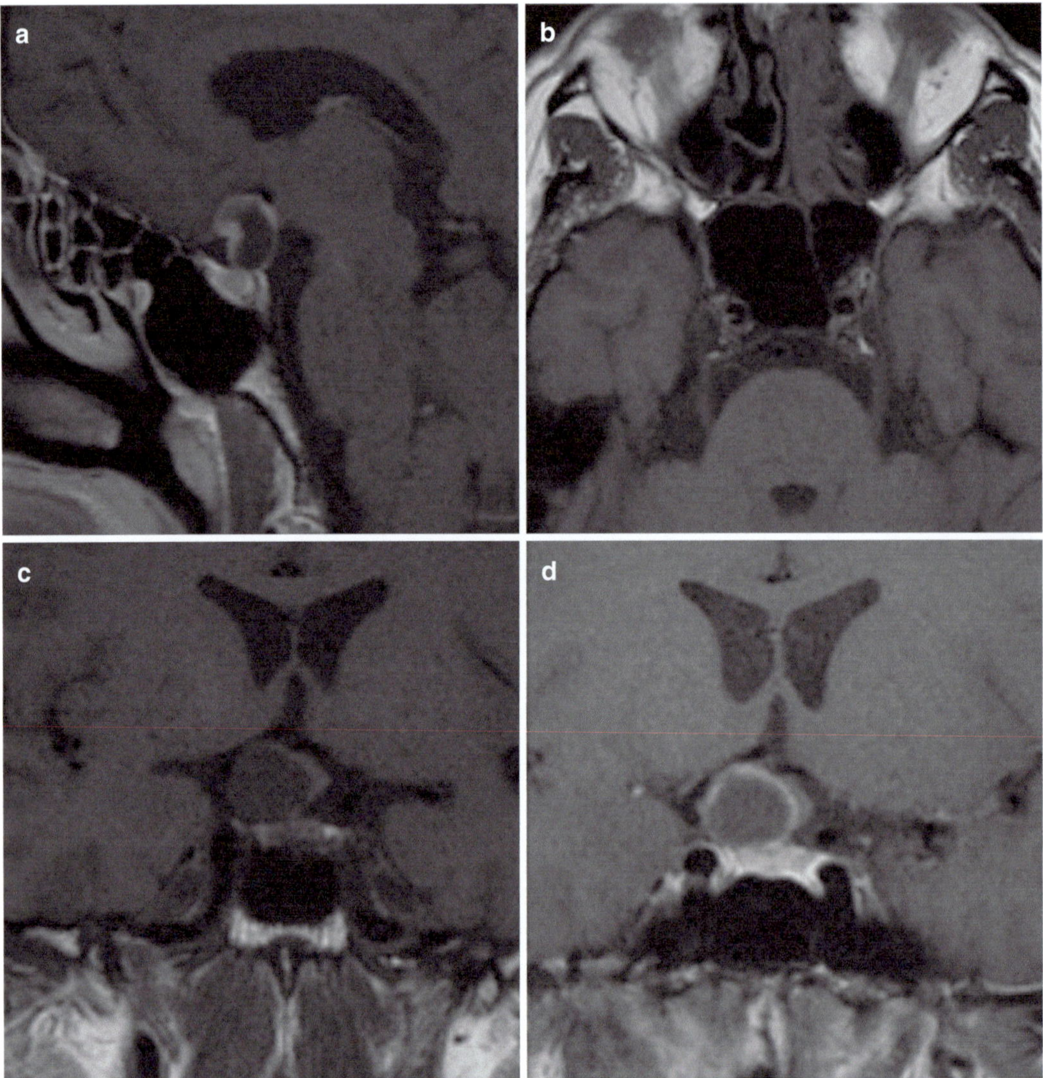

Fig. 7.3 (**a**) Sagittal post-contrast T1-weighted images showing a very well-pneumatized sphenoid sinus, (**b**) axial T1-weighted images showing the sphenoid septum that deviates to the left leading straight to the internal carotid artery, (**c**, **d**) coronal with and without contrast T1-weighted images showing the superiorly displaced chiasm and deviated stalk

obstructed) and intravenous antibiotics and hydrocortisone administered.

The images are assessed for degree of sphenoid pneumatization; the pattern of sphenoid septations; the position of optic nerves, chiasm, and pituitary stalk; and vessel position and encasement (Fig. 7.3).

A semi-sitting position is used to keep the operative field clear, but excessive head elevation is avoided. The head is turned to the right so that surgeon and patient face each other in a "conversational" attitude. The video monitor is positioned squarely over the patient's head with the navigation on the right of the patient (Fig. 7.4).

The septal flap is harvested first, based on the nasal septal branch of the sphenopalatine artery that crosses just above the choana. The septal mucosa is incised vertically just beyond the colu-

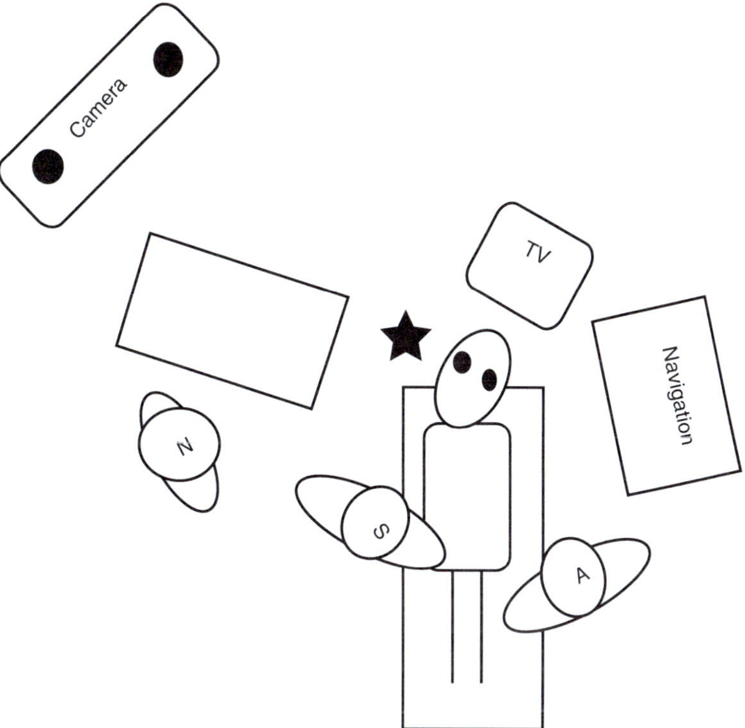

Fig. 7.4 Theater setup: surgeon (*S*) on the patient's right with endoscope monitor (*TV*) above the patient's head and navigation reference frame (*star*) and camera to the right; nurse (*N*); assistant (*A*)

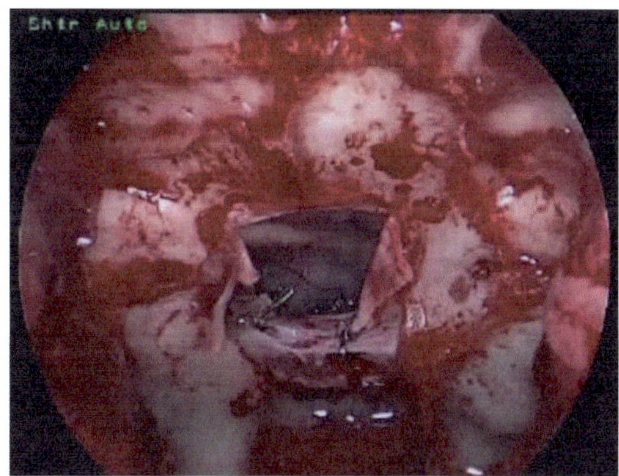

Fig. 7.5 Intraoperative image showing "I" shape of the dural opening; ligaclips are positioned at the level of the intercavernous sinus in order to control the venous bleeding. The two "doors" of dura are folded out opening the access to the suprasellar area

mellar strut and a "lollipop"-shaped flap harvested and turned down into the pharynx [16, 19, 24]. A binasal approach is used, compressing rather than removing the middle turbinate. The whole anterior wall of the sphenoid is removed, with posterior ethmoids as necessary and all septa. The mucosa of the posterior 1/3 of the nasal septum is also resected [4, 14, 13, 32]. The extent of bone removal from fossa and skull base is tailored to the individual pathology with the navigation system. The dura is opened in a capital "I" incision, across the diaphragma sellae and intercavernous sinus. The dura is thereby loose enough to control the sinus with ligaclips. The two "doors" of dura may then be folded out and the arachnoid opened (Figs. 7.5 and 7.6).

On dividing the arachnoid, the position of the optic nerves is established, by deflating the cyst if necessary. The capsule is cleared of crossing vessels and dissected from the diaphragma sellae and stalk. The inferior part of the capsule is mobilized and grasped with cup forceps. Gentle traction is used and the further attachments divided. The central capsule is then truncated and any solid component reduced with the ultrasonic aspirator. Dissection of the deeper component can then be attempted. The main determinant of whether the tumor can be completely removed or not is the degree of adhesion

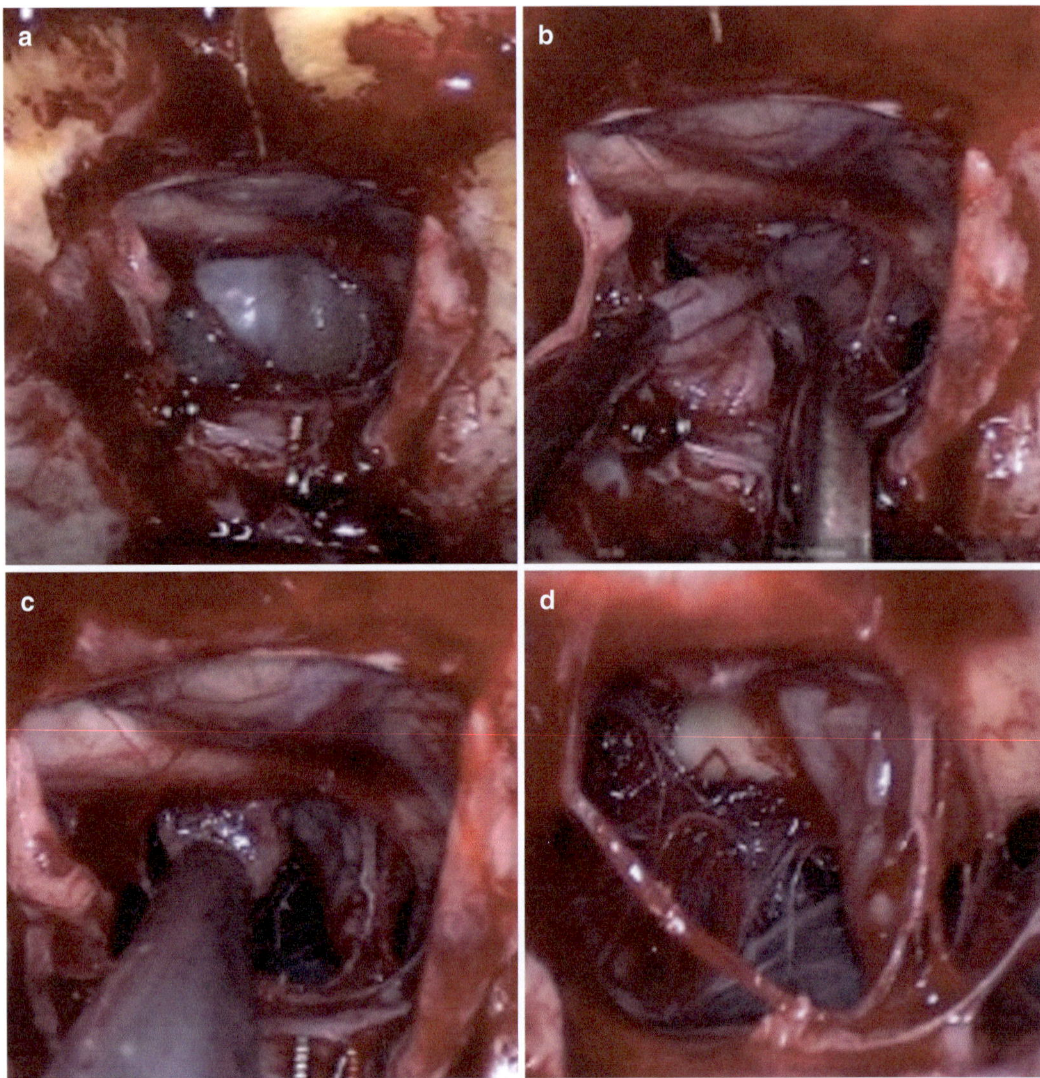

Fig. 7.6 Intraoperative image showing (**a**) the exposure of the tumor capsule, (**b**) truncating the capsule, (**c**) CUSA aspiration of the last fragment adherent to the chiasm, (**d**) final view after tumor removal

to the hypothalamus. If the capsule separates readily, then a complete removal should be possible without significant complications. If however the capsule is adherent, dissection is likely to cause neurologic deficit. Preservation of the pituitary stalk should always be attempted though in adults not at the expense of otherwise complete resection.

Regarding closure a pedicled mucosal flap is the most essential component. For best adhesion this flap should have direct contact with the bone and dural defect margins and is secured in place by spots of glue. Free fat grafts covering all edges are placed and held by sponge and ribbon gauze soaked in bismuth iodine paste.

7.8 Postoperative Management

The lumbar drain outlet height is adjusted to maintain flow at a maximum of 10 ml/h. Free drainage is continued for 5 days and the drain clamped for 24 h and removed after postural testing for a leak. The fluid balance, urine specific gravity, and serum sodium are monitored 2 hourly and DI treated with DDAVP as required. Hydrocortisone 20 mg tds is always prescribed and a 9 a.m. cortisol performed on day 3. Other hormonal assays are performed in the outpatient setting at 3–4 weeks.

7.9 Results

In the neurosurgical literature contemporary series of transcranial craniopharyngioma surgery reveals a 10-year recurrence-free survival rate of 74–81 % for gross total resection, 41–42 % for partial removal, and 83–90 % after surgery and radiotherapy [22]. A meta-analysis of the complications in CP treatment revealed new neurologic deficits in 5.1 % of patients undergoing GTR and in 2.2 % of patients undergoing fractionated radiotherapy (fXRT) or SRS alone. On multivariate analysis, GTR conferred a significant increase in the risk of neurologic deficits compared to STR + XRT. The overall rate of new endocrinopathy for all patients undergoing surgical resection of their mass was 37 %. Patients receiving GTR had over 2.5 times the rate of developing at least one endocrinopathy compared to patients receiving STR alone or STR + XRT [31]. Vascular injury was an uncommon complication of CP surgery, occurring in just two cases. Visual decline was more frequent in patient undergoing fXRT or SRS than surgery (8.5 % vs. 3.7 %, respectively) [31]. Complication rates are significantly lower for surgical teams with larger volume series. The main determinant of quality of life was found to be hypothalamic dysfunction; therefore hypothalamic-pituitary and optic nerve function preservation should be the major aims in planning the best treatment strategy [26].

In a purely endoscopic series of 64 CPs treated by the Pittsburgh group, GTR was achieved in 37.5 % of the patients. Of the 40 patients who had presented with pituitary insufficiency, pituitary function remained unchanged in 50 %, worsened in 30 %, and improved in 20 %. Approximately half of the patients suffered from postop DI. With regard to visual outcome, out of the 44 patients who had preoperative visual deficit, this improved or normalized after surgery in 86 %, remained unchanged in 5, and was transiently worse in 1. No permanent visual deterioration occurred. CSF leak was described in 23 %. No operative mortality was reported [7, 24]. The Tokyo group achieved GTR in 77.8 % of patients, STR in 18.9 %, and partial removal in 3.3 %. Postoperative hormonal disturbances were the main reported complication: 66 % of patients with normal preoperative function or partial anterior pituitary loss developed some degree of hormonal deficiencies; new DI was reported in half of the patients. Visual symptoms improved in 90.2 %. The early postoperative mortality rate was 2.2 %. CSF leakage occurred in 11 patients (5 required surgical repair) [32].

An extensive review of the literature comparing the benefits and limitations of the various approaches showed that of 3470 patients, the endoscopic cohort had a significantly greater rate of GTR (66.9 % vs. 48.3 %; $P<0.003$) and improved visual outcome (56.2 % vs. 33.1 %; $P<0.003$) compared with the open transcranial cohort. The transcranial cases carried a significantly greater rate of permanent DI, but a lower rate of new hypopituitarism compared with the transsphenoidal. The rate of CSF leakage was greater in the endoscopic (18.4 %) than in the transcranial group (2.6 %; $P<0.003$), but the transcranial group had a greater rate of seizure (8.5 % vs. 0 % in the transsphenoidal group, $P<0.003$). Hemiparesis/stroke occurred in 2.9 % of the transcranial patient, and there was also a significantly greater rate of wound or bone flap infection, but no significant difference in the rate of meningitis between groups. There was a lower rate of recurrence in the transsphenoidal cohort compared with the open cohort ($P<0.003$) [23].

7.10 Adjuvant Therapies

Even with GTR, disease-free survival is increased with radiotherapy, but there are still complications associated with radiotherapy. For known STR and observed recurrence during follow-up, radiotherapy is mandated, given via IMRT or proton beam therapy for children. Gamma knife radiotherapy may be useful but only for residual or recurrent tumor distant from the optic nerves and chiasm.

Several chemicals have been used for intracystic chemotherapy for recurrence. First reported by Leksell and Liden in 1952, beta-emitting sources, such as phosphorus-32 (32P), yttrium-90, and rhenium-186, have been tried with variable results. With 32P overall progression-free survival of 72 % and 45 % at 24 and 60 months, respectively, has been reported. 32P however does not halt the development of new cysts or the progression of solid parts [20]. Overall complete or partial cyst resolution is described in 71–88 % of cases [26]. One of the main concerns with intracystic chemotherapy is toxic effect due to subarachnoid leakage: visual and hearing loss, peritumoral edema, hypothalamic dysfunction, cerebral ischemia, hemiparesis, progressive panhypopituitarism, and death have been reported [12, 30]. The latest agent under assessment is interferon-α. This has established efficacy against squamous cell carcinoma (which shares the same embryological origin as CP) and is many times less neurotoxic than the other agents described [11, 28].

References

1. Benjamin E, Wong DK, Choa D (2004) 'Moffett's' solution: a review of the evidence and scientific basis for the topical preparation of the nose. Clin Otolaryngol Allied Sci 29(6):582–587. doi:10.1111/j.1365-2273.2004.00894.x
2. Bunin GR, Surawicz TS, Witman PA, Preston-Martin S, Davis F, Bruner JM (1997) The descriptive epidemiology of craniopharyngioma. Neurosurg Focus 3(6), e1
3. Cappabianca P, Cavallo LM (2012) The evolving role of the transsphenoidal route in the management of craniopharyngiomas. World Neurosurg 77(2):273–274. doi:10.1016/j.wneu.2011.08.040
4. Cappabianca P, Cavallo LM, de Divitiis O, Solari D, Esposito F, Colao A (2008) Endoscopic pituitary surgery. Pituitary 11(4):385–390. doi:10.1007/s11102-008-0087-5
5. Cavallo LM, Cappabianca P (2014) Craniopharyngiomas: infradiaphragmatic and supradiaphragmatic type and their management in modern times. World Neurosurg 81(5–6):683–684. doi:10.1016/j.wneu.2013.03.057
6. Cavallo LM, de Divitiis O, Aydin S, Messina A, Esposito F, Iaconetta G, Talat K, Cappabianca P, Tschabitscher M (2007) Extended endoscopic endonasal transsphenoidal approach to the suprasellar area: anatomic considerations – part 1. Neurosurgery 61(3 Suppl):24–33. doi:10.1227/01.neu.0000289708.49684.47; discussion 33–24
7. Cavallo LM, Frank G, Cappabianca P, Solari D, Mazzatenta D, Villa A, Zoli M, D'Enza AI, Esposito F, Pasquini E (2014) The endoscopic endonasal approach for the management of craniopharyngiomas: a series of 103 patients. J Neurosurg 121(1):100–113. doi:10.3171/2014.3.JNS131521
8. Cavallo LM, Prevedello D, Esposito F, Laws ER Jr, Dusick JR, Messina A, Jane JA Jr, Kelly DF, Cappabianca P (2008) The role of the endoscope in the transsphenoidal management of cystic lesions of the sellar region. Neurosurg Rev 31(1):55–64. doi:10.1007/s10143-007-0098-0; discussion 64
9. Cavallo LM, Prevedello DM, Solari D, Gardner PA, Esposito F, Snyderman CH, Carrau RL, Kassam AB, Cappabianca P (2009) Extended endoscopic endonasal transsphenoidal approach for residual or recurrent craniopharyngiomas. J Neurosurg 111(3):578–589. doi:10.3171/2009.2.JNS081026
10. Cohen M, Bartels U, Branson H, Kulkarni AV, Hamilton J (2013) Trends in treatment and outcomes of pediatric craniopharyngioma, 1975–2011. Neuro Oncol 15(6):767–774. doi:10.1093/neuonc/not026
11. Dastoli PA, Nicacio JM, Silva NS, Capellano AM, Toledo SR, Ierardi D, Cavalheiro S (2011) Cystic craniopharyngioma: intratumoral chemotherapy with alpha interferon. Arq Neuropsiquiatr 69(1):50–55
12. Fraioli MF, Moschettoni L, Catena E, Fraioli C (2010) Cystic craniopharyngioma: trans-sphenoidal surgery and intra-cystic apposition of "bleomycin wax". Acta Neurochir 152(2):293–296. doi:10.1007/s00701-009-0320-7
13. Frank F, Fabrizi AP, Frank G, Fioravanti A (1995) Stereotactic management of craniopharyngiomas. Stereotact Funct Neurosurg 65(1–4):176–183
14. Gardner PA, Kassam AB, Snyderman CH, Carrau RL, Mintz AH, Grahovac S, Stefko S (2008) Outcomes following endoscopic, expanded endonasal resection of suprasellar craniopharyngiomas: a case series. J Neurosurg 109(1):6–16. doi:10.3171/JNS/2008/109/7/0006
15. Gardner PA, Prevedello DM, Kassam AB, Snyderman CH, Carrau RL, Mintz AH (2008) The evolution of the endonasal approach for craniopharyngiomas. J Neurosurg 108(5):1043–1047. doi:10.3171/JNS/2008/108/5/1043
16. Hadad G, Bassagasteguy L, Carrau RL, Mataza JC, Kassam A, Snyderman CH, Mintz A (2006) A novel reconstructive technique after endoscopic expanded endonasal approaches: vascular pedicle nasoseptal flap. Laryngoscope 116(10):1882–1886. doi:10.1097/01.mlg.0000234933.37779.e4

17. Hoffman HJ, De Silva M, Humphreys RP, Drake JM, Smith ML, Blaser SI (1992) Aggressive surgical management of craniopharyngiomas in children. J Neurosurg 76(1):47–52. doi:10.3171/jns.1992.76.1.0047
18. Kassam AB, Gardner PA, Snyderman CH, Carrau RL, Mintz AH, Prevedello DM (2008) Expanded endonasal approach, a fully endoscopic transnasal approach for the resection of midline suprasellar craniopharyngiomas: a new classification based on the infundibulum. J Neurosurg 108(4):715–728. doi:10.3171/JNS/2008/108/4/0715
19. Kassam AB, Thomas A, Carrau RL, Snyderman CH, Vescan A, Prevedello D, Mintz A, Gardner P (2008) Endoscopic reconstruction of the cranial base using a pedicled nasoseptal flap. Neurosurgery 63 (1 Suppl 1): ONS44-52. doi:10.1227/01.neu.0000335010.53122.75; discussion ONS52-43
20. Kickingereder P, Maarouf M, El Majdoub F, Fuetsch M, Lehrke R, Wirths J, Luyken K, Schomaecker K, Treuer H, Voges J, Sturm V (2012) Intracavitary brachytherapy using stereotactically applied phosphorus-32 colloid for treatment of cystic craniopharyngiomas in 53 patients. J Neurooncol 109(2):365–374. doi:10.1007/s11060-012-0902-8
21. Kim SK, Kim YH, Park CK, Kim DG, Jung HW (2014) Extended endoscopic endonasal approach for recurrent or residual adult craniopharyngiomas. Acta Neurochir 156(10):1917–1922. doi:10.1007/s00701-014-2150-5
22. Komotar RJ, Roguski M, Bruce JN (2009) Surgical management of craniopharyngiomas. J Neurooncol 92(3):283–296. doi:10.1007/s11060-009-9841-4
23. Komotar RJ, Starke RM, Raper DM, Anand VK, Schwartz TH (2012) Endoscopic endonasal compared with microscopic transsphenoidal and open transcranial resection of craniopharyngiomas. World Neurosurg 77(2):329–341. doi:10.1016/j.wneu.2011.07.011
24. Koutourousiou M, Gardner PA, Fernandez-Miranda JC, Tyler-Kabara EC, Wang EW, Snyderman CH (2013) Endoscopic endonasal surgery for craniopharyngiomas: surgical outcome in 64 patients. J Neurosurg 119(5):1194–1207. doi:10.3171/2013.6.JNS122259
25. Miller DC (1994) Pathology of craniopharyngiomas: clinical import of pathological findings. Pediatr Neurosurg 21(Suppl 1):11–17
26. Mortini P, Gagliardi F, Boari N, Losa M (2013) Surgical strategies and modern therapeutic options in the treatment of craniopharyngiomas. Crit Rev Oncol Hematol 88(3):514–529. doi:10.1016/j.critrevonc.2013.07.013
27. Pettorini BL, Frassanito P, Caldarelli M, Tamburrini G, Massimi L, Di Rocco C (2010) Molecular pathogenesis of craniopharyngioma: switching from a surgical approach to a biological one. Neurosurg Focus 28(4), E1. doi:10.3171/2010.1.FOCUS09300
28. Pettorini BL, Inzitari R, Massimi L, Tamburrini G, Caldarelli M, Fanali C, Cabras T, Messana I, Castagnola M, Di Rocco C (2010) The role of inflammation in the genesis of the cystic component of craniopharyngiomas. Childs Nervous Syst 26(12): 1779–1784. doi:10.1007/s00381-010-1245-4
29. Shi XE, Wu B, Fan T, Zhou ZQ, Zhang YL (2008) Craniopharyngioma: surgical experience of 309 cases in China. Clin Neurol Neurosurg 110(2):151–159. doi:10.1016/j.clineuro.2007.10.013
30. Steinbok P, Hukin J (2010) Intracystic treatments for craniopharyngioma. Neurosurg Focus 28(4), E13. doi:10.3171/2010.1.FOCUS09315
31. Sughrue ME, Yang I, Kane AJ, Fang S, Clark AJ, Aranda D, Barani IJ, Parsa AT (2011) Endocrinologic, neurologic, and visual morbidity after treatment for craniopharyngioma. J Neurooncol 101(3):463–476. doi:10.1007/s11060-010-0265-y
32. Yamada S, Fukuhara N, Oyama K, Takeshita A, Takeuchi Y, Ito J, Inoshita N (2010) Surgical outcome in 90 patients with craniopharyngioma: an evaluation of transsphenoidal surgery. World Neurosurg 74(2–3):320–330. doi:10.1016/j.wneu.2010.06.014
33. Yang I, Sughrue ME, Rutkowski MJ, Kaur R, Ivan ME, Aranda D, Barani IJ, Parsa AT (2010) Craniopharyngioma: a comparison of tumor control with various treatment strategies. Neurosurg Focus 28(4), E5. doi:10.3171/2010.1.FOCUS09307
34. Yoshimoto M, Bayani J, Nuin PA, Silva NS, Cavalheiro S, Stavale JN, Andrade JA, Zielenska M, Squire JA, de Toledo SR (2006) Metaphase and array comparative genomic hybridization: unique copy number changes and gene amplification of medulloblastomas in South America. Cancer Genet Cytogenet 170(1):40–47. doi:10.1016/j.cancergencyto.2006.05.009
35. Zada G, Lin N, Ojerholm E, Ramkissoon S, Laws ER (2010) Craniopharyngioma and other cystic epithelial lesions of the sellar region: a review of clinical, imaging, and histopathological relationships. Neurosurg Focus 28(4), E4. doi:10.3171/2010.2.FOCUS09318
36. Zheng J, Fang Y, Cai BW, Zhang H, Liu W, Wu B, Xu JG, You C (2014) Intracystic bleomycin for cystic craniopharyngiomas in children. Cochrane Database Syst Rev (9):CD008890. doi:10.1002/14651858.CD008890.pub3
37. Zygourakis CC, Kaur G, Kunwar S, McDermott MW, Madden M, Oh T, Parsa AT (2014) Modern treatment of 84 newly diagnosed craniopharyngiomas. J Clin Neurosci 21(9):1558–1566. doi:10.1016/j.jocn.2014.03.005

Endoventricular Cystic Craniopharyngiomas

8

Michelangelo Gangemi

8.1 Introduction

Craniopharyngiomas are benign tumors that correspond histologically to WHO grade I. The incidence rate is 1.3 per million person-years without any sex preponderance [1].

These tumors may be predominantly cystic (with no significant solid portion), mixed (cystic and solid components), or predominantly solid [2].

On neuroimaging studies, craniopharyngioma usually presents as a cystic, calcified tumor in the suprasellar region. A cystic component can be present in up to 90 % of craniopharyngiomas [2–4].

When cystic craniopharyngioma grows up in the retrochiasmatic space, it can involve the third ventricle area [5, 6].

The clinical presentation of craniopharyngiomas involving the third ventricle includes symptoms of visual disturbance, endocrinologic disturbances, cognitive impairment, and increased intracranial pressure due to obstructive hydrocephalus.

In comparison with the high prevalence of visual and endocrine disturbances usually observed in suprasellar craniopharyngiomas (between 70 and 90 % of cases, both in adults and children) and their low prevalence of psychiatric symptoms (less than 15 %) [7, 8], intraventricular craniopharyngiomas have a much lower frequency of endocrine (27 %) and visual (28 %) disturbances and a higher presence of psychiatric abnormalities (40 %) and memory dysfunction (33 %). These differences must be related to the different positions of the tumor, which is located above the suprasellar area and involves the third ventricle floor, including the mammillary bodies, and the hypothalamus [6].

Management of craniopharyngiomas with intraventricular extension is problematic and often requires multimodal protocols. Total removal still remains the gold standard in the treatment of primary craniopharyngiomas. Excellent results have been achieved in skilled and experienced hands [3, 9].

However, the goal of complete removal can rarely be achieved without significant endocrine and neuropsychological sequelae because of the intimate relationship with delicate neurovascular structures (hypothalamus, chiasm, optic nerves, carotid arteries, and their main branches or perforating vessels). In addition the possible presence of ependymal invasion and the absence of clear-cut cleavage often suggest a less aggressive attitude. This is particularly true in recurrent cases and in very young or very old patients, who are more prone to devastating intra- and postoperative complications.

In case of subtotal or partial resections, using postoperative radiotherapy, it's possible to gain

M. Gangemi, MD
Division of Neurosurgery, Department of Neurosciences and Reproductive and Odontostomatological Sciences, Università degli Studi di Napoli Federico II, Naples, Italy
e-mail: michelangelo.gangemi@unina.it

P. Cappabianca et al. (eds.), *Midline Skull Base Surgery*, DOI 10.1007/978-3-319-21533-4_8

almost the same low rate of recurrence as in case of total resection [10]. This observation has led to the development of a policy of less surgical aggressiveness integrated in multimodal management [11, 12].

Pascual et al. [6] proposed a new topographical classification for craniopharyngiomas involving the third ventricle area. It is possible to distinguish among four theoretical relationships between the tumor and the third ventricle floor that should be considered preoperatively:

1. *Pseudo-intraventricular craniopharyngioma*: suprasellar tumor pushing the intact third ventricle floor upward
2. *Secondarily intraventricular craniopharyngioma*: suprasellar mass breaking through the third ventricle floor and invading the third ventricle cavity
3. *Non-strictly IVC*: intrinsic third ventricle floor tumor expanding within the cavity and leaving an opening in it
4. *Strictly IVC*: intraventricular mass completely located within the third ventricle cavity and with the intact floor lying below its inferior surface

The development of various neuroendoscopic surgical instruments has offered more options for endoscopic procedures in the treatment of intraventricular tumors.

In this contest transventricular neuroendoscopy has shown a great versatility playing an important part in the management of these tumors, especially for those lesions with a predominant cystic component and those growing within the third ventricle.

It has been used:

1. To fenestrate cystic tumors into the ventricular system or in the subarachnoid space (ventriculocystostomy or cystocisternostomy) [12, 13]
2. As a foraminoplasty to restore cerebrospinal fluid flow in case of hydrocephalus [14]
3. For intracavitary chemotherapy
4. To achieve gross total resection [15, 16]
5. As a first step of combined procedure [12, 13, 16, 17]

8.2 Marsupialization of the Cyst

In predominantly cystic intraventricular craniopharyngiomas, when mass effect rather than infiltration is responsible for symptoms, cyst drainage is a possible choice, especially in recurrences and for elderly patients. In this subgroup of tumors, microsurgery is burdened with a higher rate of incomplete removal and operative mortality [3, 12, 18].

Several techniques have been proposed to control the cyst volume.

The marsupialization of the cyst into the ventricles (cystoventriculostomy) allows continuous dilution of the cyst's fluid and resorption through CSF pathways [2].

A prerequisite for endoscopic fenestration is the proximity of the cystic portion of the tumor to the ventricular system.

The wide marsupialization of the cyst in both ventricles and basal cisterns, i.e., cistoventriculocisternostomy, is the procedure of choice, because it has been proven to be safe, effective, and easily repeatable in the long-term control of tumor [12].

The procedure is performed in four basic steps (Figs. 8.1 and 8.2) [19]:

1. Standard precoronal parasagittal approach to the lateral ventricle
2. Identification and puncture of the cyst's dome and complete drainage of its content by washing with Ringer's solution
3. Coagulation and resection as extensive as possible of the cyst's dome, cavity exploration, and biopsy
4. Perforation of the cyst's fundus into basal cisterns

The neuroendoscopic approach to cystic craniopharyngiomas allows control of mass effect, preservation of function, and integration with other therapeutic means (microsurgery, radiation therapy, radiosurgery).

8.3 Foraminoplasty

With the technique of foraminoplasty, a stent is placed endoscopically into the foramen of Monro with the purpose of CSF diversion, when intra-

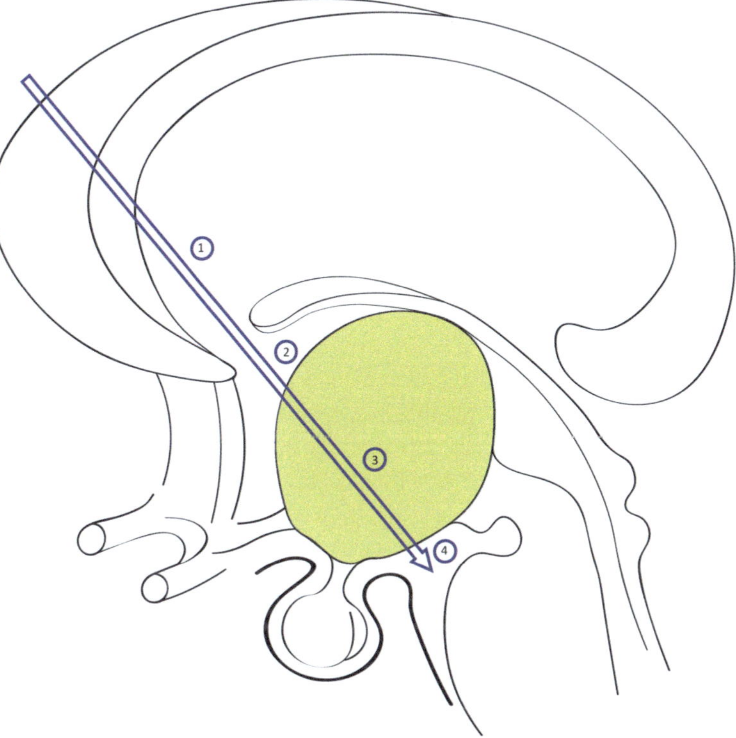

Fig. 8.1 Illustration of the marsupialization of the cyst: the *arrow* represents the trajectory of the endoscope during the surgical procedure performed in four basic steps: *1* approach to the ventricular system through a precoronal burr hole; *2* identification and puncture of the cyst's dome and complete drainage of its content; *3* exploration of the cystic cavity and biopsy of its walls; *4* perforation of the cyst's fundus into basal cisterns

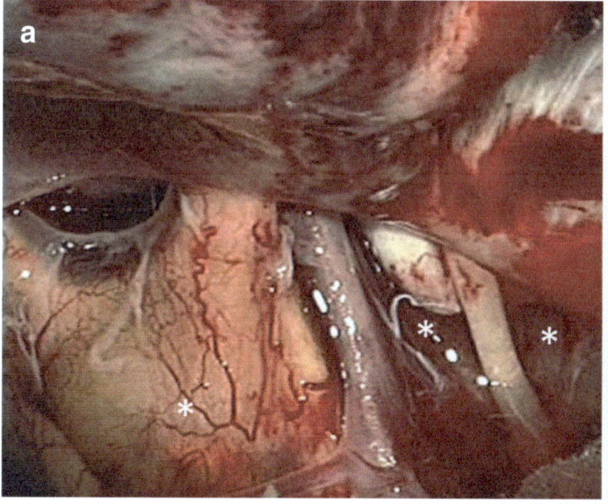

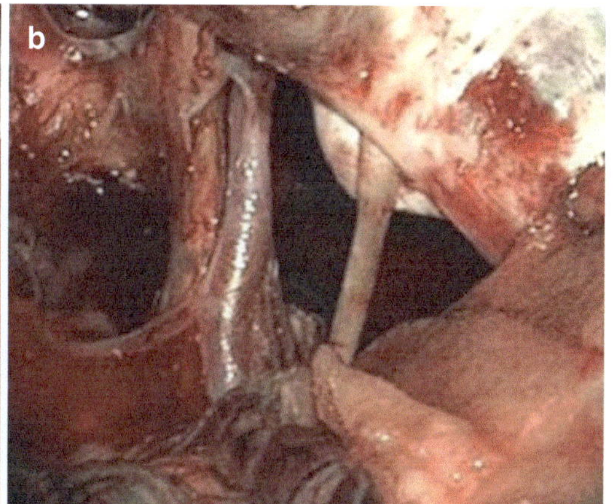

Fig. 8.2 Intraoperative images show the surgical field at the beginning (**a**) and at the end (**b**) of the procedure. The *asterisks* show the surgical corridors used in order to perform the complete removal of the tumor: the optic-oculomotor corridor to obtain the debulking of the tumor mass, the opening of the lamina terminalis to remove the retrosellar and intraventricular components, and the opening of the arachnoid of the ambient cistern medially to the tentorial incisura to remove the tumor in the posterior fossa

ventricular craniopharyngiomas cause obstructive hydrocephalus.

The endoscopic foraminoplasty technique should be considered as an optional treatment for patients who present with obstructive hydrocephalus caused by a tumor that occludes both foramina of Monro, when shunt placement or endoscopic third ventriculostomy is not practicable [14]. Depending on tumor size, this procedure could require a partial resection of the tumor to provide sufficient space for endoscopic stent placement and an endoscopic septostomy [20].

8.4 Intracavitary Chemotherapy

Several adjuvant therapies for cystic craniopharyngiomas require the placement of Ommaya reservoir systems [11]. Ommaya reservoirs could make it easier to reduce cystic volume prior to radiotherapy as the final procedure and may also be used for instillation of chemotherapeutic agents and for repeated aspirations, making the achievement of cystic control more likely.

The catheter can be safely placed under endoscopic guidance with a parallel insertion technique using a transparent ventricular sheath for the endoscope through one burr hole [21].

The burr hole is made in the right frontal region on the pupillary line anterior to the coronal suture and then the transparent peel-away sheath is inserted into the right lateral ventricle directed to the right foramen of Monro. The neuroendoscopic system is introduced into the peel-away sheath while the Ommaya reservoir catheter with a stylet is inserted running over the outer surface of the sheath itself. Its transparency allows to follow the catheter insertion under endoscopic visual control in the sheath. The catheter is introduced in the right lateral ventricle and then into the cystic tumor under endoscopic view. The catheter is then connected to a subcutaneous Ommaya reservoir; the sheath is peeled away, leaving the endoscope in the lateral ventricle, in order to enable the observation of the tip of the catheter even after sheath removal.

The advantages of using endoscopic guidance are safe fenestration of the cystic capsule under visual control, conversion of multicystic craniopharyngiomas in uniloculated cyst, avoidance of the need for multiple catheters, and the possibility of performing other neuroendoscopic procedures. Large fenestration of the cyst walls should not be performed, in order to avoid leak of neurotoxic drugs into the CSF pathways.

Nicolato et al. [22] recommend performing positive contrast CT cystography prior to administration of intracavitary drugs to exclude leakage of the contrast agent from the cyst cavity.

8.5 Endoscopic Gross Total Removal

Only a minority of small (<2 cm), cystic, purely intraventricular, noncalcified craniopharyngiomas are amenable to endoscopic resection [19, 23, 24].

Often, the solid portions arise outside the third ventricle, usually in the suprasellar area, and show an intimate relationship with the hypothalamus, optic pathway, major vessels, and perforating vessels of the cranial base; they cannot be removed without the risk of uncontrollable damage to these neurovascular structures [16]. The solid remnants, in these cases, should be later considered for microsurgery or radiation therapy [12, 14, 22].

In literature, the experience is limited and the results do not always seem to be satisfactory [15].

8.6 Combined Procedures

Marsupialization of the cystic portion of the craniopharyngiomas is often followed by additional treatments on the solid parts [11, 13, 18, 22].

Endoscopic cyst decompression and resolution of hydrocephalus before craniopharyngioma removal usually permit a delayed intervention in better clinical and technical conditions [16]. The endoscopic procedure can be performed in emergency in patients with severe and progressive visual loss or hypothalamic disorders. In most cases symptoms and signs improve and a reduced risk of the subsequent surgical tumor removal can also be anticipated, with less surgical trauma on suffering structures.

Following the collapse of the cyst, the craniopharyngioma is retracted from the brain tissue and the subsequent removal of the solid portion is technically facilitated. Thereafter the tumor can be removed through a basal approach (pterional or subfrontal) alone, often avoiding an additional superior approach (transcallosal or transcortical transventricular) to remove the intraventricular part [16].

A combined technique – endoscopic drainage followed by microsurgical removal – is an effective approach to the removal of giant cystic craniopharyngiomas in cases in which the cystic compartment bulges within the ventricular cavities and may avoid multiple craniotomies [17, 25].

As an example of combined approach, we have described a case of a giant cystic craniopharyngioma with a large extension in the posterior fossa totally removed via a two-step surgical procedure [17]. A wide stoma was performed first in the cystic lesion in the third ventricle and then in the dome bulging of the lesion extending in the posterior fossa, thus obtaining the emptying of a dense fluid content in the ventricular cavities, which was removed by endoscopic aspiration. One week later, a right pterional approach with a wider posterior subtemporal extent was performed and a complete remove of the lesion was achieved.

The combined endoscopic-microsurgical procedure offers some advantages compared to a direct microsurgical approach to the tumor, which is burdened by two main risks: firstly the risk of not being able to perform a complete resection of craniopharyngioma with a single procedure, because of its anteroposterior extent, and secondly the risk of catastrophic consequences due to an acute complete decompression. In this perspective the endoscopic approach becomes functional, reducing the symptoms of intracranial hypertension, shrinking the tumor in size, and loosening the adherences to the close-by anatomical structures making it a more easy radical removal.

Although a total resection at initial presentation is a legitimate therapeutic goal, simple endoscopic cyst fenestration and postoperative fractionated stereotactic radiotherapy are reasonable alternatives in cystic tumors that have significant hypothalamic involvement, compress the visual pathway, or obstruct the CSF flow.

References

1. Bunin GR et al (1997) The descriptive epidemiology of craniopharyngioma. Neurosurg Focus 3(6), e1
2. Spaziante R, de Divitiis E (1997) Drainage techniques for cystic craniopharyngiomas. Neurosurg Q 7: 183–208
3. Fahlbusch R et al (1999) Surgical treatment of craniopharyngiomas: experience with 168 patients. J Neurosurg 90(2):237–250
4. Margetis K, Souweidane MM (2013) Endoscopic treatment of intraventricular cystic tumors. World Neurosurg 79(2 Suppl):S19 e1–11
5. Hoffman HJ et al (1992) Aggressive surgical management of craniopharyngiomas in children. J Neurosurg 76(1):47–52
6. Pascual JM et al (2004) Intraventricular craniopharyngiomas: topographical classification and surgical approach selection based on an extensive overview. Acta Neurochir (Wien) 146(8):785–802
7. Carmel PW (1996) Brain tumors of disordered embryogenesis. In: Youmans JR (ed) Neurological surgery. WB Saunders, Philadelphia, pp 2761–2781
8. Choux M, Lena G, Genitori L (1991) Le craniopharyngiome de l'enfant. Neurochirurgie 37(Suppl 1): 59–64
9. Yasargil MG et al (1990) Total removal of craniopharyngiomas. Approaches and long-term results in 144 patients. J Neurosurg 73(1):3–11
10. Caldarelli M et al (1998) Management of recurrent craniopharyngioma. Acta Neurochir (Wien) 140(5):447–454
11. Barajas MA et al (2002) Multimodal management of craniopharyngiomas: neuroendoscopy, microsurgery, and radiosurgery. J Neurosurg 97(5 Suppl):607–609
12. Delitala A, Brunori A, Chiappetta F (2004) Purely neuroendoscopic transventricular management of cystic craniopharyngiomas. Childs Nerv Syst 20(11–12):858–862
13. Tirakotai W et al (2004) Neuroendoscopic surgery of intracranial cysts in adults. Childs Nerv Syst 20(11–12):842–851
14. Tirakotai W et al (2004) Neuroendoscopic stent procedure in obstructive hydrocephalus due to both foramina of Monro occluding craniopharyngioma: technical note. Surg Neurol 61(3):293–296; discussion 296
15. Abdullah J, Caemaert J (1995) Endoscopic management of craniopharyngiomas: a review of 3 cases. Minim Invasive Neurosurg 38(2):79–84
16. Cinalli G et al (2006) The role of transventricular neuroendoscopy in the management of craniopharyngiomas: three patient reports and review of the literature. J Pediatr Endocrinol Metab 19(Suppl 1): 341–354
17. Gangemi M et al (2009) Combined endoscopic and microsurgical removal of a giant cystic craniopharyngioma in a six-year-old boy. Clin Neurol Neurosurg 111(5):472–476
18. Locatelli D et al (2004) Endoscopic approach for the treatment of relapses in cystic craniopharyngiomas. Childs Nerv Syst 20(11–12):863–867
19. Cappabianca P et al (2008) Application of neuroendoscopy to intraventricular lesions. Neurosurgery 62(Suppl 2):575–597; discussion 597–598

20. Gaab MR, Schroeder HW (1998) Neuroendoscopic approach to intraventricular lesions. J Neurosurg 88(3):496–505
21. Mori R et al (2014) Parallel insertion endoscopic technique for precise catheter placement in cystic craniopharyngiomas. J Neurol Surg A Cent Eur Neurosurg 75(6):442–446
22. Nicolato A et al (2004) Multimodality stereotactic approach to the treatment of cystic craniopharyngiomas. Minim Invasive Neurosurg 47(1):32–40
23. Barber SM, Rangel-Castilla L, Baskin D (2013) Neuroendoscopic resection of intraventricular tumors: a systematic outcomes analysis. Minim Invasive Surg 2013:898753
24. Teo C, Nakaji P (2004) Neuro-oncologic applications of endoscopy. Neurosurg Clin N Am 15(1):89–103
25. Tirakotai W et al (2007) The role of neuroendoscopy in the management of solid or solid-cystic intra- and periventricular tumours. Childs Nerv Syst 23(6):653–658

9 Draining Techniques for Cystic Craniopharyngiomas

Alberto Delitala, Renato Spaziante, Gianluigi Zona, Andrea Brunori, Daniele Marruzzo, and Ilaria Melloni

9.1 Introduction

Microsurgical total removal still remains the gold standard in the treatment of primary craniopharyngiomas with the best long-term prognosis. Excellent results have been achieved in particularly skilled and experienced hands [1, 2]. However, the intimate relationship with delicate neurovascular structures, the frequent absence of clear-cut cleavage, and the biologically benign nature of the tumor often suggest a less aggressive attitude [3]. This is particularly true in recurrent cases and in very young or very old patients, who are more prone to devastating intra- and postoperative complications. Only 10 % of craniopharyngiomas are totally solid, while more than half are purely or predominantly cystic [1, 4, 5]. In such cases, control of mass effect, often caused by enlargement of the cystic component, may represent a suitable alternative to resection and several techniques have been proposed [4–10]. In this chapter we are going to describe two techniques for the treatment of cystic craniopharyngiomas:

1. Cysto-ventriculo-cisternostomy with neuro-endoscopic approach: drainage and wide marsupialization into CSF spaces (cysto-ventriculo-cisternostomy) are achieved to ensure mass effect control, continuous dilution, and reabsorption of the cyst's fluid. We can see that this is a more modern sump drainage [11, 12] in respect to the one performed in the past where the catheter was linked to a reservoir permanently lodged in the subgaleal space.
2. Cystosphenoidostomy (either by microsurgical or endoscopic approach): this technique allows to create a permanent communication between the cyst of the tumor and the sphenoid sinus through a silastic catheter, in order to prevent growth of the cyst due to liquid accumulation and mass effect. The catheter is easily placed through a standard transsphenoidal approach [4, 13, 14].

Electronic supplementary material The online version of this chapter (doi:10.1007/978-3-319-21533-4_9) contains supplementary material, which is available to authorized users.

A. Delitala, MD (✉) • A. Brunori, MD
D. Marruzzo, MD
Division of Neurosurgery, Department of Neurosciences "G.M. Lancisi", San Camillo-Forlanini Hospital, Rome, Italy
e-mail: alberto.delitala@tiscali.it, nchlancisi@gmail.com

R. Spaziante, MD
Department of Neurosurgery, Università degli Studi di Salerno, Salerno, Italy

G. Zona, MD • I. Melloni, MD
Department of Neurosurgery, San Martino University Hospital, Genoa, Italy

P. Cappabianca et al. (eds.), *Midline Skull Base Surgery*, DOI 10.1007/978-3-319-21533-4_9

9.2 Technique of the Cysto-Ventriculo-Cisternostomy

Between December 1996 and December 2010, 15 patients (6 males, 9 females; age range 9–73 years; average 52 years) harboring predominantly cystic craniopharyngiomas underwent neuroendoscopic exploration at our institution. The seven recurrent tumors had previously undergone: microsurgery and sump drainage (1), microsurgery and fractionated radiation therapy (3), and microsurgery alone (3). All tumors had close relationships with the ventricular system and could be classified as type c (9), type d (2), and type f (4) according to Yasargil et al. [2]. In 12 cases the cyst represented >90 % of total neoplasm's volume, while in the remaining patient, it was approximately 60–70 %. Indications for neuroendoscopy can be summarized as follows: age and poor general conditions (6 patients), recurrent tumors (7 patients), and refusal of open surgery (2 patients). All procedures were carried out by means of a 4-mm fiberoptic steerable, flexible endoscope (Codman & Shurtleff) with a single working channel. A freehand technique was used: surgical maneuvers were carried out by means of monopolar cautery, Fogarty catheter (3 French), alligator, and cup microforceps. Draining of the cyst and creation of a cysto-ventriculo-cisternostomy were obtained (patient in the supine position) as follows (Video 9.1):

1. Standard pre-coronal parasagittal burr hole and ventricular puncture by means of a "peel-away" trocar. This catheter is useful for protecting the cortex around the endoscopic tract during endoscopic procedures.
2. Identification and puncture of the cyst's dome and complete drainage of content by aspiration and washing with Ringer's solution (Fig. 9.1a).
3. Cavity exploration, biopsy, coagulation, and resection of the cyst's dome as extensively as possible.

The last steps of the procedure are perforation of the cyst's fundus into the basal cisterns (Fig. 9.1b) and positioning of the transcystic multiholed catheter with ends reaching into the cistern (caudally) and lateral ventricle (rostrally) (Fig. 9.1c). This stenting was devised in an attempt to promote continuous CSF rinsing (circulation) and prevent the cyst's reclosure. The burr hole was sealed with bone wax and the skin closed with separate sutures.

9.2.1 Results and Complications

Complete drainage was achieved in all but one patient, due to an unaccessible pouch separated from the main cavity. The mean surgical time was 126 min. There were no intraoperative complications and even the postoperative course was uneventful: surprisingly no chemical meningitis was observed and transient hyperpyrexia in three cases rapidly subsided. The mean hospital stay was 7 days. During the follow-up period (range 12–72 months; average 40 months), we observed two recurrences of the cystic portion. Both patients underwent successful repeat neuroendoscopy procedure. One died postoperatively due to unrelated causes (pulmonary embolism) while neuroradiologic examinations had shown complete drainage of the cyst. In the remaining patients, follow-up examinations have demonstrated persistent drainage and resolution of symptoms (Fig. 9.2). One patient (20-year-old man) underwent microsurgical removal of an enlarging solid nodule 9 months after endoscopy (Fig. 9.3).

9.3 Technique of Cystosphenoidostomy

Between January 1985 and June 2012, 21 patients (5 pediatric patients, age range 6–17 years, mean 11 years; 16 adults, age range 35–74 years, mean 59 years) underwent cystosphenoidostomy as surgical treatment for mainly cystic sellar craniopharyngioma. Six patients had preoperative diabetes insipidus requiring medical therapy, 16 patients had some degree of endocrine disturbance requiring hormonal substitution, and all patients had visual field defects that ranged from minimum peripheral deficits to

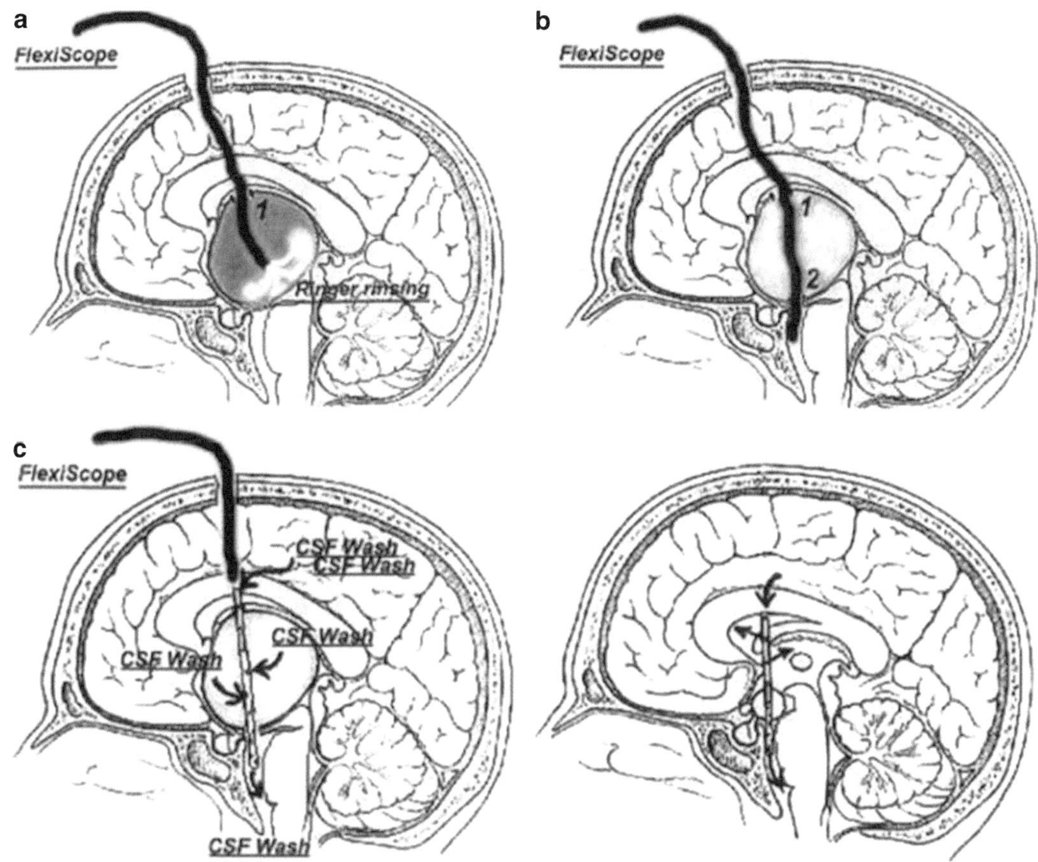

Fig. 9.1 (**a–c**) Purely neuroendoscopic, transventricular technique. (**a**) Puncture of the cyst's dome and complete drainage of content by aspiration and washing with Ringer's solution. (**b**) Perforation of the cyst's fundus into the basal cisterns. (**c**) "Stenting" of the cavity and its progressive shrinkage with time (Reproduced with permission from Delitala et al. [15])

monocular blindness in one case. All tumors had an intrasellar component, with sellar enlargement and supradiaphragmatic extension. In all cases the cyst was at least partially within the pituitary fossa. Indications for cystosphenoidostomy were recurrent tumor (6 cases), open surgery refusal (3 cases), unlikeliness of total removal basing on neuroradiological appearance (7 cases), and high anesthesiological risk in case of craniotomy (5 cases). No patients had preoperative hydrocephalus. Recurrent tumors had previously been treated with microsurgical technique either by a transcranial approach (2 cases) or a transsphenoidal approach (4 cases); 3 patients had undergone to radiotherapy as an adjuvant treatment.

Surgical technique consisted in a microsurgical or purely endoscopic transsphenoidal approach. A wide opening in the sellar floor was performed in order to expose the cyst wall. The cyst wall was incised, the contents were suctioned, and cyst walls were dissected as far as possible, taking care in avoiding any lesion to the arachnoid and cerebrospinal fluid leakage. The permanent communication with the sphenoid sinus was established through a self-securing X- or H-shaped silastic catheter, which was positioned over the sellar floor so that two arms lied within the pituitary fossa and the other two in the sphenoid sinus (Fig.9.4).

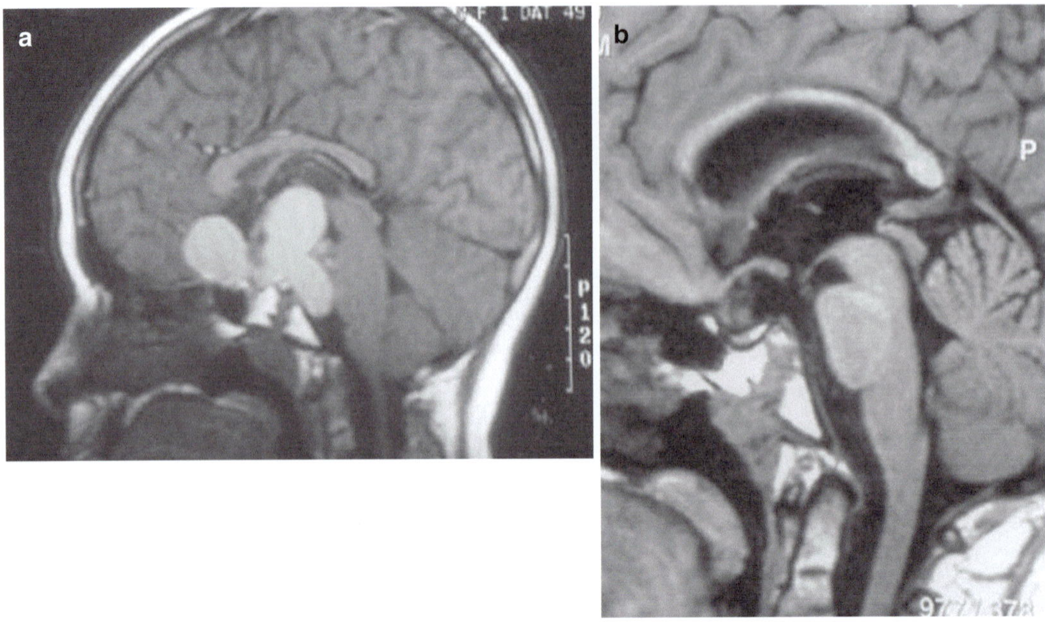

Fig. 9.2 (**a**, **b**) Patient 1: 9-year-old girl with a giant cyst recurrent after microsurgery, external radiotherapy, and sump drainage. (**a**) Pre-neuroendoscopy and (**b**) post-neuroendoscopy MRI scans at 6-year follow-up. The patient has normal visual and endocrine function (Reproduced with permission from Delitala et al. [15])

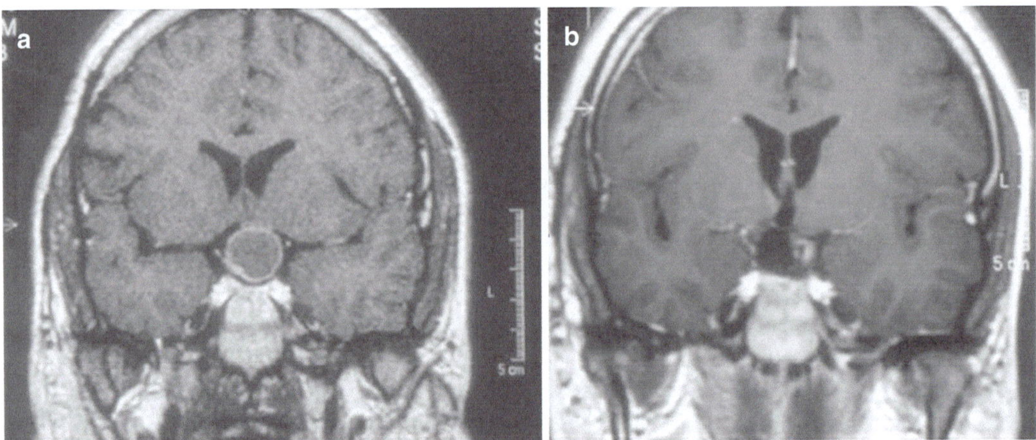

Fig. 9.3 (**a**, **b**) Patient 2: 20-year-old man with a cyst recurring after microsurgery. (**a**) Pre-neuroendoscopy and (**b**) post-neuroendoscopy MRI scans (at 22 months). The cyst did not recur and an enlarging solid subchiasmatic nodule was successfully removed by microsurgery 9 months late (Reproduced with permission from Delitala et al. [15])

9.3.1 Results and Complications

Significant cyst volume decrease was achieved in all patients and visual defects invariably improved in all cases. In one case, cystosphenoistomy was planned but intraoperatively aborted after CSF leakage was suspected. The mean surgical time was 103 min. The mean hospital stay was 5 days. One early major complication, consisting in postoperative severe hyponatremia in a patient with preoperative diabetes insipidus, was observed. We had to remove

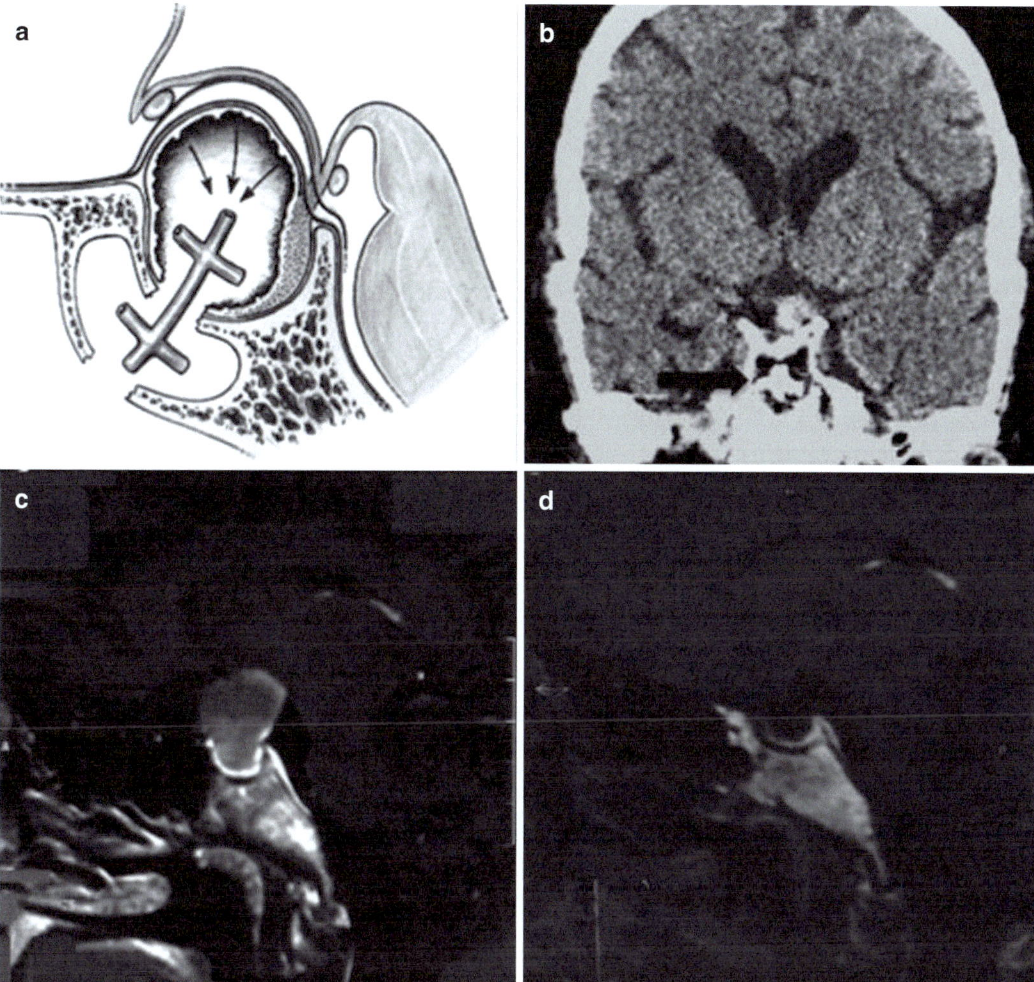

Fig. 9.4 Cystosphenoidostomy: (**a**) scheme of the technique; the homemade H-shaped silastic catheter is placed over the sellar floor, with two arms within the pituitary fossa and two arms in sphenoid sinus. (**b**) Postoperative CT scan showing catheter positioning (*arrow*). (**c**) Preoperative sagittal contrast-enhanced T1w MRI showing a large cystic intra- and suprasellar craniopharyngioma. (**d**) 3-year postoperative sagittal contrast-enhanced T1w MRI showing the cyst disappearance. No visual deficits; mild hypopituitarism under hormone replacement

the catheter in two cases, one CSF leakage that required surgical revision and one case for postoperative recurrent meningitis. Sixteen patients underwent postoperative conformational radiotherapy. In five cases we observed postoperative worsening of a previously existing endocrine disturbance. Follow-up ranged from 8 months to 20 years, and only four patients were lost at follow-up. In four cases we observed a postoperative slow growth of the solid nodule of the tumor, but in no cases a surgical excision was necessary so far.

Conclusions

The results of direct surgical attacks on craniopharyngiomas have enormously improved over the last half century. Surgical mortality has dropped from 41 % [16] before replacement therapy became available to 2 % or less in recent series [1, 2, 17]. However, a closer insight raises several issues. First of all, radicality can be achieved in only 45.7 % of transcranial procedures [1] and an overall long-term good clinical outcome in 60.3 % of patients [17]. Endocrinological sequelae are the rule and 80 % of Yasargil's patients required substitution therapy [2]. Postoperative diabetes insipidus must be accepted as a common sequela since its incidence increases 3.7 times after surgery [2, 18] and anterior pituitary function is only slightly but constantly affected [18]. More subtle neuropsychological deficits have been observed in surgically treated children in the long term [19]. Focusing on the subgroup of recurrent tumors, total removal is possible in only 21.1 % of craniotomies, and all procedures (craniotomies and transsphenoidal approach) are burdened by a 10.5 % operative mortality [1]. Finally, it must also be emphasized that these figures are quoted from some of the most successful series in the literature: craniopharyngioma is a rare tumor (1.3/million/year) [20] and it is reasonable to assume that less experienced hands would perform less brilliantly. A predominantly cystic tumor is observed in 60 % of craniopharyngioma patients [4]. Since mass effect rather than infiltration is responsible for the clinical syndrome, permanent/repeated cyst drainage seems a suitable compromise in most such cases. Fox has to be credited for the first implant of a sump drainage system in a cystic suprasellar tumor [7]. Similar experiences followed for Miles and Gutin et al. [8, 9]. In all their cases, a catheter connected to the subgaleal reservoir was positioned at craniotomy. Cysto-ventriculostomy, as proposed by Spaziante and de Divitiis, represents an evolution of these early experiences: the authors introduced the concept of marsupialization of the cyst into the ventricles, aiming at continuous dilution of the cyst's fluid and resorption through the CSF pathways [4]. They reported clinical improvement in all patients and a good outcome in the six patients available for follow-up [4]. Periodic aspiration has also been implemented with intracavitary administration of antineoplastic agents in the attempt to overcome the palliative nature of sump drainage. Although β-emitting radiocolloids and bleomycin have proven effective under certain conditions, there have also been some major drawbacks related to isotope handling and radiation damage [10, 21] and the absence of unitary protocols and fatal toxicity. In both cases treatment failures are not uncommon [4, 6, 22–24]. Fluid-filled spaces represent an ideal battlefield for neuroendoscopists: since most craniopharyngioma cysts impinge or grow into the ventricular systems (types c–f according to Yasargil's system), an endoscopic approach seems a suitable option. Minimum invasiveness, a radical cyst drainage, and wide marsupialization into CSF fluid spaces under direct visual control represent clear-cut advantages over other draining techniques. Indeed in the last decade, different institutes have published endoscopic treatment of cystic craniopharyngioma [3, 5, 12, 25] On the other hand, we never attempted nor in the light of our experience recommend an endoscopic resection of solid components due to the risk of uncontrollable damage to neurovascular structures. We prefer to remove as much of the relatively avascular dome and leave behind basal tumor remnants that can later be considered for radiation therapy. In our hands, the neuroendoscopic management of cystic craniopharyngiomas has proven to be safe, repeatable, and effective in the midterm, and it should be especially considered in recurrent tumors and in very young or very old patients. No intraoperative or postoperative complications related to surgery were observed, including chemical meningitis, probably due to careful rinsing of all debris. On the other hand, it must be emphasized that neuroendoscopy is oncologically palliative and not compatible with further intracavitary treatments, which require a sealed cavity. The recurrence rate is undetermined, but seems unrelated to surgical aggressiveness. In only two of our cases, reclosure and filling of the cyst led to clinical symptoms several months after the first procedure and was probably due to insufficient dome stripping. Systematic cisternostomy and stenting of the internal cyst create an additional outflow route to the intracystic CSF circulation and can limit the need for further procedures. Remote recurrence of craniopharyngiomas has been related to intraoperative transplant or CSF spreading [26], and therefore cysto-ventriculo-cisternostomy should in theory be at risk. However, seeding represents an exceptional event, with only eight cases reported to date in the world literature. All of these cases occurred after open surgery with the manipulation of solid, more cellular tumors. The surgical treatment of craniopharyngiomas is extremely challenging and often success requires a multimodal approach. Dealing with mostly cystic tumors can be deceiving since the microsurgical approach ensures drainage, but only seldom radicality, since stripping of the capsule away from the hypothalamus and major vessels is highly risky. Simple drainage has therefore been achieved by puncture and aspiration. The neuroendoscopic approach represents a major advance compared with classic draining techniques, since emptying is obtained under direct vision and operativity of the instrument allows a partial resection of the capsule for diagnostic purposes and especially wide marsupialization. Perforation into the basal cisterns and stenting are measures to prevent reclosure and recurrence, and other therapeutic modalities (microsurgery, radiosurgery, fractionated external radiation therapy) can later be scheduled to eradicate solid remnants, if indicated. A purely endoscopic approach as a first choice is an alternative to microsurgery, in selected cases. Case selection must be based on anatomo-surgical (cystic/solid rate, Yasargil's type) and clinical (primary/recurrent, age, conditions) considerations: in such cases, if tumor control and satisfactory reintegration into the appropriate social setting are the goals, endoscopy cannot be overlooked.

Cystosphenoidostomy has been proved to be a safe and effective palliative treatment for cystic craniopharyngiomas. In particular, it allows significant reduction of mass effect and resolution of symptoms caused by compressive mechanisms, even if it does not affect tumor growth, and it can be combined to other treatment, such as radiotherapy or radiosurgery, aimed to control tumor progression. This technique can be easily proposed to patients whose tumor has a major cystic component that can be reached through a transsphenoidal approach, without a cisternal layer interposing between the tumor and the sellar floor. Even tumors whose cysts have a voluminous suprasellar development may be approached, as the cyst content is usually fluid and can be simply suctioned [4]. The only absolute contraindication to cystosphenoidostomy is intraoperative CSF leakage detection, as the connection may sustain a permanent CSF fistula, with subsequent intracranial hypotension and alarming infectious sequelae. However, it is mainly a low-risk procedure, as it avoids manipulation of neurovascular structures, provides indirect decompression of optic nerves and chiasm, and has a low incidence of pituitary stalk damage and subsequent diabetes insipidus [13, 14]. Furthermore, cystosphenoidostomy has been proven to be effective and safe even in children, in which hypothalamic damage due to tumor compression or surgical manipulation can induce deplorable long-term sequelae [13].

Some sentences of this chapter are taken from *Delitala A, et al. Purely neuroendoscopic transventricular management of cystic craniopharyngiomas. Child's Nervous System 2004; 20:858–862* with kind permission from Springer Science+Business Media and with authorization of the authors.

References

1. Fahlbush R, Honegger J, Paulus W, Huk W, Buchfelder M (1999) Surgical treatment of craniopharyngiomas: experience with 168 patients. J Neurosurg 90: 237–250
2. Yasargil MG, Curcic M, Kis M, Siegenthaler G, Teddy PJ, Roth P (1990) Total removal of craniopharyngiomas. J Neurosurg 73:3–11
3. Tirakotai W, Hellwig D, Bertalanffy H, Riegel T (2007) The role of neuroendoscopy in the management of solid or solid-cystic intra- and periventricular tumours. Childs Nerv Syst 23(6):653–658
4. Spaziante R, de Divitiis E (1997) Drainage techniques for cystic craniopharyngiomas. Neurosurg Q 7: 183–208
5. Pettorini BL, Tamburrini G, Massimi L, Caldarelli M, Di Rocco C (2009) Endoscopic transventricular positioning of intracystic catheter for treatment of craniopharyngioma. Technical note. J Neurosurg Pediatr 4(3):245–248

6. Broggi G, Giorgi C, Franzini A, Servello D, Solero CL (1989) Preliminary results of intracavitary treatment of craniopharyngioma with bleomycin. J Neurosurg Sci 33:145–148
7. Fox JL (1967) Intermittent drainage of intracranial cyst via the subcutaneous Ommaya reservoir. J Neurosurg 27:272–273
8. Gutin PH, Klemme WM, Lagger RL, MacKay AR, Pitts LH, Hosobuchi Y (1980) Management of the unresectable cystic craniopharyngioma by aspiration through an Ommaya reservoir drainage system. J Neurosurg 52:36–40
9. Miles J (1977) Sump drainage: a palliative manoeuvre for the treatment of craniopharyngioma. J Neurol Neurosurg Psychiatry 40:120–126
10. Shapiro B, Fig LM, Gross MD (1999) Intracavitary therapy of craniopharyngiomas. Q J Nucl Med 43:367–374
11. Abdullah J, Camaert J (1995) Endoscopic management of craniopharyngiomas: a review of 3 cases. Minim Invasive Neurosurg 38:79–84
12. Nakamizo A, Inamura T, Nishio S, Inoha S, Ishibashi H, Fukui M (2001) Neuroendoscopic treatment of cystic craniopharyngioma in the third ventricle. Minim Invasive Neurosurg 44:85–87
13. Zona G, Spaziante R (2006) Management of cystic craniopharyngioma in children by a transsphenoidal approach. J Pediatr Endocrinol Metab 19(Suppl 1):381–388
14. Rilliet B, Vernet O, Pica A (2005) The Geneva and Lausanne (French-speaking Switzerland) experience: in favor of the transsphenoidal approach when feasible. Childs Nerv Syst 21(8–9):725–728
15. Delitala A, Brunori A, Chiappetta F (2004) Purely neuroendoscopic transventricular management of cystic craniopharyngiomas. Childs Nerv Syst 20:858–862
16. Gordy PG, Peet MM, Kahn EA (1949) The surgery of craniopharyngioma. J Neurosurg 6:503–517
17. Duff JM, Meyer FB, Ilstrup DM, Laws ER, Schleck CD, Scheitauer BW (2000) Long term outcomes for surgically resected craniopharyngiomas. Neurosurgery 46:291–305
18. Honegger J, Buchfelder M, Fahlbush R (1999) Surgical treatment of craniopharyngiomas: endocrinological results. J Neurosurg 90:251–257
19. Carpentieri SC, Waber DP, Scott RM (2001) Memory deficits among children with craniopharyngiomas. Neurosurgery 49:1053–1058
20. Bunin GR, Surawicz TS, Witman PA, Preston-Martin S, Davis F, Bruner J (1998) The descriptive epidemiology of craniopharyngioma. J Neurosurg 89:547–551
21. Voges J, Sturm V, Lehrke R, Treuer H, Gauss C, Berthold F (1997) Cystic craniopharyngioma: long term results after intracavitary irradiation with stereotactically applied colloidal B-emitting radioactive sources. Clinical study. Neurosurgery 40:1992–1998
22. Haisa T, Ueki K, Yoshida S (1994) Toxic effects of bleomycin on the hypothalamus following its administration into a cystic craniopharyngioma. Br J Neurosurg 8:747–750
23. Savas A, Erdem A, Tun K, Kanpolat Y (2000) Fatal toxic effect of bleomycin on brain tissue after intracystic chemotherapy for craniopharyngioma: case report. Neurosurgery 46:213–217
24. Takahashi H, Nakazawa S, Shimura T (1985) Evaluation of postoperative intratumoral injection of bleomycin for craniopharyngioma in children. J Neurosurg 62:120–127
25. Buchfelder M, Schlaffer SM, Lin F, Kleindienst A (2013) Surgery for craniopharyngioma. Pituitary 16:18–25
26. Ito M, Jamshidi J, Yamanaka K (2001) Does craniopharyngioma metastasize? Case report and review of the literature. Neurosurgery 48:933–936

10 Rathke's Cleft Cyst: Endoscopic Endonasal Transsphenoidal Approach

Felice Esposito

10.1 Introduction

Cysts of the Rathke's cleft or pouch are benign, nonadenomatous lesions of the sellar and supra-parasellar areas, which are included in the differential diagnosis with other cystic lesions in such regions, such as craniopharyngiomas, arachnoid cysts, epidermoid cysts, cystic pituitary adenomas, etc. The pathogenesis of Rathke's cleft cysts (RCCs) remains controversial: cuboidal or ciliated columnar epithelial cells line the majority of RCCs, and the leading theory is that they represent remnants from the incomplete obliteration of Rathke's pouch during embryological development [1]. As a matter of fact, the Rathke's pouch represents a superiorly directed evagination from the stomodeum of the 4-week-old human embryo, which becomes entirely obliterated with the exception of its cranial portion by the seventh week of gestation. The anterior wall of the remaining small cavity forms the anterior lobe of the pituitary gland (adenohypophysis), and its posterior wall proliferates much less to become the pars intermedia of the gland. The posterior lobe and the pituitary stalk form from an inferiorly directed evagination from the diencephalon, which meets the Rathke's pouch at the level of the sella turcica.

Indeed, residual clefts of Rathke's pouch may persist, and a residual cavity between the anterior and posterior lobes may be commonly found even in the adult life as small fluid cysts. Such facts explain the reason why growing RCCs, when intrasellar or intra-suprasellar, typically split the gland, pushing and compressing the adenohypophysis anteriorly and the neurohypophysis posteriorly in sagittal MRI images. There are several routine autopsy studies that describe the finding of asymptomatic cysts of the Rathke's pouch in up to 13–33 % of normal pituitary glands and, actually, account for the 2–9 % of all the intracranial tumors removed via a transsphenoidal approach [2–16].

Typically, RCCs are lined with cuboidal or columnar epithelial cells, often ciliated, and include mucin-secreting goblet cells, which stain positively by the periodic acid-Schiff method. Stratified or pseudostratified squamous epithelium may also be present and may rest on a collagenous connective tissue stroma. However, since stratified squamous epithelial cells (like those typically seen in craniopharyngiomas) are sometimes noted to line a portion of RCCs, some authors have speculated that RCCs and craniopharyngiomas have continuum of cystic sellar lesions [1].

Electronic supplementary material The online version of this chapter (doi:10.1007/978-3-319-21533-4_10) contains supplementary material, which is available to authorized users.

F. Esposito
Division of Neurosurgery, Department of Biomedical Sciences, Dentistry, and Morphological and Functional Imaging, University of Messina, Via Consolare Valeria 1, Messina 98125, Italy
e-mail: esposito.felice@gmail.com; fesposito@unime.it

P. Cappabianca et al. (eds.), *Midline Skull Base Surgery*, DOI 10.1007/978-3-319-21533-4_10

In most instances RCCs remain asymptomatic, remaining located within the sella or even extending into the suprasellar space or, conversely, arising as purely suprasellar lesions. Indeed, symptomatic RCCs have historically been felt to be uncommon, determining mass effect on the surrounding structures causing endocrinological and/or neurological dysfunction. Symptomatic patients may present with headaches, visual disturbance, hyperprolactinemia, and/or varying degrees of hypopituitarism. In such cases, RCCs require surgical removal [1, 6–8, 10, 11, 13, 17–19].

10.2 Endoscopic Endonasal Transsphenoidal Approach to RCCs

RCCs are characterized based on preoperative and postoperative magnetic resonance (MR) findings and categorized as (a) purely intrasellar, (b) intrasellar/suprasellar, or (c) purely suprasellar [1]. Therefore, the optimal surgical strategy varies according to both clinical status and cyst volume and location. Furthermore, during the last 20 years, with the advent, refinement, and widespreading of the endoscopic endonasal technique for removing pituitary lesion, this technique has been advocated for the treatment of different sellar and suprasellar lesions, including the Rathke's cleft cyst [5, 9, 15, 16, 20–22]. More recently, the introduction of the endoscopic endonasal "extended" approaches permitted to access the suprasellar area thanks to the additional removal of the tuberculum sellae and posterior portion of the sphenoidal planum, rendering amenable the excision of purely suprasellar lesions, traditionally removed via a transcranial route only [23].

As a matter of fact, the surgical treatment of the RCCs can be performed via a "standard" endoscopic endonasal approach for those lesions that are purely intrasellar or intra-/suprasellar, whereas patients with supraglandular cysts may be candidate to transtuberculum transplanum "extended" approach.

The procedure is typically performed using a rigid 0° endoscope, 18 cm in length and 4 mm in diameter (Karl Storz Endoscopy, Tuttlingen, Germany), as the sole visualizing tool. The 30–45° angled endoscopes are usually employed to explore large intra-suprasellar tumor residual cavities. The details of the surgical procedures have been already described in previous publications [20, 23–25]. However, there are significant differences in the surgical management of the RCC with an intra- or intra-suprasellar location and those with a purely suprasellar location, so that we will analyze relative peculiar features separately.

10.2.1 Intra-suprasellar RCCs

The nasal and sphenoidal steps of the procedure are performed following the same principles of the standard pituitary approach for pituitary adenomas: a binarial 3–4 hands technique is usually adopted; as for standard pituitary surgery, no middle turbinate is routinely removed in both nostrils; they are simply lateralized with an elevator and are repositioned back at the end of the procedure. In purely intrasellar RCC, the sellar floor is extensively removed down to the clival recess to grant proper maneuverability of the surgical instruments inside the sella. Anyway, it can be useful to preserve a reliable extradural plane undermining the bony edges, in order to allow an effective extradural closure of the sellar floor in case of intraoperative CSF leak. After the opening of the dura mater, one may directly access the cyst or may first see the normal pituitary gland, since, usually, the adenohypophysis is pushed anteriorly by the cyst. Though, the cyst is entered and emptied and any floating part of the cyst wall is taken out by sharp maneuvers, in order to have the histopathological confirm of the diagnosis. As the residual cavity is wide enough, the endoscope is inserted inside the residual cavity: by continuous irrigation through the irrigation sheath, the so-called diving technique is performed, which is a similar technique used by laparoscopic surgeons in creating the pneumoperitoneum [26]. This permits the removal of any cystic content remnant eventually adherent to the cyst wall. Should the cyst wall be tightly adherent to the pituitary tissue, the dissection maneuvers should be limited or even avoided in order to lower the chance of causing any postoperative further impairment of the pituitary function. At the end of the procedure, no sellar closure is performed, unless an intraoperative CSF leak occurred [27].

10.2.2 Purely Suprasellar RCCs

In purely suprasellar RCCs, the sellar cavity is usually not enlarged and an endoscopic endonasal transtuberculum/transplanum approach is needed to access the suprasellar area. As already described elsewhere [20–23, 25, 28], the approach is realized through both nostrils with a middle turbinectomy on one side, resection of the posterior portion of the nasal septum and a wider anterior sphenoidotomy. Owing that RCCs content is in most cases fluid, large bone opening over the planum sphenoidale is usually not required and extensive drilling at the level of the medial opto-carotid recess or over the planum sphenoidale is not mandatory [29]. The cyst is usually clearly identified after the dura opening. Such maneuver usually causes the creation of a large CSF leakage, since the anterior part of the cyst wall is surrounded by or even intimately adherent to the arachnoid of the suprasellar cistern; the remaining part of the cyst wall can be attached to the pituitary stalk – which is usually pushed contralaterally – the superior hypophyseal arteries and/or the optic chiasm. In such cases it is of utmost importance to avoid tractions in order to prevent injuries to these neurovascular structures. Bimanual microsurgical dissection is performed while dealing with the anatomical structures in the suprasellar area: one surgeon works bimanually, with either sharp and blunt instruments, to dissect, if easily possible and remove the cyst wall, while a second surgeon drives dynamically the endoscope.

Concerning the reconstruction of the skull base and dural defects, the techniques vary according to the surgical procedure adopted and the grade of the intraoperative CSF leak [27]. In case of a standard approach without any evidence of intraoperative CSF leakage, no reconstruction is usually performed; anyway, a single layer of dural substitute can be placed extradurally in order to close the dural opening. Should a CSF leak occur, especially in cases of extended approaches with the creation of a large CSF leak, one of the reliable methods for the reconstruction is the intradural filling of the dead space with a gasket-seal extradural closure of the osteodural defect eventually supported by a pedicled nasoseptal flap [27, 30–32].

10.2.3 Outcome

10.2.3.1 Extent of Resection, Clinical Symptoms, and Recurrence Rate

In terms of the extent of resection, a gross total removal can be defined as a condition of complete cyst content evacuation with cyst wall removal, while subtotal removal is usually intended as the cyst drainage with eventual partial removal or even a simple biopsy of the cyst wall. One should always balance the opportunity to seek a total removal of the cyst wall with the possibility of creating new postoperative hormonal deficits of either the anterior or the posterior gland and also injury of the neurovascular structures, thus risking the creation of a new visual deficit or the worsening of any preoperative visual impairment. On the other side, a subtotal removal poses higher risks of cyst recurrence. It should be noted that, usually, a standard approach is reserved for the treatment of a purely intrasellar or intra- and suprasellar cysts, while the extended endoscopic surgical techniques are adopted for the removal of those cysts with a purely suprasellar location or to remove the suprasellar component of intra-suprasellar cysts. Having such principles in mind, the most common occurrence in case of RCCs is the subtotal removal. As a matter of fact, the simple cyst emptying with a limited removal of any nonadherent cyst wall as specimens for the histopathological diagnosis is usually sufficient to improve or even resolve the preoperative symptoms, mainly related with the mass effect due to the cyst enlargement. Indeed, in many clinical series on RCCs, the most common presenting symptom – i.e., headache – resolves in the majority of cases [1, 6–9, 11, 12, 15, 16, 19, 21, 22]. Besides, the visual symptoms may improve with simple cyst content evacuation, while the creation of new visual deficits with the endoscopic endonasal approach is rare [6, 33].

Concerning the endocrine outcome, it should be noted that symptomatic RCCs predominantly occur in women; however, this may simply reflect a detection bias as irregular menses often trigger an endocrine evaluation [1]. Anyway, preoperative endocrine deficits are those that more inconstantly improve postoperatively. In some series an anterior pituitary insufficiency has been reported to improve in roughly half of the patients, while in others such symptoms are recorded to not improve at all [1, 6–9, 11, 12, 15, 16, 19, 21, 22]. Conversely, the creation of new hormonal deficits has been reported in a more consistent way; the occurrence of new anterior pituitary insufficiency and also diabetes insipidus (either transient or permanent) is a fairly common evidence, especially when the surgeon attempts to extensively remove the cyst wall. It is worth of note that patients with the higher chances of new hormonal deficiencies usually have suprasellar RCCs that are intimately attached to the pituitary stalk, making their removal considerably more challenging [1]. Also the rate of delayed hyponatremia has been described to be higher (17 %) in RCCs than the 2–17 % rate reported after transsphenoidal surgery for pituitary adenomas [1]. Delayed hyponatremia after pituitary surgery is generally attributed to the syndrome of inappropriate secretion of antidiuretic hormone (SIADH). It is possible that a higher rate of hyponatremia after RCC surgery may result from the closer anatomical association of RCC with the pituitary stalk and neurohypophysis [1].

Concerning the possibility of cyst recurrence, several authors have concluded that a relatively high rate of recurrence may indicate a link between RCCs and craniopharyngiomas, while the extent of resection of the cyst wall was not associated with an increased rate of recurrence, founding no differences in recurrence rates between radical and subtotal resections [34].

It can be concluded that the removal of a different Rathke's cleft cyst can benefit from the adaptability of the endoscopic endonasal approach, having the possibility of extending the surgical route to the tuberculum sellae and the posterior sphenoid in those cases where the cyst cannot be effectively drained via a standard transsphenoidal corridor or when the cyst is purely located in the suprasellar area. As well, the cyst wall total removal does not represent a key step to gain the resolution of the pathology; it can be thought reasonable to leave a residual behind when it is tightly attached to the surrounding neurovascular structures [20]. Particularly, there is no conclusive evidence that a more aggressive resection of the cyst wall can result in a lower risk of recurrence (Figs. 10.1, 10.2, 10.3 and 10.4).

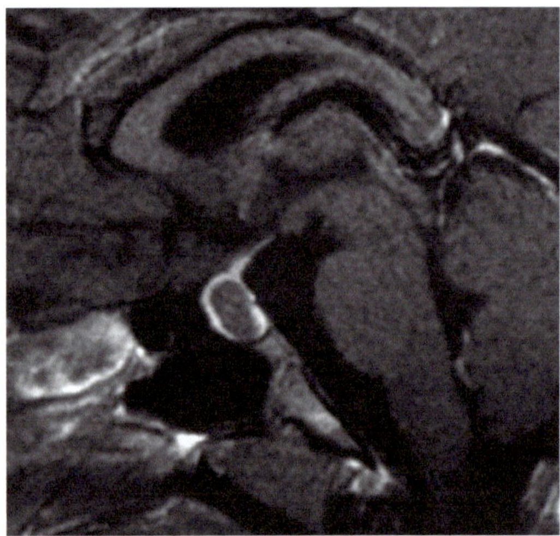

Fig. 10.1 Contrast-enhanced sellar MRI, sagittal image: typical appearance of a Rathke's cleft cyst. The cyst has split the pituitary gland: the adenohypophysis has been moved and compressed anteriorly, and the neurohypophysis has been moved and compressed posteriorly. The cystic content does not show contrast enhancement

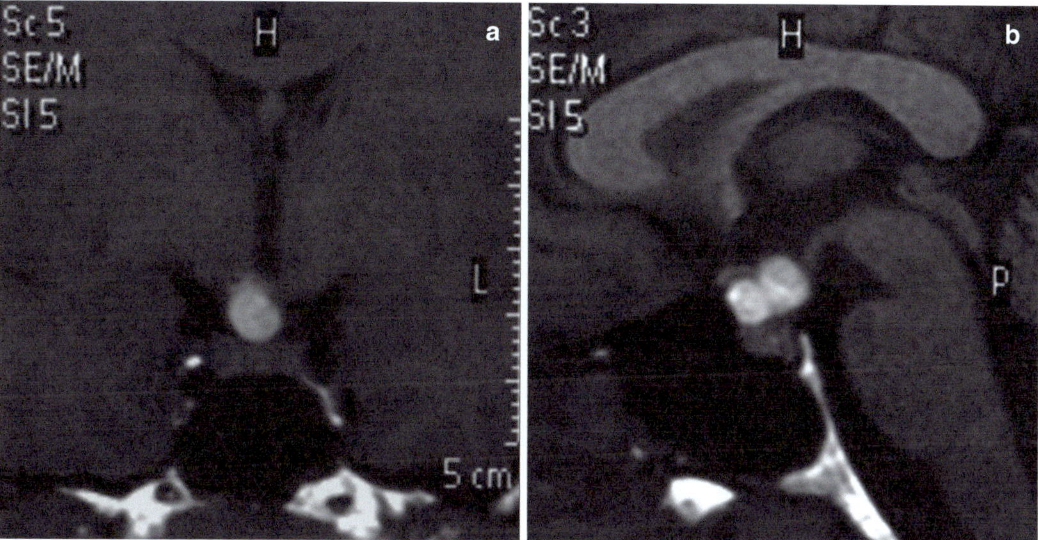

Fig. 10.2 (**a**) Sagittal and (**b**) coronal MRI scan showing an intra- and suprasellar Rathke's cleft cyst

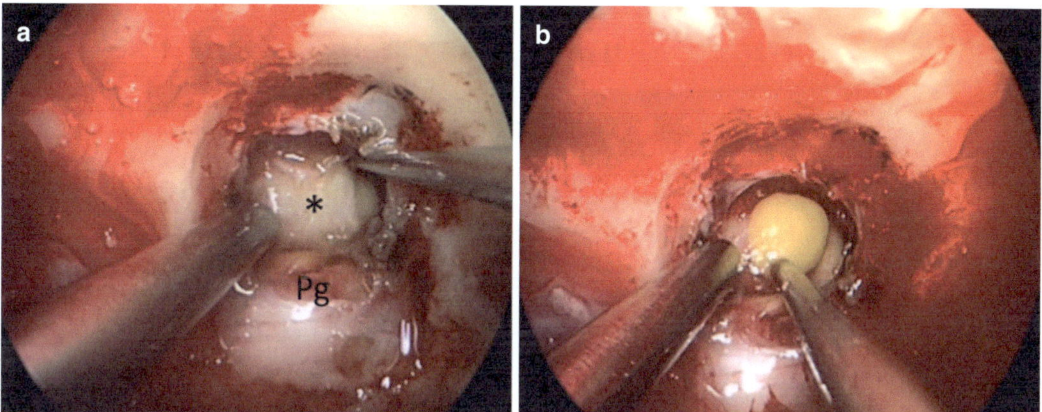

Fig. 10.3 (**a**) After the opening of the dura mater, the cyst can be seen posterosuperiorly to the adenohypophysis pushed anteriorly by the cyst. (**b**) The cyst is entered and emptied. *Pg* pituitary gland (adenohypophysis), * Rathke's cleft cyst

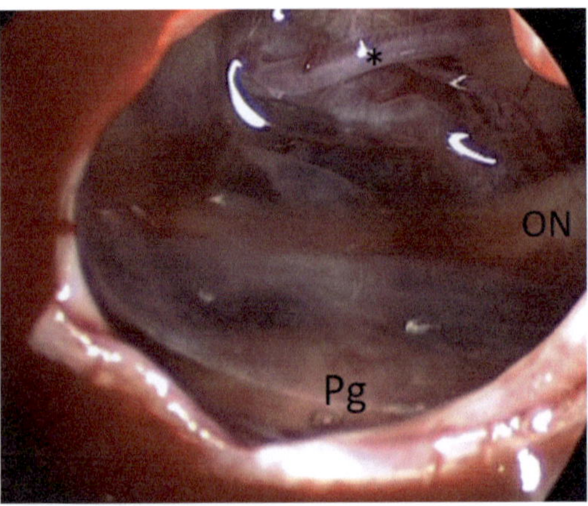

Fig. 10.4 Endoscopic endonasal closeup view of the residual Rathke's cleft cyst cavity: note the prolapsed suprasellar arachnoid through the incompetent diaphragma sellae. *Pg* pituitary gland, *ON* optic nerve, * Heubner's artery

References

1. Cohan P, Foulad A, Esposito F, Martin NA, Kelly DF (2004) Symptomatic Rathke's cleft cysts: a report of 24 cases. J Endocrinol Invest 27(10):943–948
2. Arai T, Horiguchi K, Saeki N, Oka H, Saito T, Takahashi-Fujigasaki J, Sakamoto H, Kato N, Dobashi H, Tanaka T, Hasegawa Y, Abe T (2011) Surgical treatment of a calcified Rathke's cleft cyst with endoscopic extended transsphenoidal surgery–case report. Neurol Med Chir (Tokyo) 51(7):535–538
3. Brassier G, Morandi X, Tayiar E, Riffaud L, Chabert E, Heresbach N, Poirier JY, Carsin-Nicol B (1999) Rathke's cleft cysts: surgical-MRI correlation in 16 symptomatic cases. J Neuroradiol 26(3):162–171
4. Ceylan S, Koc K, Anik I (2009) Extended endoscopic approaches for midline skull-base lesions. Neurosurg Rev 32(3):309–319; discussion 318–309. doi:10.1007/s10143-009-0201-9
5. Dusick JR, Esposito F, Kelly DF, Cohan P, DeSalles A, Becker DP, Martin NA (2005) The extended direct endonasal transsphenoidal approach for nonadenomatous suprasellar tumors. J Neurosurg 102(5):832–841
6. el-Mahdy W, Powell M (1998) Transsphenoidal management of 28 symptomatic Rathke's cleft cysts, with special reference to visual and hormonal recovery. Neurosurgery 42(1):7–16; discussion 16–17
7. Fan J, Peng Y, Qi S, Zhang XA, Qiu B, Pan J (2013) Individualized surgical strategies for Rathke cleft cyst based on cyst location. J Neurosurg 119(6):1437–1446. doi:10.3171/2013.8.JNS13777
8. Fan MC, Wang QL, Wang JF, Deng WS, Li LD, Wang ZH, Sun P (2012) Surgical treatment of symptomatic Rathke's cleft cysts: clinical features, therapy considerations and outcomes. Chin Med J (Engl) 125(16):2919–2924
9. Frank G, Sciarretta V, Mazzatenta D, Farneti G, Modugno GC, Pasquini E (2005) Transsphenoidal endoscopic approach in the treatment of Rathke's cleft cyst. Neurosurgery 56(1):124–128; discussion 129
10. Jahangiri A, Molinaro AM, Tarapore PE, Blevins L Jr, Auguste KI, Gupta N, Kunwar S, Aghi MK (2011) Rathke cleft cysts in pediatric patients: presentation, surgical management, and postoperative outcomes. Neurosurg Focus 31(1):E3. doi:10.3171/2011.5.FOCUS1178
11. Kim E (2012) Symptomatic Rathke cleft cyst: clinical features and surgical outcomes. World Neurosurg 78(5):527–534. doi:10.1016/j.wneu.2011.12.091
12. Laws ER, Kanter AS (2004) Rathke cleft cysts. J Neurosurg 101(4):571–572; discussion 572. doi:10.3171/jns.2004.101.4.0571
13. Potts MB, Jahangiri A, Lamborn KR, Blevins LS, Kunwar S, Aghi MK (2011) Suprasellar Rathke cleft cysts: clinical presentation and treatment outcomes. Neurosurgery 69(5):1058–1068; discussion 1068–1057. doi:10.1227/NEU.0b013e318228bcea
14. Trifanescu R, Ansorge O, Wass JA, Grossman AB, Karavitaki N (2012) Rathke's cleft cysts. Clin Endocrinol (Oxf) 76(2):151–160. doi:10.1111/j.1365-2265.2011.04235.x
15. Xie T, Hu F, Yu Y, Gu Y, Wang X, Zhang X (2011) Endoscopic endonasal resection of symptomatic Rathke cleft cysts. J Clin Neurosci 18(6):760–762. doi:10.1016/j.jocn.2010.10.014
16. Zada G (2011) Rathke cleft cysts: a review of clinical and surgical management. Neurosurg Focus 31(1):E1. doi:10.3171/2011.5.FOCUS1183
17. Benveniste RJ, King WA, Walsh J, Lee JS, Naidich TP, Post KD (2004) Surgery for Rathke cleft cysts: technical considerations and outcomes. J Neurosurg 101(4):577–584. doi:10.3171/jns.2004.101.4.0577
18. Han SJ, Rolston JD, Jahangiri A, Aghi MK (2014) Rathke's cleft cysts: review of natural history and surgical outcomes. J Neurooncol 117(2):197–203. doi:10.1007/s11060-013-1272-6
19. Koutourousiou M, Grotenhuis A, Kontogeorgos G, Seretis A (2009) Treatment of Rathke's cleft cysts: experience at a single centre. J Clin Neurosci 16(7):900–903. doi:10.1016/j.jocn.2008.10.007
20. Cavallo LM, Prevedello D, Esposito F, Laws ER, Dusick JR, Messina A, Jane JA, Kelly DF, Cappabianca P (2008) The role of the endoscope in the transsphenoidal management of cystic lesions of the sellar region. Neurosurg Rev 31(1):55–64. doi:10.1007/S10143-007-0098-0
21. Jahangiri A, Potts M, Kunwar S, Blevins L, El-Sayed IH, Aghi MK (2014) Extended endoscopic endonasal approach for suprasellar Rathke's cleft cysts. J Clin Neurosci 21(5):779–785. doi:10.1016/j.jocn.2013.07.023
22. Madhok R, Prevedello DM, Gardner P, Carrau RL, Snyderman CH, Kassam AB (2010) Endoscopic endonasal resection of Rathke cleft cysts: clinical outcomes and surgical nuances. J Neurosurg 112(6):1333–1339. doi:10.3171/2009.10.JNS09348

23. Cappabianca P, Cavallo LM, Esposito F, de Divitiis O, Messina A, de Divitiis E (2008) Extended endoscopic endonasal approach to the midline skull base: the evolving role of transsphenoidal surgery. In: Pickard JD, Akalan N, Di Rocco C et al (eds) Advances and technical standards in neurosurgery. Springer, Wien New York, pp 152–199
24. Cappabianca P, Cavallo LM, de Divitiis E (2004) Endoscopic endonasal transsphenoidal surgery. Neurosurgery 55(4):933–940; discussion 940–941
25. de Divitiis E, Cavallo LM, Cappabianca P, Esposito F (2007) Extended endoscopic endonasal transsphenoidal approach for the removal of suprasellar tumors: part 2. Neurosurgery 60(1):46–58; discussion 58–59
26. Locatelli D, Canevari FR, Acchiardi I, Castelnuovo P (2010) The endoscopic diving technique in pituitary and cranial base surgery: technical note. Neurosurgery 66(2):E400–E401; discussion E401. doi:10.1227/01.NEU.0000363746.84763.A5
27. Esposito F, Dusick JR, Fatemi N, Kelly DF (2007) Graded repair of cranial base defects and cerebrospinal fluid leaks in transsphenoidal surgery. Neurosurgery 60(2):ONS1–ONS9
28. Kassam A, Snyderman CH, Mintz A, Gardner P, Carrau RL (2005) Expanded endonasal approach: the rostrocaudal axis. Part I. Crista galli to the sella turcica. Neurosurg Focus 19(1):E3:1–E3:12
29. de Notaris M, Solari D, Cavallo LM, D'Enza AI, Ensenat J, Berenguer J, Ferrer E, Prats-Galino A, Cappabianca P (2012) The "suprasellar notch," or the tuberculum sellae as seen from below: definition, features, and clinical implications from an endoscopic endonasal perspective. J Neurosurg 116(3):622–629. doi:10.3171/2011.11.JNS111162
30. Cavallo LM, Messina A, Esposito F, de Diviths O, Dal Fabbro M, de Diviths E, Cappabianca P (2007) Skull base reconstruction in the extended endoscopic transsphenoidal approach for suprasellar lesions. J Neurosurg 107(4):713–720. doi:10.3171/Jns-07/10/0713
31. Leng LZ, Brown S, Anand VK, Schwartz TH (2008) "Gasket-seal" watertight closure in minimal-access endoscopic cranial base surgery. Neurosurgery 62(5 Suppl 2):ONSE342–ONSE343; discussion ONSE343. doi:10.1227/01.neu.0000326017.84315.1f 00006123-200805002-00010 [pii]
32. Cappabianca P, Esposito F, Magro F, Cavallo LM, Solari D, Stella L, de Divitiis O (2010) Natura Abhorret a Vacuo-use of fibrin glue as a filler and sealant in neurosurgical "dead spaces". Technical note. Acta Neurochir (Wien) 152(5):897–904. doi:10.1007/S00701-009-0580-2
33. Cappabianca P, Cavallo LM, Esposito F, De Divitiis O, Messina A, De Divitiis E (2008) Extended endoscopic endonasal approach to the midline skull base: the evolving role of transsphenoidal surgery. Adv Tech Stand Neurosurg 33:151–199
34. Aho CJ, Liu C, Zelman V, Couldwell WT, Weiss MH (2005) Surgical outcomes in 118 patients with Rathke cleft cysts. J Neurosurg 102(2):189–193. doi:10.3171/jns.2005.102.2.0189

11 Frontotemporal Approach

Oreste de Divitiis, Crescenzo Capone, Teresa Somma, Andrea Elefante, Pierpaolo Di Lorenzo, Paolo Cappabianca, and Peter A. Winkler

11.1 Indications

"Craniopharyngioma" is the name introduced by Cushing for tumors derived "from epithelial rests ascribable to an imperfect closure of the hypophysial or craniopharyngeal duct" [12]. It may arise anywhere along the craniopharyngeal duct: 4 % are purely intrasellar, 21 % are sellar-suprasellar, and 75 % are suprasellar alone, often with extension up into the third ventricle [24].

The primary treatment of craniopharyngiomas is surgical excision. Two main different options could be used by the neurosurgeon to remove the lesion: the low route via microsurgical or endoscopic transsphenoidal approach and the high route via different types of craniotomies. Lesions with significant supra- and parasellar extension, especially when mostly solid, are treated preferably with surgery through intracranial corridors. The pterional approach is the most versatile access to the majority of craniopharyngiomas. It offers different working channels: between the two optic nerves, between the optic nerve and the carotid artery (ICA), and between the ICA and the oculomotor nerve. In particular, tumors extending broadly into the third ventricle or arousing primarily in the third ventricle represent the greatest surgical challenge. The most used and safe corridor to reach such lesions is the approach via the lamina terminalis. The lamina terminalis is a transparent whitish membrane at the base and front of the brain, which forms most of the anterior wall of the third ventricle. Its fenestration, after the retraction of the anterior communicating artery complex, allows the direct access to the anterior part of the third ventricle [15, 28]. Furthermore, this is the best transcranial approach in two particular conditions: pre-fixed chiasm and chiasm in post-fixed position due to a retrochiasmatic tumor.

Electronic supplementary material The online version of this chapter (doi:10.1007/978-3-319-21533-4_11) contains supplementary material, which is available to authorized users.

O. de Divitiis, MD (✉) • C. Capone, MD
T. Somma, MD • P. Cappabianca, MS
Division of Neurosurgery,
Department of Neurosciences, Reproductive and Odontostomatological Sciences,
Università degli Studi di Napoli "Federico II", Naples, Italy
e-mail: oreste.dedivitiis@unina.it

A. Elefante, MD
Neuroradiology Unit,
Department of Advanced Biomedical Sciences,
Università degli Studi di Napoli "Federico II", Naples, Italy

P. Di Lorenzo, MD, PhD
Division of Legal Medicine,
Department of Advanced Biomedical Sciences,
Università degli Studi di Napoli "Federico II", Naples, Italy

P.A. Winkler, MD
Department of Neurosurgery,
Christian Doppler Klinik,
Paracelsus Medical University,
Salzburg, Austria

P. Cappabianca et al. (eds.), *Midline Skull Base Surgery*, DOI 10.1007/978-3-319-21533-4_11

11.2 Neuroradiology

The role of neuroimaging is to provide the neurosurgeon the understanding of the lesion by means of a full pattern of preoperative informations, location, extent, and relationships of the craniopharyngioma to the distorted normal anatomy and, above all, to decide the best way to approach the tumor. Radiologic evaluation of craniopharyngiomas includes computed tomography (CT), magnetic resonance imaging (MRI) and, in order to obviate the need for invasive cerebral angiography, magnetic resonance angiography (MRA). MRI is the gold standard for evaluating hypothalamic-pituitary-related endocrine diseases, above all, for the diagnosis of craniopharyngiomas. Advanced MRI techniques, including diffusion-weighted imaging (DWI), MR spectroscopy (MRS), and perfusion-weighted imaging (PWI), may be helpful to provide a further definition of the tumor's features [5, 23, 30, 57]. From an imaging standpoint, craniopharyngiomas are typically described as calcified, solid, and/or cystic lesions, typically with a lobular shape. The majority of craniopharyngiomas involve the suprasellar space, with 40–53 % of the cases exhibiting some intrasellar involvement [35].

MRI patterns of craniopharyngiomas vary with cyst contents (Fig. 11.1). Craniopharyngioma cysts containing serous fluid are typically hypointense on T1-weighted sequences and variably hyperintense on T2-weighted and FLAIR ones. Mucoid cysts show hyperintensity both on T1-weighted [6, 32] and on T2-weighted and FLAIR sequences [19, 23, 57], reflecting its heterogeneous contents. Sometimes it may not be easy to differentiate cysts from acute hemorrhages. Indeed, GRE T2*-weighted sequence is useful in demonstrating calcification, or possibly demonstrating blood products (Fig. 11.1). The solid tumor portions and the cyst wall usually enhance after contrast administration [37, 40] (Figs. 11.1 and 11.2). MRI has a pivotal role in differentiating the anatomical variants and the different patterns of chiasm distortion caused by suprasellar tumors. The growth of the tumor in the suprasellar area causes different patterns of chiasm distortions. In the preoperative planning, it is of critical importance to distinguish a condition of pre-fixed or post-fixed chiasm. In the first case, chiasm is pushed forward by a retrochiasmatic craniopharyngioma, whether in the second there is a prechiasmatic tumor which pushes upward and backward the chiasm, representing the best anatomical variation for performing the transcranial approach to the lesion (Fig. 11.2). Craniopharyngiomas occasionally extend into the anterior, middle, or posterior fossa and may invade the floor or walls of the third ventricle (Fig. 11.3). Hydrocephalus is observed in up to 38 % of cases and is a more common finding in children (Fig. 11.3) [16, 56]. Noncalcified solid craniopharyngiomas may have radiological features that are indistinguishable from those of other suprasellar neoplasms, including chiasmatic hypothalamic gliomas, germinomas, pituitary macroadenomas, meningiomas, and epidermoids. DWI, proton MRS, and PWI can provide additional information which are helpful in differential diagnosis of sellar/parasellar tumors. DWI is useful in the differential diagnosis if an epidermoid or a meningioma is suspected, as they show low ADC values, while craniopharyngiomas may have variable patterns of diffusivity depending upon the character of the cyst fluid (Fig. 11.4) [35]. Proton MRS allows to demonstrate a unique spectroscopic pattern that differentiates these tumors [45]. Craniopharyngiomas show dominant peak in the quote of lactate or lipids, characteristic of the cholesterol and lipid constituents, and only a few other metabolites. On the other hand, gliomas demonstrate choline, N-acetylaspartate, and creatine, with an increased ratio of choline to N-acetylaspartate compared with normal brain tissue. Pituitary adenomas show either choline peaks or no metabolites at all. PWI shows high rCBV (relative cerebral blood volume) in squamous-papillary type of craniopharyngiomas and low rCBV in adamantinomatous type. Conversely, other sellar and parasellar tumors as meningiomas, macroadenomas, and gliomas usually show relatively high perfusion patterns [5]. MRA with its post-processing reconstructions can be further useful to complete the neuroradiological preoperative briefing,

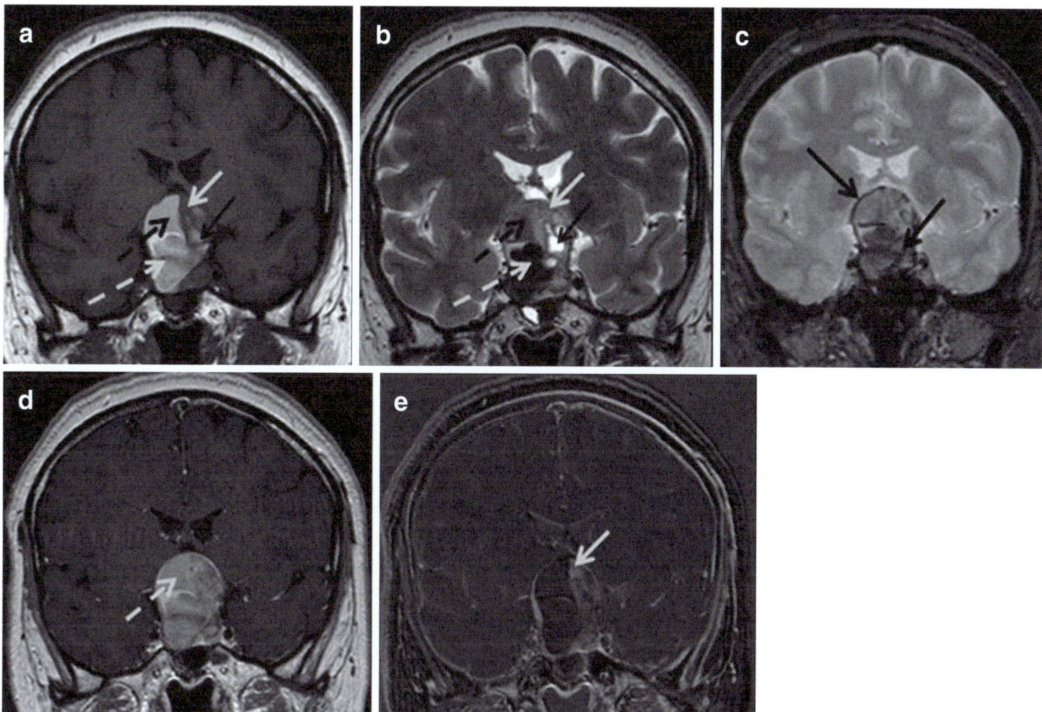

Fig. 11.1 MRI study in a 39-year-old woman. MRI study without contrast-medium administration: (**a**) coronal spin-echo T1-weighted (T1WI), (**b**) coronal turbo-spin-echo T2-weighted (T2WI) and (**c**) coronal gradient-echo T2* sequences. MRI study after contrast-medium administration: (**d**) coronal spin-echo T1-weighted (T1WIC+) and (**e**) coronal subtracted spin-echo T1 sequences. MRI study shows a large and heterogeneous intra- and supra-sellar mass, with a solid and mostly peripheral portion and multiple cystic components. The solid portion is nearly isointense with cortex both on T1WI and T2WI (*white arrows*), with intense nodular (*black arrows*) and rim enhancement after contrast-medium administration. The cystic portion is strongly heterogeneous: right intra- (*dashed white arrows*) and supra-sellar (*dashed black arrows*) components appear hyperintense on T1WI and hypointense on T2WI, for hyperproteic and hypercolesterinic content; the other ones show hyperintense signal both on T1WI and T2WI, for hyperproteic content. GRE T2* sequence shows strongly hypointense peripheral rim and internal septa, associated to the presence of hemosiderinic debris

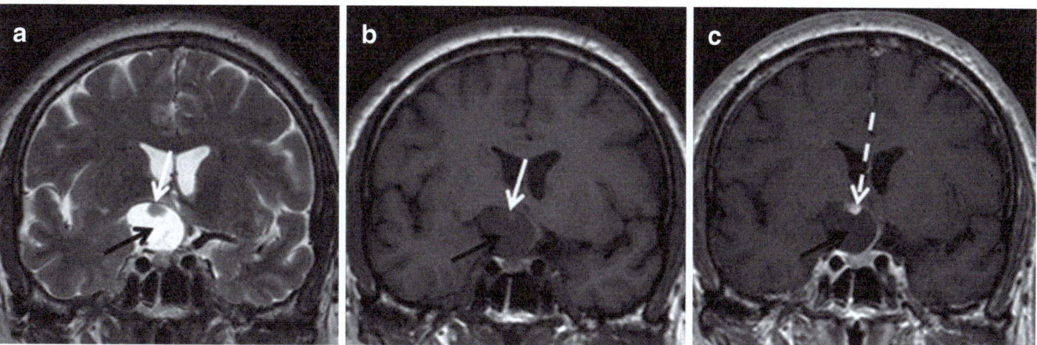

Fig. 11.2 MRI study in a 57-year-old man. (**a**) Turbo-spin-echo T2-weighted sequence (T2WI), (**b**) coronal spin-echo T1-weighted sequence (T1WI) and (**c**) coronal spin-echo T1-weighted sequence after contrast-medium administration (T1WIC+). MRI study shows a large and lobulated supra-sellar mass, which pushes upward and backward the chiasm. It has a large cystic portion, which is hyperintense in T2WI and hypointense in T1WI (*black arrows*), and a mural tumor nodule located in its cranial portion, which is isointense with cortex (*white arrows*). T1WIC+ shows the thin enhancing tumor rim with a small tumor nodule (*dashed white arrows*)

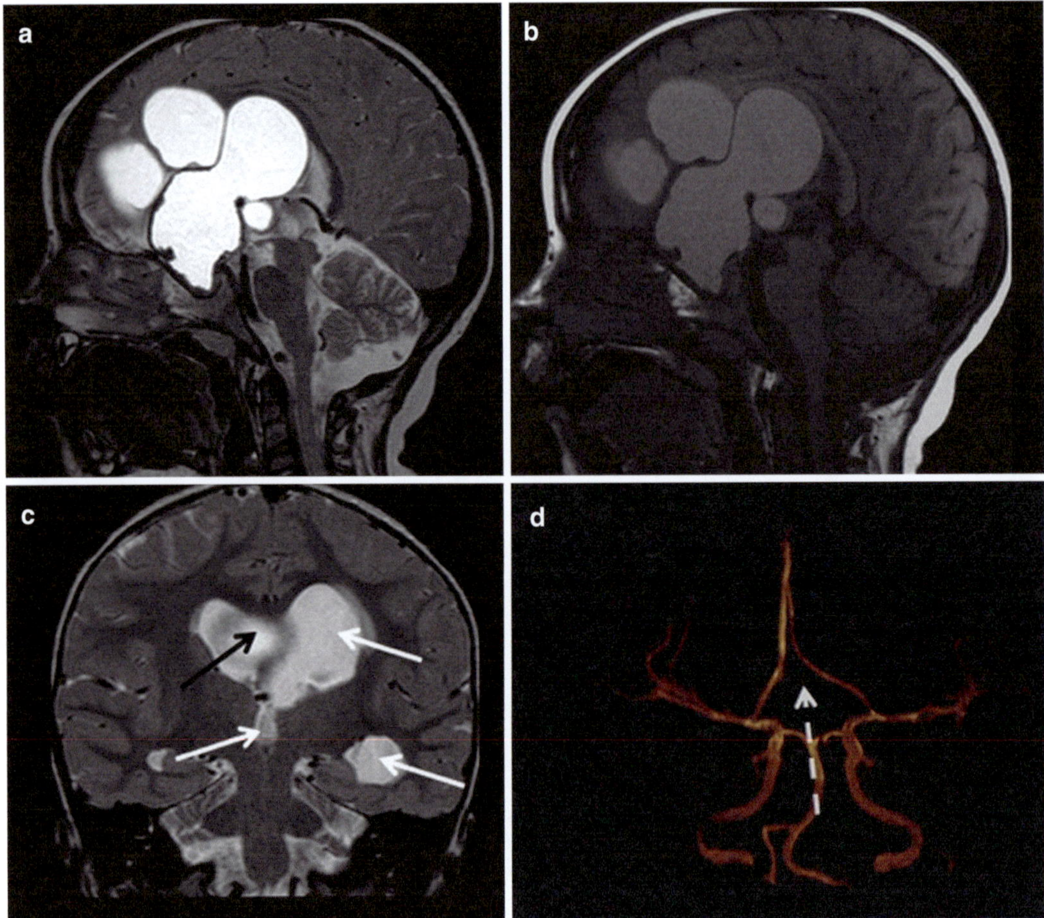

Fig. 11.3 MRI study in a 4-year-old boy. (**a**) Sagittal turbo-spin-echo T2-weighted (T2WI) and (**b**) sagittal spin-echo T1-weighted (T1WI) sequences. (**c**) Coronal turbo-spin-echo T2-weighted (T2WI) and (**d**) maximum intensity projection (MIP) reconstruction of MRA study. MRI study shows a large and heterogeneous intra- and suprasellar mass with extension to anterior cranial fossa. Coronal T2WI shows triventricular hydrocephalus (*white arrows*) caused by the mass (*black arrow*). MIP reconstruction shows distortion of A1 segments of anterior cerebral arteries, which are wide apart (*dashed white arrow*)

making the neurosurgeon aware of the relationship between the craniopharyngioma and the cavernous sinuses or the adjacent vascular structures as well (Fig. 11.3).

Postoperative follow-up with MRI is essential. The main focus of postsurgical evaluation is the determination of the presence and extent of residual tumor. In addition, MRI plays a pivotal role in the evaluation of the potential surgical complications. These include hypothalamic injury, with associated endocrine abnormalities, injury to the pituitary gland, and vascular injury including pseudoaneurysm formation of adjacent structures.

Computed tomography (CT) has a complementary role in the identification of intralesional calcifications and in the evaluation of bone structures prior to transsphenoidal surgery [23, 49, 57]. Non-enhanced CT scan usually shows a suprasellar and often intrasellar mass with hypodense solid and cystic components [57]. CT also shows calcifications in 90 % of adamantinomatous craniopharyngiomas, while papillary ones rarely calcify [49]. CT may show secondary changes in the skull base, such as enlargement of the sella turcica and/or erosion of the dorsum sella. Additionally, anatomy of the sphenoid

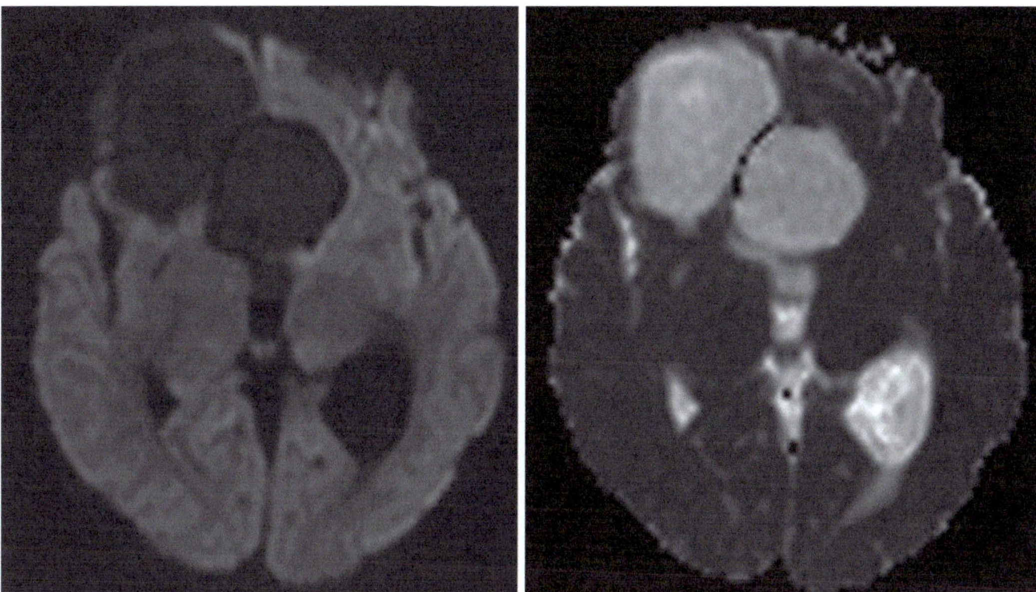

Fig. 11.4 MRI study in a 4-year-old boy. DWI study shows no restriction of the large and plurilobulated mass

sinus can be evaluated to recognize the presence of pneumatized sinus, thus giving the neurosurgeon an essential hint to choose the right surgical approach between transsphenoidal and transcranial surgeries [30].

11.3 Anatomy of the Approach

The frontotemporal region is a complex anatomical area; therefore, it is important to fix some anatomical remarks.

The soft tissue covering this area comprises five layers: skin, subcutaneous tissue, galea aponeurotica, loose connective tissue, and pericranium. These five layers are covered by an outermost horny layer, variable in thickness, while the subcutaneous tissue is made of derma and fatty tissue, which is thicker over the zygomatic arch; therefore, the thickness of the scalp varies from 4 to 9 mm.

In the temporal region, the galea pericranium is called temporoparietal fascia and is considered part of the superficial muscle-aponeurotic system. This fascia is attached in an arched fashion to the superior temporal line, to the lateral surface of the frontozygomatic process and to medial surface of the zygoma. Inside it, it is possible to identify the superficial temporal artery and the frontotemporal branches of the facial nerve.

The loose connective tissue is located directly beneath the fascia and is composed of connective tissue which becomes thin and fatty in correspondence of the zygoma, thus making the first fat pad in continuity with the subcutaneous fat below the zygomatic arch [2].

The pericranium, at the level of the superior temporal line, splits into two layers, a deeper one, beneath the temporal muscle, in contact with the temporal squama, and the other more superficial, covering the muscle and called temporal fascia. Furthermore, this layer splits into two separate laminae, superficial and deep, which enclose the superficial temporal fat pad. Between the fascia and the temporalis muscle, there is another fat pad that forms a sort of pillow, provided of vessels and nerves and variable in thickness, from very thick to extremely thin. Some authors consider another fascia, defined innominate fascia, or parotid temporal fascia closely adherent to the superficial temporal layer [1, 54].

In order to avoid postoperative cosmetic deficits, the knowledge of the anatomy of the superficial temporal artery and the facial nerve is essential.

The superficial temporal artery is a terminal branch of the external carotid artery, running close to the tragus within the subcutaneous tissue and bifurcating in the temporal region 2 cm above the zygomatic arch. The frontal branch gives rise to many twigs in the frontal area and finally anastomoses with the supraorbital artery of the ophthalmic artery. The parietal branch supplies the parietal, temporal, and occipital areas, anastomosing with the contralateral parietal branch and the posterior auricular and occipital arteries. Its collateral arteries are the transverse artery of the face, the temporal artery, and the zygomatic-orbital artery. The superficial temporal artery could be a useful landmark indicating the position of the frontal nerve that runs 1 cm caudal and parallel to its frontal branch [55].

The facial nerve divides into temporal and zygomatic branches within the parotid gland. The temporal branch of the facial nerve is located in the same plane as the superficial fat pad, both being in the subgaleal space; however, the presence of a sizable twig of the middle division of the temporal branch of the facial nerve (frontal ramus) going into the intrafascial space and then entering the frontalis muscle has been described [2]. The temporal branch pierces the parotid-masseteric fascia below the zygomatic arch and then immediately divides into its terminal branches: anterior, middle, and posterior [54]; in particular, the point where the temporal branch of the facial nerve gives off the anterior and middle rami is located 2–2.5 cm anterior to the tragus (range, 1.5–3.5 cm). The anterior ramus innervates the corrugator supercilii and orbicularis oculi muscles, while the middle one (frontal ramus) innervates the frontalis muscle; the posterior ramus, which innervates auricular and tragus muscles, does not have any practical importance in man [2]. In particular the general course of the frontal ramus, as described by Pitanguy and Ramos (Pitanguy line), begins 0.5 cm below the tragus and extends 1.5 cm above the lateral aspect of the eyebrow [38]. At the inferior border of the zygoma, it is deep to the temporoparietal fascia, then becomes superficial to the periosteum of the arch, and at the superior edge of the zygomatic arch, it is found in close proximity to the deep temporal fascia [48]. The branches of the facial nerve and its rami, which are variable in number, cross at the middle third of the zygomatic arch and may cover up more than half the length of the arch [4, 22].

The pterion is a region in the temporal fossa, localized about 4.0 cm above the zygomatic arch and 3.5 cm behind the frontozygomatic arch; it is defined as an H-shaped small circular area made by the junction of four bones: frontal, parietal, temporal, and sphenoid [29, 42, 44]. It is a meeting point of skull base, calvarium, and the skeleton part of facial anatomy and therefore has a different morphology [18]. Murphy defined four types of pteria: sphenoparietal, frontotemporal, epipteric, and stellate; the sphenoparietal and frontotemporal pteria present the straight line between the ends of the suture as the center of the pterion, while for the other types, the center is the smallest circle encompassing the edge of all bones (Fig. 11.5) [33]. This point is a landmark for the anterior branch of the middle meningeal artery, Broca's motor speech area to the left, insula, and the Sylvian cerebral fissure [50]; the pterion is also commonly used as an important guide for age estimation and sex determination in archeologically and forensic specimens [27].

Once performed, the pterional craniotomy, which would be detailed and described in the next paragraph, and the arachnoidal dissection with microsurgical technique, it is possible to expose and visualize the neurovascular structures of the anterior cranial fossa. Among them it is relevant to focus on the lamina terminalis. It is a translucent whitish membrane, made by a thin sheet of gray matter covered by a pial layer. It is at the base and front of the brain and forms most of the anterior wall of the third ventricle, together with the optic chiasm and the anterior commissure [41]. It is a triangular structure: the height is calculated as the distance between the midportion of the posterosuperior surface of the chiasm and the anterior commissure, while the base is the distance between the medial edges of the optic tracts (Fig. 11.6) [15]. It runs from the midportion of the superior surface of the optic chiasma to the inferior surface of the anterior commissure medially and the pillars of the fornix laterally, leaving

Fig. 11.5 The four types of pterional bone by Murphy's classification: (**a**) epipteric, (**b**) sphenoparietal, (**c**) frontotemporal, and (**d**) stellate. In (**a**) and (**d**) morphotypes, the pterion is the smallest circle encompassing the edge of other bones; in (**b**) and (**c**) morphotypes, the center of pterion is represented by the straight line between the ends of the sutures

a small cleft called optic recess, between the upper half of the chiasm and the lamina. The lamina has not a direct relationship to the hypothalamus, but it is closely laterally related to it [51].

The lamina terminalis cistern is located in the anterior incissural space, above the optic chiasm and delimitated superiorly by the rostrum of the corpus callosum, posteriorly by the lamina terminalis, and laterally by the portions of the medial surfaces of the frontal lobes. Important vascular structures are contained in the lamina terminalis cistern and are intimately related to the lamina terminalis: both A_1 tracts and the proximal A_2 tracts of the anterior cerebral arteries, the anterior communicating artery, perforating vessels, both recurrent Heubner arteries, both fronto-orbital arteries, arteries running to the hypothalamus, and anterior communicating and anterior cerebral

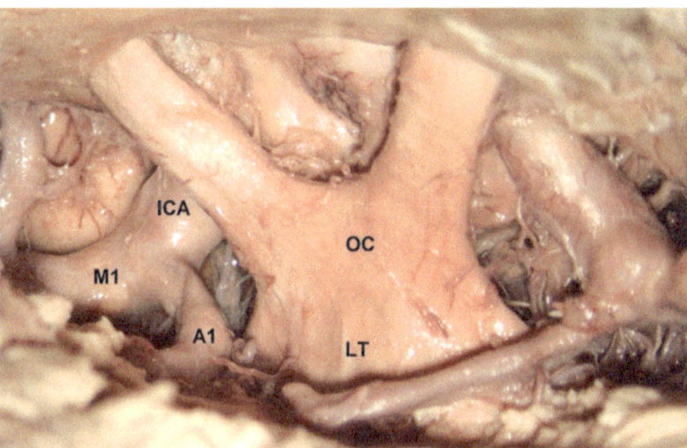

Fig. 11.6 The lamina terminalis (*LT*) seen after pterional craniotomy. It is at the base and front of the brain and forms most of the anterior wall of the third ventricle together with the optic chiasma (*OC*) and anterior commissure. Laterally, it is possible to identify the distal part of the internal carotid artery (*ICA*), the A1 tract of the anterior cerebral artery (*A1*), and the M1 portion of the middle cerebral artery (*M1*)

veins. In particular, the anterior cerebral artery, in its A_2 portion, passes in front of the lamina terminalis and the anterior wall of the third ventricle, reaching the rostrum of the corpus callosum in the anterior portion of the callosum cistern. The perforating vessels arise from the anterior cerebral and anterior communicating arteries and reach the hypothalamus through the optic chiasm and the infundibulum, or pass through the lamina terminalis to enter the wall of the third ventricle [15]. A pericallosal artery arising from the anterior communicating artery sometimes passes upward in front of the lamina terminalis, reaching the rostrum of the corpus callosum (Fig. 11.7) [3, 15].

The optic chiasm is a quadrilateral X-shaped structure, situated at the bottom of the brain, immediately below the hypothalamus. It is possible to describe three anatomical variations in the relationship between the optic chiasm and the sella turcica: the so-called normo-fixed variant, overlies the diaphragma sellae; the pre-fixed variant, located above the tuberculum sellae; and the post-fixed variant, situated superior to the dorsum sellae [39].

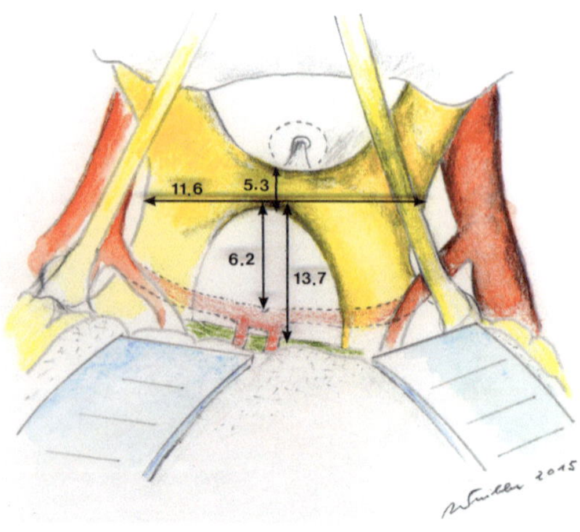

Fig. 11.7 The artistic drawing showing the relations, with related measurements, among the lamina terminalis, the optic chiasma, and the anterior communicating artery complex

11.4 Technique

A variety of operative approaches have been described as the optimal treatment for craniopharyngiomas, including the subfrontal, pterional, bifrontal interhemispheric, and transcallosal approaches [17, 28, 46, 52]. All the intracranial approaches are performed with the operating microscope, usually under moderate to high magnification. More recently the extended endoscopic endonasal transsphenoidal approach provides a new option for the treatment of craniopharyngiomas [7, 9, 10, 13, 14, 25]. Surgical adjuncts, including the ultrasonic aspirator and neuronavigation, should be available and utilized when appropriate.

The widely recognized advantage of the frontotemporal craniotomy is the enhanced exposure of deep neurovascular structures, which offers a shorter and wider view of the surgical target.

Moreover, the frontotemporal craniotomy offers the shortest and most direct route to the suprasellar region and, with splitting of the Sylvian fissure, minimizes or eliminates retraction of normal brain [53].

The patient is positioned supine on the surgical table with the legs flexed. The head is turned to the side contralateral to the approach about 30–60°, according to the exposure required, and secured to the Mayfield-Kees pin headrest. The single-pin arm is placed on the homolateral side: we use to fix it behind the ear, above the mastoid process, within the parietal bone. The two-pin arm is fixed on the contralateral site: the anterior pin inside the frontal bone, behind the hairline, near the pupillary line, and the posterior placed over the parietal bone, on the superior temporal line. The neurosurgeon has to prevent any penetration in the temporal muscle, which would increase instability of the head and postoperative displeasure. The vertex of the head is then tilted down 10–15°, so that the malar eminence is almost the highest edge of the surgical field. Once the patient is well fixed to the operating table, it is important to raise the thorax 10–15°, which ensures the reduction of venous distension, since the head is marginally above the level of the heart.

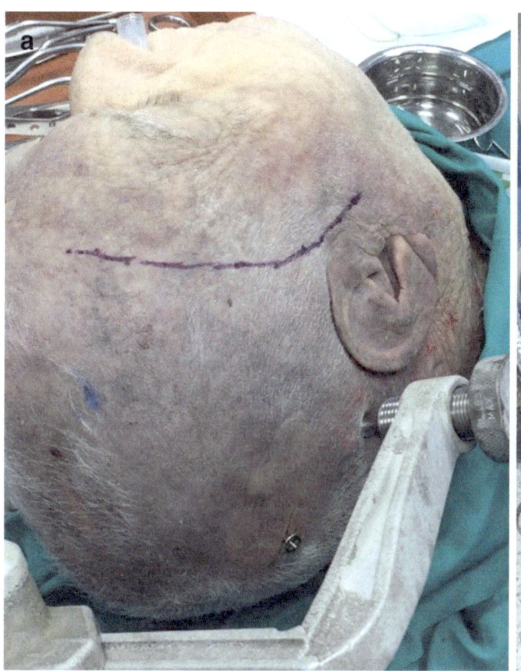

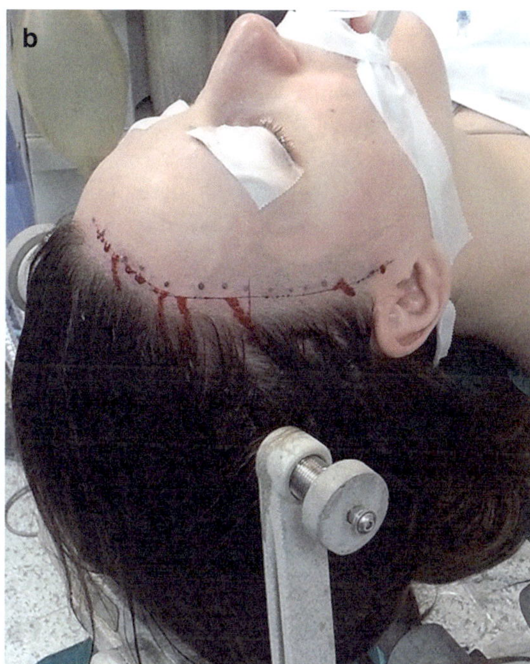

Fig. 11.8 (**a**) Cadaver positioning (**b**): patient positioning. The head is turned to the side contralateral to the approach by about 45° and the vertex is tilted down 12° so that the malar eminence is almost the highest edge of the surgical field. Mayfield-Kees pin headrest is blocked in this way: single-pin arm is fixed behind the ear, above the mastoid process; two-pin arm fixed on the contralateral site with the anterior pin placed over the frontal bone, behind the hairline, near to the pupillary line and the posterior pin inside the parietal bone

During these procedures the surgeon must not overstretch the neck, to prevent venous drainage damage, as well as of the esophagus and trachea. Moreover, it is important to keep safe the cervical portion of the spine from any extreme rotation.

Correct positioning ensures an optimal viewing angle of the central cranial base, thus minimizing the use of spatulae on the cerebral lobes and providing the surgeon a natural retraction of frontal lobe (falling from the orbital roof) and temporal lobe (coming out from the sphenoid ridge) (Fig. 11.8).

Cautious disinfection of the skin and draping has to be performed before starting surgery.

The skin incision for the standard frontotemporal approach is performed in the standard fashion for a pterional craniotomy as described by Yasargil et al. [54]. A relaxing skin incision should be made in order to avoid inadvertent penetration of the pericranium and temporal fascia over the frontal and the temporal regions, respectively. It starts from the frontal region, and it is made in short segments, using a smooth dissector to prevent damage to the close neurovascular structures. Moreover, we suggest the use of Raney clips to manage the scalp hemostasis.

The galea and pericranium are reflected in one layer over the frontal bone (Fig. 11.9), and the skin flap is reflected anteriorly over the deep temporal fascia up to where the fat pad is visible through it. Before dissecting the temporal muscle, some important landmarks should be taken into account: the frontal branch of facial nerve, the zygomatic arch, the superior temporal line, and the supraorbital foramen. This latter, when identified, serves as a landmark for most medial extent of the dissection over the orbital edge.

Particular attention must be paid to the frontal branch of the facial nerve, as it is the most vulnerable neural structure during the exposure [2, 21, 34, 43]. It is important to perform blunt subgaleal dissection always to avoid harming the facial nerve and the superficial temporal artery (Fig. 11.10).

Once the galeocutaneous layer has been dissected, three different methods of temporal muscle dissection can be performed: interfascial, subfascial, or submuscular.

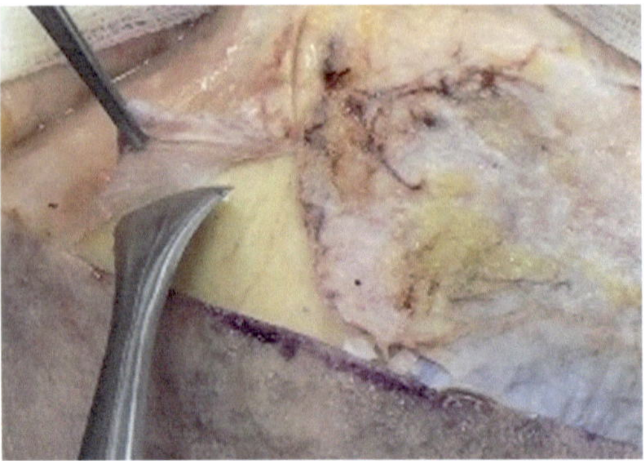

Fig. 11.9 Galea and pericranium are reflected in one layer over the frontal bone. The skin flap is reflected anteriorly over the deep temporal fascia up to where the fat pad is visible through it

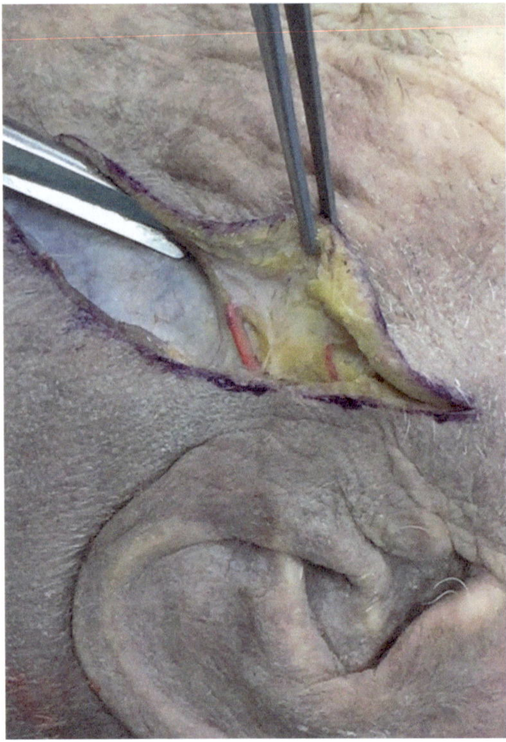

Fig. 11.10 Blunt subgaleal dissection in the preauricular area. It is possible to identify the frontal branch of the facial nerve and the superficial temporal artery beginning 0.5 cm below the tragus and extending 1.5 cm above the lateral aspect of the homolateral eyebrow (Pitanguy line)

In our experience, the risk of injury to the frontotemporal branch of the facial nerve is lower with the submuscular approach and offers a valid alternative to the interfascial technique [11].

To expose the temporal fascia, scalp and temporal submuscular dissection is performed with careful attention to anatomical landmarks in the subgaleal plane. When it is possible to detect the superficial layer of the temporal fascia, the temporal muscle is cut and dissected free from the temporal bone, leaving the temporal fascia with its fat envelope in situ, covering the muscle. It is important to follow the posterior-to-anterior direction of the fibers near the zygoma, going along the superior temporal line, to avoid tearing the muscle from the deeper part of the temporal fossa. Monopolar coagulation should be avoided to prevent atrophy of the temporal muscle, due to loss of the vascular supply. Once fishhooks are fixed to the muscle, the bony temporal surface is clearly exposed (Fig. 11.11).

The pterional craniotomy is performed with one burr hole alongside the squama temporalis, just under the temporal muscle, where the bony surface is thinner, in order to provide a better aesthetic outcome (Fig. 11.12). A craniotome is then

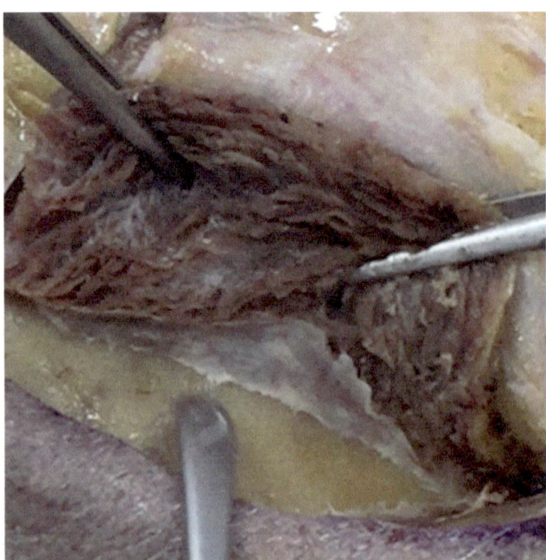

Fig. 11.11 The temporal muscle is dissected following the posterior-to-anterior direction of the fibers

inserted into the burr hole, and the craniotomy is realized upward in a curvilinear fashion, over the parietal bone, finishing over the spheno-temporal suture. Then, we prefer to finalize the craniotomy using a high-speed drill, to groove the bone over the zygomatic-sphenoidal suture and then spanning the greater wing of the sphenoid near the line of the zygoma. This method assures a sharp and safe fracture line across the sphenoid when raising the bone flap.

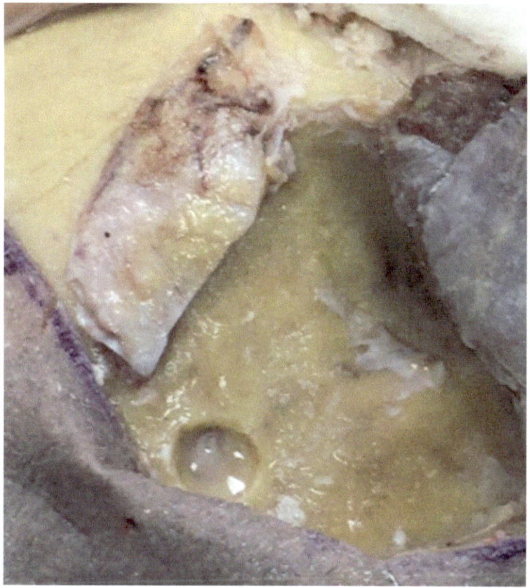

Fig. 11.12 The single burr hole performed alongside the thin squama temporalis, just under the temporalis muscle

The bone flap is elevated carefully and the dura has to be detached from the inner surface with a blunt dissector (Fig. 11.13). When the flap has been removed, the lesser wing of the sphenoid is drilled down to optimize the most basal trajectory to the skull base and obtain a wider operative corridor and a shorter distance to the tumor. Surgical microscope magnification is crucial to flatten the orbital roof with a diamond burr, and great caution has to be paid to prevent unplanned damage to surrounding structures.

Once the sphenoid wing is drilled off, the incision of the orbitotemporal periosteal fold (OTPF, also known as the meningo-orbital band or the frontotemporal dural fold) is performed (Fig. 11.14) [20]. This procedure allows a wider opening of the space between the frontal dura

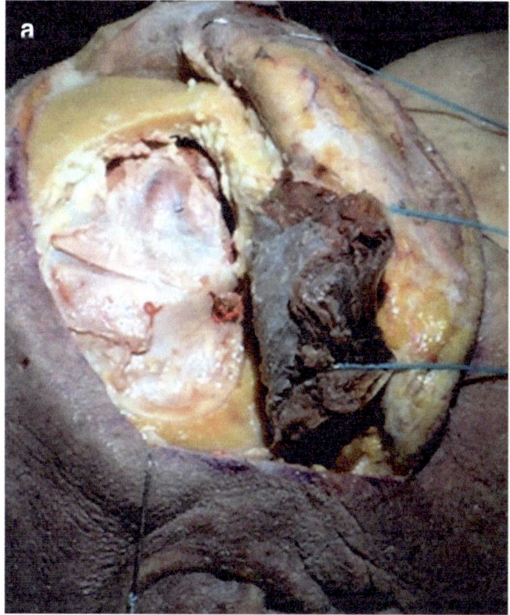

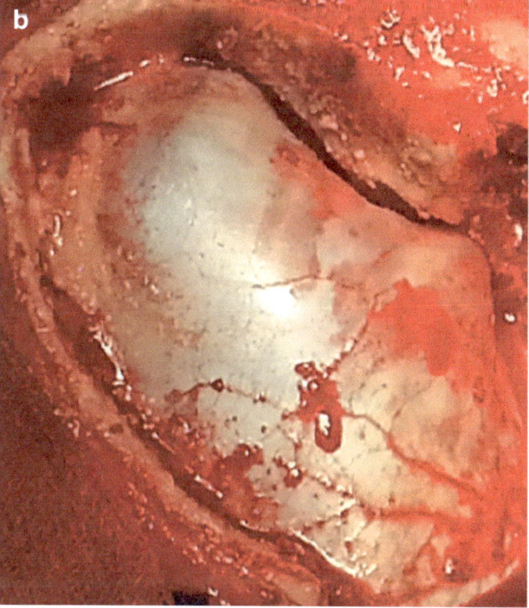

Fig. 11.13 (**a**) Cadaver, (**b**) patient. Temporal muscle is fixed by fishhooks. It is possible to observe the curvilinear fashion craniotomy performed from the parietal bone to the sphenotemporal suture. After the removal of the bone flap and the drilling of the large sphenoidal wing, it is possible to see the dura covering the temporal and frontal lobes and the Sylvian fissure

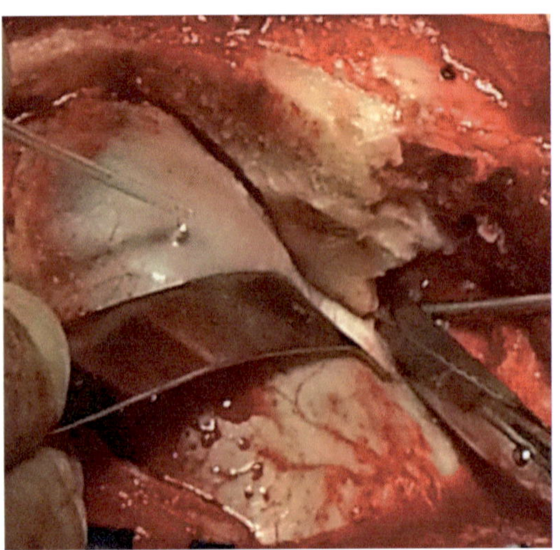

Fig. 11.14 Incision of the orbitotemporal periosteal fold with microsurgical technique, holding the dural surface in safe position

and the orbital apex, thus providing a proper and easier drilling of the anterior clinoid process [26].

Now the dura can be opened. The incision is made in a flap-wise semicircular microscope assisted fashion. The dural flap is reflected toward the greater sphenoidal wing previously drilled off, to improve the parasellar visualization and then retracted using 3/0 Vicryl stitches. A slight retraction of the frontal lobe allows exposure of the carotid, lamina terminalis cisterns, Sylvian fissure, inferior frontal gyrus, superior temporal gyrus, and middle temporal gyrus. Early release of cerebrospinal fluid from these cisterns allows optimal brain relaxation and minimizes the use of spatulae.

The dissection of the Sylvian fissure is typically undertaken in a distal-to-proximal direction.

Beginning at the level of the opercular part of the inferior frontal gyrus, the dissection extends following the axis of the middle cerebral artery, to avoid parenchymal harm. Bipolar coagulation has to be avoided to prevent arachnoidal plane adhesions (Fig. 11.15).

Opening of the Sylvian fissure can be facilitated using planes. Toth's water dissection is a gentle microsurgical method that works better than a "destructive knife" [31]. The "water jet dissection technique" described by Toth et al. [47] is a very simple and effective method, not requiring any expensive devices, but just low pressure water. Once the cistern has been opened, it is possible to early visualize the ICA with its bifurcation and the optic nerve.

When retracting the frontal lobe, the surgeon should avoid excessive displacement and stretching of the olfactory nerve. So, we eventually recommend to perform a sharp microsurgical dissection of the olfactory nerve from its arachnoidal envelope, since it is fully mobilized from a proximal-to-distal direction, to early identify the olfactory bulb (Fig. 11.16) [8].

These maneuvers maximize the exposure of the skull base by allowing the frontal lobe to be spatuled away from the orbit. Once this step has been completed, dural take-up sutures can be placed circumferentially to minimize bleeding from the epidural space. Working in the prechiasmatic, optico-carotid, and carotid-tentorial triangles, it is crucial to maintain an arachnoidal plane between the intact tumor and the neurovascular structures.

It is then possible the fenestration and the drainage of the fluid contained in the cysts and the debulking of solid components of the tumor. We suggest to always take care in preserving the capsule of a craniopharyngioma. Once these steps are completed, by working in the parachiasmal spaces and maintaining arachnoidal planes, it is possible to progressively dissect the tumor free from the optic nerves, the inferior side of the optic chiasm, and the carotid artery and its branches. Manipulation of the optic nerves, chiasm, and tracts should be minimized, since these structures can be injured by traction over the sharp, fixed edge of the dura proprium. Both the optic nerves and/or the chiasm may be pinched between the anterior cerebral artery above and the tumor below.

An attempt is always made to identify and preserve the pituitary stalk. When the stalk cannot be separated from the tumor, it is sectioned as distally as possible. After the tumor is dissected free with microsurgical technique from the entire circle of Willis, the pituitary stalk, and the optic apparatus, the capsule is grasped and, with continuous traction and blunt dissection, the gliotic plane is developed, which allows the tumor to be

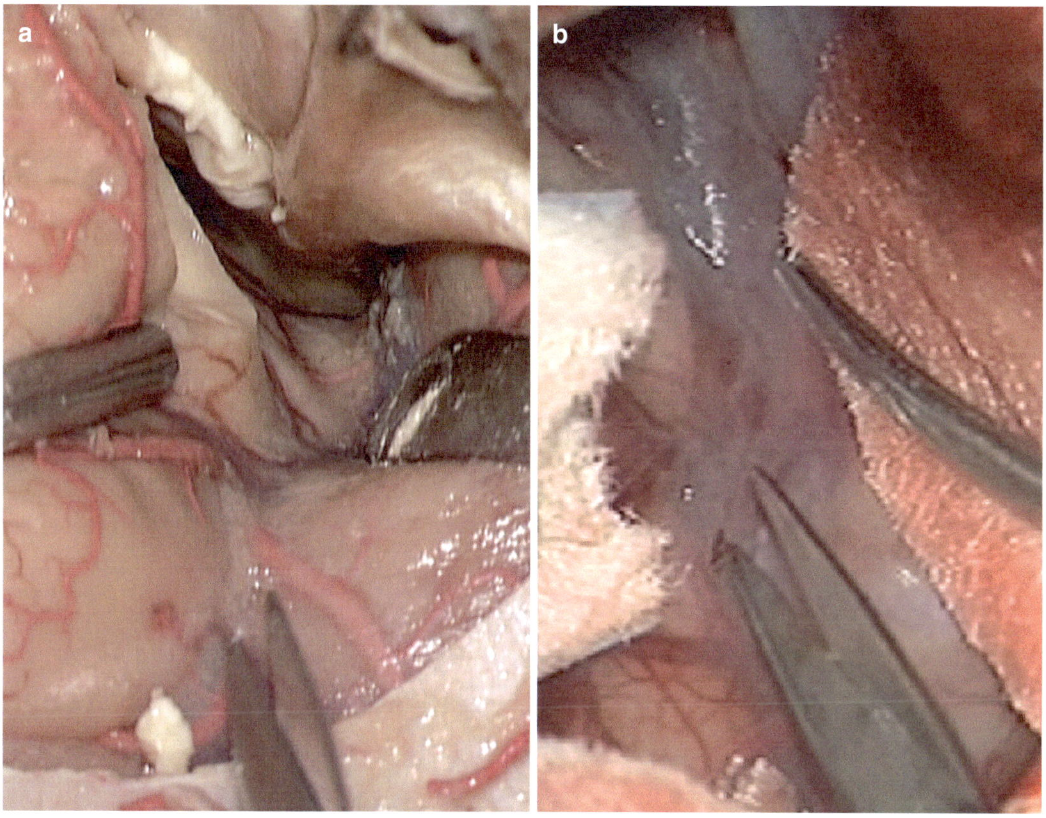

Fig. 11.15 (**a**) Cadaver, (**b**) patient. Dissection of the Sylvian fissure. It is performed in a distal-to-proximal direction, from the opercular part of the inferior frontal gyrus following the axis of the middle cerebral artery

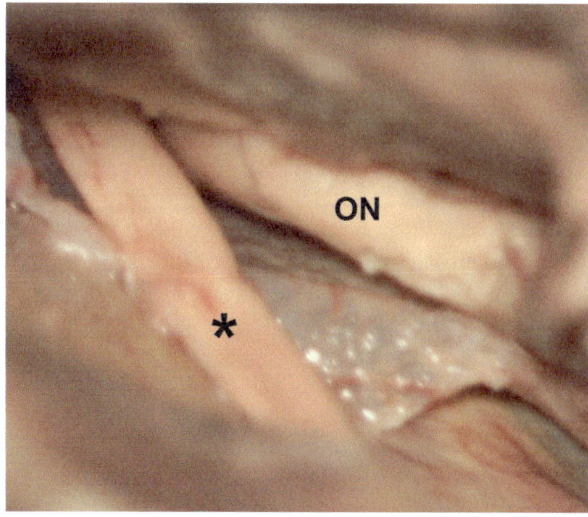

Fig. 11.16 After the retraction of the frontal lobe, it is possible to see the olfactory nerve (*) and the optic nerve (*ON*)

delivered from its attachment to the hypothalamus in the region of the tuber cinereum. After the tumor has been cleared, the whole cleavage plane must be observed for possible remnants. Endoscopic techniques allow to visualize around surgical tight corridors without brain retraction: the main advantage is to reach structures otherwise hidden.

If the tumor extends into the third ventricle or has a significant retrochiasmatic component, it can be approached through the lamina terminalis, by performing a fenestration in its lowest portion on the midline, immediately above the chiasm (Fig. 11.17). To complete the surgical tumor removal, we take advantage of the endoscopic technique for exploring the surgical field. The endoscopes 0°, 30°, and 45° are carefully introduced along the previous Sylvian access, and once the chiasm is identified, it reaches the third ventricle through the lamina terminalis, identifying tumor remnants that are subsequently removed by microsurgical technique.

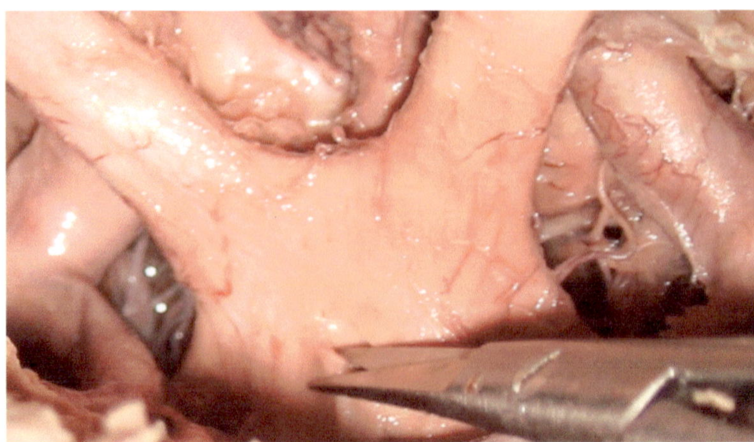

Fig. 11.17 Lamina terminalis is included in lowest portion on the midline, immediately above the chiasma

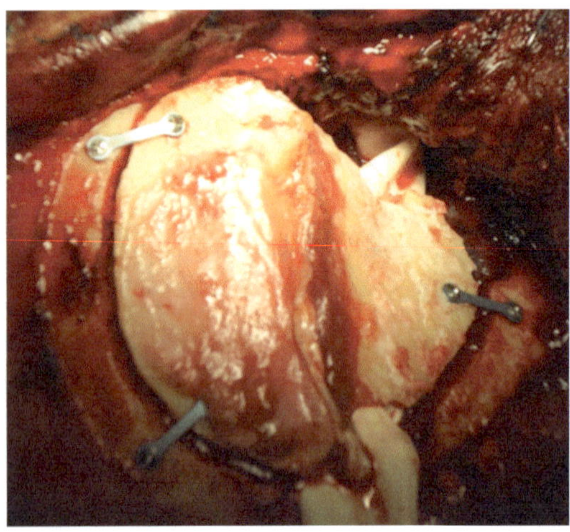

Fig. 11.18 The bone operculum is fixed by plates and screws in the cranial region

If the tumor extends into the sella turcica, it could be necessary to remove the posterior planum sphenoidale and tuberculum sellae to access properly the sella [36] or a combined endoscopic endonasal approach can be planned.

After tumor removal, carefully hemostasis has to be performed. The dura mater is sutured with 4/0 stitches. The suture should be watertight, and it is usually performed using the surgical microscope. After water-injection-verify, the spots not perfectly closed can be sealed by placing galea patches or etherologus materials with fibrin glue.

The bone operculum is fixed by titanium plates and screws and the temporal muscle is sutured with 2/0 Vicryl stitches by running suture (Fig. 11.18).

Underskin and skin layers are sutured respectively with 3/0 Vicryl stitches and 2/0 Nylon stitches. The wound can be closed by performing a tight running suture.

To prevent any formation of subcutaneous blood collection, a small vacuum drainage is placed in subgaleal space, which is removed on POD 3.

Acknowledgement The editors wish to thank Peter A. Winkler for the original drawing prepared for this chapter.

References

1. Agarwal CA, Mendenhall SD 3rd, Foreman KB, Owsley JQ (2010) The course of the frontal branch of the facial nerve in relation to fascial planes: an anatomic study. Plast Reconstr Surg 125(2):532–537. doi:10.1097/PRS.0b013e3181c82e9d
2. Ammirati M, Spallone A, Ma J, Cheatham M, Becker D (1993) An anatomicosurgical study of the temporal branch of the facial nerve. Neurosurgery 33(6):1038–1043; discussion 1044
3. Apuzzo MLJ, Litofsky NS (1993) Surgery in and around the anterior third ventricle. In: Brain surgery: complication avoidance and management. Churchill Livingstone, New York, pp 541–579
4. Bernstein L, Nelson RH (1984) Surgical anatomy of the extraparotid distribution of the facial nerve. Arch Otolaryngol 110(3):177–183
5. Bladowska J, Zimny A, Guzinski M, Halon A, Tabakow P, Czyz M, Czapiga B, Jarmundowicz W, Sasiadek MJ (2013) Usefulness of perfusion weighted magnetic resonance imaging with signal-intensity curves analysis in the differential diagnosis of sellar and parasellar tumors: preliminary report. Eur J Radiol 82(8):1292–1298. doi:10.1016/j.ejrad.2013.01.033

6. Brassier G, Morandi X, Tayiar E, Riffaud L, Chabert E, Heresbach N, Poirier JY, Carsin-Nicol B (1999) Rathke's cleft cysts: surgical-MRI correlation in 16 symptomatic cases. J Neuroradiol 26(3):162–171
7. Cappabianca P, Cavallo LM, Esposito F, De Divitiis O, Messina A, De Divitiis E (2008) Extended endoscopic endonasal approach to the midline skull base: the evolving role of transsphenoidal surgery. Adv Tech Stand Neurosurg 33:151–199
8. Cardali S, Romano A, Angileri FF, Conti A, La Torre D, de Divitiis O, d'Avella D, Tschabitscher M, Tomasello F (2005) Microsurgical anatomic features of the olfactory nerve: relevance to olfaction preservation in the pterional approach. Neurosurgery 57(1 Suppl):17–21; discussion 17–21
9. Cavallo LM, de Divitiis O, Aydin S, Messina A, Esposito F, Iaconetta G, Talat K, Cappabianca P, Tschabitscher M (2007) Extended endoscopic endonasal transsphenoidal approach to the suprasellar area: anatomic considerations – part 1. Neurosurgery 61:ONS-24–ONS-34
10. Cavallo LM, Frank G, Cappabianca P, Solari D, Mazzatenta D, Villa A, Zoli M, D'Enza AI, Esposito F, Pasquini E (2014) The endoscopic endonasal approach for the management of craniopharyngiomas: a series of 103 patients. J Neurosurg 121(1):100–113. doi:10.3171/2014.3.JNS131521
11. Coscarella E, Vishteh AG, Spetzler RF, Seoane E, Zabramski JM (2000) Subfascial and submuscular methods of temporal muscle dissection and their relationship to the frontal branch of the facial nerve. Technical note. J Neurosurg 92(5):877–880. doi:10.3171/jns.2000.92.5.0877
12. Cushing H (1932) The craniopharyngiomas. In: Intracranial tumors: notes upon a series of two thousand verified cases with surgical mortality percentages pertaining thereto. Charles C Thomas, Springfield, pp 93–98
13. de Divitiis E, Cappabianca P, Cavallo LM (2002) Endoscopic transsphenoidal approach: adaptability of the procedure to different sellar lesions. Neurosurgery 51(3):699–705; discussion 705–707
14. de Divitiis E, Cavallo LM, Cappabianca P, Esposito F (2007) Extended endoscopic endonasal transsphenoidal approach for the removal of suprasellar tumors: Part 2. Neurosurgery 60(1):46–58; discussion 58–59
15. de Divitiis O, Angileri FF, d'Avella D, Tschabitscher M, Tomasello F (2002) Microsurgical anatomic features of the lamina terminalis. Neurosurgery 50(3):563–569; discussion 569–570
16. Elliott RE, Hsieh K, Hochm T, Belitskaya-Levy I, Wisoff J, Wisoff JH (2010) Efficacy and safety of radical resection of primary and recurrent craniopharyngiomas in 86 children. J Neurosurg Pediatr 5(1):30–48. doi:10.3171/2009.7.PEDS09215
17. Fahlbusch R, Honegger J, Paulus W, Huk W, Buchfelder M (1999) Surgical treatment of craniopharyngiomas: experience with 168 patients. J Neurosurg 90(2):237–250
18. Feng WF, Qi ST, Huang SP, Huang LJ (2005) [Surgical treatment of anterior circulation aneurysm via pterion keyhole approach]. Di Yi Jun Yi Da Xue Xue Bao 25(12):1546–1548, 1551
19. Freeman MP, Kessler RM, Allen JH, Price AC (1987) Craniopharyngioma: CT and MR imaging in nine cases. J Comput Assist Tomogr 11(5):810–814
20. Froelich SC, Aziz KM, Levine NB, Theodosopoulos PV, van Loveren HR, Keller JT (2007) Refinement of the extradural anterior clinoidectomy: surgical anatomy of the orbitotemporal periosteal fold. Neurosurgery 61(5 Suppl 2):179–185; discussion 185–176. doi:10.1227/01.neu.0000303215.76477.cd
21. Gonzalez LF, Crawford NR, Horgan MA, Deshmukh P, Zabramski JM, Spetzler RF (2002) Working area and angle of attack in three cranial base approaches: pterional, orbitozygomatic, and maxillary extension of the orbitozygomatic approach. Neurosurgery 50(3):550–555; discussion 555–557
22. Gosain AK, Sewall SR, Yousif NJ (1997) The temporal branch of the facial nerve: how reliably can we predict its path? Plast Reconstr Surg 99(5):1224–1233; discussion 1234–1226
23. Harwood-Nash DC (1994) Neuroimaging of childhood craniopharyngioma. Pediatr Neurosurg 21:2–10
24. Jane JA Jr, Laws ER (2006) Craniopharyngioma. Pituitary 9:323–326
25. Koutourousiou M, Gardner PA, Fernandez-Miranda JC, Tyler-Kabara EC, Wang EW, Snyderman CH (2013) Endoscopic endonasal surgery for craniopharyngiomas: surgical outcome in 64 patients. J Neurosurg 119(5):1194–1207. doi:10.3171/2013.6.JNS122259
26. Lehmberg J, Krieg SM, Meyer B (2014) Anterior clinoidectomy. Acta Neurochir 156(2):415–419; discussion 419. doi:10.1007/s00701-013-1960-1
27. Lovejoy CO, Meindl RS, Mensforth RP, Barton TJ (1985) Multifactorial determination of skeletal age at death: a method and blind tests of its accuracy. Am J Phys Anthropol 68(1):1–14. doi:10.1002/ajpa.1330680102
28. Maira G, Anile C, Rossi GF, Colosimo C (1995) Surgical treatment of craniopharyngiomas: an evaluation of the transsphenoidal and pterional approaches. Neurosurgery 36(4):715–724
29. Moore KL, Dalley AF (1999) Clinically oriented anatomy, 4th edn. Lippincott Williams & Wilkins, Baltimore, pp 836–842
30. Morana G, Maghnie M, Rossi A (2010) Pituitary tumors: advances in neuroimaging. Endocr Dev 17:160–174. doi:10.1159/000262537
31. Nagy L, Ishii K, Karatas A, Shen H, Vajda J, Niemela M, Jaaskelainen J, Hernesniemi J, Toth S (2006) Water dissection technique of Toth for opening neurosurgical cleavage planes. Surg Neurol 65(1):38–41; discussion 41. doi:10.1016/j.surneu.2005.08.025
32. Naylor MF, Scheithauer BW, Forbes GS, Tomlinson FH, Young WF (1995) Rathke cleft cyst: CT, MR, and pathology of 23 cases. J Comput Assist Tomogr 19(6):853–859
33. Oguz O, Sanli SG, Bozkir MG, Soames RW (2004) The pterion in Turkish male skulls. Surg Radiol Anat 26(3):220–224. doi:10.1007/s00276-003-0210-2

34. Oikawa S, Mizuno M, Muraoka S, Kobayashi S (1996) Retrograde dissection of the temporalis muscle preventing muscle atrophy for pterional craniotomy. Technical note. J Neurosurg 84(2):297–299. doi:10.3171/jns.1996.84.2.0297
35. Osborn A (2012) Osborn's brain: imaging, pathology and anatomy. Amirsys Pub, Salt Lake City
36. Patterson RH Jr, Danylevich A (1980) Surgical removal of craniopharyngiomas by the transcranial approach through the lamina terminalis and sphenoid sinus. Neurosurgery 7(2):111–117
37. Pigeau I, Sigal R, Halimi P, Comoy J, Doyon D (1988) MRI features of craniopharyngiomas at 1.5 tesla. A series of 13 cases. J Neuroradiol 15(3):276–287
38. Pitanguy I, Ramos AS (1966) The frontal branch of the facial nerve: the importance of its variations in face lifting. Plast Reconstr Surg 38(4):352–356
39. Renn WH, Rhoton AL Jr (1975) Microsurgical anatomy of the sellar region. J Neurosurg 43(3):288–298
40. Rennert J, Doerfler A (2007) Imaging of sellar and parasellar lesions. Clin Neurol Neurosurg 109(2):111–124. doi:10.1016/j.clineuro.2006.11.001
41. Rhoton AL Jr (1987) Microsurgical anatomy of the third ventricular region. In: Surgery of the third ventricle. Williams & Wilkins, Baltimore, pp 92–167
42. Saxena RC, Bilodi AK, Mane SS, Kumar A (2003) Study of pterion in skulls of Awadh area–in and around Lucknow. Kathmandu Univ Med J 1(1):32–33
43. Spetzler RF, Lee KS (1990) Reconstruction of the temporalis muscle for the pterional craniotomy. Technical note. J Neurosurg 73(4):636–637. doi:10.3171/jns.1990.73.4.0636
44. Standring S, Ellis H, Healy JC, Johnson D (2005) Gray's anatomy, 39th edn. Elsevier Churchill Livingstone, Philadelphia, pp 442–471
45. Sutton LN, Wang ZJ, Wehrli SL, Marwaha S, Molloy P, Phillips PC, Zimmerman RA (1997) Proton spectroscopy of suprasellar tumors in pediatric patients. Neurosurgery 41(2):388–394; discussion 394–385
46. Tomita T, McLone DG (1993) Radical resections of childhood craniopharyngiomas. Pediatr Neurosurg 19(1):6–14
47. Toth S, Vajda J, Pasztor E, Toth Z (1987) Separation of the tumor and brain surface by "water jet" in cases of meningiomas. J Neurooncol 5(2):117–124
48. Trussler AP, Stephan P, Hatef D, Schaverien M, Meade R, Barton FE (2010) The frontal branch of the facial nerve across the zygomatic arch: anatomical relevance of the high-SMAS technique. Plast Reconstr Surg 125(4):1221–1229. doi:10.1097/PRS.0b013e3181d18136
49. Tsuda M, Takahashi S, Higano S, Kurihara N, Ikeda H, Sakamoto K (1997) CT and MR imaging of craniopharyngioma. Eur Radiol 7(4):464–469. doi:10.1007/s003300050184
50. Urzi F, Iannello A, Torrisi A, Foti P, Mortellaro NF, Cavallaro M (2003) Morphological variability of pterion in the human skull. Ital J Anat Embryol 108(2):83–117
51. Yamamoto I, Rhoton AL Jr, Peace DA (1981) Microsurgery of the third ventricle: part I. Microsurgical anatomy. Neurosurgery 8(3):334–356
52. Yasargil MG (1996) Craniopharyngiomas. In: Microneurosurgery IVB: microneurosurgery of CNS tumors. Thieme Medical Publishers, New York, pp 205–216
53. Yasargil MG, Curcic M, Kis M, Siegenthaler G, Teddy PJ, Roth P (1990) Total removal of craniopharyngiomas. Approaches and long-term results in 144 patients. J Neurosurg 73(1):3–11
54. Yasargil MG, Reichman MV, Kubik S (1987) Preservation of the frontotemporal branch of the facial nerve using the interfascial temporalis flap for pterional craniotomy. Technical article. J Neurosurg 67(3):463–466. doi:10.3171/jns.1987.67.3.0463
55. Youssef AS, Ahmadian A, Ramos E, Vale F, van Loveren HR (2012) Combined subgaleal/myocutaneous technique for temporalis muscle dissection. J Neurol Surg Part B Skull Base 73(6):387–393. doi:10.1055/s-0032-1326778
56. Zacharia BE, Bruce SS, Goldstein H, Malone HR, Neugut AI, Bruce JN (2012) Incidence, treatment and survival of patients with craniopharyngioma in the surveillance, epidemiology and end results program. Neuro Oncol 14(8):1070–1078. doi:10.1093/neuonc/nos142
57. Zimmerman RA (1990) Imaging of intrasellar, suprasellar, and parasellar tumors. Semin Roentgenol 25(2):174–197

Supraorbital Approach

12

Masahiro Tanji, Ibironke Ogunbameru, Garni Barkhoudarian, and Daniel F. Kelly

Abbreviations

CSF	Cerebrospinal fluid
EEA	Endonasal endoscopic approach
ICA	Internal carotid artery
MRI	Magnetic resonance imaging
SO	Supraorbital eyebrow approach
SRT	Stereotactic radiotherapy

12.1 Introduction

Craniopharyngiomas represent one of the most challenging brain tumors to treat. Surgical removal is the primary treatment, but complete removal is possible in only 50–70 % of cases. The surgical goal is maximal safe tumor removal with reversal of neurological deficits and complication avoidance. In recent years, minimally invasive keyhole approaches have been increasingly used to remove these tumors that may arise in the sellar, suprasellar, and parasellar regions. Of these approaches, the two most commonly used are the extended endonasal endoscopic transsphenoidal route and the supraorbital (SO) eyebrow craniotomy. Although both approaches may be appropriate for a given patient, in many cases, one route offers a better opportunity for safe and maximal tumor removal.

The most common growth pattern of craniopharyngiomas is into the retrochiasmal suprasellar space with displacement of the optic chiasm into a prefixed or superior location; this pathoanatomy facilitates endonasal endoscopic removal by allowing one to pass under the chiasm directly into the retrochiasmal space. In contrast, for craniopharyngiomas with extrasellar extensions lateral to the supraclinoid carotid arteries and/or into the anterior cranial fossa, a transcranial approach may be required. Given that a majority of craniopharyngiomas arise in the retrochiasmal space, the endonasal endoscopic route is our most commonly used approach for craniopharyngiomas. However, for craniopharyngiomas that require a craniotomy, the SO approach offers a potentially less-invasive alternative to the traditional pterional, cranio-orbito-zygomatic or bifrontal approaches. In our series of craniopharyngioma surgeries over the last 7 years, approximately 25 % had an SO approach while the remainder had an endonasal endoscopic approach.

Using an incision within the eyebrow and a small craniotomy that is flush with the orbital roof, the SO approach offers a direct anterolateral

Electronic supplementary material The online version of this chapter (doi:10.1007/978-3-319-21533-4_12) contains supplementary material, which is available to authorized users.

M. Tanji, MD • I. Ogunbameru, MD
G. Barkhoudarian, MD • D.F. Kelly, MD (✉)
Brain Tumor Center & Pituitary Disorders Program, John Wayne Cancer Institute and Saint John's Health Center, 2200 Santa Monica Blvd., Santa MoniCA CA 90404, USA
e-mail: kellyd@jwci.org

P. Cappabianca et al. (eds.), *Midline Skull Base Surgery*, DOI 10.1007/978-3-319-21533-4_12

subfrontal trajectory to the ipsilateral frontal fossa, orbitofrontal lobe, a wide medial portion of the contralateral frontal fossa, parasellar and suprasellar regions, Sylvian fissure, and the anterior aspect of the medial temporal lobe. The SO approach abides by the keyhole principle, of a small well-placed craniotomy that allows relatively wide access to deeper lesions with minimal need for fixed brain retraction. The potential advantages of this approach over conventional transcranial approaches include shorter operative times, reduced extent of scalp, muscle and bone dissection, reduced postoperative pain, a shorter hospital stay, and satisfactory cosmetic outcomes. Despite these potential benefits, the SO approach is technically demanding and poses similar risks and some additional challenges compared to conventional craniotomies and skull base approaches. There are some limitations in terms of exposure and maneuverability that are particularly important to consider before using this approach. With those cautions, the SO approach is considered ideal for removal of many suprasellar craniopharyngiomas, particularly those with extrasellar far lateral and anterior extensions. The use of endoscopy in addition to microscope further extends the range and versatility of this keyhole approach and is considered an essential adjunct for allowing safe and maximal tumor removal.

Herein, we discuss the key selection factors for using the SO approach in patients with a craniopharyngioma and detail technical aspects of the approach, highlighting potential pitfalls and methods of complication avoidance. The endonasal endoscopic and other approaches to craniopharyngiomas are discussed in other chapters in Part II.

12.2 Indications for Supraorbital Approach

The choice of a specific approach takes into consideration numerous factors including the tumor size, location, invasiveness, prior treatments, and the symptom of the patient [1, 2]. Based on our experience and others, the endonasal route is preferred for most retrochiasmal craniopharyngiomas and those lesions that are predominantly sellar [1–3] (Fig. 12.1). In contrast, for those craniopharyngiomas that are predominantly prechiasmal or with prominent lateral extensions, the supraorbital route may be preferred [1–3]. The SO approach provides excellent access for tumors that extend well lateral to the supraclinoid carotid arteries, an area that is difficult to safely access with the endonasal route. In some complex tumors with both prechiasmal and retrochiasmal extensions, either route may be appropriate. In addition, performing simultaneously an SO and an endonasal approach can be considered for lesions in which residual tumor would be anticipated if only one or the other approach were done [4]. The SO approach may also be used in young children with small nasal cavities and poorly pneumatized sinuses. Extremely narrow bilateral internal carotid artery (ICA) distance, the presence of severe sinusitis, and the presence of cavernous ICA aneurysms are relative contraindications of endonasal endoscopic approach and favor the SO approach (Fig. 12.2).

In patients with prior surgery with or without radiation, the SO approach may offer a more favorable route for recurrent craniopharyngiomas than the endonasal approach (Fig. 12.2) [5]. In addition to providing a trajectory that potentially avoids or minimizes dissection through scar tissue, the SO approach has the advantage of a simplified skull base reconstruction with a lower risk of postoperative CSF leak in the setting of recurrent tumors. The extensive scar tissue from the prior endonasal route or a nasoseptal flap in previously irradiated patients in whom the risk of postoperative CSF leak was thought to be relatively high can weigh favorably toward use of the SO approach (Table 12.1).

Regarding the side of approach, preoperative visual assessment and tumor location are key factors guiding the side of surgical approach. In general, if the tumor is predominantly located eccentrically to one side, approaching from that ipsilateral side is recommended. However, if the tumor is predominantly medial to an optic nerve in the prechiasmatic space, or under an optic nerve, approaching the lesion from the contralateral eyebrow may be advantageous.

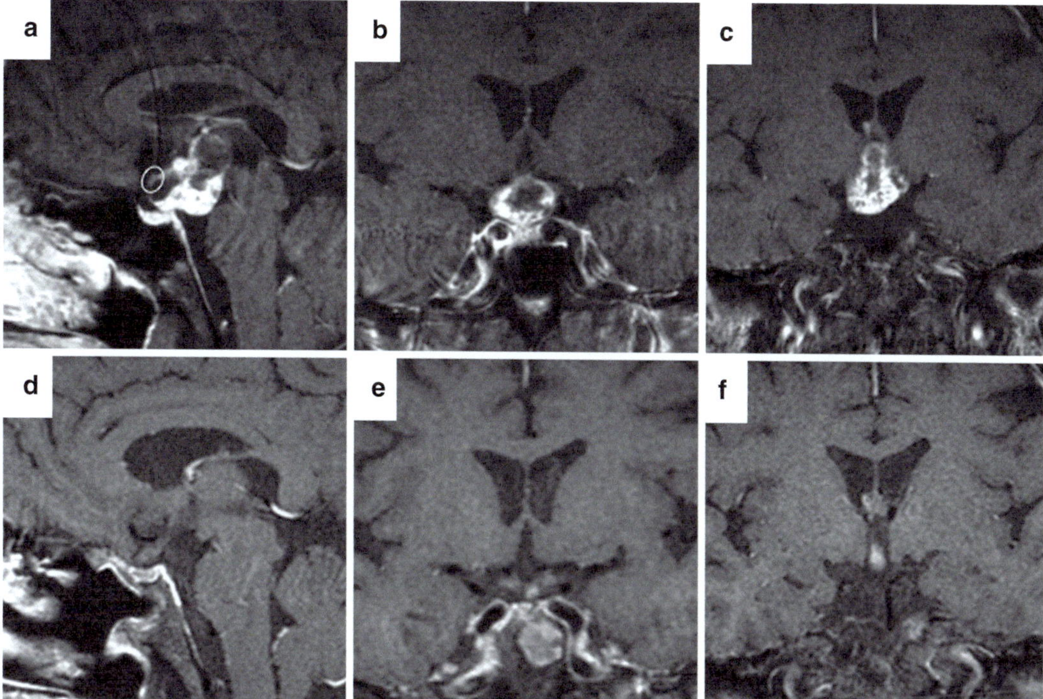

Fig. 12.1 MRI of a 52-year-old man with a visual loss and panhypopituitarism with a typical retrochiasmal craniopharyngioma. He underwent uneventful endonasal endoscopic gross total tumor resection. He is currently doing well more than 2 years after surgery with improved vision and on full pituitary hormone replacement therapy. *Top row*: Preoperative sagittal (**a**), and coronal (**b**, **c**) post-gadolinium MRI scans showing large cystic tumor extending into retrochiasmal and suprasellar space. *Circle* in **a** indicates position of the optic chiasm. *Bottom row*: Images **d–f** show corresponding 1-year postoperative sagittal and coronal MRIs confirming gross total tumor resection without evidence of recurrence.

This contralateral trajectory may avoid scar tissue from an original craniotomy and gives better access to the inferomedial aspect of the contralateral optic nerve. If there is prior severe or complete loss of vision in one eye, the approach may be optimally performed on this side in order to preserve the remaining eye. As detailed below, the size and extent of frontal sinus pneumatization is also a consideration in choosing the best side of approach with the choice being preferably to avoid entering the frontal sinus.

From 2007, we had 33 operations for 30 patients with craniopharyngiomas. Among the 33 operations, 9 operations were performed by the SO approach for 7 patients (27 % of total operations and 23 % of total patients). The remaining 23 operations were done by endonasal endoscopic approach and 1 operation by temporal craniotomy. Among the seven patients treated by SO approach, two patients had an SO for their first and only operation, and the remaining five patients had a previous endonasal endoscopic approach or a previous craniotomy. Two patients had a repeat SO approach.

12.3 Neuroradiology

Prior to surgery, the preoperative MRI including sellar/pituitary protocol must be carefully studied to determine which approach, endonasal endoscopic, SO, or alternative approach, is most suitable. The key anatomical relationships and structures to ascertain are the locations of the optic chiasm and nerves, the infundibulum, the pituitary gland, the circle of Willis vessels, and whether the tumor reaches the hypothalamus. The location and extent of the tumor will dictate

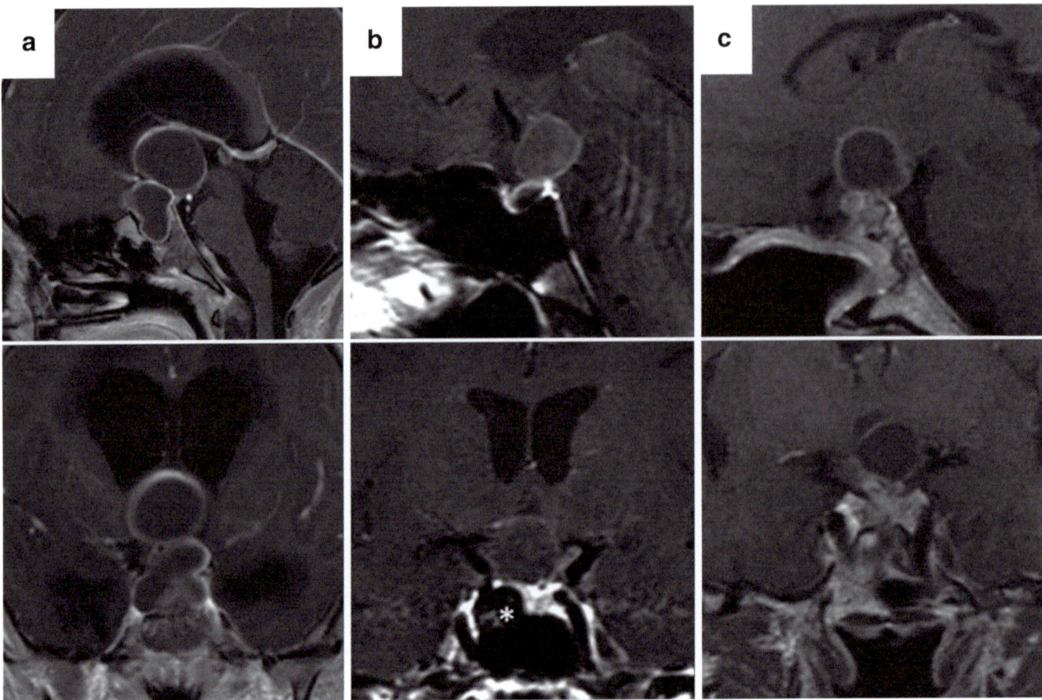

Fig. 12.2 Examples of MRIs of three patients who underwent the SO approach: (**a**): 6-year-old pediatric patient with small nostrils, and extensive cystic and solid craniopharyngioma with suprasellar and suprachiasmatic extension. (**b**) A 71-year-old woman with coexisting cavernous sinus and sellar aneurysm (*asterisk*) (**c**): A 51-year-old man who underwent prior endonasal endoscopic surgery and radiation with residual tumor and growing suprachiasmatic tumor cyst

Table 12.1 Advantages, disadvantages, and possible indications of the SO approach versus the endonasal route

	SO approach	Endonasal
Advantages	Enhanced exposure of lesions lateral to ICA Simplified skull base repair with reduced postoperative CSF leak	Enhanced exposure of sella and retrochiasmal area No brain retraction Enhanced view of the superior hypophyseal arteries
Disadvantages	Limited access to the retrochiasmal area compared to endonasal Brain retraction (rarely)	Restricted lateral access beyond ICAs and optic nerves Narrower surgical corridor More demanding skull base repair
Possible indications	Prechiasmal and suprachiasmal craniopharyngiomas Craniopharyngiomas with prominent lateral extension beyond ICAs Prior history of transsphenoidal surgery, transcranial surgery, and/or radiotherapy in whom there is extensive scar tissue and possibly limited endonasal options for skull base repair Young pediatric patients (<5 years old) with small nostrils and poorly pneumatized paranasal sinuses Cavernous sinus/intrasellar aneurysm	Most retrochiasmal craniopharyngiomas Sellar craniopharyngiomas

the likelihood of success with an SO approach or the potential need for a larger alternative craniotomy or endonasal route. Axial, coronal, and sagittal MRI sequences should be carefully reviewed to determine the lateral and anterior extent of the lesion. Probably the most important factor in choice of approach is the tumor location in relation to the optic chiasm and optic nerves (Figs. 12.1 and 12.2). This anatomical relationship is typically best appreciated on sagittal sellar images and T2-weighted coronal sellar images, but all sequences should be reviewed to provide the best possible three-dimensional understanding of the tumor. Although a pre-fixed optic chiasm may be a relative contraindication to the SO approach, in such cases, the SO approach still allows access through the lamina terminalis to tumor within the retrochiasmal space and third ventricle. Craniopharyngiomas with lateral extension beyond the supraclinoid carotid arteries or large anterior extensions are often best approached via the SO approach or the pterional route. Extension into the middle cranial fossa may necessitate a traditional pterional or minipterional craniotomy; however, in most cases, the SO route allows excellent access to the Sylvian fissure and the medial temporal lobe region.

Coronal and sagittal MRI sequences demonstrate the superior extent of the lesion, as well as involvement of the sella and sphenoid sinus. Craniopharyngiomas with significant sellar expansion are typically best approached via an endonasal endoscopic approach. Likewise, lesions with significant superior extension that extend into the third ventricle typically require the inferior-to-superior trajectory provided by the endonasal corridor; rarely such tumors can also be approached via an interhemispheric transventricular approach. Significant superior midline extension is a relative contraindication to the SO approach, as the flat trajectory along the floor of the frontal fossa may not provide access to the superior extent of the tumor.

Finally, the size and lateral extent of the frontal sinus should be considered in the approach decision. A large lateral extension of the frontal sinus may discourage one from using the SO approach, but in general this is only an issue in a minority of cases. If the planned craniotomy will likely enter the lateral edge of the sinus, then one should plan accordingly by prepping the patient for a possible abdominal fat graft or, less frequently, use of a pericranial flap to rotate over the defect.

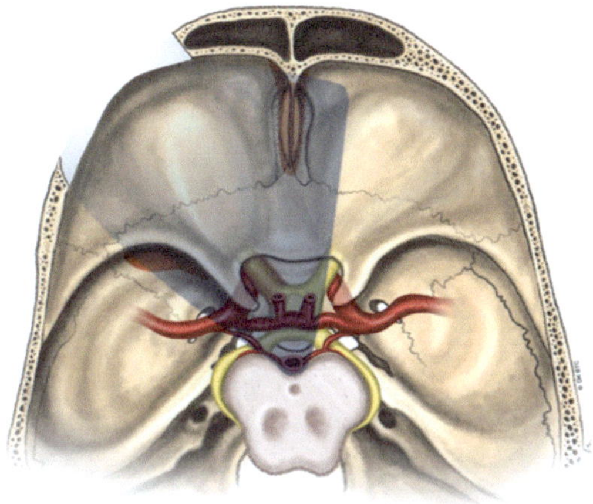

Fig. 12.3 Artistic drawing showing the extent of exposure of the SO approach: *shaded areas* including cribriform plate area, inferior space directly under ipsilateral optic nerve, ipsilateral medial middle fossa, and medial temporal lobe are difficult to visualize without endoscopy

12.4 Anatomy of the Approach

12.4.1 Anatomical Studies on SO Approach

By the SO approach, the field of view includes the ipsilateral frontal fossa, including the olfactory groove and planum, a portion of the medial contralateral frontal fossa, ipsilateral basal frontal lobe and frontal pole, the ipsilateral proximal Sylvian fissure, the medial temporal lobe, the lateral wall of cavernous sinus, the ipsilateral third nerve, the optico-carotid cistern, the suprasellar region including the optic chiasm and nerves (but only the medial and superior aspect of the contralateral optic nerve), the suprachiasmatic cistern, the perimesencephalic/interpeduncular cistern, the lamina terminalis, both supraclinoid carotid arteries, both A1 segments, the anterior communicating artery, both A2 segments, and the pituitary stalk (Fig. 12.3).

Additional dissection through the optico-carotid or carotid-oculomotor windows will expose the ventral brainstem, the basilar artery and ipsilateral posterior cerebral artery, and posterior communicating arteries and perforators.

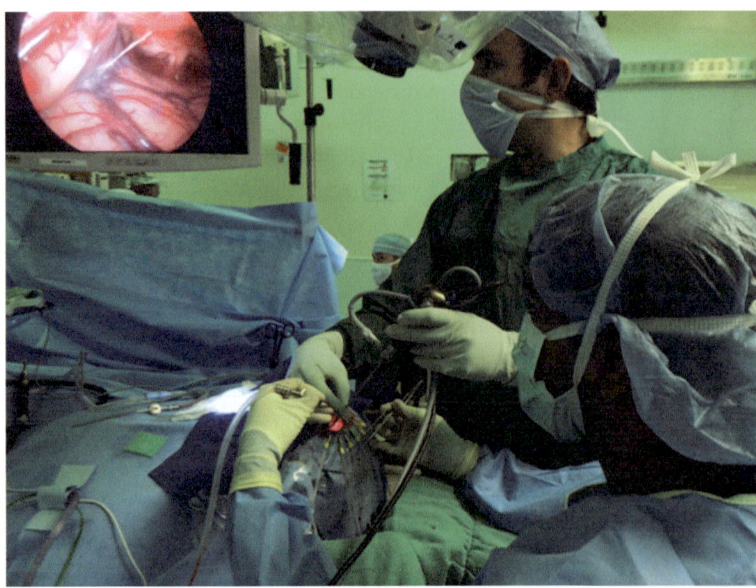

Fig. 12.4 Intraoperative photo showing a two-surgeon team using a rigid endoscope in the SO approach for visualization; the endoscope is being "driven" by an assistant allowing two-handed surgery by the primary surgeon

When necessary, the SO approach can be used to reach as far posteriorly and inferiorly to the ventral brainstem and top third of the clivus.

Recent anatomical studies have compared the surgical exposure afforded by the keyhole SO approach to standard transcranial approaches [6, 7]. Results showed that the working space deep within the surgical field obtained with the keyhole SO approach is similar to [7] or greater than [6] that obtained by the standard pterional approach. In contrast, the angular exposure appears to be increased with the orbitozygomatic approach or pterional approach due to the more extensive bony removal obtained [7]. Indeed, the pterional and orbitozygomatic craniotomy were able to offer significantly better angles of work in both the vertical and horizontal planes [7]. Similarly, other authors have shown that removal of the orbital rim in the transorbital keyhole approach increases the inferior projection of the inferior boundary of the craniotomy [6].

However, these measurements were performed using the surgical microscope. The introduction of the rigid endoscope to the SO approach either as an adjunctive visualization technique [1, 8, 9] or as the sole imaging modality [10] appears to broaden the surgical exposure without the need for additional bony removal or brain retraction (Fig. 12.4). The panoramic and multidirectional view obtained with the endoscope appears to lessen the need for the larger external openings afforded by conventional craniotomies [8, 10] (Fig. 12.5). With the use of a 30° or 45° angled endoscope, one can also visualize into areas not well seen with the microscope, including the cribriform plate region, under the ipsilateral optic nerve, along part of the ipsilateral medial sphenoid wing, over the tuberculum sellae into the pituitary fossa, and over the dorsum sellae into the prepontine cistern.

12.5 Surgical Technique

12.5.1 Overview, Instrumentation, and Monitoring

Several authors, including our group [1, 2, 5], have previously described the technical steps of the SO approach with subtle variations [3, 4, 11–14]. For all cases of craniopharyngiomas, intraoperative neuronavigation and evoked potential monitoring are used. Image guidance is helpful in evaluating the anticipated surgical trajectory and in mapping the frontal sinus. Evoked potential monitoring is helpful for cranial nerve monitoring and to monitor for any potential vascular compromise during surgery. The Doppler probe should also be available for all cases, as many if not most craniopharyngiomas will often abut or

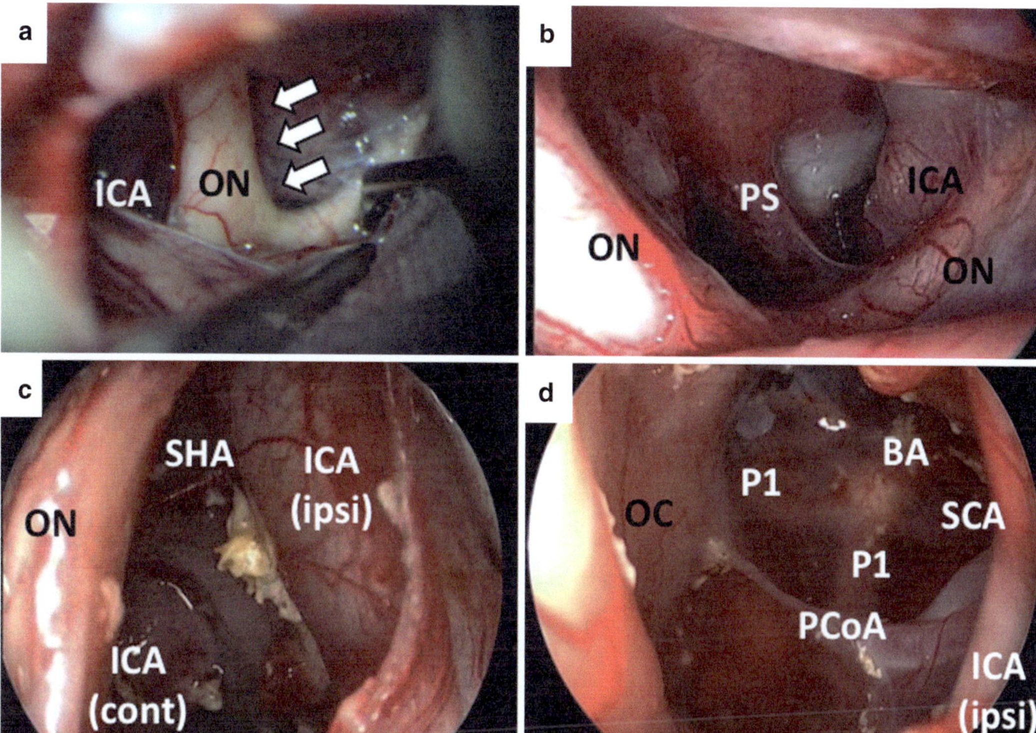

Fig. 12.5 Operative views of SO approach: (**a**) Right SO approach with microscope. *Arrow* indicates the blind spot under the ipsilateral optic nerve. (**b**) Endoscopic view of the right SO approach. Note the contralateral ICA and the PS though the prechiasmal space. (**c**, **d**) Endoscopic view of the left SO approach through the ipsilateral optico-carotid space after subtotal removal of recurrent suprasellar craniopharyngioma. In **c**, blind area behind the ipsilateral optic nerve by microscope is well visualized by endoscope. In **d**, deeper endoscopic view is provided through optico-carotid space. Posterior circulation is well visualized. The area under the optic chiasm is also visualized. *SHA* superior hypophyseal artery, *BA* basilar artery, *ICA* internal carotid artery, *OC* optic chiasm, *ON* optic nerve, *PCoA* posterior communicating artery, *PS* pituitary stalk, *P1* P1 segment of posterior cerebral artery, *SCA* superior cerebellar artery

encase at least one of the circle of Willis vessels [15]. Low-profile micro-instrumentation is essential to allow maximal maneuverability through the relatively narrow SO corridor. Most instruments should be bayoneted or pistol grip in design. Finally, 0°, 30° and 45° 4 mm rigid endoscopes should be available on all cases.

12.5.2 Positioning and Preparation

Proper positioning is necessary to optimize the reach of the SO approach. As previously described, the patient is placed in the supine position and the head fixated in a Mayfield head holder [3]. The table is placed in mild reverse Trendelenburg, and the head is elevated above the level of the heart to enhance venous drainage. The neck is slightly extended with the head above the heart level, and the head is rotated to the contralateral side between 20° and 30° depending on the location of the tumor and its pattern of extension. Head extension, with the vertex angled back toward the floor, is an important maneuver that allows gravity to work in the surgeon's favor and obviates the need for fixed retraction in opening the subfrontal corridor through which the surgeon will operate [3].

Once the patient is positioned, neuronavigation is registered and the location of the frontal sinus relative to the eyebrow incision and the planned craniotomy is determined. In planning the eyebrow incision, the lateral aspect of the frontal sinus is marked with a surgical pen and the supraorbital notch is palpated. The incision is then marked within the eyebrow extending from

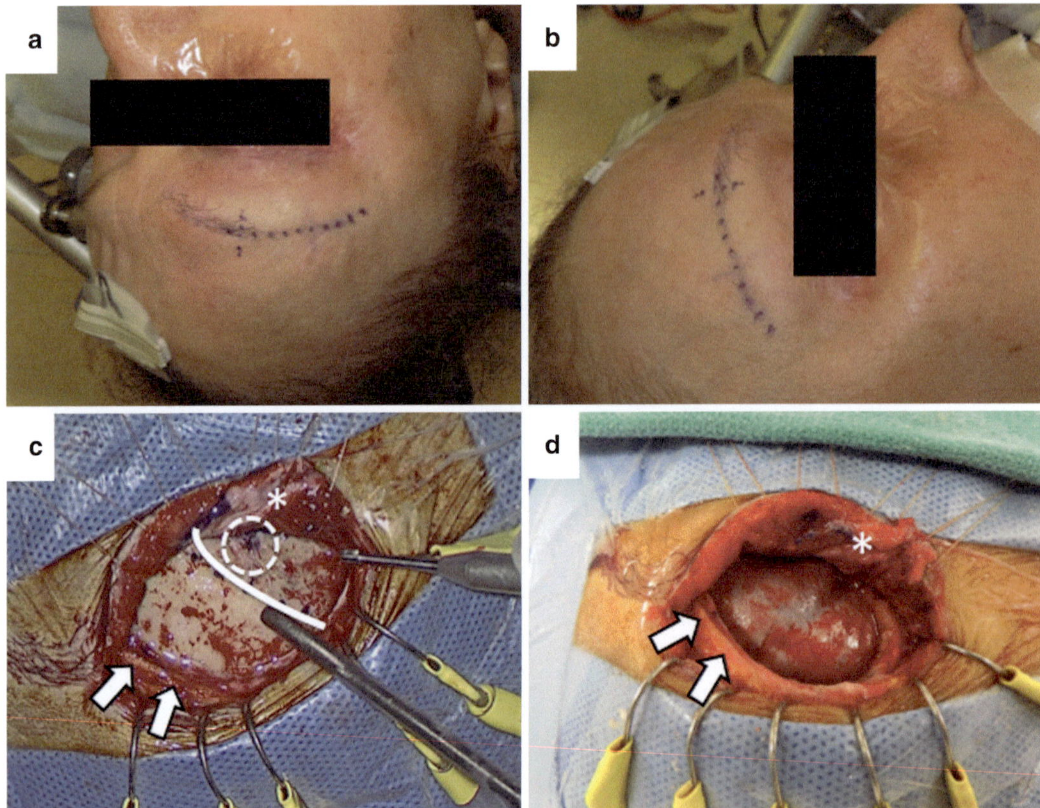

Fig. 12.6 Skin incision and craniotomy of right SO approach: (**a**, **b**) Eyebrow incision is marked from just medial to supraorbital notch extending laterally to eyebrow termination. (**c**) *Asterisk* indicates the pericranial flap reflected with sutures. *Arrow* indicates the course of the exposed supraorbital nerve. *White line* shows the superior temporal line. *Dotted circle* indicates the position of the keyhole. (**d**) Craniotomy showing dural exposure. The inner table of the inferior edge of the craniotomy and any protuberances of the orbital roof are drilled flat prior to dural opening

just medial to the supraorbital notch and coursing laterally to the lateral termination of the eyebrow. Note that the exposure must allow access to the area immediately below the superior temporal line since that is where the burr hole will be placed.

12.5.3 Skin Incision and Craniotomy

The skin incision is made within the middle of the eyebrow, and care is taken to identify and preserve the supraorbital nerve at the medial aspect of the opening (Fig. 12.6). In patients with relatively short eyebrows, the lateral extent of the incision may need to extend up to 1 cm beyond the eyebrow in a skinfold along the frontozygomatic process. The incision extension should not extend more than 13 mm lateral to the zygomatic process in order to prevent injury to the frontalis muscle branch of the facial nerve [16]. If the eyebrow is very thin, the skin incision can be made in a crease or a previous scar of the supraorbital area [17]. In general, to maximize preservation of the supraorbital nerve, the supraorbital notch represents the medial extent of the incision. As the medial extent of the incision is taken deeper toward the pericranium, the supraorbital nerve should be anticipated and protected. In some cases, careful drilling of the nerve's bony encasement can be performed, thus allowing the surgeon to gently mobilize it medially and away from the main operative field.

The subgaleal plane is then dissected superiorly while preserving the underlying pericranium. The skin flap is reflected superiorly and is maintained in position with multiple fishhooks to evenly distribute the pressure on the superior skin edge. Inferior reflection of the frontal and orbital muscles should be sufficient to expose the supraorbital rim but gentle enough to prevent periorbital hematoma. The pericranium is incised as superiorly as possible to fashion a U-shaped pericranial flap that extends laterally over the superior temporal line and into temporalis fascia. This flap is reflected inferiorly along the supraorbital rim and is kept tense with sutures and humid with a wet cloth to prevent shrinkage and desiccation. In preparation for the burr hole, a short segment of temporalis fascia and muscle are released at the superior temporal line and then retracted inferiorly and laterally with fishhooks to expose the keyhole below and posterior to the frontozygomatic process.

A single burr hole is placed below the superior temporal line and posterior to the standard keyhole. A supraorbital half-moon-shaped bone flap measuring approximately 20 mm in height by 20–25 mm in length is made which is flush with the orbital roof but does not include the orbital rim (Fig. 12.6c, d). Once the bone flap is removed, the underlying dura is dissected from the orbital roof. Prior to dural opening, the inner table of the inferior edge of the craniotomy and any protuberances of the orbital roof are drilled flat with a high-speed drill. This maneuver is essential to optimize the flat surgical trajectory along the frontal floor, as even small boney ridges may significantly impair the line of sight to deeper regions. For cosmetic reasons, care must be taken not to drill up to the superficial cortical bone on the inferior craniotomy border. If the frontal sinus is entered, it is not cranialized and can be covered with Gelfoam® (Pfizer) during the tumor removal.

12.5.4 The Dural Opening and Approach to the Lesion

The dura is opened in a C-shape manner with its base toward the orbital rim and reflected inferiorly. The dural flap is kept moist and under tension throughout the case to prevent shrinking and allow for a watertight closure.

The rest of the procedure is performed under microscopic visualization and intermittent use of endoscopy. The frontal lobe is protected with strips of Telfa® (American Surgical Company). The main anatomical structure at this point becomes the olfactory tract on the inferior surface of the frontal lobe, and it is followed back to the ipsilateral optic nerve. The arachnoid overlying the optic, opticocarotid, and carotid cisterns is sharply opened with egress of CSF and further brain relaxation. A brain spatula may be placed initially over the frontal lobe to gently retract the frontal lobe. With egress of CSF, the brain rapidly becomes well relaxed and the retractor is generally not needed. This step of CSF drainage may require patience, particularly if the brain is "full." However, as CSF egress proceeds, the surgical corridor will open. Any forceful retraction of the frontal lobe is to be avoided. Additional dissection of the arachnoid at the base of the frontal lobe over the interface with the optic chiasm and within the proximal Sylvian fissure will further free the frontal lobe from the basal cisterns and temporal lobe and allow it to fall away with gravity.

12.5.5 Tumor Removal

Depending upon the location of the craniopharyngioma, tumor in the suprasellar space, prechiasmatic space, the optico-carotid cistern region, or further laterally along the Sylvian fissure should all now be accessible. Tumor in these areas is then approached, and surgery proceeds using standard microsurgical technique depending on the site and size of the craniopharyngioma. For large craniopharyngiomas with multiple cystic components, draining the cysts as an initial part of the procedure will help reduce pressure on the optic apparatus and aid with brain relaxation and exposure. In general, care must be taken in assessing tumor involvement of any of the number of surrounding neurovascular structures mentioned above. Of particular concern are the carotid artery and its branches and the optic apparatus. To anticipate and preserve bilateral superior hypophyseal arteries arising from medial supraclinoid carotid arteries is mandatory.

The position of the optic chiasm and pituitary stalk must be carefully assessed. Craniopharyngiomas often are very adherent to the optic apparatus and pituitary stalk, and a workable surgical plane between the tumor and hypothalamus is often not present. If tumor is located in predominantly retrochiasmal region, trans-lamina terminalis route can also be used to access tumor in this region and the third ventricle. Proximal Sylvian fissure dissection is done as needed when the lateral extension of the tumor extends to the middle fossa, requiring dissection of the capsule and the medial temporal lobe. Dense adhesion to the hypothalamus is saved.

In cases of prior transsphenoidal or transcranial surgery, significant scar tissue in the arachnoid over the optic apparatus is often noted, requiring careful dissection using microsurgical techniques and the frequent use of Doppler ultrasound to confirm the surrounding vessels that might be hidden under the scar tissue. Anterior cerebral arteries are often elevated and pushed posteriorly. If significant scarring around the optic apparatus exists, approaching the tumor through the gyrus rectus may sometimes be needed.

The 0° and 30° endoscopes are used intermittently to provide a panoramic perspective of the surgical anatomy. The endoscope often allows one to better define tumor-vascular relationships along the outer recesses of the suprasellar space. Small tumor remnants or infiltration directly visualized by endoscopy may be missed on intraoperative MRI or may be considered as postoperative changes on follow-up imaging [18]. Therefore, endoscopic visualization is strongly encouraged for all SO cases. Visualization of more lateral areas is improved, without the need of additional dissection or retraction. Particularly in the setting of craniopharyngiomas, assessment of the surgical field for tumor remnants with the endoscope gives the best chance of identifying residual tumor that can be addressed before terminating the procedure [9, 10]. The endoscope is particularly helpful for visualizing tumor remnants under the ipsilateral optic nerve and tract which is a relative "blind spot" of the SO approach given that its trajectory is in direct alignment with the optic nerve [1, 8]. In case of an extremely narrow corridor, the 2.7 mm endoscope may be useful to inspect the area.

One important caveat, however, is that unlike in endonasal surgery in which the operating corridor is the nose and sinuses, in the SO approach, the corridor is the frontal fossa with all its critical neurovascular structures. It is critical in intracranial skull base endoscopy to be constantly mindful of the endoscope and instrument locations. Wielding the endoscope and multiple instruments safely in this confined space must be done with utmost caution and care, as the endoscopic view is blind behind the lens.

12.5.6 Closure

Due to the unique location of the eyebrow incision, a cosmetically pleasing closure is essential. After tumor removal and hemostasis is achieved, the dura is closed in a watertight fashion. The medial bone edge of the craniotomy is inspected to confirm that the frontal sinus has not been entered or that a frontal sinus breach has been adequately repaired. A large piece of collagen sponge (Helistat® or Duragen® – Integra LifeSciences) is placed over the dura with redundant collagen extending over the bony edges. The bone flap is repositioned and secured with a lateral burr hole cover and a straight plate spanning the medial edge of the craniotomy (Fig. 12.7). When replacing the bone flap, the more cosmetically noticeable gap at the superior aspect of the craniotomy should be minimized. Gaps between the bone flap and calvarium are filled with collagen sponge in order to minimize visible scalp depressions in the supraorbital region. Temporalis muscle and fascia and the attached pericranial flap are reflected back into anatomical position and re-approximated over the bone flap with absorbable sutures. Similarly, scalp incision is closed with absorbable galeal and subcutaneous stitches. A final running 5-0 absorbable subcuticular skin stitch is then placed to evenly approximate the skin edges. After undraping, pressure is applied over the incision until the patient is extubated and breathing comfortably to prevent the formation of a pseudomeningocele.

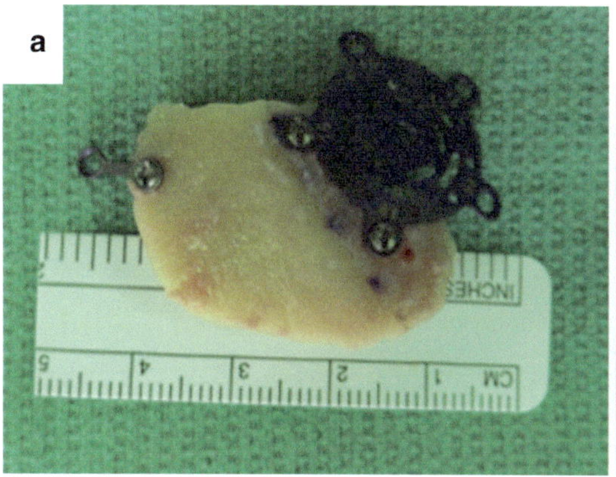

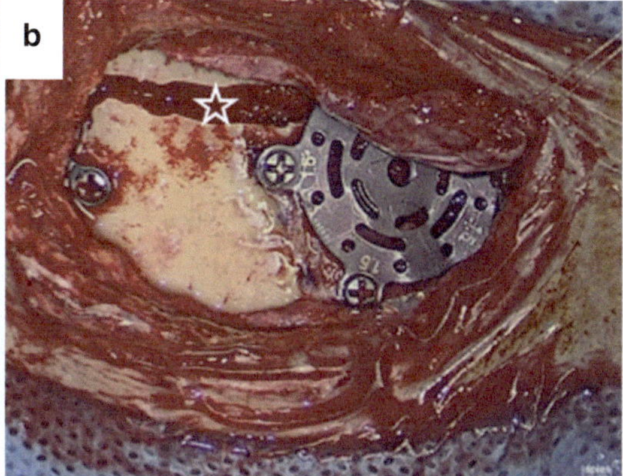

Fig. 12.7 Bone flap and closure: (**a**) A right-sided bone flap with titanium plates. (**b**) A right-sided bone flap is positioned and secured with a lateral burr hole cover and a straight plate spanning the medial edge of the right-sided craniotomy. Note that for cosmesis, the bone flap is pushed superiorly, so it is flush with supraorbital calvarium leaving no gap along the forehead; the bone gap (*star*) on the inferior edge of the craniotomy is generally well-hidden by the eyebrow. This gap can also be filled in with collagen or bone cement

In cases where the frontal sinus has been breached, closure can be performed in three ways depending upon the size of the defect. For small defects, placement of collagen sponge against the opening with the bone flap directly opposed against the defect is typically effective. For larger defects, abdominal fat should be placed within sinus opening and the lateral aspect of the sinus, and reinforced with collagen, tissue glue, and the bone flap. Alternatively for larger defects, the repair with fat can be further reinforced with the pericranial flap rotated over the defect. This last option is less desirable from a cosmetic standpoint. After addressing the frontal sinus, the closure then proceeds as described above.

12.6 Possible Complications and Their Avoidance

While the SO approach carries little approach-related morbidity, it is associated with a unique set of potential complications. Transient forehead numbness from injury to the supraorbital nerve is a common event in the early postoperative period but is rarely permanent, being reported in up to 7.5 % of patients in some series [3]. Transient frontalis weakness from injury or stretching of the frontalis branch of the facial nerve can be seen immediately after surgery and is also typically transient, although lasting frontalis paresis has been reported in up to 5.5 % of patients [3]. Both of these complications may be avoided by careful planning of the incision and meticulous soft tissue dissection. The supraorbital nerve is readily identifiable as it courses from the orbit through the supraorbital notch at the medial aspect of the eyebrow incision. Although the frontalis branch of the facial nerve may be more difficult to identify, the risk of injury can be reduced by minimizing the lateral extent of the incision.

CSF rhinorrhea may occur if the frontal sinus is violated and inadequately repaired. This complication has been reported in up to 4 % of patient [3] and can [3] be avoided by carefully planning the craniotomy lateral to the lateral-most edge of the frontal sinus. However, if the sinus is entered, it should be carefully repaired. In all cases, the medial aspect of the craniotomy should be thoroughly inspected to determine if there is sinus entry. As mentioned above, a small frontal sinus breach may be repaired with bone wax with an overlay of collagen sponge. Larger frontal sinus breaches may require packing with fat or muscle as well as with a pericranial flap and collagen sponge reinforcement. Because the soft tissue dissection of the eyebrow approach does create a small potential space low over the frontal bone, postoperative pseudomeningocele formation is a possible complication if a watertight dural closure is not achieved. Application of pressure over the incision while the patient is being extubated may reduce the incidence of this potential complication.

Overall, because the SO approach utilizes a small incision and involves minimal temporalis dissection, scalp pain, temporalis atrophy, and difficulty with mastication are rarely observed.

12.7 Illustrative Cases

Case 1

A 71-year-old woman reported a 3-month history of progressive peripheral visual loss and headache. MRI revealed a 16×18 mm retrochiasmal suprasellar cystic lesion causing severe compression of the optic chiasm and posterior displacement of the infundibulum (Fig. 12.8). The patient's pituitary hormonal studies were normal except for mild hyperprolactinemia. There was evidence of a right cavernous flow void; MRA confirmed a right cavernous carotid artery aneurysm which appeared to be entirely contained within the cavernous sinus and sella. To avoid the potential manipulation of the cavernous sinus aneurysm, a left SO approach was chosen. Pseudocapsule of the lesion was entered with large windows made into it. However, there were multiple perforators adherent to the tumor capsule. Considering the patient's age and perforators, no attempt was made for complete removal. The pathological diagnosis was craniopharyngioma. Postoperatively her visual fields were full. She subsequently had stereotactic radiotherapy (SRT). Two years after craniotomy and SRT, the residual mass has shrunken and remains stable in size.

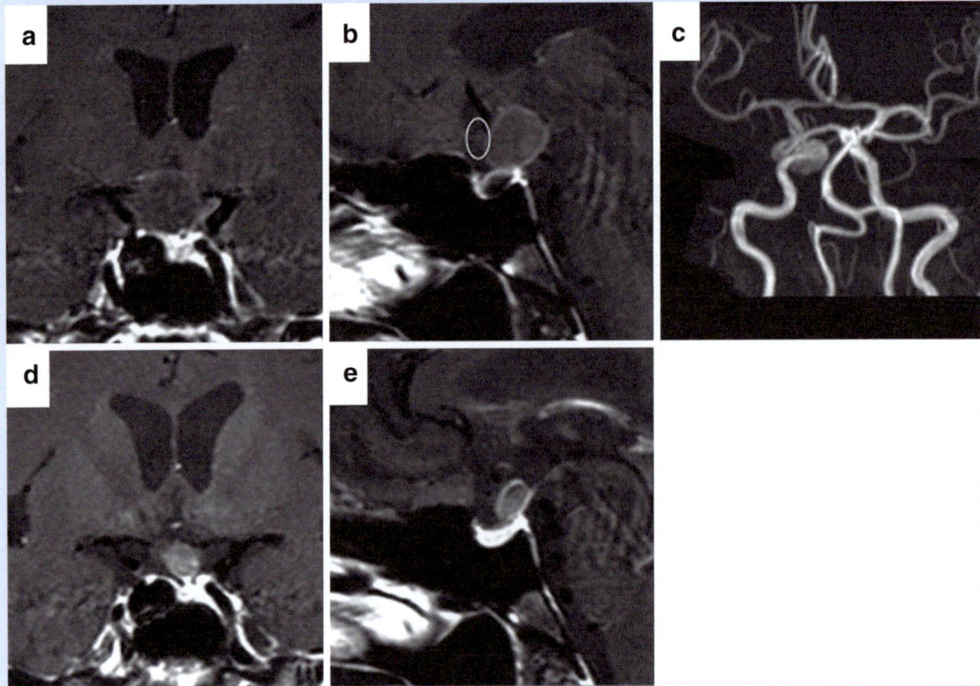

Fig. 12.8 Case illustration 1. Craniopharyngioma in a 71-year-old woman with progressive visual loss. Preoperative coronal (**a**) and sagittal (**b**) postgadolinium MRI scans showing large cystic tumor in suprasellar area. Note the flow void in the right cavernous sinus and sella (the *circle* represents the location of the optic chiasm). MR angiography (**c**) reveals right cavernous sinus ICA aneurysm. Two-year postoperative coronal (**d**) and sagittal (**e**) postgadolinium MRI showing persistent regression of cystic craniopharyngioma. See text for additional clinical history

Case 2

A 46-year-old woman developed progressive loss of vision and worsening headaches over 2 months. MRI of the brain showed a heterogeneously enhancing and partially cystic suprasellar tumor attached to the pituitary stalk, which was pushed posteriorly. The cystic lesion was multi-lobulated, being larger anteriorly and optic chiasm was markedly compressed (Fig. 12.9). She underwent a left SO craniotomy, cyst decompression, and tumor debulking. The tumor was partially calcified and densely adherent to the left aspect of the chiasm and left optic nerve and tract. She did well after surgery with visual improvement and no new endocrinopathy. She underwent SRT and at 5 years after surgery has a stable small residual tumor.

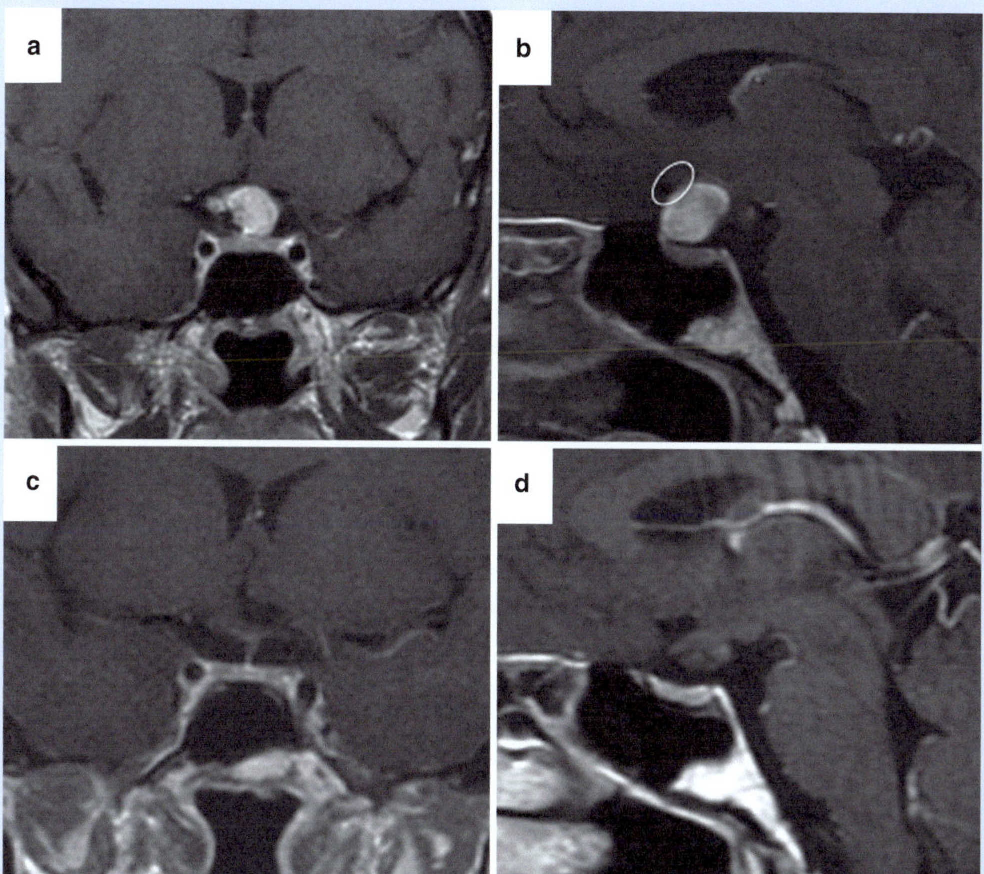

Fig. 12.9 Case illustration 2. Craniopharyngioma in a 46-year-old woman with progressive visual loss. Preoperative coronal (**a**) and sagittal (**b**) postgadolinium MRI scans showing large cystic tumor in suprasellar area (the *circle* represents the location of the optic chiasm). Five-year post-surgery and post-SRT, coronal (**c**), and sagittal (**d**) post-gadolinium MRI showing persistent cyst regression. See text for additional clinical history

Case 3

A 51-year-old man with multiple previous therapies for a retrochiasmal craniopharyngioma treated elsewhere including endonasal resection and postoperative CSF leak repair with a ventriculoperitoneal shunt. He had developed craniopharyngioma cyst progression in the retrochiasmatic and third ventricular space. His visual fields had progressively deteriorated. Considering the scar tissue from his previous endonasal approach, he underwent left SO approach. There was significant scar tissue around the optic nerves and chiasm. He had a trans-lamina terminalis decompression of the craniopharyngioma cyst. Given the multiple dense adhesions to the optic apparatus and hypothalamus, no attempt was made to remove a significant portion of the cyst wall. He had an uneventful postoperative course. His initial postoperative MRI showed good decompression of the large tumor cyst (Fig. 12.10 and Video 12.1).

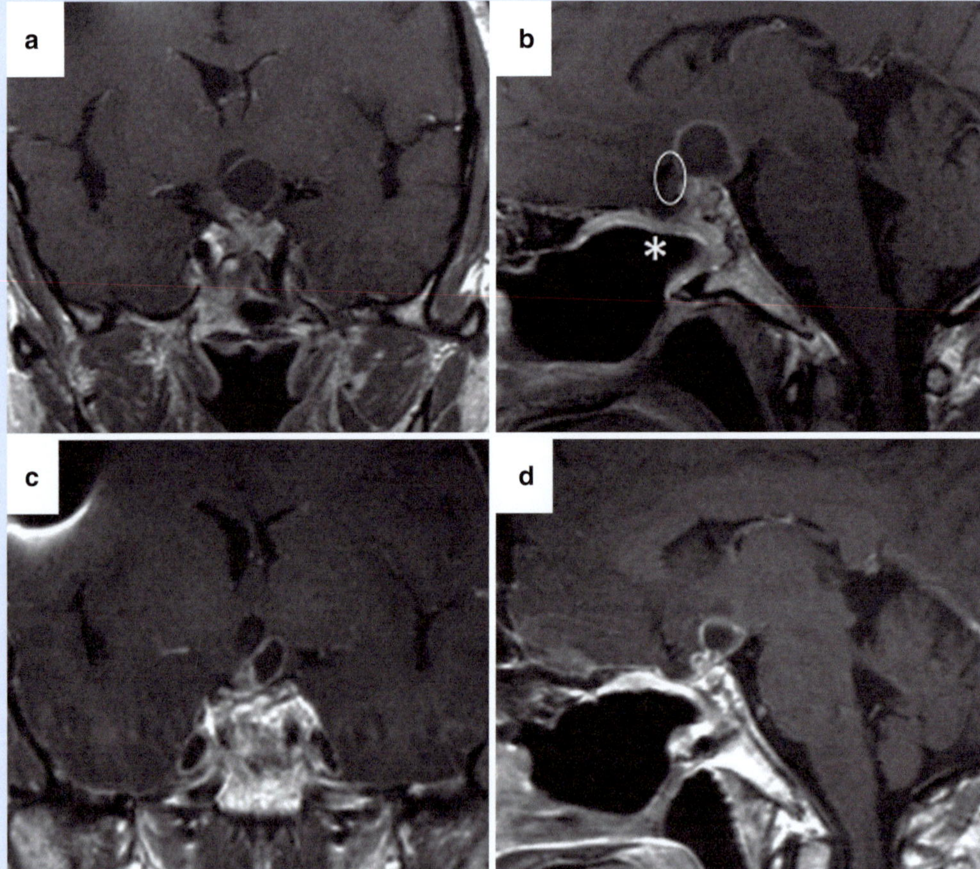

Fig. 12.10 Case illustration 3. Recurrent craniopharyngioma in a 51-year-old man. Preoperative coronal (**a**) and sagittal (**b**) postgadolinium MRI scans showing large cystic tumor in suprasellar area. *Asterisk* indicates the nasal septal flap utilized for the previous endonasal endoscopic surgery (the *circle* represents the location of the optic chiasm). Postoperative day 1 coronal (**c**) and sagittal (**d**) postgadolinium MRI showing cyst collapse. See text for additional clinical history

Case 4

A 6-year-old boy with progressive visual loss and lethargy was found to have left optic atrophy and right-sided papilledema. MRI showed a large 4 cm multilobulated cystic and solid craniopharyngioma arising from the suprasellar cistern with sellar extension. A larger retroinfundibular cystic component obliterated the third ventricle and caused severe obstructive hydrocephalus. Preoperatively he had low thyroid and cortisol levels consistent with secondary hypothyroidism and adrenal insufficiency. Given his small nostrils and sinonasal corridor, he underwent right SO approach with temporary external ventricular drainage. At surgery, after opening the large suprasellar and retrochiasmatic tumor cysts, a near complete removal of the tumor capsule was accomplished with preservation of the infundibulum. Postoperatively, he had a marked improvement in vision and overall alertness and well-being. He did require full anterior and posterior pituitary hormone replacement. His postoperative MRI 3 months after the surgery showed no obvious residual tumor and resolution of obstructive hydrocephalus (Fig. 12.11).

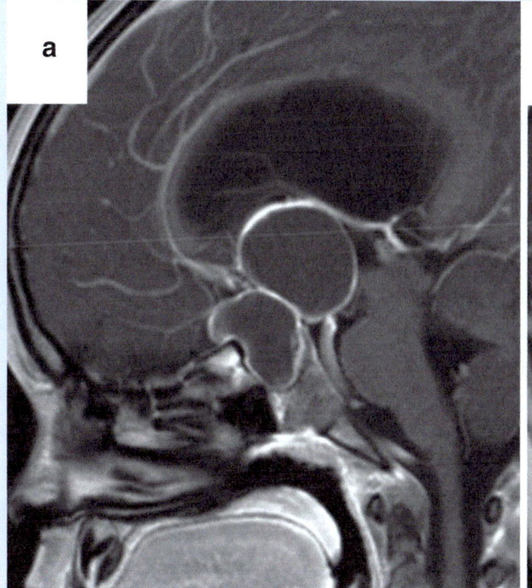

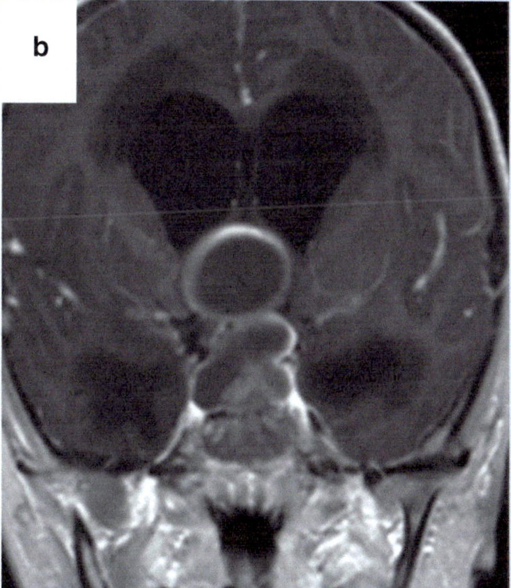

Fig. 12.11 Case illustration 4. Six-year-old patient with small sinonasal structures and extensive cystic and solid craniopharyngioma with suprasellar and retrochiasmatic extension. Preoperative sagittal (**a**) and coronal (**b**) post-gadolinium MRI scans showing large multicystic tumor in suprasellar and retrochiasmatic area with obstructive hydrocephalus. Three-month postoperative sagittal (**c**) and coronal (**d**) post-gadolinium MRI after right SO craniotomy showing no obvious residual tumor and resolution of obstructive hydrocephalus. See text for additional clinical history

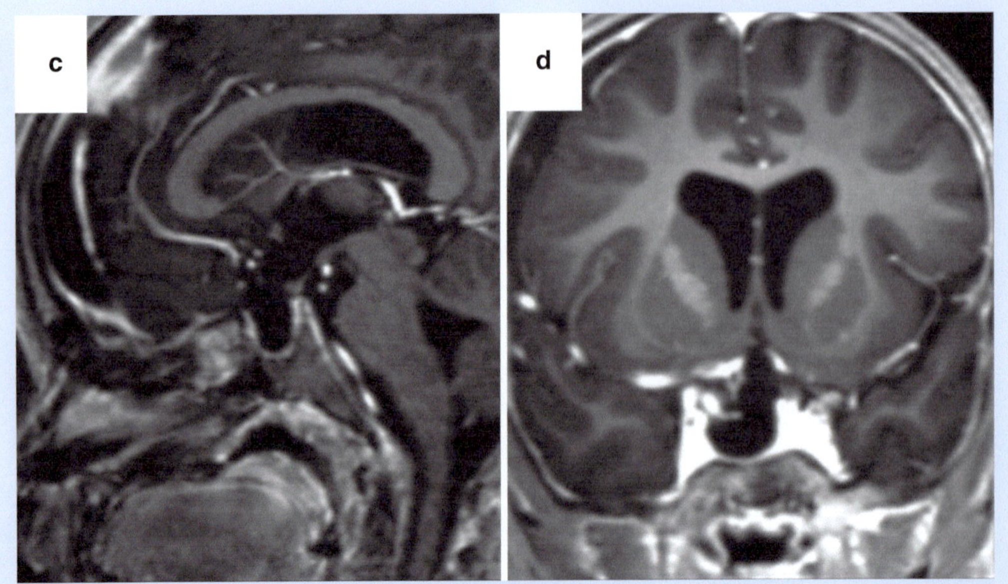

Fig. 12.11 (continued)

12.8 Additional Therapy for Residual or Recurrent Craniopharyngioma

Although total resection of craniopharyngiomas has been advocated by some, it is associated with a higher morbidity and mortality [19, 20]. Consequently, we opt for subtotal removal if dense adhesions to neurovascular structures and hypothalamus are present [21–23]. Given the effectiveness of stereotactic radiotherapy (SRT) and stereotactic radiosurgery (SRS), these modalities are frequently employed for residual and/or recurrent craniopharyngiomas; these modalities are further discussed in Chap. 14.

Conclusions

The SO approach is a minimally invasive keyhole technique that offers wide access to the anterior skull base and parasellar region by exploiting the subfrontal corridor. Endoscopy expands the reach of this approach by providing a more panoramic assessment of the parasellar space and maximizing safe tumor removal. The SO approach is an excellent alternative to the endonasal approach for certain craniopharyngiomas, particularly those with frontal and lateral extensions. The major advantage of the SO approach over the endonasal route is a simplified skull base closure and reduced risk of postoperative CSF leak. It should also be considered as an effective alternative route for recurrent or residual suprasellar craniopharyngiomas previously treated by conventional craniotomy or transsphenoidal surgery. The unique location of the eyebrow incision demands meticulous cosmetic closure. With proper technique, excellent cosmetic results are routine.

References

1. Fatemi N, Dusick JR, de Paiva Neto MA, Malkasian D, Kelly DF (2009) Endonasal versus supraorbital keyhole removal of craniopharyngiomas and tuberculum sellae meningiomas. Neurosurgery 64(5 Suppl 2):269–284; discussion 284–266. doi:10.1227/01.NEU.0000327857.22221.53
2. Wilson DA, Duong H, Teo C, Kelly DF (2014) The supraorbital endoscopic approach for tumors.

World Neurosurg 82(1–2):e243–e256. doi:10.1016/j.wneu.2013.02.002
3. Reisch R, Perneczky A (2005) Ten-year experience with the supraorbital subfrontal approach through an eyebrow skin incision. Neurosurgery 57(4 Suppl):242–255
4. van Lindert EJ, Grotenhuis JA (2009) The combined supraorbital keyhole-endoscopic endonasal transsphenoidal approach to sellar, perisellar and frontal skull base tumors: surgical technique. Minim Invasive Neurosurg 52(5–6):281–286. doi:10.1055/s-0029-1242776
5. McLaughlin N, Ditzel Filho LF, Shahlaie K, Solari D, Kassam AB, Kelly DF (2011) The supraorbital approach for recurrent or residual suprasellar tumors. Minim Invasive Neurosurg 54(4):155–161. doi:10.1055/s-0031-1284401
6. Beretta F, Andaluz N, Chalaala C, Bernucci C, Salud L, Zuccarello M (2010) Image-guided anatomical and morphometric study of supraorbital and transorbital minicraniotomies to the sellar and perisellar regions: comparison with standard techniques. J Neurosurg 113(5):975–981. doi:10.3171/2009.10.JNS09435
7. Figueiredo EG, Deshmukh V, Nakaji P, Deshmukh P, Crusius MU, Crawford N, Spetzler RF, Preul MC (2006) An anatomical evaluation of the mini-supraorbital approach and comparison with standard craniotomies. Neurosurgery 59(4 Suppl 2):ONS212–ONS220; discussion ONS220. doi:10.1227/01.NEU.0000223365.55701.F2
8. Perneczky A, Fries G (1998) Endoscope-assisted brain surgery: part 1–evolution, basic concept, and current technique. Neurosurgery 42(2):219–224; discussion 224–225
9. Zheng X, Liu W, Yang X, Gong J, Shen F, Shen G, Shen H, Zheng X, Fu W (2007) Endoscope-assisted supraorbital keyhole approach for the resection of benign tumors of the sellar region. Minim Invasive Ther Allied Technol 16(6):363–366. doi:10.1080/13645700701625955
10. Kabil MS, Shahinian HK (2005) Application of the supraorbital endoscopic approach to tumors of the anterior cranial base. J Craniofac Surg 16(6):1070–1074; discussion 1075
11. Czirjak S, Nyary I, Futo J, Szeifert GT (2002) Bilateral supraorbital keyhole approach for multiple aneurysms via superciliary skin incisions. Surg Neurol 57(5):314–323; discussion 323–324
12. Hayhurst C, Teo C (2011) Tuberculum sella meningioma. Otolaryngol Clin North Am 44(4):953–963, viii–ix. doi:10.1016/j.otc.2011.06.012
13. Jallo GI, Bognar L (2006) Eyebrow surgery: the supraciliary craniotomy: technical note. Neurosurgery 59(1 Suppl 1):ONSE157–ONSE158; discussion ONSE157–ONSE158. doi:10.1227/01.NEU.0000220045.23743.80
14. Mitchell P, Vindlacheruvu RR, Mahmood K, Ashpole RD, Grivas A, Mendelow AD (2005) Supraorbital eyebrow minicraniotomy for anterior circulation aneurysms. Surg Neurol 63(1):47–51; discussion 51. doi:10.1016/j.surneu.2004.02.030
15. Dusick JR, Esposito F, Malkasian D, Kelly DF (2007) Avoidance of carotid artery injuries in transsphenoidal surgery with the Doppler probe and micro-hook blades. Neurosurgery 60(4 Suppl 2):322–328; discussion 328–329. doi:10.1227/01.NEU.0000255408.84269.A8
16. Lin Y, Zhang W, Luo Q, Jiang J, Qiu Y (2009) Extracranial microanatomic study of supraorbital keyhole approach. J Craniofac Surg 20(1):215–218. doi:10.1097/SCS.0b013e318191cf8a
17. Reisch R, Perneczky A, Filippi R (2003) Surgical technique of the supraorbital key-hole craniotomy. Surg Neurol 59(3):223–227
18. Nimsky C, Ganslandt O, Hofmann B, Fahlbusch R (2003) Limited benefit of intraoperative low-field magnetic resonance imaging in craniopharyngioma surgery. Neurosurgery 53(1):72–80; discussion 80–81
19. Yasargil MG, Curcic M, Kis M, Siegenthaler G, Teddy PJ, Roth P (1990) Total removal of craniopharyngiomas. Approaches and long-term results in 144 patients. J Neurosurg 73(1):3–11. doi:10.3171/jns.1990.73.1.0003
20. Zhou ZQ, Shi XE (2004) Changes of hypothalamus-pituitary hormones in patients after total removal of craniopharyngiomas. Chin Med J (Engl) 117(3):357–360
21. Baskin DS, Wilson CB (1986) Surgical management of craniopharyngiomas. A review of 74 cases. J Neurosurg 65(1):22–27. doi:10.3171/jns.1986.65.1.0022
22. Puget S, Garnett M, Wray A, Grill J, Habrand JL, Bodaert N, Zerah M, Bezerra M, Renier D, Pierre-Kahn A, Sainte-Rose C (2007) Pediatric craniopharyngiomas: classification and treatment according to the degree of hypothalamic involvement. J Neurosurg 106(1 Suppl):3–12. doi:10.3171/ped.2007.106.1.3
23. Van Effenterre R, Boch AL (2002) Craniopharyngioma in adults and children: a study of 122 surgical cases. J Neurosurg 97(1):3–11. doi:10.3171/jns.2002.97.1.0003

13 Transcallosal Approach

Filippo Flavio Angileri, Francesca Granata, and Francesco Tomasello

13.1 Indications

The transcallosal approach is indicated for craniopharyngiomas that are primarily located in the third ventricle cavity with a significant expansion into the superior-posterior part of the ventricular cavity. Relationship with the third ventricle floor should be identified preoperatively. In some cases craniopharyngiomas displace upward the roof of the ventricle. These tumors are basically those described as type IV in the Kassam classification based on the tumor growth and the position of the infundibulum [1]. In other cases tumor grows primarily inside the third ventricle cavity, displacing downward the hypothalamus. Tumors can be dissected through both foramina of Monro even if, in some cases, a subchoroidal or interforniceal route may help in the dissection of the posterior pole of the tumor. The interforniceal route carries the risk of bilateral fornices' damage with devastating neurologic consequences for memory and cognitive postoperative performances. In case of a cystic cavum pellucidum, the so-called cavum vergae, this anatomical variation produces itself a corridor between fornices to access the roof of the third ventricle without adjunctive neural splitting and, thus, providing enough space for a safe and effective dissection and tumor removal. Hydrocephalus is not a prerequisite for the transcallosal route, while it is mandatory for the transcortical approach. Lesions involving supra- and parasellar cisterns are not resectable by the transcallosal route. If the tumor has a significant portion into the parasellar cisterns, a translamina-terminalis approach through an anterolateral (pterional) or anterior (frontal mono- or bilateral) craniotomy should be considered to resect this portion and its eventual extension into the anterior portion of the third ventricle. A combined translamina-terminalis and transcallosal approach may be indicated for craniopharyngiomas extending into the supra- and parasellar lesion with a significant portion reaching the middle and superior portion of third ventricle cavity [2].

The presence of a cystic lesion may influence the choice of the approach. Usually, emptying the cystic portion of the lesions may help in the dissection allowing an early decompression and facilitating the dissection from neural structures.

13.2 Neuroradiology

Craniopharyngiomas are tumors that arise from remnants of the craniopharyngeal duct and they may occur anywhere along the stalk from the

Electronic supplementary material The online version of this chapter (doi:10.1007/978-3-319-21533-4_13) contains supplementary material, which is available to authorized users.

F.F. Angileri, MD (✉) • F. Granata, MD
F. Tomasello, MD
Division of Neurosurgery, Department of Neurosciences, University of Messina, Messina, Italy
e-mail: fangileri@unime.it

P. Cappabianca et al. (eds.), *Midline Skull Base Surgery*, DOI 10.1007/978-3-319-21533-4_13

hypothalamus to the pituitary gland [3]. Infrequently, the lesions are entirely within the sella or in the third ventricle [4]. However, at the time of diagnosis, a majority of craniopharyngiomas involve the third ventricle to some degree [5]. Craniopharyngiomas vary greatly in size, from a few millimeters to several centimeters in diameter. They may be largely cystic, mixed solid cystic, or entirely solid. More than 90 % of adamantinomatous craniopharyngiomas present cysts and calcified foci [3]. The papillary type of the tumor is more often solid with less common incidence of calcification [6].

Computed tomography (CT scan) diagnostic approach is very useful to confirm the presence of tumor calcifications. The calcifications may be a thin, circumferential rim around the cyst or chunks of calcium within the solid part of the tumor [3]. Ninety percent of craniopharyngiomas enhance after the intravenous administration of iodinated contrast medium [3].

On magnetic resonance imaging (MRI), the cystic portion of the tumor may present high or low signal intensity on T1-weighted images. The hyperintensity on T1-weighted images may reflect the protein or cholesterol content of the "motor oil-like" fluid found in the tumor cysts [3, 6].

On T2-weighted images, including fluid attenuated inversion recovery (FLAIR) sequence, both cystic and solid parts of the lesion tend to have high signal intensity. Tumor calcifications are often not detected on fast spin-echo (FSE) sequence, but they stand out particularly on a susceptibility sequence such as gradient-recalled echo (GRE)

GRE sequences are also mandatory to evaluate an intratumoral hemorrhage or a superficial CSN siderosis due to the chronic bleeding of a craniopharyngioma [7].

After gadolinium-DTPA administration, the solid part of the tumor and the thin wall of the cyst nearly always enhance [3]. The enhancement of the solid portion may be either uniform or patchy and heterogeneous. Enhancement patterns in a given tumor are similar on both CT and MR [6].

FLAIR sequence can be useful in delineating cystic portions of tumor, hyperintense vs. loculated portions of the third ventricle, or other CSF spaces, iso- or hypointense [6].

Diffusion-weighted imaging (DWI) can be useful in the differential diagnosis if an epidermoid is suspected. Typically, epidermoid cysts present very high signal intensity on DWI images.

Preoperative MRI examination should include FSE high-resolution T1- and T2-weighted sagittal and coronal sections. After Gd administration, FSE T1-weighted sagittal and coronal imaging or a volumetric acquisition (mprGE) should be performed. Additional sequences such as FLAIR, GRE, or DWI may be helpful in answering specific questions [6]. Sagittal sections are indispensable to evaluate the topographic extension of craniopharyngioma, especially in regard to pre- or retrochiasmatic site of the lesion and of third ventricle involvement.

On sagittal MRI images, the mammillary body angle (MBA) is assessable; MBA is the angle formed by the intersection of a plane tangential to the base of 1 of the mammillary bodies with the plane tangential to the floor of the fourth ventricle (Fig. 13.1) [5]. The evaluation of the mammillary body displacement, by measurement of the MBA, represents a reliable neuroradiological sign that could be used to discriminate the intraventricular involvement in patients with craniopharyngioma. An acute MBA (<60°) is indicative of a primary tuberal-intraventricular topography, whereas an obtuse MBA (>90°) denotes a primary suprasellar CP position [5].

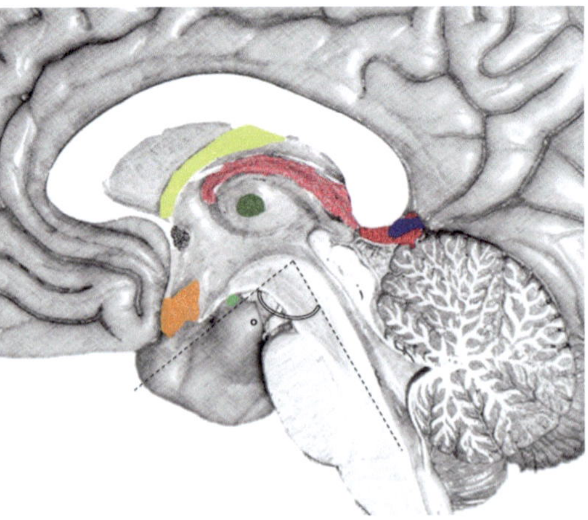

Fig. 13.1 Schematic drawing showing the mammillary body angle (MBA); MBA is the angle formed by the intersection of a plane tangential to the base of 1 of the mammillary bodies with the plane tangential to the floor of the fourth ventricle

13.3 Anatomy of the Approach

Anatomy of the interhemispheric fissure may widely influence feasibility and challenges in planning a transcallosal approach. The presence, number, and size of bridging veins should be carefully evaluated preoperatively. Even small bridging veins running from the frontal cerebral lobe to the superior sagittal sinus should be preserved to avoid postoperative edema and infarction leading to disastrous clinical outcome. After wide dissection of the interhemispheric fissure, both pericallosal and calloso-marginal arteries should be identified as anatomical landmarks before performing the callosotomy. The corpus callosum appears as a pale white-colored and hypovascular structure, usually well distinct from the cortex of the cingulate gyrus. A small incision along the sagittal plane, usually 15–20 mm, on the corpus callosum revealed the lateral ventricle chamber. At this point the thalamostriate and septal vein come into view. This step is mandatory to identify the foramen of Monro and, even more important, to be oriented in the discrimination of the left lateral ventricle from the right one. Posteriorly, thalamostriate and septal veins join each other to form the internal cerebral vein. On the lateral ventricle floor, the choroidal plexus hides the choroidal fissure, where the internal cerebral vein runs. Opening of the choroidal fissure may increase the third ventricle exposure allowing access of the middle and posterior portion of the third ventricle. The third ventricle is a deep-seated, narrow, vertically oriented, median cavity. Its roof goes from the suprapineal recess posteriorly to the foramen of Monro anteriorly, and it is formed by two thin membranous layers of tela choroidea, a layer of blood vessels between these sheets, and a neural layer formed by the fornix. The body of the fornix forms the anterior part of the roof, and the crura and hippocampal commissure form the posterior one. The velum interpositum is the space that contains the vascular layer, composed of the two medial posterior choroidal arteries and their branches and internal cerebral veins and their tributaries. The upper layer of the tela choroidea is attached to the lower surface of the fornix and the lower wall contacts the stria medullaris thalami and extends along the superomedial border of the thalamus, from the foramen of Monro to the habenular commissure; the posterior part of the lower wall is attached to the superior surface of the pineal gland. The paired strands of choroid plexus are attached to the lower layer of tela choroidea.

The floor extends from the optic chiasm to the opening of the aqueduct of Sylvius posteriorly; between those structures, the infundibulum of the hypothalamus, the tuber cinereum, the mammillary bodies, the posterior perforated substance (located in a space limited anteriorly and laterally by the optic chiasm and tracts, and posteriorly by the cerebral peduncles), and the part of the tegmentum of the midbrain located above the medial aspect of the cerebral peduncles are comprised. The posterior part of the floor extends posterior and superior to the medial part of the cerebral peduncles and superior to the tegmentum of the midbrain.

The boundaries of the anterior wall are formed by the optic chiasm, the optic recess, the lamina terminalis (a thin sheet of gray matter and pia matter that connect the chiasm with the rostrum of corpus callosum), anterior commissure (a 1.5–6 mm anterior-posterior diameter bundle of fibers that crosses the midline in front of the columns of the fornix), foramina of Monro, and the columns of the fornix. The lamina terminalis fills the interval between the anterior commissure and the optic chiasm [8]. The lamina attaches to the midportion of the superior surface of the chiasm, leaving a small cleft between the upper half of the chiasm and the lamina, called the optic recess.

The posterior wall, that extends from the suprapineal recess to the aqueduct of Sylvius, contains the habenular commissure, the pineal body and its recess, and the posterior commissure. The pineal gland projects posteriorly into the quadrigeminal cisterns and is concealed by the splenium of the corpus callosum above, the thalamus laterally, and the quadrigeminal plate and the vermis of the cerebellum inferiorly.

13.4 Technique

The patient is placed in supine position with the head in a neutral position, slightly flexed, and fixed in a three-pin Mayfield-Kees headholder.

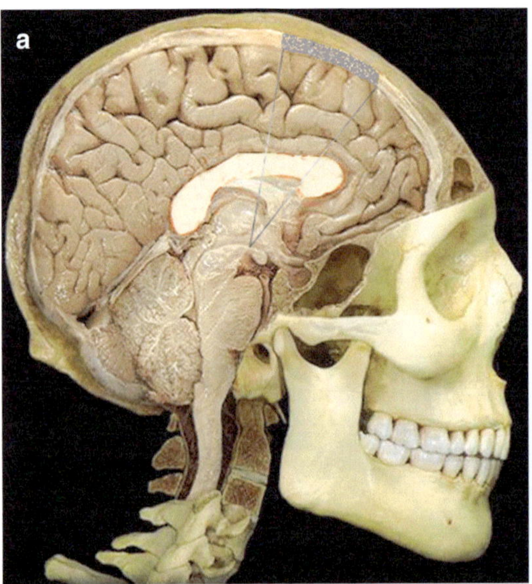

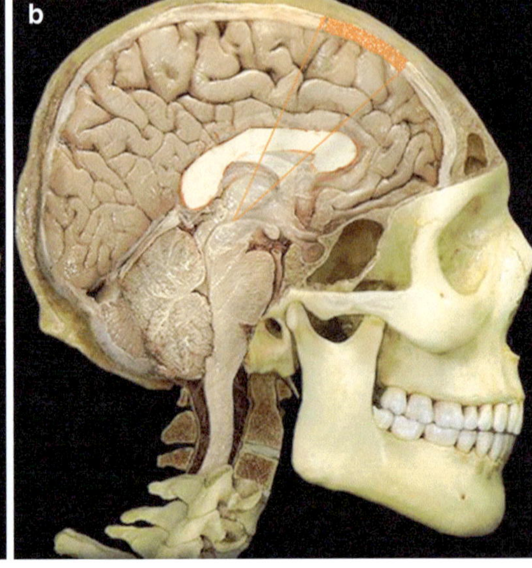

Fig. 13.2 (**a**, **b**) Schematic drawing showing the position of craniotomy flap to access the third ventricle cavity. (**a**) Standard 2/3 anteriorly and 1/3 posteriorly to the coronal suture. (**b**) More anterior craniotomy with posterior margin on coronal suture to access a more posterior portion of the third ventricle cavity

Some authors propose a lateral position with the operative side down to let the frontal lobe fall by gravity from the midline, avoiding unnecessary retraction during the interhemispheric fissure dissection. In our opinion the neutral position allows a better orientation in the midline and an improved cerebral venous outflow, while a strict microsurgical technique using sharp dissection and early CSF release minimize retraction damage to the frontal lobe. The approach is usually performed on the right side. An inverse U-shaped laterally based skin incision is usually performed 2/3 anteriorly and 1/3 posteriorly to the coronal suture. The skin incision can be placed more anteriorly to obtain a better exposure of the posterior portion of the third ventricle avoiding unnecessary manipulation of the prerolandic frontal lobe (Fig. 13.2). The use of neuronavigation to identify bridging veins may help in tailoring the position of skin incision and bone flap. The bone flap should be designed to expose the superior sagittal sinus in the midline. Usually a partial exposition of the sinus is enough to allow a direct access into the interhemispheric fissure, thus avoiding frontal lobe retraction. Before opening the dura, bridging vein position should be verified by means of neuronavigation. ICG video angiography may help in this task [9]. Dural opening is performed according to the bridging vein anatomy and with the base on the sagittal sinus. All the bridging veins should be carefully preserved. In some instances the bridging veins enter into a dural duplication before reaching the SSS. Careful incision of these dural duplications improves vein mobilization and access into the interhemispheric fissure. At this point sharp dissection is mandatory to widely open the fissure. Using cottonoids at the extreme anterior and posterior portion of the dissected fissure may help in maintaining it open avoiding the use of retractors. In case of tensive hydrocephalus, interhemispheric dissection may be very difficult; in such condition positioning of a ventricular catheter through the exposed frontal cortex may help in obtaining enough brain relaxation, facilitating arachnoidal dissection. Corpus callosum is a whitish, relatively avascular structure usually clearly different from the cortex of the cingulate gyrus. The correct identification of the pericallosal and calloso-marginal arteries is mandatory adjunctive landmarks. At this point, with the aid of the bipolar tips, a sagittal 15–20 mm wide

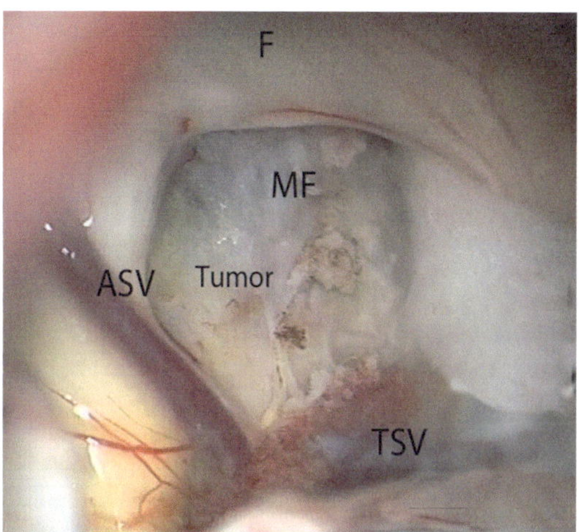

Fig. 13.3 Intraoperative view showing landmarks to be oriented inside the lateral ventricle cavity. *F* fornix, *MF* foramen of Monro, *ASV* anterior septal vein, *TSV* thalamostriate vein

incision is performed in the anterior portion of the corpus callosum. A transverse (coronal) callosal incision has been proposed by some authors especially in case of azygos anterior cerebral artery, with regard to neural fibers sparing [10]. In our experience, according to most other authors, the sagittal incision allows a wide exposure without permanent neuropsychological impairment. This deficit is most consequence of bilateral fornices manipulation more than callosal incision. The thickness of the corpus callosum is widely variable according to the preexisting hydrocephalus. Entering the lateral ventricle cavity allows further CSF outflow and brain relaxation. At this point a retractor may help in maintaining the fissure and callosal split opened to improve access to the deeper operative field. As soon as the lateral ventricle cavity is entered, orientation is granted by identification of foramen of Monro and thalamostriate vein. In the right lateral ventricle, the thalamostriate vein runs from the foramen to the right, while in the left lateral ventricle, it runs to the left (Fig. 13.3). If no vein is visualized, then a *cavum septum pellucidum* has been entered.

Access to third ventricle cavity is granted by one or both foramina of Monro. The foramen of Monro on the right side is usually firstly explored. In most cases tumor is already visible and it should be carefully and sharply dissected from the fornix (Video 13.1).

At this point the craniopharyngioma is debulked and then dissected from the lateral walls of the third ventricle. As soon as the tumor is debulked, its posterior pole comes into view. If this is not possible or excessive traction is needed, we suggest to perform a choroidal fissure opening. Low-voltage coagulation of the choroid plexus improves visualization and identification of the choroidal fissure. Splitting is performed with an anterior to posterior trajectory. Two different techniques have been proposed: opening the choroidal fissure on the thalamic side, retracting the fornix and attaching choroid plexus medially [11], and opening the forniceal side with lateral displacement of the fornix and the choroid plexus [12] (Fig. 13.4). The latter technique reduces the risk of damage to thalamostriate and caudate veins and improves third ventricular exposure compared with opening the forniceal side of the fissure. In fact, because of the retraction of the choroid plexus toward the midline with the fornix, there are more structures inhibiting access to the third ventricle [12]. Another trajectory to improve visualization and control of the posterior portion of the third ventricle is the use of the interforniceal corridor. The interforniceal approach is performed by splitting the midline forniceal raphe with subsequent perforation of the diencephalic roof along the plane between the two fornix bodies. In our experience this route should be limited in cases where a cavum septum pellucidum is identified. This anatomical variation usually widens the interforniceal space giving an easy access through the roof of the third ventricle, avoiding the risk of bilateral forniceal damage leading to severe postoperative memory and neuropsychological impairment. It is very important to stay on the midline because all neurovascular structures, such as body of the fornix, ICV, and choroidal arteries, are laterally placed.

Once the craniopharyngioma dissection from the fornices and lateral walls of the third ventricle has been completed, adherences with the floor should be identified and sharply dissected. In some cases it is impossible to identify a dissection plane between the tumor and the floor of the third ventricle. In these cases a subtotal resection should be considered to avoid catastrophic damage to the hypothalamus.

At the end of the resection, careful hemostasis should be achieved because even a small clot may cause postoperative CSF pathway obstruction leading to acute hydrocephalus. Gentle compression and use of hemostatic agents, such as thrombin gelatin matrix, may be very helpful at this step. Bipolar coagulation should be avoided. To prevent ventricular obstruction, irrigation is used to wash out blood that may collected in the ventricles. Endoscopic exploration may help in looking for residual tumor and checking CSF flow. Finally, ventricle cavities are filled with solution to limit postoperative intracranial hypotension (Fig. 13.5).

An external ventricular catheter is left in the lateral ventricle for approximately 48 h postoperatively to monitor intracranial pressure and check patency of the ventricular system [13].

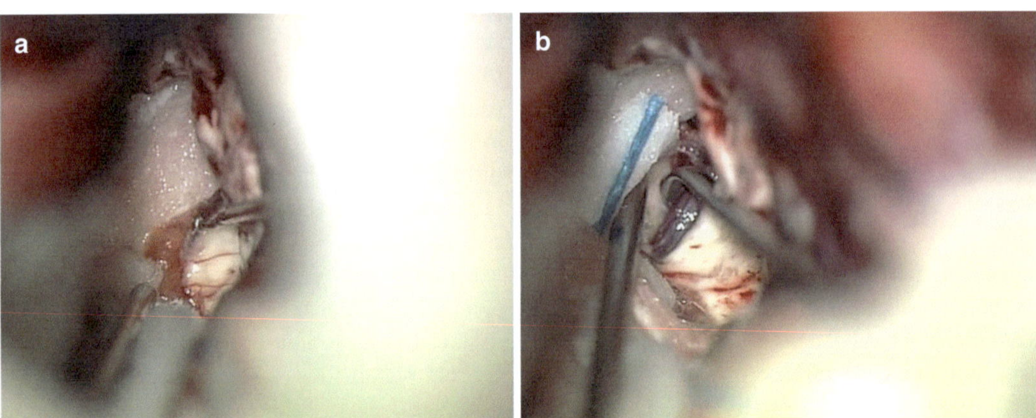

Fig. 13.4 (**a**, **b**) Intraoperative view showing splitting of the choroidal fissure. (**a**) Identification of choroidal fissure behind the choroidal plexus. (**b**) Opening the forniceal side with lateral displacement of the fornix

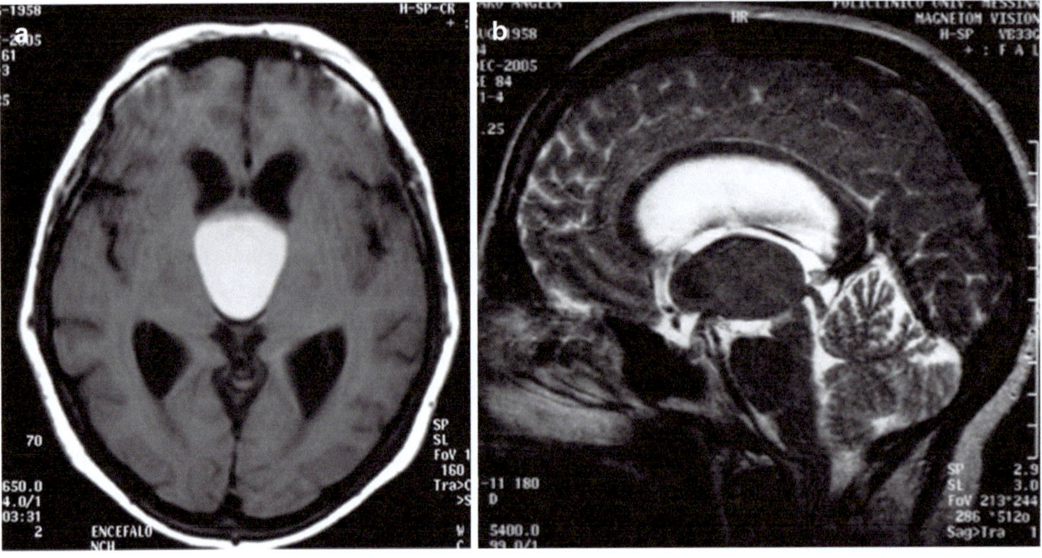

Fig. 13.5 (**a–f**) Pre- (**a–c**) and postoperative (**d–f**) MRI of a large third ventricle craniopharyngioma

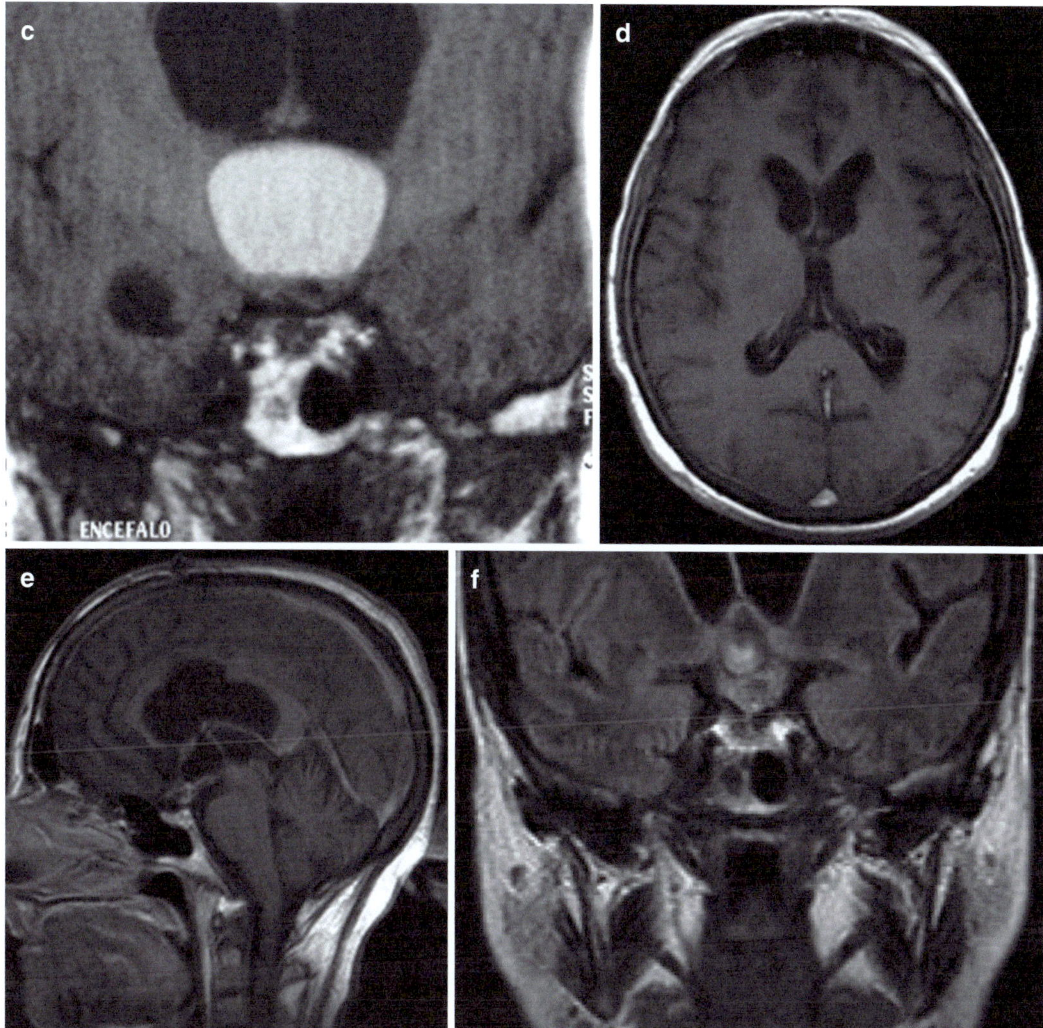

Fig. 13.5 (continued)

References

1. Kassam AB, Gardner PA, Snyderman CH, Carrau RL, Mintz AH, Prevedello DM (2008) Expanded endonasal approach, a fully endoscopic transnasal approach for the resection of midline suprasellar craniopharyngiomas: a new classification based on the infundibulum. J Neurosurg 108(4):715–728. doi:10.3171/JNS/2008/108/4/0715
2. Yasargil MG (1996) In: Yasargil MG (ed) Intraventricual tumors: Microneurosurgery, vol IV B. Thieme, Stuttgart, pp 313–338
3. Barchovich AJ (1996) Brain tumors of childhood. In: Barchovich AJ (ed) Pediatric neuroradiology, 2nd edn. Lippincott-Raven Publishers, Philadelphia, pp 321–437
4. Kucharczyk W, Montanera W, Becker L (1996) The sella turcica and parasellar region. In: Atlas WS (ed) Magnetic resonance imaging of the brain and spine, 2nd edn. Raven Press, New York, pp 871–930
5. Pascual JM, Prieto R, Carrasco R, Barrios L (2013) Displacement of mammillary bodies by craniopharyngiomas involving the third ventricle: surgical-MRI correlation and use in topographical diagnosis. J Neurosurg 119(2):381–405. doi:10.3171/2013.1.JNS111722
6. Curran JG, O'Connor E (2005) Imaging of craniopharyngioma. Childs Nerv Syst 21(8–9):635–639. doi:10.1007/s00381-005-1245-y

7. Tosaka M, Sato K, Amanuma M, Higuchi T, Arai M, Aishima K, Shimizu T, Horiguchi K, Sugawara K, Yoshimoto Y (2015) Superficial siderosis of the central nervous system caused by hemorrhagic intraventricular craniopharyngioma: case report and literature review. Neurol Med Chir (Tokyo) 55(1):89–94
8. de Divitiis O, Angileri FF, d'Avella D, Tschabitscher M, Tomasello F (2002) Microsurgical anatomic features of the lamina terminalis. Neurosurgery 50(3):563–569; discussion 569–570
9. Nussbaum ES, Defillo A, Nussbaum L (2012) The use of indocyanine green videoangiography to optimize the dural opening for intracranial parasagittal lesions. Neurosurgery 70(1 Suppl Operative):61–63; discussion 63–64. doi:10.1227/NEU.0b013e31822ecfeb
10. Mazza M, Di Rienzo A, Costagliola C, Roncone R, Casacchia M, Ricci A, Galzio RJ (2004) The interhemispheric transcallosal-transversal approach to the lesions of the anterior and middle third ventricle: surgical validity and neuropsychological evaluation of the outcome. Brain Cogn 55(3):525–534. doi:10.1016/j.bandc.2004.03.005
11. Viale GL, Turtas S (1980) The subchoroid approach to the third ventricle. Surg Neurol 14(1): 71–74
12. Ulm AJ, Russo A, Albanese E, Tanriover N, Martins C, Mericle RM, Pincus D, Rhoton AL (2009) Limitations of the transcallosal transchoroidal approach to the third ventricle. J Neurosurg 111(3):600–609. doi:10.3171/2008.7.JNS08124
13. Tomasello F, Cardali S, Angileri FF, Conti A (2013) Transcallosal approach to third ventricle tumors: how I do it. Acta Neurochir 155(6):1031–1034. doi:10.1007/s00701-013-1714-0

Radiotherapy and Radiosurgery

14

Giuseppe Minniti and Claudia Scaringi

14.1 Introduction

Surgery is the primary treatment modality for patients with craniopharyngiomas. Complete surgical excision is associated with a 5-year tumor growth control of 70–90 % in either adult or pediatric series [1, 2]. For uncompleted resected craniopharyngiomas, local control can be improved with the use of radiotherapy (RT) [3–5]. A few retrospective studies have demonstrated that partial resection followed by RT may provide outcomes comparable to those achieved with complete resection with lower incidence of toxicity as compared with aggressive surgery [6–9]. Modern RT has seen technical advances in all aspects of treatment with better immobilization, imaging, treatment planning, and dose delivery. In the last two decades, stereotactic radiation techniques, either stereotactic radiosurgery (SRS) or fractionated stereotactic radiotherapy (FSRT), have been employed in patients with craniopharyngioma with the aim of treating less normal brain and minimizing the long-term consequences of conventional RT while improving its effectiveness. In addition, there is a renewed interest in particle therapy with protons and ions, because of their physical and biological properties.

G. Minniti, MD (✉)
Radiation Oncology Unit, Department of Radiation Oncology, Sant' Andrea Hospital, University Sapienza, Via di Grottarossa 1035, Rome 00189, Italy

Department of Neuroscience, Neuromed Institute, Pozzilli (IS), Italy
e-mail: gminniti@ospedalesantandrea.it; giuseppeminniti@libero.it

C. Scaringi, MD
Radiation Oncology Unit, Department of Radiation Oncology, Sant' Andrea Hospital, University Sapienza, Via di Grottarossa 1035, Rome 00189, Italy

14.2 Conventional Radiotherapy

Retrospective studies in patients with residual and recurrent craniopharyngiomas have demonstrated benefit in local tumor control and survival following conventional conformal RT using doses of 50–55 Gy in 1.8–2.0 Gy fractions [3, 5–7, 10–18] (Table 14.1). In a series of 173 patients with craniopharyngioma treated at the Royal Marsden Hospital with external beam RT, the 10- and 20-year progression-free survival (PFS) rates were 83 and 79 %, and the respective overall survival (OS) rates were 77 and 66 %, at a median follow-up of 12 years [11]. Visual field defects and visual acuity improved after RT in 36 % and 30 % of patients, respectively, with no patient developing radiation optic neuropathy. In another retrospective series of 87 patients with residual or recurrent craniopharyngioma, Pemberton et al. [3] reported 10- and 20-year PFS rates of 78 % and 66 % and OS rates of 86 % and 76 %, respectively. A similar 10-year tumor

P. Cappabianca et al. (eds.), *Midline Skull Base Surgery*, DOI 10.1007/978-3-319-21533-4_14

Table 14.1 Summary of published studies on fractionated radiotherapy for craniopharyngioma

Authors	Patient no	Type of RT	Median dose Gy	Follow-up months	Tumor control (%)
Flickinger et al. [10]	21	CRT	60	7.3 years	95 at 10 years
Regine et al. [12]	58	CRT	56–62	17 years	82 at 10 years
Rajan et al. [11]	173	CRT	50	12 years	83 at 10 years
Hetelekidis et al. [6]	37	CRT	54	49	86 at 10 years
Mark et al. [13]	25	CRT	46–63	8 years	96 at 5 years
Habrand et al. [14]	37	CRT	50	98	56.5 at 10 years
Merchant et al. [15]	15	CRT	54	72	94 at 5 years
Varlotto et al. [16]	24	CRT	60	12 years	89 at 10 years
Stripp et al. [7]	76	CRT	55	7.6 years	84 at 10 years
Moon et al. [17]	50	CRT	54	12.8 years	91 at 10 years
Pemberton et al. [3]	87	CRT	43	8 years	77 at 10 years
Merchant et al. [18]	28	CRT	55	36	90 at 3 years
Masson-Cote et al. [5]	53	CRT	50	86	69 at 10 years
Selch et al. [19]	16	FSRT	50.4	28	75 at 3 years
Schulz-Ertner et al. [20]	26	FSRT	52.2	43	100 at 10 years
Minniti et al. [21]	39	FSRT	50	40	92 at 5 years
Combs et al. [22]	40	FSRT	52.2	98	100 at 10 years
Hashizume et al. [23]	10	FSRT	33	25.5	100
Kanesaka et al. [24]	16	FSRT	30	52	82.4 at 3 years
Harrabi et al. [25]	55	FSRT	52.2	128	92 at 10 years
Fritzek et al. [26]	15	FSRT/PBT	56.9 CGE	13.1 years	85 at 10 years
Luu et al. [27]	16	PBT	50.4–59.4 CGE	60.2	93

RT radiotherapy, *CRT* conventional radiotherapy, *FSRT* fractionated stereotactic radiotherapy, *PBT* proton beam therapy, *CGE* cobalt gray equivalent

control and survival rates ranging from 56 % to 95 % and from 65 % to 100 %, respectively, have been reported in the majority of published series [3, 5–7, 10–18].

The optimal dose of irradiation and timing of RT for patients with craniopharyngiomas is still matter of debate. Although a few reports have shown a better tumor control for doses >55 Gy [10, 13, 16], a comparable 5-year tumor control >90 % has been showed with doses of 50–54 Gy given in daily fractions of 1.7–1.8 Gy [3, 5, 6, 14], suggesting that such doses may achieve a similar tumor control as for higher doses, possibly decreasing the incidence of late radiation-induced toxicity. Another debated issue is the optimal timing of RT after surgical resection of a craniopharyngioma. A few pediatric studies have suggested that RT given immediately after surgery provides better local control than RT given at tumor recurrence [12, 28]. For adult patients, tumor control and survival are apparently similar when RT is administered postoperatively or at recurrence [3, 7, 17]. In clinical practice, early postoperative RT is usually reserved for patients with residual tumor after limited surgery; however, patients with complete resection may continue surveillance without immediate irradiation.

RT for patients with craniopharyngiomas may be associated with long-term toxicity. The most frequent complication is represented by the development of hypopituitarism; a new pituitary deficit or worsening of a partial hypopituitarism has been reported in 20–60 % of irradiated patients after 5–10 years [10–16], and this proportion is likely to increase with longer follow-up. Other toxicities, including radiation optic neuropathy and other cranial deficits, cerebrovascular events [11, 12, 29], and second malignant neoplasms [6, 8, 12, 14] are reported in less than 3–5 % of patients. Although the potential detrimental effect of RT on neurocognitive function especially in young patients is of concern, a few studies, using formal neurocognitive testing, showed no significant neurocognitive decline in patients with craniopharyngioma after radiation therapy [15, 18, 30]. In contrast, other factors such as extensive surgery, hydrocephalus at diagnosis, and shunt insertion have been associated with worse neurocognitive outcome [18, 30].

14.3 Stereotactic Techniques

Stereotactic RT is a further refinement of 3D conformal RT. Improved immobilization is achieved with either a frame-based or a frameless mask stereotactic system with submillimetric accuracy of patient repositioning. Radiation dose can be delivered as single-fraction SRS, as multifraction SRS (2–5 fractions), and as FSRT when a conventional fractionation of 1.8–2.0 Gy per fraction is used. SRS can be delivered using a modified linear accelerator (Linac SRS), a Gamma Knife (GK SRS), or a CyberKnife device (CK SRS).

Improved local control in patients with craniopharyngioma undergoing FSRT has been shown in several studies [19–25] (Table 14.1). In a series of 39 patients treated at the Royal Marsden Hospital with FSRT using a dose of 50 Gy in 30 fractions, the 5-year actuarial tumor control and survival rates were 92 % and 100 %, respectively [21]. Similarly, Combs et al. [22] reported 10-year local control and survival rates of 100 % in a series of 40 patients treated with FSRT using doses of 54 Gy in 30 fractions. In another series of 55 patients treated with FSRT, Harrabi et al. [25] showed 10-year local control and OS rates of 92 % and 83 %, respectively, at a median follow-up of 128 months. Overall, the reported results indicate that FSRT is an effective treatment option for craniopharyngiomas of any size. In the respect of the limited follow-up data in most published studies, FSRT is a safe treatment modality, associated with a relatively low toxicity. The main reported late effect of treatment is the development of hypopituitarism, with a new hormonal deficit in up to 40 % of treated patients at 5 years. Other complications are rarely observed, suggesting that the use of stereotactic irradiation could further reduce the toxicity observed with conventional RT.

SRS may represent a convenient treatment option for patients with small tumors not in close proximity (0–3 mm) to the optic pathway. One of the most widely chosen treatment modalities to deliver SRS is the GK [31]. In its most used version, an array of 201 cobalt sources are arranged in a hemisphere and focused using a collimator helmet onto a central point (isocenter). This results in a spherical dose distribution of 4–18 mm diameter. For larger irregularly shaped tumors, the best tumor conformality is achieved by different combinations of number, aperture, and position of the collimators using a multiple isocenter technique. During treatment, the patient is immobilized with a head frame fixed to the outer skull, allowing a positioning accuracy of <1 mm.

Several studies have reported the safety and efficacy of GK SRS in patients with residual or recurrent craniopharyngiomas after surgery [32–38] (Table 14.2). In a study of 98 patients treated with GK SRS, Kobayashi et al. [34] reported a tumor control rate of 79.6 % at a median follow-up of 65 months. In another series of 35 patients with craniopharyngiomas, Saleem et al. [38] observed a local control of 88.5 % at a median follow-up of 22 months, and similar findings have been reported by others [32, 33, 35–37]. Overall, local control rates ranging from 34 to 94 % using median marginal doses of 11–16 Gy are reported in seven studies including 286 patients (Table 14.2).

The most commonly observed complication following SRS for craniopharyngiomas is the development of new hypopituitarism, with an incidence ranging between 0 and 38 % in the different series. The main limitation to the use of SRS is the proximity of tumor to the optic pathway. Visual deficits are observed in up to 20 % of patients, although a few series report lower complication rates [35–37]. A well-defined dose-dependent risk of radiation optic neuropathy exists following single doses of irradiation. The reported incidence of radiation-induced optic neuropathy after SRS is about 2 % for doses of 8–12 Gy and becomes >10 % for doses of 12–15 Gy [25, 32–34]. In current clinical practice, SRS to doses of 15–16 Gy may represent a convenient approach to patients

Table 14.2 Summary of published studies on SRS for craniopharyngioma

Authors	Patient no	Type of SRS	Marginal dose Gy	Follow-up months	Tumor control (%)
Chung et al. [32]	31	GK SRS	12	36	87
Ulfarsson et al. [33]	21	GK SRS	3–25	17 years	34
Kobayashi et al. [34]	98	GK SRS	11	65	79.6
Yomo et al. [35]	18	GK SRS	11.6	24	94
Niranjan et al. [36]	46	GK SRS	13	62	68 at 5 years
Xu et al. [37]	37	GK SRS	14.5	50	67 at 5 years
Saleem et al. [38]	35	GK SRS	11.5	22	88.5
Lee et al. [39]	11	CK SRS	21.6[a]	15.4	91
Iwata et al. [40]	43	CK SRS	13–25[a]	40	85

SRS stereotactic radiosurgery, *GK* Gamma Knife, *CK* CyberKnife
[a]Dose delivered in 2–5 radiosurgical fractions

with small- and moderate-sized residual craniopharyngiomas not in close proximity to optic chiasm and nerves. By contrast, there is no restriction to the size of craniopharyngiomas suitable for FSRT, since the delivered total doses are within tolerance of normal brain structures, including the optic apparatus.

More recently, the CyberKnife (CK) robotic system has been employed for performing frameless SRS [41]. The device consists of a small linear accelerator mounted on a robotic arm. The robotic arm has 6° of freedom of movement, allowing a highly precise delivery of radiation from multiple angles directly to the tumor. The CK has x-ray cameras that monitor and correct target position continually during treatment. Only a few studies have investigated the outcomes of CK SRS in craniopharyngioma (Table 14.2). In a series of 11 patients with tumors in close proximity to the optic pathways, treated with doses of 20–25 Gy in 3–5 fractions, Lee et al. [39] reported a 2-year local control of 91 %, with no development of hormonal deficits or radiation-induced optic neuropathy. In another series of 43 patients treated with single-fraction (14 Gy) or multi-fraction (16–25 Gy in 2–5 fractions) SRS, Iwata et al. [40] reported a 3-year tumor control rate of 85 % at a median follow-up of 40 months. One patient developed hypopituitarism, while no cases of visual deterioration were reported. While these results are promising, the efficacy of hypofractionated treatment schedules in terms of tumor control and reduced risk of radiation-related adverse effects as compared to single-fraction SRS and FSRT remains to be investigated.

14.4 Intracavitary Radiotherapy

Intracavitary irradiation with radioisotopes (brachytherapy) has been employed for craniopharyngiomas with a significant cystic component [42], or, more frequently, for residual or recurrent disease after surgery and/or RT. The treatment requires stereotactical insertion of a beta-emitting isotope directly into the cyst. The advantage is that by delivering a high dose of radiation into the lining of the cyst, the secretory epithelium is destroyed, causing the cyst to collapse [43]. Beta radiation has a tissue penetration range of few millimeters, which means that the dose gradient falls off rapidly with distance from the source. As a result, the maximum dose is delivered to the target site, while the tissues surrounding the cyst receive a very small dose of radiation. The radioisotopes are delivered using colloid or microspheres as carriers to prevent systemic adsorption. Several radionuclides have been assessed in the past decades, and currently, the most widely used are phosphorus-32 ([^{32}P]) and yttrium-90 ([^{90}Y]) [42].

A few studies reporting the use of intracavitary RT for cystic craniopharyngiomas report tumor control rates of 67–100 % [44–49], with a relatively low rate of complications, including visual deterioration, hormone deficiencies, and perforation of adjacent vessels [44–46, 49–51].

14.5 Proton Radiotherapy

Proton RT has seen an increasing role in the treatment of children and adolescents with brain tumors with the aim of reducing the potential long-term side effects of radiation. The principal characteristic of protons is the deposit of little energy until the end of their range (Bragg peak), with the highest energy deposition in the tumor volume and low dose to the surrounding normal tissues [52]. A few series have evaluated the efficacy of proton beam therapy in patients with craniopharyngioma [26, 27, 53] (Table 14.1). In a small series of 15 pediatric and adult patients treated with a combination of proton and photon irradiation, Fitzek et al. [26] observed 10-year survival and local control rates of 72 % and 85 %, respectively, using median dose of 56.9 cobalt gray equivalent (CGE; 1 proton gray = 1.1 CGE). Two patients developed visual deterioration after RT, whereas no patient developed panhypopituitarism. In another series of 16 patients aged 7–34 years treated with proton beam RT using doses of 50.4–59.4 CGE, Luu et al. [27] reported a local control of 93 % at a median follow-up of 60.2 months with no significant long-term toxicity. Currently, published results on RT of craniopharyngiomas do not indicate that proton irradiation is superior to photon-based stereotactic radiation techniques in terms of local control and potential reduction of long-term toxicity.

References

1. Mortini P, Gagliardi F, Boari N et al (2013) Surgical strategies and modern therapeutic options in the treatment of craniopharyngiomas. Crit Rev Oncol Hematol 88:514–529
2. Buchfelder M, Schlaffer SM, Lin F et al (2013) Surgery for craniopharyngioma. Pituitary 16:18–25
3. Pemberton LS, Dougal M, Magee B et al (2005) Experience of external beam radiotherapy given adjuvantly or at relapse following surgery for craniopharyngioma. Radiother Oncol 77:99–104
4. Jeon C, Kim S, Shin HJ et al (2011) The therapeutic efficacy of fractionated radiotherapy and gamma-knife radiosurgery for craniopharyngiomas. J Clin Neurosci 18:1621–1625
5. Masson-Cote L, Masucci GL, Atenafu EG et al (2013) Long-term outcomes for adult craniopharyngioma following radiation therapy. Acta Oncol 52:153–158
6. Hetelekidis S, Barnes PD, Tao ML et al (1993) 20-year experience in childhood craniopharyngioma. Int J Radiat Oncol Biol Phys 27:189–195
7. Stripp DC, Maity A, Janss AJ et al (2004) Surgery with or without radiation therapy in the management of craniopharyngiomas in children and young adults. Int J Radiat Oncol Biol Phys 58:714–720
8. Schoenfeld A, Pekmezci M, Barnes MJ et al (2012) The superiority of conservative resection and adjuvant radiation for craniopharyngiomas. J Neurooncol 108:133–139
9. Lo AC, Howard AF, Nichol A et al (2014) Long-term outcomes and complications in patients with craniopharyngioma. the British Columbia Cancer Agency experience. Int J Radiat Oncol Biol Phys 88:1011–1018
10. Flickinger JC, Lunsford LD, Singer J et al (1990) Megavoltage external beam irradiation of craniopharyngiomas: analysis of tumor control and morbidity. Int J Radiat Oncol Biol Phys 19:117–122
11. Rajan B, Ashley S, Gorman C et al (1993) Craniopharyngioma–a long-term results following limited surgery and radiotherapy. Radiother Oncol 26:1–10
12. Regine WF, Mohiuddin M, Kramer S (1993) Long-term results of pediatric and adult craniopharyngiomas treated with combined surgery and radiation. Radiother Oncol 27:13–21
13. Mark RJ, Lutge WR, Shimizu KT et al (1995) Craniopharyngioma: treatment in the CT and MR imaging era. Radiology 197:195–198
14. Habrand JL, Ganry O, Couanet D et al (1999) The role of radiation therapy in the management of craniopharyngioma: a 25-year experience and review of the literature. Int J Radiat Oncol Biol Phys 44:255–263
15. Merchant TE, Kiehna EN, Sanford RA et al (2002) Craniopharyngioma: the St. Jude Children's Research Hospital experience 1984–2001. Int J Radiat Oncol Biol Phys 53:533–542
16. Varlotto JM, Flickinger JC, Kondziolka D et al (2002) External beam irradiation of craniopharyngiomas: long-term analysis of tumor control and morbidity. Int J Radiat Oncol Biol Phys 54:492–499
17. Moon SH, Kim IH, Park SW et al (2005) Early adjuvant radiotherapy toward long-term survival and better quality of life for craniopharyngiomas–a study in single institute. Childs Nerv Syst 21:799–807
18. Merchant TE, Kiehna EN, Kun LE et al (2006) Phase II trial of conformal radiation therapy for pediatric patients with craniopharyngioma and correlation of surgical factors and radiation dosimetry with change in cognitive function. J Neurosurg 104:94–102
19. Selch MT, DeSalles AA, Wade M et al (2002) Initial clinical results of stereotactic radiotherapy for the treatment of craniopharyngiomas. Technol Cancer Res Treat 1:51–59

20. Schulz-Ertner D, Frank C, Herfarth KK et al (2002) Fractionated stereotactic radiotherapy for craniopharyngiomas. Int J Radiat Oncol Biol Phys 54:1114–1120
21. Minniti G, Saran F, Traish D et al (2007) Fractionated stereotactic conformal radiotherapy following conservative surgery in the control of craniopharyngiomas. Radiother Oncol 82:90–95
22. Combs SE, Thilmann C, Huber PE et al (2007) Achievement of long-term local control in patients with craniopharyngiomas using high precision stereotactic radiotherapy. Cancer 109:2308–2314
23. Hashizume C, Mori Y, Kobayashi T (2010) Stereotactic radiotherapy using Novalis for craniopharyngioma adjacent to optic pathways. J Neurooncol 98:239–247
24. Kanesaka N, Mikami R, Nakayama H et al (2012) Preliminary results of fractionated stereotactic radiotherapy after cyst drainage for craniopharyngioma in adults. Int J Radiat Oncol Biol Phys 82:1356–1360
25. Harrabi SB, Adeberg S, Welzel T et al (2014) Long term results after fractionated stereotactic radiotherapy (FSRT) in patients with craniopharyngioma: maximal tumor control with minimal side effects. Radiat Oncol 9:203
26. Fitzek MM, Linggood RM, Adams J et al (2006) Combined proton and photon irradiation for craniopharyngioma: long-term results of the early cohort of patients treated at Harvard Cyclotron Laboratory and Massachusetts General Hospital. Int J Radiat Oncol Biol Phys 64:1348–1354
27. Luu QT, Loredo LN, Archambeau JO et al (2006) Fractionated proton radiation treatment for pediatric craniopharyngioma: preliminary report. Cancer J 12:155–159
28. Lin LL, El Naqa I, Leonard JR et al (2008) Long-term outcome in children treated for craniopharyngioma with and without radiotherapy. J Neurosurg Pediatr 1:126–130
29. Di Pinto M, Conklin HM, Li C et al (2012) Learning and memory following conformal radiation therapy for pediatric craniopharyngioma and low-grade glioma. Int J Radiat Oncol Biol Phys 84: e363–e369
30. Liu AK, Bagrosky B, Fenton LZ et al (2009) Vascular abnormalities in pediatric craniopharyngioma patients treated with radiation therapy. Pediatr Blood Cancer 52:227–230
31. Yamamoto M (1999) Gamma knife radiosurgery: technology, applications, and future directions. Neurosurg Clin N Am 10:181–202
32. Chung WY, Pan DH, Shiau CY et al (2000) Gamma knife radiosurgery for craniopharyngiomas. J Neurosurg 93:47–56
33. Ulfarsson E, Lindquist C, Roberts M et al (2002) Gamma knife radiosurgery for craniopharyngiomas: long-term results in the first Swedish patients. J Neurosurg 97:613–622
34. Kobayashi T, Kida Y, Mori Y et al (2005) Long-term results of gamma knife surgery for the treatment of craniopharyngioma in 98 consecutive cases. J Neurosurg 103:482–488
35. Yomo S, Hayashi M, Chernov M et al (2009) Stereotactic radiosurgery of residual or recurrent craniopharyngioma: new treatment concept using Leksell gamma knife model C with automatic positioning system. Stereotact Funct Neurosurg 87:360–367
36. Niranjan A, Kano H, Mathieu D et al (2010) Radiosurgery for craniopharyngioma. Int J Radiat Oncol Biol Phys 78:64–71
37. Xu Z, Yen CP, Schlesinger D et al (2011) Outcomes of Gamma Knife surgery for craniopharyngiomas. J Neurooncol 104:305–313
38. Saleem MA, Hashim AS, Rashid A et al (2013) Role of gamma knife radiosurgery in multimodality management of craniopharyngioma. Acta Neurochir Suppl 116:55–60
39. Lee M, Kalani MY, Cheshier S et al (2008) Radiation therapy and CyberKnife radiosurgery in the management of craniopharyngiomas. Neurosurg Focus 24:E4
40. Iwata H, Tatewaki K, Inoue M et al (2012) Single and hypofractionated stereotactic radiotherapy with CyberKnife for craniopharyngioma. J Neurooncol 106:571–577
41. Dieterich S, Gibbs IC (2011) The CyberKnife in clinical use: current roles, future expectations. Front Radiat Ther Oncol 43:181–194
42. Cáceres A (2005) Intracavitary therapeutic options in the management of cystic craniopharyngioma. Childs Nerv Syst 21:705–718
43. Shapiro B, Fig LM, Gross MD (1999) Intracavitary therapy of craniopharyngiomas. Q J Nucl Med 43:367–374
44. Pollock BE, Lunsford LD, Kondziolka D et al (1995) Phosphorus-32 intracavitary irradiation of cystic craniopharyngiomas: current technique and long-term results. Int J Radiat Oncol Biol Phys 33:437–446
45. Voges J, Sturm V, Lehrke R et al (1997) Cystic craniopharyngioma: long-term results after intracavitary irradiation with stereotactically applied colloidal beta-emitting radioactive sources. Neurosurgery 40:263–270
46. Hasegawa T, Kondziolka D, Hadjipanayis CG et al (2004) Management of cystic craniopharyngiomas with phosphorus-32 intracavitary irradiation. Neurosurgery 54:813–822
47. Shahzadi S, Sharifi G, Andalibi R et al (2008) Management of cystic craniopharyngiomas with intracavitary irradiation with 32P. Arch Iran Med 11:30–34
48. Barriger RB, Chang A, Lo SS et al (2011) Phosphorus-32 therapy for cystic craniopharyngiomas. Radiother Oncol 98:207–212
49. Kickingereder P, Maarouf M, El Majdoub F et al (2012) Intracavitary brachytherapy using stereotactically

applied phosphorus-32 colloid for treatment of cystic craniopharyngiomas in 53 patients. J Neurooncol 109:365–374
50. Van den Berge JH, Blaauw G, Breeman WA et al (1992) Intracavitary brachytherapy of cystic craniopharyngiomas. J Neurosurg 77:545–550
51. Julow J, Backlund EO, Lányi F et al (2007) Long-term results and late complications after intracavitary yttrium-90 colloid irradiation of recurrent cystic craniopharyngiomas. Neurosurgery 61:288–296
52. Durante M, Loeffler JS (2010) Charged particles in radiation oncology. Nat Rev Clin Oncol 7:37–43
53. Beltran C, Roca M, Merchant TE (2012) On the benefits and risks of proton therapy in pediatric craniopharyngioma. Int J Radiat Oncol Biol Phys 82:e281–e287

Part III

Arachnoid Cysts

15 Endoscopic Endonasal Transsphenoidal Approach

Felice Esposito

15.1 Introduction

Although intracranial and/or spinal arachnoid cysts are fairly frequent and, most of the time, are asymptomatic, sellar or sellar/suprasellar arachnoid cysts (SACs) are relatively rare and, when symptomatic, are even more rare. Overall, SACs represent only approximately 1 % of intracranial space-occupying masses, and sellar arachnoid cysts comprise roughly 3 % of all intracranial ACs [1, 2]. In a recent survey of the pertinent English and French literature, McLaughlin et al. report the occurrence of symptomatic SACs in only 76 patients, including their own [1].

Such condition needs to be distinguished from the far more common evenience of the empty sella and, therefore, from its clinically evident counterpart, i.e., the empty sella syndrome. Even though the pathophysiology of sellar arachnoid cysts remains controversial, according with some authors, SACs, especially if communicating with the subarachnoid space, may represent one of the forms of the empty sella conditions. As a matter of fact, a possible physiopathological explanation states that sellar arachnoid cysts result from a defective diaphragma sellae through which the basal arachnoid membrane herniates [1]. However, SACs represent more an arachnoid diverticulum that may remain patent and be responsible for communication between the subarachnoid space and the cyst's cavity, qualifying SACs as communicating [1, 3–5]. The communication through which the arachnoid membrane herniates may close, creating a noncommunicating cyst [1, 3–5].

A second hypothesis has been proposed by Meyer et al. [6] and reported also by McLaughlin et al. [1]. They stated that SACs develop in the same fashion as other intracranial arachnoid cysts, such as between the arachnoid layers, as an arachnoid diverticulum originating above the diaphragma sellae and then expanding through its aperture or developing from a subdiaphragmatic arachnoid layering [1, 6]. Such possible explanation has been strengthened by the evidence of the presence of arachnoid tissue below the diaphragma sellae [7, 8]. Such authors have shown that the basal arachnoid membrane covering the diaphragma sellae extends also inferiorly, along the pituitary stalk at a variable distance. However, an intrasellar arachnoid cyst may potentially arise from one of these arachnoid sleeves, and the cerebrospinal fluid may penetrate via a ball-valve mechanism and favor expansion similarly as for other intracranial arachnoid cysts [1].

Electronic supplementary material The online version of this chapter (doi:10.1007/978-3-319-21533-4_15) contains supplementary material, which is available to authorized users.

F. Esposito, MD, PhD
Division of Neurosurgery, Department of Biomedical Sciences, Dentistry, and Morphological and Functional Imaging, University of Messina, Via Consolare Valeria 1, Messina 98125, Italy
e-mail: fesposito@unime.it; esposito.felice@gmail.com

P. Cappabianca et al. (eds.), *Midline Skull Base Surgery*, DOI 10.1007/978-3-319-21533-4_15

Being nonneoplastic lesions, SACs may become clinically eloquent because of the mass effect they may produce on the adjacent neurovascular structures and on the pituitary gland. As a matter of fact, like other benign cystic lesions of the sellar area (i.e., Rathke's cleft cysts), sellar arachnoid cysts can be serendipitously discovered and, therefore, may not require any surgical treatment; conversely, they can be diagnosed because of the occurrence of headache and/or endocrinopathy and/or visual impairment they may provoke, thus requiring a surgical intervention for decompressive purposes. Even though the presurgical management of patients with SACs is similar to those with other cystic lesions of the sellar area (clinical history, neurological examination, sellar imaging, endocrinological and ophthalmological evaluation), their surgical management and outcomes may be quite different [3, 9, 10].

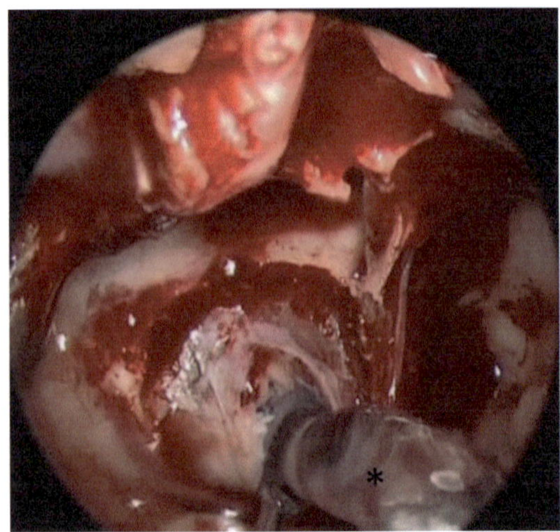

Fig. 15.1 After the small dural opening, the cyst content can be drained. *Arachnoid cyst content

15.2 Preoperative and Postoperative Assessment

Standard endocrinological assessment investigating the pituitary function is fundamental for the correct indication for the surgical treatment of SACs. Preoperative or postoperative pituitary dysfunction includes anterior gland axis deficiencies of hypoadrenalism, hypothyroidism, hypogonadism, and IGF-I deficiency, as well as posterior lobe dysfunction of diabetes insipidus. The standard hormonal assays include the evaluation of levels for plasma adrenocorticotropic hormone and serum cortisol, thyroid-stimulating hormone and thyroxine, luteinizing hormone, follicle-stimulating hormone, testosterone in men and estradiol in women, growth hormone, and IGF-I. Since several of the patients already present long-standing hormonal deficiencies, although subclinical, such condition needs to be correctly diagnosed and properly treated before surgery. The posterior pituitary function should be assessed as well, especially in the early postoperative period. In order to do that, all patients should be monitored for diabetes insipidus, although temporary, based on urine volume and urine specific gravity (a value of urine specific gravity below 1005 indicated the occurrence of diabetes insipidus). It is possible that the pituitary stalk compression my cause increased levels of prolactin as well as hyponatremia [1, 11–13].

Preoperative visual function assessment is also of fundamental importance in the surgical decision-making process. Either the visual acuity or formal visual field testing should be included in the routinary preoperative and postoperative tests of patients with SACs.

All patients should undergo preoperative and postoperative sellar magnetic resonance imaging with and without gadolinium, including early postoperative MR imaging (i.e., on postoperative day 1 or 2) and then subsequent MR study at 3-month postsurgery and yearly thereafter. A presumptive diagnosis of sellar arachnoid cyst is made when the MR imaging shows the signal of the cystic content similar to that of the normal CSF on all sequences and there is absence of abnormal enhancement in the cyst wall (Fig. 15.1).

15.3 Surgical Treatment of Sellar or Sellar/Suprasellar Arachnoid Cysts

When needed, the surgical treatment of SACs has mainly involved the marsupialization of the cyst's wall via a transsphenoidal route or, less frequently, through a craniotomy. Compared with transcranial approach, the transsphenoidal approach appears to provide a more direct and safer access to such cystic lesions. Nevertheless, the transcranial route may be still taken into account for the managements of SACs greater than 3–4 cm, with a relatively large suprasellar component, where a reliable communication between the cyst and the subarachnoid space exists, being responsible of the possible cyst recurrence after the simple transsphenoidal marsupialization.

Various techniques of cyst fenestration have been described. While some authors advocate a simple drainage of the cystic content through a limited opening of the sellar dura and the subsequent closure of the sural defect [1, 14], others have advocated the excision of the cyst's membranes either partially or entirely and/or to enlarge the communication between the cyst cavity and the suprasellar subarachnoid space [4].

Since SACs are nonneoplastic CSF-filled lesions that produce symptoms because of their volume and their mass effect over the surrounding structures, an effective and safe treatment of these lesions in most cases is the simple fenestration of the cyst wall with the emptying of the fluid content with the possibility to deflate the cyst and reduce the compression on the adjacent organs.

In such settings and in most cases, the standard endoscopic endonasal transsphenoidal approach represents the optimal surgical strategy for the marsupialization of SACs.

Anyway, one of the most important aspects in the transsphenoidal management of intra-suprasellar arachnoid cysts is to determine whether they communicate with the subarachnoid space, so differentiating the communicating from the noncommunicating SACs. This is almost always not possible based on the preoperative imaging studies. One empiric method is to scrutinize the refilling of the sellar cavity after it has been emptied, confirming the communication of the cyst with the subarachnoid space. Nevertheless, this might not occur in all cases as the communication may be very small, and even after the marsupialization of the cyst, a CSF leak may not be visible. Endoscopic exploration of the sellar cavity may facilitate the identification of an eventual communication of the cyst with the subarachnoid space using angled scopes (30° and 45°), which permit a panoramic exploration of the entire cyst wall allowing in many instances localization of the communication, if any. Small intrasellar cysts are usually noncommunicating, while in the larger intra-suprasellar arachnoid cysts, a communication with the subarachnoid space, even if very small, is usually present. An indirect sign of communication between the arachnoid cyst and the subarachnoid space may be the presence of small air bubbles behind the cyst wall [14].

15.3.1 Technique

The procedure is typically performed using a rigid 0° endoscope, 18 cm in length, and 4 mm in diameter (Karl Storz Endoscopy, Tuttlingen, Germany), as the sole visualizing tool. The 30–45° angled endoscopes are usually employed to explore the cystic cavity after its emptying. The nasal and sphenoidal steps of the procedure are performed following the same principles of the standard pituitary approach for pituitary adenomas [14–17]. A binostril 3–4 hand technique is usually adopted; as for standard pituitary surgery, the middle turbinate is not routinely removed but, rather, simply lateralized with an elevator and is repositioned back at the end of the procedure. After a wide sphenoidotomy and sellar bone opening, a relatively small dural opening is performed that is large enough to work through

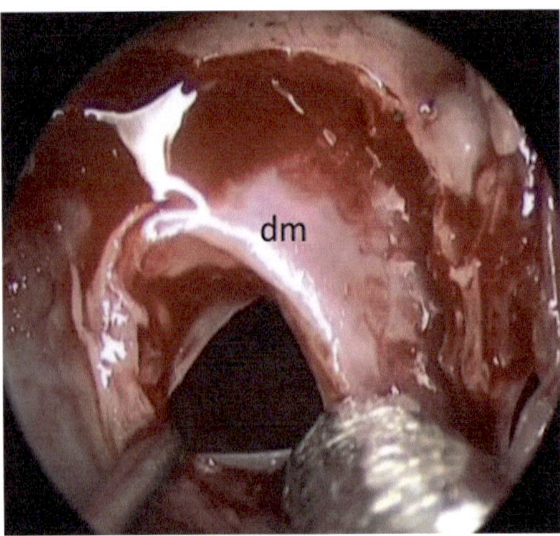

Fig. 15.2 The endoscope can be advanced inside the cavity of the cyst. *dm* dura mater

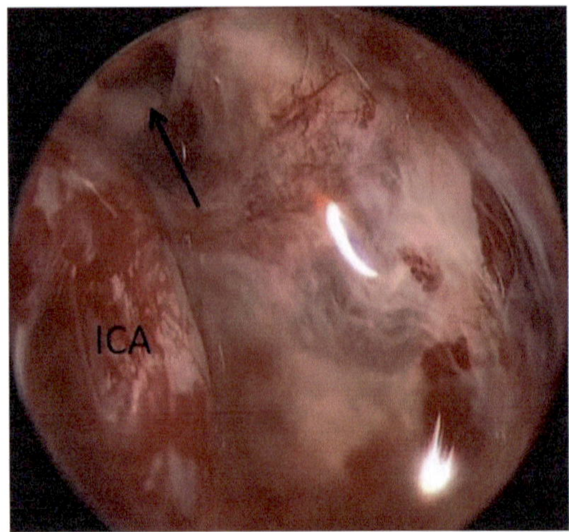

Fig. 15.3 Endoscopic endonasal close-up view of the arachnoid cyst cavity: note the communication with the suprasellar subarachnoid space (*arrow*). *ICA* internal carotid artery

and pass a 4-mm rigid endoscope but is not so large to not extend to the inferior sellar pole or the lateral sellar edges so that a dural margin will remain circumferentially to help hold the possible reconstruction materials in position. Care should also be taken to selectively open the dura only, while not penetrating the pituitary gland; should the gland be pushed anteriorly, a vertical gland incision may be needed to enter the cyst [1]. The cyst membrane is then punctured with a spinal needle or opened sharply with microscissors or with a microblade, causing the clear CSF immediately pouring forth (Figs. 15.1 and 15.2). A small fragment may be taken from the anterior cystic membrane, if any is recognizable, and the specimen is sent to pathology for the histopathological diagnosis. An inspection of the cystic cavity is performed using the 0° endoscope and subsequently with the angled scopes (30° and 45°) to visualize the lateral, posterior, and superior cyst walls, making sure the lesion is not a cystic tumor and looking for potential communication of the cyst with the subarachnoid space (Fig. 15.3). Anyway, most of the time, soon after the cyst drainage, the superior and lateral portions of the cyst collapse, making the intracystic exploration more difficult. In such cases, it can be effectively employed the so-called diving technique, popularized by Locatelli et al. [18]. Such maneuver is a similar technique used by laparoscopic surgeons in creating the pneumoperitoneum: the endoscope is inserted inside the residual cavity, and the continuous irrigation through the irrigation sheath permits the temporary reflating of the cyst cavity, allowing a more complete inspection from its inside. During such maneuvers, enlarging the possible communication into the subarachnoid space should be avoided, which may cause the transformation of a possible low-flow CSF leak into a high-flow CSF outflow, which is far more difficult to treat. Nevertheless, the insertion of the infundibulum into the diaphragma should be carefully inspected, as defects may be present in this location, and although small, they may be a site for postoperative CSF leak [1, 4]. Furthermore, any attempt to dissect the cyst wall off of the pituitary gland should be avoided, given the risk of worsening pituitary dysfunction [1, 14].

A key step of the endoscopic endonasal transsphenoidal treatment of sellar or sellar/suprasellar arachnoid cysts is the avoidance of their recurrence and, in case of communicating cysts, the prevention of the postoperative CSF leak. Thus, the dead space left by the emptying of the cyst, even though it may be partially reduced by the collapse of the cyst walls, needs to be completely filled, since “Natura abhorret a vacuo”

("Nature abhors a vacuum") [19, 20]. Several different materials have been proposed as "filler" of the sellar dead space, either autologous, heterologous, or synthetic [19–25]. If a definitive diaphragmatic defect is visualized, the tissue graft filling should, whether possible, partially obliterate this defect. Indeed, the filling should be sized enough to not overpack the sella, thus causing excessive optic apparatus compression. It is believed that the filling of the cyst cavity prevents the sella from refilling with CSF in the short period, while it likely induces scar formation to the diaphragma and parasellar arachnoid, recreating the natural partition between the sella and subarachnoid space in the longer period [1]. Subsequently, the dura should be reconstructed, and one of the reliable methods for the reconstruction is the extradural closure of the defect eventually supported by a pedicled nasoseptal flap [19, 20, 23, 26]. A Valsalva maneuver is performed to ascertain effectiveness of the reconstruction, and tissue glue is applied over the reconstruction with the double function of sealing the reconstruction and holding the materials in place [20]. The use of the lumbar drain is debated, and it may be reserved to those cases where an intraoperative CSF leak of high grade (Grade 3) is evident [20].

15.4 Outcome

Although SACs have a benign nature, being non-neoplastic lesions, transsphenoidal treatment of sellar ACs has been associated with the occurrence of serious complications including visual loss [27], postoperative CSF leak [3, 4, 9, 14, 27–29], and meningitis [6, 14, 27, 29].

On the other part, the endoscopic endonasal marsupialization of SACs has been associated with the postoperative improvement of the symptoms in a relatively high percentage of patients. Besides the case described by Spaziante et al. [27], most of the patients with preoperative visual symptoms improved postoperatively (67–100 %) [4, 6, 10, 14]. Pituitary dysfunctions have been also reported to improve postoperatively in a large percentage of operated patients with preoperative anterior pituitary defective endocrinopathies and/or hyperprolactinemia [1, 4, 6, 10, 14]. Nevertheless, new postoperative endocrine symptoms may occur and have been reported in up to 15 % of cases [4, 6]. Finally, headache has been reported to improve in up to circa 50 % of patients [4, 10, 14].

References

1. McLaughlin N, Vandergrift A, Ditzel Filho LF, Shahlaie K, Eisenberg AA, Carrau RL, Cohan P, Kelly DF (2012) Endonasal management of sellar arachnoid cysts: simple cyst obliteration technique. J Neurosurg 116(4):728–740. doi:10.3171/2011.12.JNS11399
2. Miyamoto T, Ebisudani D, Kitamura K, Ohshima T, Horiguchi H, Nagahiro S (1999) Surgical management of symptomatic intrasellar arachnoid cysts–two case reports. Neurol Med Chir (Tokyo) 39(13):941–945
3. Baskin DS, Wilson CB (1984) Transsphenoidal treatment of non-neoplastic intrasellar cysts. A report of 38 cases. J Neurosurg 60(1):8–13
4. Dubuisson AS, Stevenaert A, Martin DH, Flandroy PP (2007) Intrasellar arachnoid cysts. Neurosurgery 61(3):505–513; discussion 513. doi:10.1227/01.NEU.0000290896.69825.40
5. Hornig GW, Zervas NT (1992) Slit defect of the diaphragma sellae with valve effect: observation of a "slit valve". Neurosurgery 30(2):265–267
6. Meyer FB, Carpenter SM, Laws ER Jr (1987) Intrasellar arachnoid cysts. Surg Neurol 28(2):105–110
7. Song-tao Q, Xi-an Z, Hao L, Jun F, Jun P, Yun-tao L (2010) The arachnoid sleeve enveloping the pituitary stalk: anatomical and histologic study. Neurosurgery 66(3):585–589. doi:10.1227/01.NEU.0000365371.50165.06
8. Campero A, Troccoli G, Martins C, Fernandez-Miranda JC, Yasuda A, Rhoton AL Jr (2006) Microsurgical approaches to the medial temporal region: an anatomical study. Neurosurgery 59(4 Suppl 2):ONS279–ONS307; discussion ONS307-278. doi:10.1227/01.NEU.0000223509.21474.2E
9. Iqbal J, Kanaan I, Al Homsi M (1999) Non-neoplastic cystic lesions of the sellar region presentation, diagnosis and management of eight cases and review of the literature. Acta Neurochir (Wien) 141(4):389–397; discussion 397–388
10. Shin JL, Asa SL, Woodhouse LJ, Smyth HS, Ezzat S (1999) Cystic lesions of the pituitary: clinicopathological features distinguishing craniopharyngioma, Rathke's cleft cyst, and arachnoid cyst. J Clin Endocrinol Metab 84(11):3972–3982
11. Hsu YJ, Chau T, Yang SS, Tsai WS, Lin SH (2003) Rathke's cleft cyst presenting with hyponatremia

and transient central diabetes insipidus. Acta Neurol Scand 107(5):382–385
12. Sivakumar W, Cole CD, Couldwell WT (2011) Rathke cleft cyst presenting with hyponatremia: an unusual presentation. Neurosurg Focus 31(1):E4. doi: 10.3171/2011.4.FOCUS1180
13. Son JH, Fujimaki T, Tsuchiya Y, Ishii T, Takagi K, Nakagomi T (2005) Pituitary cyst presenting with hyponatremia and increased secretion of brain natriuretic peptide. Case report. J Neurosurg 103(6):1092–1094. doi:10.3171/jns.2005.103.6.1092
14. Cavallo LM, Prevedello D, Esposito F, Laws ER, Dusick JR, Messina A, Jane JA, Kelly DF, Cappabianca P (2008) The role of the endoscope in the transsphenoidal management of cystic lesions of the sellar region. Neurosurg Rev 31(1):55–64. doi:10.1007/S10143-007-0098-0
15. Cappabianca P, Cavallo LM, de Divitiis E (2004) Endoscopic endonasal transsphenoidal surgery. Neurosurgery 55(4):933–940; discussion 940–941
16. Cappabianca P, Cavallo LM, Esposito F, de Divitiis O, Messina A, de Divitiis E (2008) Extended endoscopic endonasal approach to the midline skull base: the evolving role of transsphenoidal surgery. In: Pickard JD, Akalan N, Di Rocco C et al (eds) Advances and technical standards in neurosurgery. Springer, Wien New York, pp 152–199
17. de Divitiis E, Cavallo LM, Cappabianca P, Esposito F (2007) Extended endoscopic endonasal transsphenoidal approach for the removal of suprasellar tumors: part 2. Neurosurgery 60(1):46–58; discussion 58–59
18. Locatelli D, Canevari FR, Acchiardi I, Castelnuovo P (2010) The endoscopic diving technique in pituitary and cranial base surgery: technical note. Neurosurgery 66(2):E400–E401; discussion E401. doi:10.1227/01.NEU.0000363746.84763.A5
19. Cappabianca P, Esposito F, Magro F, Cavallo LM, Solari D, Stella L, de Divitiis O (2010) Natura Abhorret a Vacuo-use of fibrin glue as a filler and sealant in neurosurgical "dead spaces". Technical note. Acta Neurochir (Wien) 152(5):897–904. doi:10.1007/S00701-009-0580-2
20. Esposito F, Dusick JR, Fatemi N, Kelly DF (2007) Graded repair of cranial base defects and cerebrospinal fluid leaks in transsphenoidal surgery. Neurosurgery 60(2):ONS1–ONS9
21. Cappabianca P, Cavallo LM, Valente V, Romano I, D'Enza AI, Esposito F, de Divitiis E (2004) Sellar repair with fibrin sealant and collagen fleece after endoscopic endonasal transsphenoidal surgery. Surg Neurol 62(3):227–233; discussion 233
22. Cappabianca P, Esposito F, Cavallo LM, Messina A, Solari D, di Somma LGM, de Divitiis E (2006) Use of equine collagen foil as dura mater substitute in endoscopic endonasal transsphenoidal surgery. Surg Neurol 65(2):144–149. doi:10.1016/J.Surneu.2005.08.023
23. Cavallo LM, Messina A, Esposito F, de Diviths O, Dal Fabbro M, de Diviths E, Cappabianca P (2007) Skull base reconstruction in the extended endoscopic transsphenoidal approach for suprasellar lesions. J Neurosurg 107(4):713–720. doi:10.3171/Jns-07/10/0713
24. Kelly DF, Oskouian RJ, Fineman I (2001) Collagen sponge repair of small cerebrospinal fluid leaks obviates tissue grafts and cerebrospinal fluid diversion after pituitary surgery. Neurosurgery 49(4):885–889; discussion 889–890
25. Esposito F, Becker DP, Villablanca JP, Kelly DF (2005) Endonasal transsphenoidal transclival removal of prepontine epidermoid tumors: technical note. Neurosurgery 56(2 Suppl):E443
26. Leng LZ, Brown S, Anand VK, Schwartz TH (2008) "Gasket-seal" watertight closure in minimal-access endoscopic cranial base surgery. Neurosurgery 62(5 Suppl 2):ONSE342–ONSE343; discussion ONSE343. doi:10.1227/01.neu.0000326017.84315.1f 00006123-200805002-00010 [pii]
27. Spaziante R, de Divitiis E, Stella L, Cappabianca P, Donzelli R (1981) Benign intrasellar cysts. Surg Neurol 15(4):274–282
28. Saeki N, Tokunaga H, Hoshi S, Sunada S, Sunami K, Uchino F, Yamaura A (1999) Delayed postoperative CSF rhinorrhea of intrasellar arachnoid cyst. Acta Neurochir (Wien) 141(2):165–169
29. Esposito F, Cappabianca P, Fusco M, Cavallo LM, Bani GG, Biroli F, Sparano A, de Divitiis O, Signorelli A (2008) Collagen-only biomatrix as a novel dural substitute examination of the efficacy, safety and outcome: clinical experience on a series of 208 patients. Clin Neurol Neurosurg 110(4):343–351. doi:10.1016/J.Clineuro.2007.12.016

Endoscopic Treatment of Arachnoid Cysts

16

Giuseppe Cinalli, Pietro Spennato, Giuliana Di Martino, Giuseppe Mirone, and Daniele Cascone

Arachnoid cysts are a congenital malformation, secondary to splitting or duplication of the arachnoid that becomes filled with CSF [1]. They typically arise within the arachnoidal cisterns, in most cases in the middle fossa at the sylvian fissure (30–50 %). Ten percent arise on the hemisphere convexity, 10 % in the suprasellar cistern, 10 % in the quadrigeminal cistern, 10 % in the cerebellopontine angle, and 10 % in the midline of the posterior fossa [1]. Midline cysts (suprasellar, interhemispheric, quadrigeminal, and posterior fossa) are usually associated with hydrocephalus and present earlier in life, usually during the first 10 years.

Symptomatic cysts typically present with local mass effect on neural tissue, obstruction of CSF flow, and macrocephaly in younger children. Most frequent symptoms are headache, head bobbing, focal neurologic deficits, seizures, and psychomotor retardation. An increased risk of posttraumatic extradural and subdural hematomas/hygromas is associated to the presence of the cyst. In symptomatic cysts, indication for treatment is clear. In infants, a pathologic increase (symmetric and asymmetric) in head circumference is a surgical indication. However, considerable debate continues to exist in the management of asymptomatic, incidentally discovered cysts. Because of the concern for impairment of brain development, in the pediatric population, treatment should always be recommended at the time of discovery unless the cyst is of a small size with minimal distortion of surrounding tissues and has been discovered incidentally [2, 3]. Cysts that distort surrounding neural tissues may be responsible for alteration in cerebral blood flow, thus explaining the atrophy often observed in the adjacent neural tissue.

Multiple surgical strategies have been developed in the management of symptomatic arachnoid cysts. These include endoscopic resection of the cyst wall with establishment of communication between the cyst and the contiguous CSF pathway (ventricles or basal cisterns), craniotomy with microsurgical fenestration, and shunting of the cyst in the peritoneum. The advantage of neuroendoscopy is that it avoids major surgical procedures, such as craniotomy with the risk of some major complications, and it avoids shunt dependence with all of the shunt-related problems [4, 5]. The choice between shunt and neuroendoscopy must be made on the basis of neuroradiological imaging to detect an area of contiguity between the cyst wall and the ventricular ependyma or subarachnoid spaces. This should be opened under endoscopic control to allow continuous drainage of the cyst. To avoid

G. Cinalli, MD (✉) • P. Spennato, MD
G. Di Martino, MD • G. Mirone, MD
Department of Pediatric Neurosurgery, Santobono-Pausilipon Children's Hospital, Naples, Italy
e-mail: giuseppe.cinalli@gmail.com

D. Cascone, MD
Pediatric Neuroradiology, Santobono-Pausilipon Children's Hospital, Naples, Italy

P. Cappabianca et al. (eds.), *Midline Skull Base Surgery*, DOI 10.1007/978-3-319-21533-4_16

reclosure of the stoma, large openings, at least 10–15 mm in diameter with removal of cyst wall fragments, should be performed [5]. The success rate (control of symptoms and cyst size without other surgical procedures) amounts for 71–81 % in endoscopic series [5–9]. The treatment is usually easier when the cyst obstructs the CSF pathway and hydrocephalus is associated, due to the possibility of working in larger spaces.

Surgical technique and results vary according to the location of the cysts. Best results have been achieved with suprasellar cysts. On the contrary, in case of arachnoid cysts of the middle fossa, indication to endoscopy is controversial. The arterial vessels of the Sylvian fissure may course within the medial wall of the cyst in proximity of the sites where fenestrations should be made. Therefore, some authors prefer microsurgery to endoscopic surgery for the arachnoid cysts in this location.

For infants with large hemispheric arachnoid cysts, the success rate of endoscopic fenestration appears to be less favorable than in older children [10]; however, in young children also, shunting is burdened by high rate of failure, and therefore, a neuroendoscopic approach should be advocated if possible. The possible need of a secondary cyst-peritoneal shunting in case of neuroendoscopy failure is always discussed prior to the intervention [10].

16.1 Middle Fossa Cyst

The middle fossa is the most common location for arachnoid cysts. These cysts may be responsible of a wide range of signs or symptoms, which include headache, focal neurological deficits, macrocrania, and hydrocephalus. They may also present with "functional" symptoms such as seizures and developmental delay [12].

16.1.1 Indication for Surgery

Indication for surgery in case of middle fossa cyst is highly debated. In the presence of symptoms and signs related to the cyst (headache, intracranial hypertension, macrocrania, hydrocephalus, focal neurological deficits), indication for surgery is clear. In case of "functional" symptoms, such as epilepsy and neurodevelopmental delay, indication for surgery is less clear. Some authors [12] suggest efficacy in postoperative seizure control and improvement in development, although direct clinical correlation of these symptoms to the cysts may be tenuous. In the series of Di Rocco et al. [13], patients with seizures were treated only if they also presented headache and/or macrocrania and/or focal neurology and/or progressive increase in size of the cyst. They observed good outcome of seizures in these patients. On the contrary, patients with developmental delays did not improve. In our opinion, patients with functional symptoms and mass effect on neuroradiological imaging are candidates for surgery, especially if they are young babies, with the aim to allow better brain development.

The debate of indication for surgery in asymptomatic young children with very large cyst with mass effect is still open. In our opinion, the younger the patient, the stronger is the indication for surgery.

In the recent paper of Choi et al. [15], the reasons for surgery (endoscopic or microsurgical fenestration) were categorized into three groups. In one group, surgery was necessary because the symptoms were related to the cyst (hydrocephalus, intracranial hypertension). In the second group, the symptoms were ambiguous, thought to be correlated with the cyst (headache, dizziness, large head, abnormality of skull, seizures, strabismus, or developmental delay). The patients in the third group presented minimal or no clinical symptoms, but underwent surgery with the expectation of improvement of abnormal findings in radiological or other examinations (huge cyst or enlarging cyst on follow-up image, abnormality in neuropsychologic tests, severe perfusion defect of adjacent brain parenchyma in single-photon emission computed tomography – SPECT). Interestingly, while the improvement rate in the first group was satisfactory, in the second group (the cases that showed ambiguous correlations between cysts and symptoms), it was very low. The improvement rate in this category was only 11 %, while the complication rate was as high as 43 %. In the third group, the radiological appearance of the cyst improved in 50 % of patient, and abnormality of neuropsychological tests improved in 35 %, while in no patients, there was improvement in SPECT evaluation. Therefore, they suggest surgical interventions only for those patients with symptoms indisputably related to the cyst.

Risk of traumatic hemorrhage after head injury is well known in patients with middle fossa cyst. However, surgery appears not to reduce the risk of traumatic hemorrhage. Surgery should not be proposed to prevent traumatic hemorrhage.

16.1.2 Selection of Candidates to Endoscopic Procedure Versus Alternative Treatments

Careful evaluation of preoperative imaging is crucial for considering endoscopy in case of intracranial cysts. Best evaluation is by MRI, especially with the modern CISS or DRIVE sequences that offer extraordinary contrast between CSF and brain parenchyma. The Prerequisite for safe endoscopic fenestration is the presence of enough space to safely reach the site of fenestration and the presence of a thin, not vascularized membrane to be fenestrated. In case of middle fossa cyst, microsurgical fenestration is also a straightforward procedure, with low operative risk and no need to cross the brain parenchyma. The choice between microsurgical and endoscopic fenestration should be well pondered: a minimal invasive procedure should be chosen only if it offers the same safety and the same success rate. Middle fossa cysts are usually classified in accordance with the Galassi classification [14]: type I cysts are small, spindle shaped, and limited to anterior middle cranial fossa; type II cysts show superior extension along sylvian fissure with displacement of the temporal lobe; type III cysts are large and fill the whole middle cranial fossa, with displacement of not only the temporal lobe but also the frontal and parietal lobes. Type I cysts are usually asymptomatic and only rarely treatment is necessary. In case of indication for surgery, endoscopic approach is not the ideal treatment, because the space for endoscopic maneuvers is limited. Moreover, it is necessary to cross the brain parenchyma to reach the cyst. Microsurgical fenestration is the best option in this kind of cysts. Type II and III cysts are very large with enough space for the endoscope to reach the target. The choice between endoscopic and microsurgical fenestration should be based on the appearance of the chiasmatic and interpeduncular cisterns on MRI. In case of large cisterns with thin membranes and enough space between carotid artery and optic nerve and/or tentorial notch and third cranial nerve, endoscopic surgery should be considered a valid option; otherwise, microsurgical fenestration should be preferred. Microsurgical techniques allow safer dissection of deep, thick membranes near vital structures, such as carotid artery and its branches, optic nerve, oculomotor nerves, and brain stem. In every case, the surgeon following endoscopic inspection of the deep membranes of the cyst should be ready to convert his procedure into microsurgery. This should be well explained to the patients and/or their parents in the informed consent. Several factors should be considered before performing endoscopic fenestration. Once within the cyst, the arterial vessels of the Sylvian fissure can be seen coursing the medial wall. They can be followed down to the basal cisterns, where the fenestrations can be made. The membrane of these cysts may be rich in collagen and can be difficult to penetrate, so that scissors or sharp instruments can be used to cut an opening. Often, the stoma should be enlarged with sharp instruments with some risks for the vessels of the Sylvian fissure. Open surgical procedures permit bimanual manipulation and the use of regulated suction to manipulate such thick and vascularized arachnoid membranes. Bleeding can be more easily controlled with traditional methods such as bipolar cautery and topical application of hemostatic agents (Fig. 16.1a–f).

Shunting, as the first surgical procedure, should be avoided in middle fossa cysts, because of the well-known risk common to all shunts (infection, mechanical dysfunction) and the

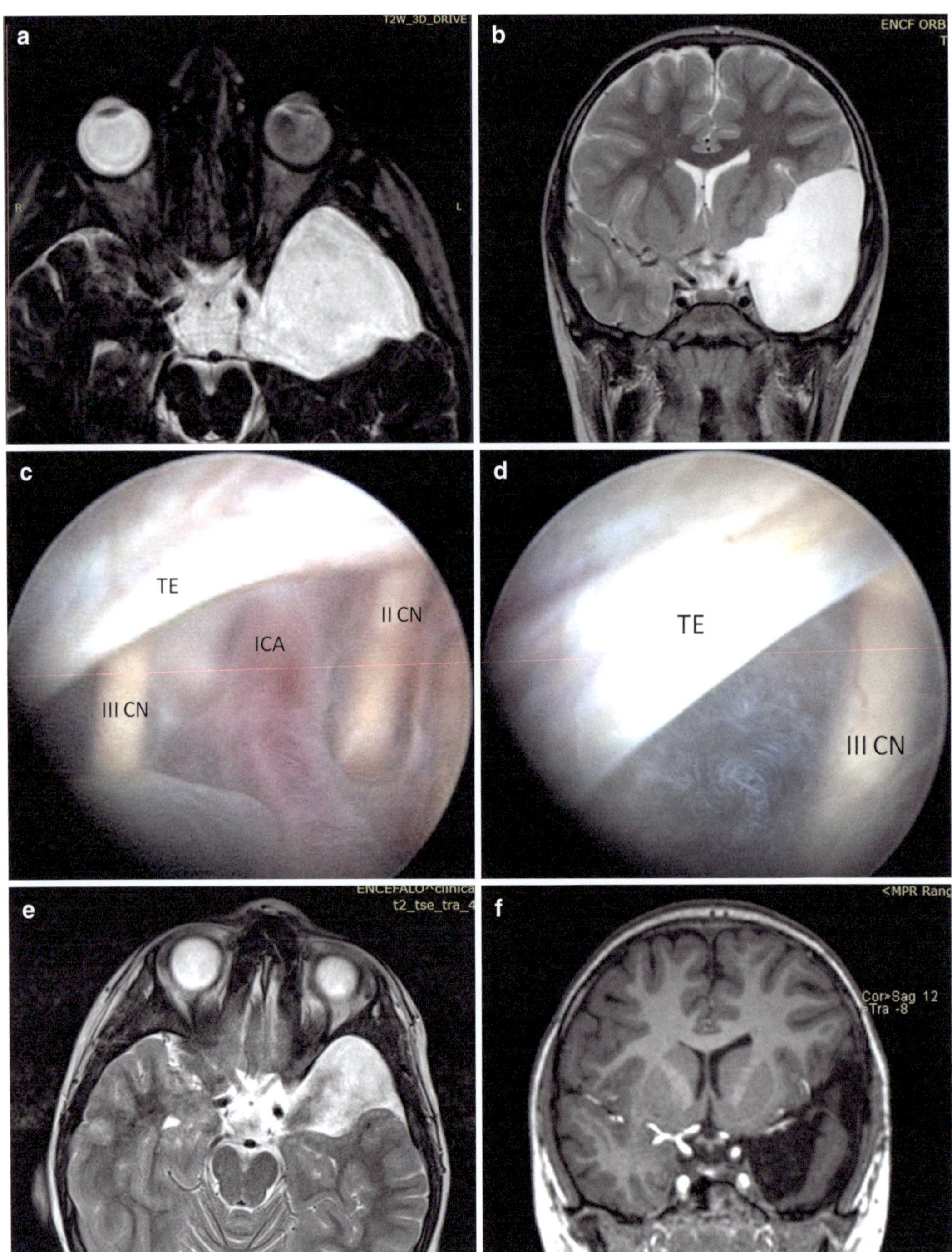

Fig. 16.1 (**a**) Arachnoid cyst of the middle fossa. Note the inner layer bulging medially behind the carotid artery. (**b**) Same patient as shown in (**a**), coronal view, where a large area of possible fenestration is easily identified. (**c**) Endoscopic view, where nerves and arteries are easily identified through the translucent layer of the cyst and delimitate areas of fenestration. (**d**) A safe, posterior window of fenestration is identified between the free edge of the tentorium and the third cranial nerve. (**e**, **f**) Postoperative MRI showing good flow artifact behind the carotid artery on axial T2 turbo spin echo sequences (**e**) and reduction of the cyst volume on coronal T1 (**f**)

higher probability of overdrainage, with slit cyst syndrome and secondary Chiari malformation that can be challenging to treat.

16.1.3 Authors' Preferred Surgical Technique

We use a surgical technique similar to those described by Di Rocco et al. [13] and Spacca et al. [12]. The aim of the procedure is to establish communication between the cyst and interpeduncular or carotid cistern (cyst-cisternostomy). The site of fenestration is between the optic nerve and the carotid artery, between the carotid artery and the oculomotor nerve, and between the third nerve and the free edge of tentorium. Electromagnetic neuronavigation is a very useful tool in order to choose the optimal entry point and to plan the best trajectory. It also provides real-time control of the endoscope position. The patient is positioned supine with the head tilted contralaterally. A small incision is performed over the temporal muscle behind the hairline. A burr hole is drilled directly above the cyst, avoiding residual cerebral mantle. The dura mater is opened with a knife to favor dural closure at the end of the procedure. A 30° free-hand rigid scope (Storz ®, Tuttlinger, Germany) is inserted within the cyst. The landmarks for the orientation are the free edge of the tentorium, the sylvian fissure with the arterial trunks, and the cranial nerves. The site of fenestration is decided on the basis of the aspect of the deep membrane (thickness and transparency). Usually the safest site is between the tentorial edge and the third cranial nerve. It allows to reach the interpeduncular cistern with good visualization of the basilar artery. Whenever possible, several holes within the deep membranes are performed. Based on the experience of Karabagli, multiple perforations are associated with decreased risk of cyst regrowth [19]. The best way to fenestrate the membranes is using Tulium LASER coagulation and forceps. Scissors should be used with great caution, because of the risk of arterial bleeding from small vessels. The stoma is also enlarged using the double-balloon catheter (neuro-balloon catheter from Integra Neurosciences®, Antipolis, France). Care is taken to open all layers. The cyst-cistern communication is considered satisfactory when it is possible to directly view the basilar artery and cerebrospinal fluid (CSF) pulsation through the fenestration. At the end of the procedure, the endoscope is removed. The dura mater is closed. The muscular fascia and the superficial layers are sutured in a standard fashion.

16.1.4 Follow-Up

CT scan or MRI is obtained until 24 h following operation to exclude major complication, in particular subdural effusion. MRI is planned in the first few weeks to confirm the presence of a flow artifact through the fenestration.

After hospital discharge, the patients are regularly controlled (clinical examination and brain MRI) 3 and 6 months and 1, 2, and 3 years after surgery.

Postoperative radiological appearance is very variable: in most successful cases, the cysts remain unchanged, or with minimal reduction of mass effect on surrounding tissue. The flow of CSF through the cyst- cisternostomies is confirmed by signal voids around ICA or tentorial edge on postoperative T2-weighted coronal MR imaging studies (*flow artifact*). There is no concordance between clinical and radiological outcome: patients who show radiological improvement not always demonstrate a corresponding improvement of clinical symptoms, especially if the reason for surgery was not clearly related to the cyst. Conversely, the patients who show clinical improvement, not always have radiological improvement [15].

Disappearance of the cyst following fenestration is very rare. In Choi's series [15], the cyst disappeared in 4/39 cases (10 %) and significantly decreased in 16/39. Sometimes the decrease of the cyst may be associated with the increase in size of the ventricles (especially at the level of the temporal horn) and presence of subdural fluid collection.

16.1.5 Complications

The main complication of the endoscopic series is subdural hygroma, with an incidence as high as 40 % of cases [4, 13, 15, 17]. This complication also occurs in microsurgical series and often requires surgical treatment with subduro-peritoneal shunt.

Leakage of CSF is another important complication, which has been reported to occur in 3.9–6 % of patients both in endoscopic and microsurgical series [16, 18]. Often, patients with CSF leaks are younger than 1 year of age and need a CSF diversion procedure.

Other surgical-related complications are subcutaneous collection, CSF infection, and third cranial nerve palsy.

16.1.6 Results

Good clinical outcome with complete recovery or significant improvement has been achieved in more than 90 % of cases in several series [12, 13, 19]. Relief of headache and other neurological deficits was obtained in all series but that of Choi et al. [15], in which headache was not always related to the presence of the cyst. These data are similar to those achieved by Levy et al. [18] following microsurgical fenestration. In the series of Choi et al. [15], the results are not so satisfactory, especially in infants, where the rate of surgical failure (need for additional operations such as a shunt or a second fenestration procedure) was 50 % (3/6). These results were also noted by others, so that some authors consider cyst-peritoneal shunt more effective in the infant group. In our opinion, the advantage of being shunt-free overcomes the risk of second surgery in the infant population, in which also the shunt-related problems (high rate of shunt revision, lifelong shunt dependency, overdrainage, and even brain herniation) are more frequent.

A second line of repeat endoscopy, craniotomy, or shunt may be considered in case of failures. In recurrent middle fossa cysts, we rarely perform repeat endoscopy and we prefer to offer craniotomy and microsurgical fenestration in case of absent flow artifact on neuroimaging (with the aim to achieve larger fenestrations of the deep membranes). If the fenestration appears to be patent on neuroimaging but symptoms are still present, cyst-peritoneal shunt is the preferred option, especially in younger children.

In conclusion, recent reports indicate that increasing number of authors prefer endoscopic approach as the first-line management of middle fossa arachnoid cysts [12, 13, 19–21]. However, larger randomized series are needed to identify the real advantages in managing middle fossa cysts by endoscopy, rather than alternative techniques (Table 16.1).

16.2 Suprasellar Cysts

Endoscopic surgery has radically changed the management of deep-seated arachnoid cyst. Patients with arachnoid cysts in the suprasellar region, especially if associated with hydrocephalus,

Table 16.1 Review of case series for pure neuroendoscopic treatment of middle fossa cysts

Authors	Cohort size	Results	Complications
Elhammady et al. [20]	6	Six successful	Subdural hygroma ($n=3$)
Di Rocco et al. [13]	17	Two recurrences	Venous bleeding ($n=1$)
Spacca et al. [12]	40	Satisfactory outcome reported in 92.5 % cases; cyst reduction in 72.5 % of cases; 10 % requiring second procedure	Subdural hygroma ($n=4$)
El-Ghandour [22]	32	Clinical improvement reported in 87.5 % cases; reduction in cyst size in 71.9 % cases; three cases of recurrence	Subdural hygroma ($n=2$), CN III palsy ($n=1$)
Karabagli and Etus [19]	20	Eighteen successful cases (in three endoscopy was repeated); two failures (CP shunt)	Asymptomatic subdural hygroma ($n=1$)

From Choudhri et al. [10], modified

are ideal candidates to endoscopic surgery, which allows wide fenestration of the cyst, both in the ventricular system and in the cisternal spaces [8], avoiding major surgical procedures, such as craniotomy and transcallosal approach. For this kind of cysts, endoscopic surgery is the treatment of choice, considering repeat endoscopy in case of failures and reserving shunting only to refractory cases. Typically, the suprasellar cysts elevate the floor of the third ventricle, often appearing just under the body of the lateral ventricle. Hydrocephalus due to obstruction of the CSF pathways either at the foramen of Monro or at the level of the cerebral aqueduct is often associated. Miyajima et al. [23] identified two different types of suprasellar arachnoid cyst, according to the position of the basilar artery. In the first type, the basilar artery is inside the cyst. They speculated that these cysts arise from invagination of the membrane of Liliequist. In the second type, the basilar artery is pushed posteriorly by the cyst. Their interpretation was that these cysts arise from cystic dilatation of the interpeduncular cistern.

16.2.1 Indication for Surgery

Suprasellar cysts are rare. They represent 8–15 % of all intracranial cysts. Treatment is indicated in case of symptomatic cysts or in case of coexisting hydrocephalus. The majority of cysts become symptomatic in early childhood, usually presenting with hydrocephalus and symptoms and signs of increased intracranial hypertension. Other frequent symptoms are visual field defects/impaired visual acuity (about 30 % of cases) and endocrinological disorders (about 60 % of cases) secondary to compression of the chiasm and hypothalamic-pituitary axis. Head bobbing in children is a rare feature, but quite typical of suprasellar cyst. Recurrent seizures are also indication for surgery.

Incidentally discovered cysts are usually not candidates for surgery, even if demonstration of cyst growth or the presence of neural compression, especially in children, should be an indication for consideration of surgical treatment to allow the potentially normal development and function of the adjacent brain [11].

16.2.2 Selection of Candidates to Endoscopic Procedure Versus Alternative Treatments

The location of the suprasellar may favor a different surgical treatment compared with cysts in other locations. The cysts are always in close relationship with the third ventricle; so, in case of sufficient ventricular dilatation, endoscopic treatment is the treatment of choice [24]. Usually, the cyst can be approached from the ventricles through a standard precoronal burr hole. Shunt placement is no longer suggested because of the need for foreign body implantation and the concomitant risk of shunt infection, failure, or lifelong shunt dependence. It should be reserved only to refractory cases.

Open surgical approaches are associated with a relatively higher surgical morbidity compared with endoscopic procedures and have success rate that does not exceed 70 % [11]. Microsurgery, through a subfrontal or pterional approach, should be reserved to those few cases not associated with ventricular dilatation. In the very rare cases in which the cyst expands from the suprasellar region to reach laterally the temporal fossa, the cyst can be approached with endoscope from a temporal burr hole, even if hydrocephalus is absent.

Different techniques have been advocated for endoscopic fenestration of suprasellar cysts. Some have advocated fenestration only of the apical membrane, usually at the level of the Monro foramen, between the ventricle and the cyst (ventriculocystostomy). Others suggested to also perform concurrent basilar fenestration toward prepontine cistern (cyst-cisternostomy), realizing a ventriculocystocisternostomy (VCC). Decq et al. demonstrated by MR-imaged CSF flow dynamics the importance of fenestrating suprasellar cysts both in the ventricles and in the basal cisterns, to prevent secondary closure of the opening and recurrence of symptoms [8]. The passage of CSF pulse waves in the cyst's cavity through sufficiently large windows in a "bipolar" fashion lowers the risk of re-formation of the cyst's membrane [8, 11]. Multiple fenestrations into all arachnoid cisterns that are accessible should lead to a lower rate of recurrence at long-term follow-up than do less aggressive methods, such as single fenestration [11]. Also the more recent paper from Maher and Goumnerova [24], which summarized their experience with 44 published cases, concluded that endoscopic ventriculocystocisternostomy is more effective than ventriculocystostomy.

16.2.3 Authors' Preferred Surgical Technique

Our surgical technique is similar to that described by Kirollos et al. [11]. Under general anesthesia, a frontal burr hole is drilled 3–4 cm from the midline (usually on the right side, or on the larger side, in case of asymmetrical ventricular dilatation) and on the coronal suture. The ideal position of the entry point and the best trajectory is selected on the basis of preoperative MR imaging. Neuronavigation is useful but usually not mandatory in standard cases, unless the ventricular system is small. The lateral ventricle is tapped, and the endoscope is directed toward the foramen of Monro, where the dome of the cyst is usually protruding into the third ventricle and comes into view. A fenestration is made between the cyst and the ventricle with various techniques, and we prefer to use Tulium LASER coagulation and scissors. Wide fenestration, at least 10 mm in diameter, is achieved, with coagulation of the apical portion of the cyst and removal of the cyst wall if possible. The cyst is then entered with the endoscope to visualize the basal wall of the third ventricle and the position of the basilar artery (inside the cyst, or outside the cyst, pushed toward the brain stem). It is usually possible to observe all the anatomical structures around the interpeduncular cistern through the thin inner layer of the arachnoid cyst, such as the basilar artery, internal carotid artery, posterior communicating arteries, pituitary stalk, optic chiasm, and third cranial nerves. Several openings into the basal prepontine cistern should be created, usually between basilar artery and third cranial nerves from both sides. The openings can be done using a probe without the application of any current and enlarged with balloon catheters. The endoscope is then advanced through the fenestration to visualize the neurovascular structures in the basal cisterns and to ensure the creation of adequate communication between the cyst and the subarachnoid space.

In the rare cases in which suprasellar cyst expand laterally toward the temporal fossa, the cyst can be approached directly through a temporal burr hole, like middle fossa cyst. Once inside the cyst with the endoscope, a cyst-cisternostomy can be performed in standard fashion, trying to make multiple perforations, on both sides of the basilar artery (Figs. 16.2a, b and 16.3a–j).

16.2.4 Follow-Up

The follow-up is similar to middle fossa cyst: a neuroradiological investigation (preferably MRI) is obtained until 24 h following operation. The presence of flow artifact through the fenestration at MRI should be addressed before discharge from the hospital. After hospital discharge, the patients are regularly controlled 3 and 6 months and 1, 2, and 3 years after surgery.

The reduction in arachnoid cyst size following endoscopy, also for cysts in this location, is variable. The indications for further intervention depend on the persistence of the patient's symptoms and not upon the appearance of the cyst on postoperative imaging [11].

Endocrinological disorders usually persist following treatment despite the satisfactory decrease in volume of the cyst [11].

16.2.5 Complications and Results

Reported complication rate is very low in this kind of surgery [10], with few addressed cases of ventriculitis and subdural hygromas. The success rate is high. Maher and Goumnerova [24] in their review calculated a success rate (no need for subsequent surgical procedures) of 86 % when only ventriculocystostomy (VC) was performed, and that increased to 92 % when ventriculocystocisternostomy (VCC) was performed as first procedure.

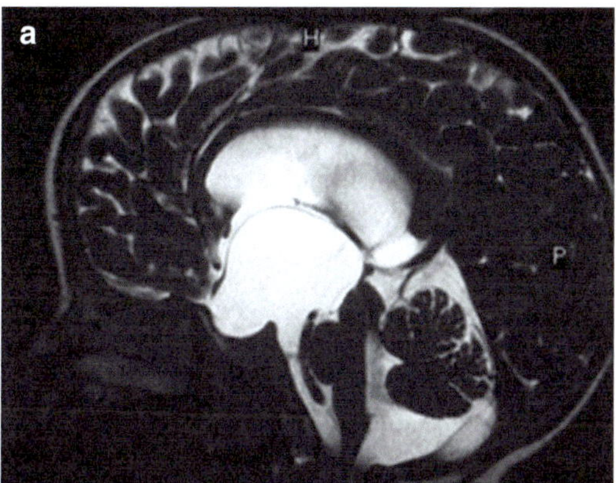

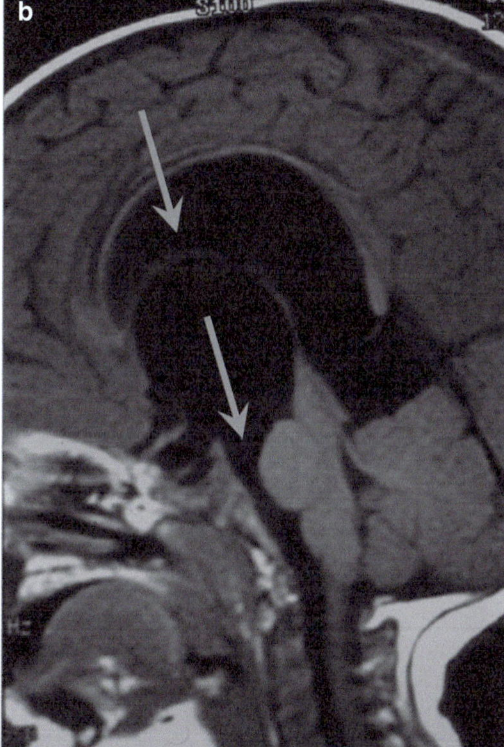

Fig. 16.2 (**a**) Type 1 suprasellar cyst, bulging into the third ventricle and occluding both foramina of Monro and the inlet of the aqueduct. (**b**) Surgical trajectory (*arrows*) for ventriculocystostomy and cyst-cisternostomy through a coronal burr hole

They analyzed separately the success rate of VC or VCC, when they were performed following a prior shunt treatment. VC alone was successful in 64 % of cases, while VCC was successful in 88 %.

Recently, Rizk et al. [25] reported a long-term clinical follow-up of six patients treated with endoscopic techniques, with an average of 46.5 months. Apart from one patient who developed ventriculitis that was successfully treated with antibiotics and temporary external drainage, no patients suffered recurrence of symptoms, abnormal imaging findings, or any sequelae of the surgical intervention.

In conclusion, endoscopic treatment of suprasellar cysts is safe and effective and should be considered in each case with compatible anatomy, in patients already treated with shunts and also in case of failure of the first endoscopic procedure. In these cases, larger fenestrations, with removal of cyst wall, especially at the level of the basal membrane, should be done by experienced neuroendoscopists.

16.3 Interhemispheric Cysts

Interhemispheric arachnoid cysts are congenital malformations usually associated with complete or partial agenesis of corpus callosum. They should be distinguished from other types of cystic lesions that can occur in the interhemispheric fissure and are part of more complex brain malformation, such as holoprosencephaly, diencephalic cyst with upward extension of the third ventricle, and porencephalic cyst. These cystic malformations are in communication with the ventricular system, do not need specific treatment, and have a very bad cognitive prognosis [26, 27].

Sometimes they can be confused with convexity cysts with interhemispheric extension (Fig. 16.4a). Often interhemispheric cysts are associated with ventricular enlargement. Various mechanisms are implicated: downward displacement of the foramina of Monro, obstruction of the aqueduct, or impairment of the resorption mechanism over the convexity.

Generally, interhemispheric cysts are diagnosed in the first year of life. Head enlargement, seizures, and psychomotor retardation are the most frequent presenting symptoms. These symptoms, however, may also result from the associated malformations (agenesis of the corpus callosum, gyral abnormality, and neuronal heterotopia). The cysts can be diagnosed antenatally, during routine ultrasound evaluation. They can remain silent for many years (Fig. 16.4b, c).

16.3.1 Indication for Surgery

As for cysts in other locations, surgery is indicated in case of symptomatic cysts. For patients with progressive signs of increased intracranial pressure or progressive cyst or ventricle enlargement, surgery is indisputably indicated. The indication for surgery is less established in patients with epilepsy and psychomotor retardation that can be attributed to the associated brain malformation. Usually, in young children with large cyst, associated to ventricular dilatation, surgery should be considered also in the absence of specific symptoms. Asymptomatic patients, for whom a conservative treatment is chosen, require

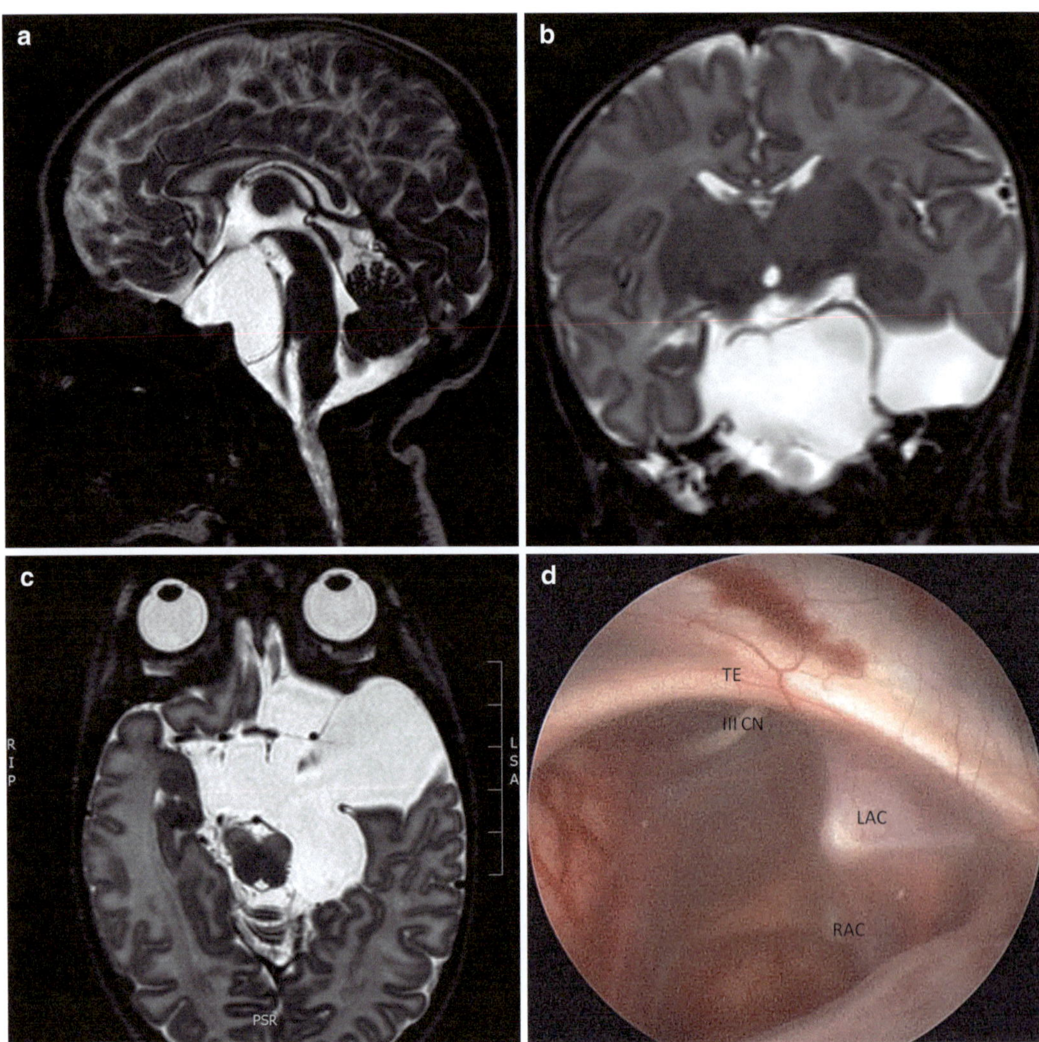

Fig. 16.3 Type 2 suprasellar cyst with lateral extension as seen on T2 sagittal (**a**), T2 coronal (**b**), and T2 axial (**c**) magnetic resonance. Endoscopic view of the skull base area chosen for fenestration (**d**). Following fenestrations, the stretching of the cranial nerves has decreased (**e**). Endoscopic views of the posterior fossa cisterns (**f**, **g**) through the fenestrations. Postoperative MRI showing significant decrease of the cyst size on sagittal (**h**), coronal (*arrow* indicate flow artifact through the stomy) (**i**), and axial (**j**) T2-weighted images

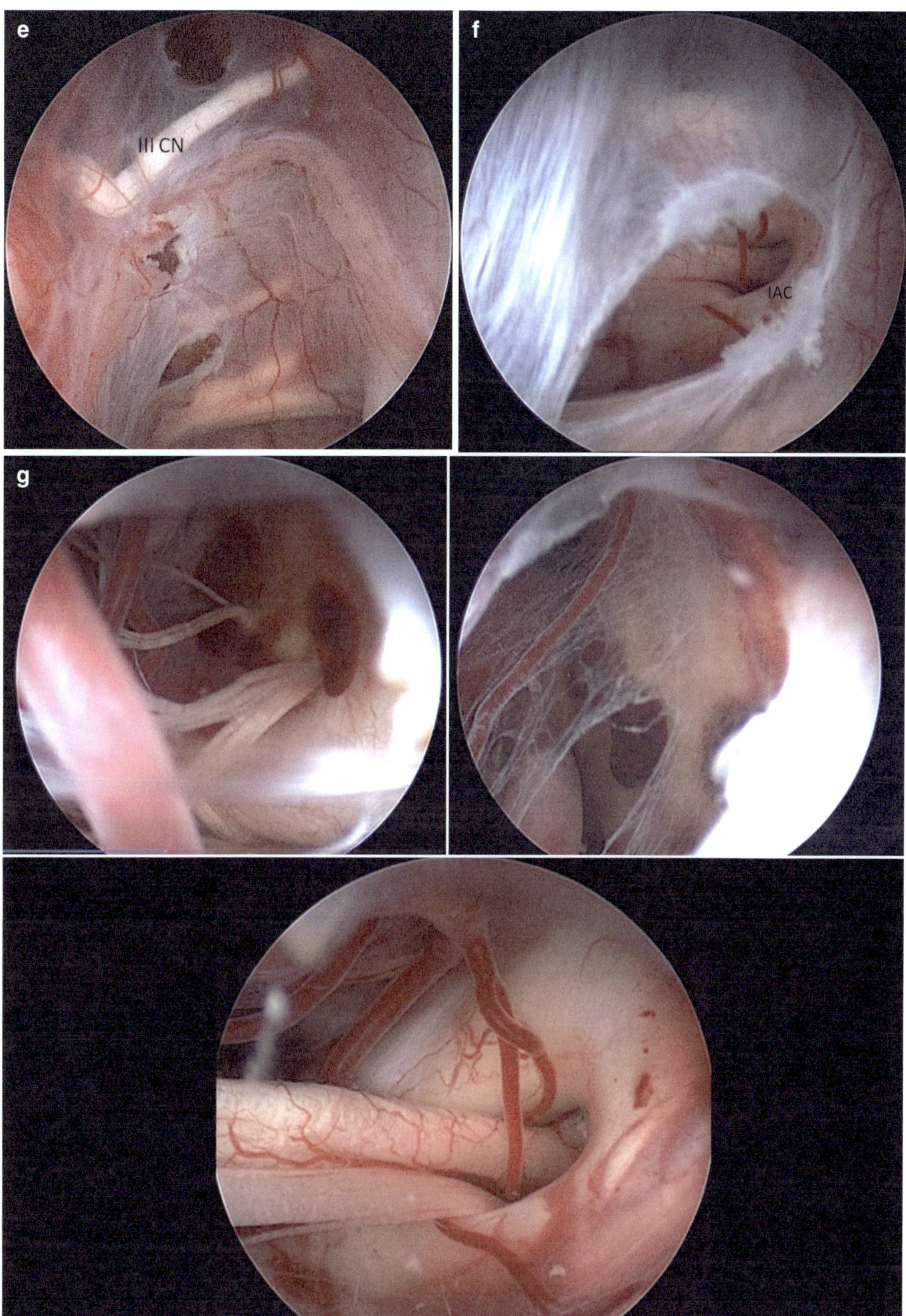

Fig. 16.3 (continued)

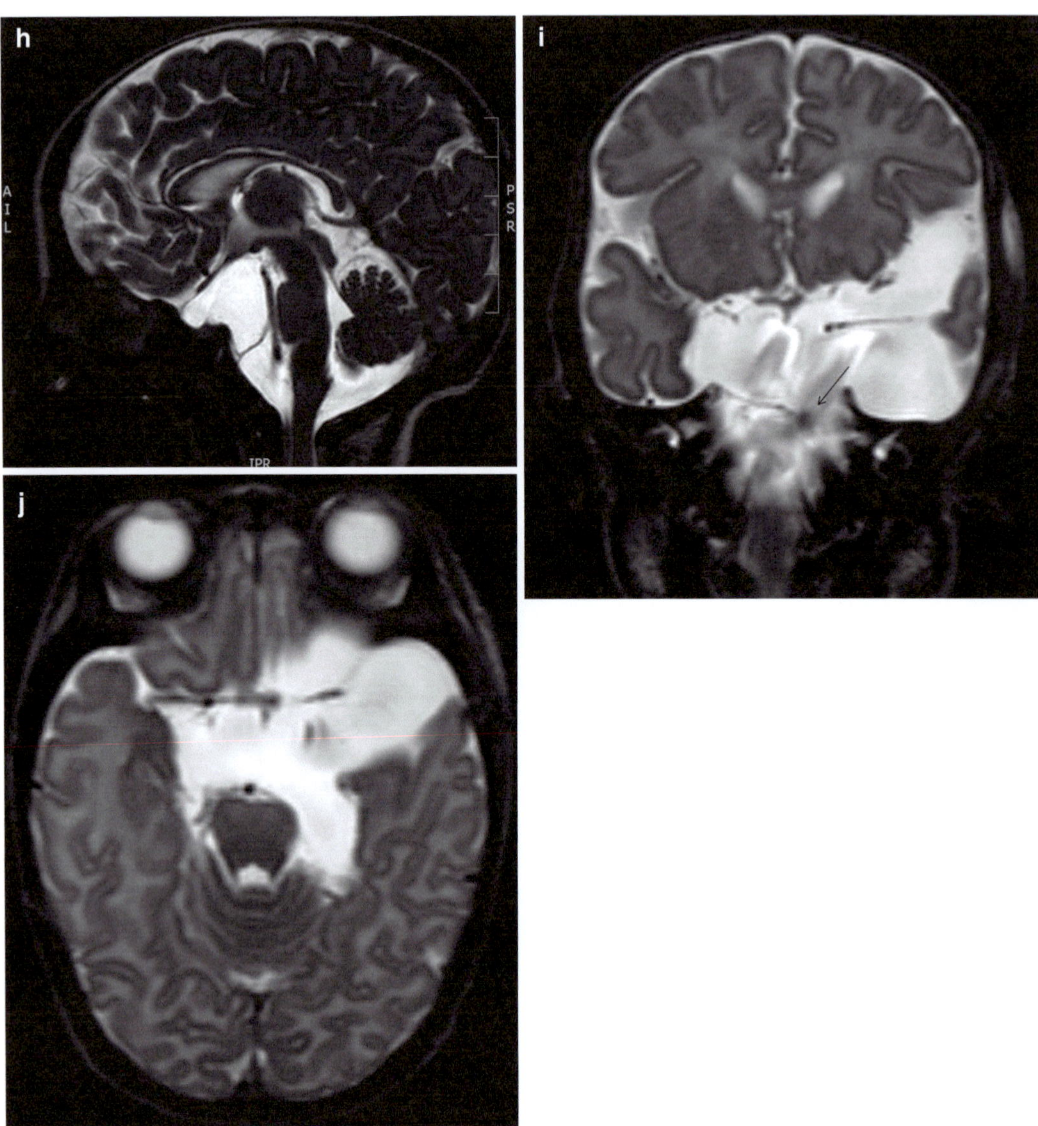

Fig. 16.3 (continued)

a close psychometric and neuroradiological follow-up, especially in the first year of life.

16.3.2 Selection of Candidates to Endoscopic Procedure Versus Alternative Treatments

According with Mori classification [26], Mori distinguished two types of arachnoid cyst in the interhemispheric fissure: unilateral parasagittal cysts and midline cysts. In the first case, the cysts have unilateral extension, are usually discovered in older children, and are not associated with corpus callosum agenesis. Usually, there is no contiguity between this kind of cysts and the third ventricle or other part of the ventricular system. Moreover, these cysts are not associated with hydrocephalus. The best option for these cysts, which usually reach the convexity, is microsurgery with excision of the lining membranes. It is a straightforward procedure, similar to removal

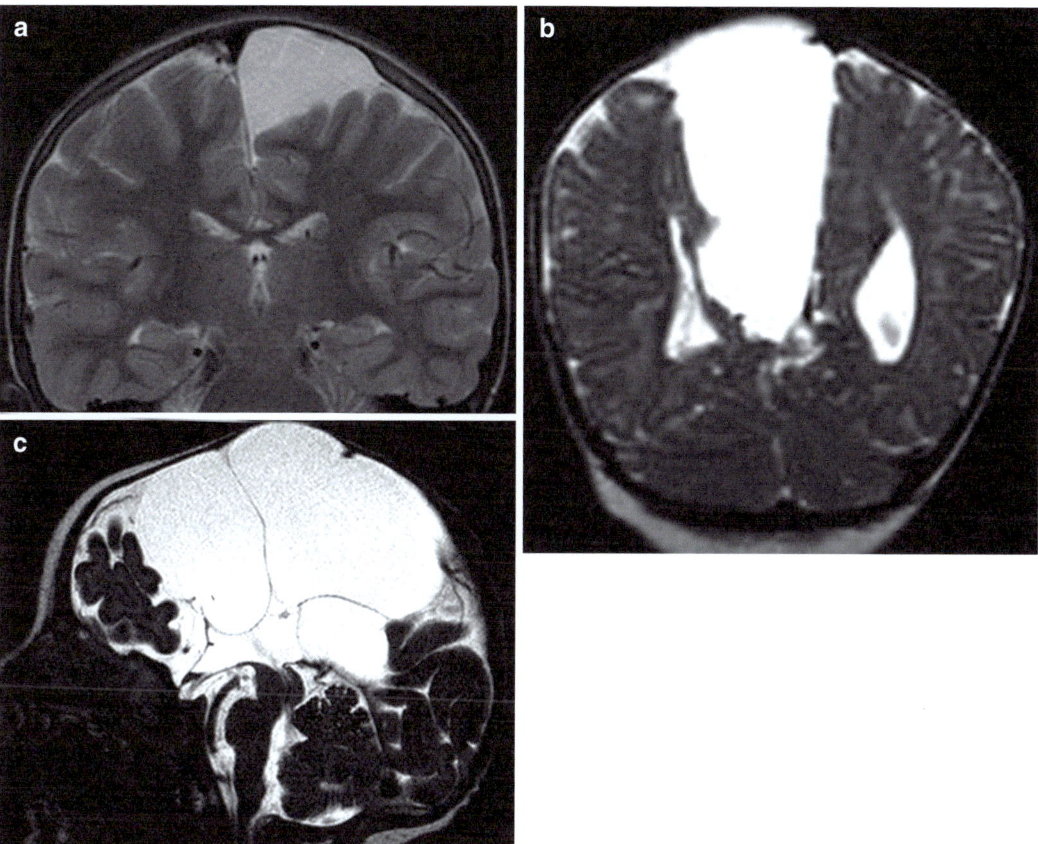

Fig. 16.4 (**a**) Convexity cyst with parasagittal expansion. Interhemisperic cyst associated with corpus callosum agenesis on coronal view (**b**) and sagittal view (**c**)

of arachnoid cysts over the convexity. On the contrary, midline cysts are more complex cyst often multiloculated, discovered in neonates and infants, and associated with agenesis of corpus callosum and ventricular dilatation. They usually expand inside the ventricular system, from which are separated by thin membranes. Due to the absence of the corpus callosum, the most frequent site of contiguity between the cyst and the ventricles is at the level of the roof of the third ventricle. The third ventricle, in fact, is often the final target of fenestration. In midline cyst, endoscopy is usually the best choice, because it allows simplification of multiloculated cysts, fenestration of the cyst with the ventricular system and the subarachnoid space of the interhemispheric/quadrigeminal cistern. In selected cases, third ventriculostomy can also be performed, to treat the associated hydrocephalus and to reduce the chance of stoma reclosure as discussed for suprasellar cysts. Craniotomy with cyst membrane excision, and creation of communication with the subarachnoid cisternal spaces and/or the ventricular system, is a major surgical procedure, with higher rate of complications, especially in neonates. Experience with open surgery is limited [26, 28], with not negligible rate of failure and secondary shunting. Shunting of the cyst was the best option prior to development of endoscopy. It is associated with low operative risk but also by all the well-known complications of the shunts in the long period, such as occlusions, inadequate drainage, and infection [28]. Moreover, in multiloculated cyst and in case of associated hydrocephalus, single cyst catheter may not be sufficient [29].

16.3.3 Authors' Preferred Surgical Technique

The goal of endoscopic surgery is to create communication between the cyst and the ventricular system (cyst-ventriculostomy) and/or the cyst and the cisternal space (cyst-cisternostomy). Surgical planning begins with careful evaluation of preoperative neuroradiological investigations (in particular MRI with DRIVE and CSF flow study) in order to detect the thinner point of the cyst walls where the stoma should be created and the multiple membranes, in case of multiconcamerated cysts. Neuronavigation is mandatory, because of the very distorted anatomy, to place the burr hole and to guide the endoscope through the target. Major vessels of the basal cisterns, the pericallosal arteries, the free edge of the tentorium, and the choroid plexus may be useful orientating landmarks.

Usually the most simple option is to penetrate first in the cyst, through a paramedian burr hole (drilled in the frontal, parietal, or occipital region, according to the location of the cyst), and hence, after recognition of the membranes to be perforated, to perform endoscopic fenestration in standard fashion. We prefer to use Tulium LASER coagulation and removal of large fragments of membranes. Also, the wall of the ventricle is usually a thin membrane. After entering the ventricle, the ependyma is easily recognized. In most cases of frontal and parietal interhemispheric cysts, associated to corpus callosum agenesis, the final target is the third ventricle. If the third ventricle is large enough, it is often possible to add a third ventriculostomy, in standard fashion, so to realize a ventriculocystocisternostomy. In case of posteriorly located interhemispheric cyst, the third ventricle is difficult to reach, and fenestration can be performed toward the interhemispheric fissure or lamina quadrigeminal cistern (cyst-cisternostomy) and toward an enlarged occipital horn of the lateral ventricle. Also in these cases, navigation is mandatory (Fig. 16.5a–e).

Postoperative imaging is essential to assess the patency of the stomas and the patency of the subarachnoid spaces in which the CSF is diverted after the endoscopic procedure.

They are also important to detect possible complications related to the rapid decrease of the cyst volume, such as subdural hygromas.

16.3.4 Complications and Results

The endoscopic experience in the treatment of interhemispheric cysts is limited. Our group reported a small series of seven patients [30] affected by interhemispheric cysts associated with corpus callosum agenesis. Complete success (control of hydrocephalus and of the cyst size with no further surgical procedures) was achieved in five cases (71 %). Partial successes were achieved in the remaining two cases: one patient was endoscopically reoperated with success 1 year later because of closure of the stoma. The remaining patient required implantation of a lumboperitoneal shunt for persistence of subcutaneous CSF collection over the burr hole. The lumboperitoneal shunt was successfully removed without recurrence of the pseudomeningocele 8 months after insertion.

Subdural collection developed in three patients; in only one case, it was managed with insertion of subduro-peritoneal shunt. This was uneventfully removed 4 months later. No patients were shunt dependent at the end of follow-up. Neurodevelopmental evaluation performed in six patients showed normal intelligence (IQT>80) in three patients, mild developmental delay (IQT range 50–80) in two patients, and persistence of severe developmental delay (IQT<50) in one patient, who had undergone surgery when he was 12 years old. Similar satisfactory results were achieved by Giannetti et al. [31], who reported another small series of five patients. They avoided shunt in all very cases and reordered two complications: one subdural hygroma (treated with subduro-peritoneal shunt) and one CSF fistula (treated with lumbar puncture).

16.4 Quadrigeminal Cysts

Arachnoid cysts originated in the quadrigeminal cistern represent only the 10 % of all intracranial cysts. They are not homogeneous but have different extension toward surrounding regions,

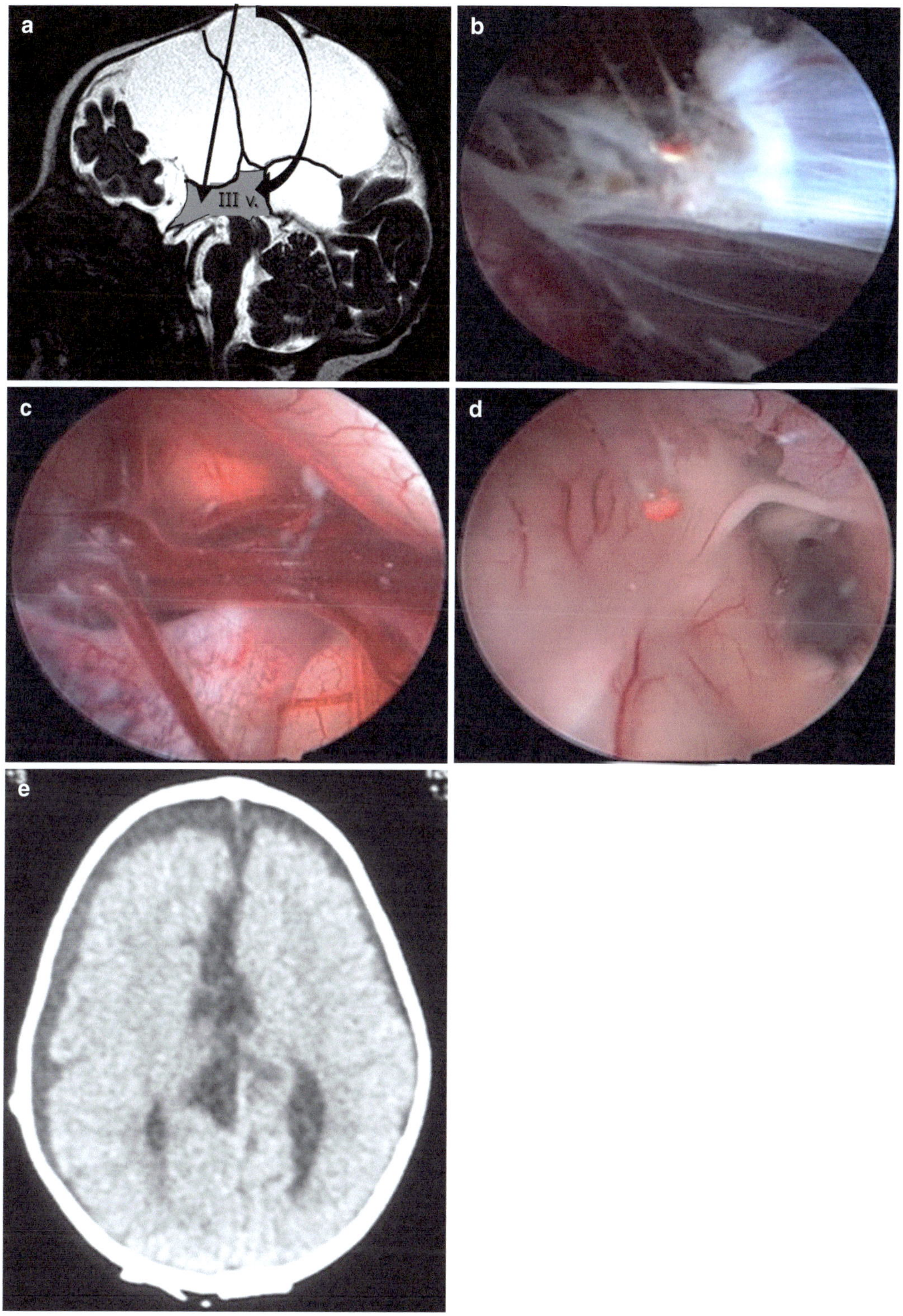

Fig. 16.5 (**a**) Surgical plan for the patient shown on Fig. 16.4. Cyst membranes are open using Thullium laser (**b**). Endoscopic view of the two internal cerebral veins and of Galen complex (**c**). Endoscopic view of the third ventricle (**d**), note the clear ependyma and the two mammillary bodies. Postoperative CT scan (**e**) showing reduction of the cyst volume

according to the presence of loci minoris resistentiae, such as the region of the trigone cranially, the supracerebellar cistern caudally, the third ventricle anteriorly, and the ambient cisterns laterally. Most of them extend both in the supratentorial (at the level of the trigone) and the infratentorial regions (in the supracerebellar cistern) (type I). More rarely, they have only infratentorial extension, in the supracerebellar or supraretrocerebellar regions (type II), or lateral extension in the ambient cisterns toward the temporal lobe (type III) (Fig. 16.6a–c) [16, 27]. Because of their intimate relationship with the dorsal midbrain, quadrigeminal cysts produce distortion or compression of the cerebral aqueduct at an early stage [27]. Symptoms are usually related to the associated hydrocephalus

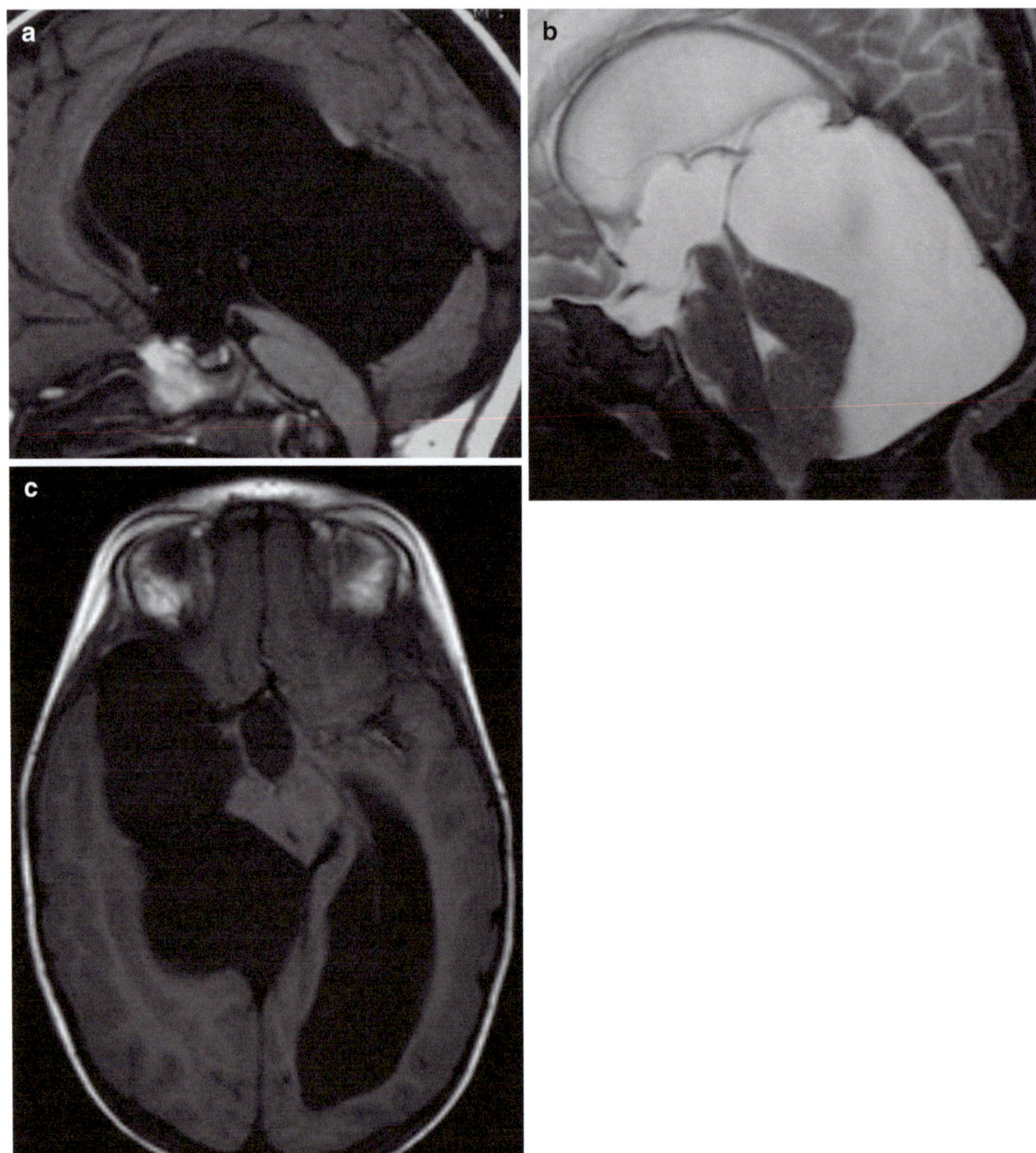

Fig. 16.6 Arachnoid cysts of the quadrigeminal cistern. Type 1 (**a**) has a dumbbell shape and occupies equal volume in the supra and infratentorial space. Type 2 (**b**) is mostly confined to the infratentorial space, in the retrocerebellar or supracerebellar space. Type 3 (**c**) presents a very significant lateral expansion through the choroidal fissure

(macrocrania, headache, vomiting, lethargy, papilledema) and/or compression of the dorsal midbrain (impairment of upward gaze and other ocular disorders).

16.4.1 Indication for Surgery

Large quadrigeminal cyst usually need treatment, because they distort CSF pathways at an early stage and become symptomatic. Untreated cysts may lead to macrocephaly and neurodevelopment delay. Only small cysts not associated with hydrocephalus and with minimal distortion of the aqueduct can be managed conservatively, with close clinical and radiological follow-up, especially in young children.

Careful evaluation of MR preoperative exams should be made in order to distinguish quadrigeminal cysts from pulsion diverticula, which are formed by herniation of the medial wall of the ventricular atrium into the quadrigeminal cistern through the tentorial hiatus in case of severe triventricular hydrocephalus. Anatomically the diverticula are not cysts but communicate with the ventricles; therefore, the treatment is different: endoscopic third ventriculostomy (ETV), curing the hydrocephalus, is usually sufficient to resolve also the associated diverticula, without additional procedures at the level of the quadrigeminal cistern.

16.4.2 Selection of Candidates to Endoscopic Procedure Versus Alternative Treatments

Because quadrigeminal cysts are almost invariably associated with hydrocephalus, endoscopic treatment is usually technically feasible because of the possibility of working in large spaces and the presence of an area of contiguity between the cyst wall and the ventricular ependyma (at the level of the trigone of the lateral ventricle, or at the level of the posterior third ventricle) or subarachnoid spaces. Third ventriculostomy can be also performed (Fig. 16.7a, b) [8, 32–34].

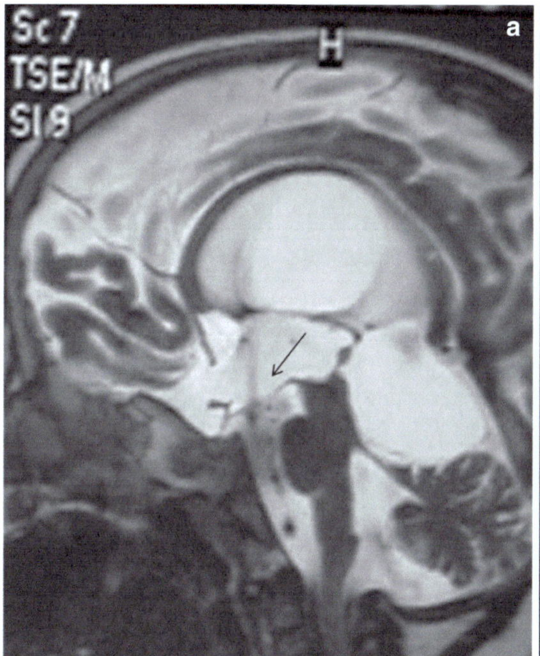

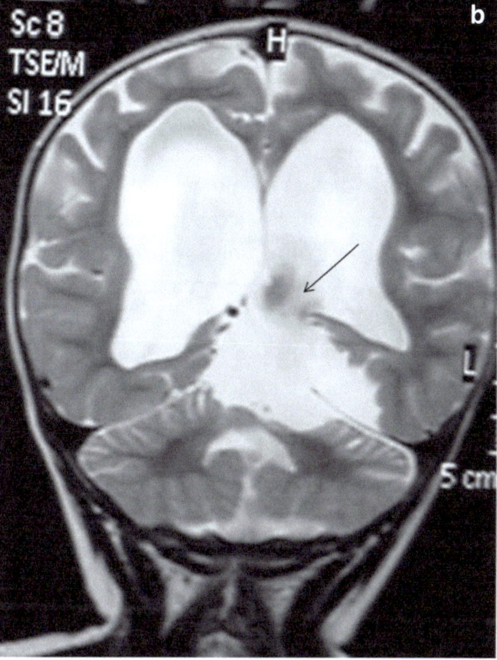

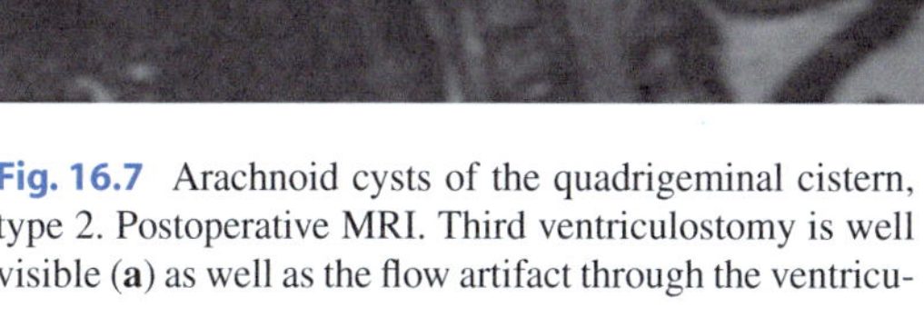

Fig. 16.7 Arachnoid cysts of the quadrigeminal cistern, type 2. Postoperative MRI. Third ventriculostomy is well visible (**a**) as well as the flow artifact through the ventriculocystostomy on coronal cuts (**b**), performed through the lateral ventricle following coronal approach. *Arrows* indicate flow artifact through the stomy

Extrinsic aqueductal stenosis arising from long-standing compression by the cyst may persist despite cyst opening.

Endoscopy can be also considered an alternative to shunt revision in patients already shunted, in order to remove the shunt, or to simplify the shunt system in those patients in whom only one compartment expands (the cyst or the ventricular system), while the other is adequately drained [16, 27].

16.4.3 Authors' Preferred Surgical Technique

In the most frequent presentation (type I), the cyst extends upward in the lateral ventricle, thinning the floor of the ventricular trigone. In these cases, a standard precoronal burr hole is indicated and the upper pole of the cyst, which appears below the ependyma medial to the choroid plexus, can be fenestrated (lateral ventricle –cystostomy). Neuronavigation is useful but not mandatory. The side of incision should be chosen according to the position of the internal cerebral veins: the cyst, in fact, has usually an asymmetric expansion, and the cerebral veins are displaced contralaterally. The ependyma and the cyst wall can be opened by monopolar or bipolar laser coagulation; the fenestration can be enlarged by grasping forceps and 3-F Fogarty balloon or double-balloon catheter (Lighttouch balloon; Integra Neuroscience, Biot, France). To avoid reclosure of the stoma, large openings, at least 10–15 mm in diameter, should be performed. After decompression of the arachnoid cyst, the endoscope can be advanced through the foramen of Monro to perform a standard endoscopic third ventriculostomy. Fenestration of the deep wall of the cyst, if ETV is successfully performed, seems to not add significant advantages.

In case of cysts bulging in the posterior aspect of the third ventricle (type II), a precoronal trans-Monro approach to the third ventricle allows fenestration of both the anterior wall of the cyst (third ventricle – cystostomy) and the floor of third ventricle. In this case, a steerable endoscope should be preferred, allowing both fenestrations through the same burr hole. With a rigid endoscope, a more anterior burr hole should be drilled, to reach the posterior part of the third ventricle: cyst fenestration and ETV can be both performed only when the ventricular system and the foramen of Monro are markedly dilated.

In the case of laterally extending cysts in the ambient cistern (type III), (Fig. 16.8a–h) a parietal burr hole with the patient head rotated 90° on the contralateral side is usually indicated to approach the lateral ventricle at the level of the trigone. The upper pole of the cyst will appear just in front of the endoscope. In these cases, third ventriculostomy cannot be performed; therefore, further fenestration of the deep wall in the basal cistern (usually in the cisterna ambiens) should be attempted. In type III cyst, neuronavigation is very useful, to plan the correct entry point and to guide the endoscope toward the target in the basal cistern.

16.4.4 Results

In the last decades, endoscopic treatment has become the first-line option in the treatment of quadrigeminal cysts in several centers all around the world [11, 32–39]. The results are very encouraging results, especially when double fenestration was performed (ventriculocystostomy + third ventriculostomy, ventriculocystocisternostomy, double ventriculocystostomy).

In our series of 14 cases [30], double fenestration was realized in 12 cases, with only one failure (success rate 91 %). All seven cases in which only ventriculocystostomy was performed failed and required a second procedure (repeat endoscopy or shunting).

In our experience, the patients, already shunted, who present with cysts enlarging, despite functioning VP shunts, were the most difficult to treat. The shunts were externalized, and the drainage bag progressively elevated to obtain enough space to allow safe endoscopic navigation. However, their ventricular system was not so compliant and there were symptoms of increased ICP before dilation occurred. The endoscopic procedure was uneventful in only one out of three cases. In the remaining two cases (one of these was complicated by venous bleeding from the cyst walls and also from the third ventricular floor) the cysts recurred and the shunts were reimplanted.

In conclusion, neuroendoscopic approaches can be considered an effective alternative to traditional methods in the management of quadrigeminal cistern cysts either in primary presentation or in patients presenting with shunt malfunction. In case of failure, because of the high success rate also in secondary cases, endoscopic reoperation can be considered before considering alternative treatments. The indications for further intervention depend on the persistence of the patient's symptoms and progressive enlargement of the cyst on postoperative imaging at follow-up.

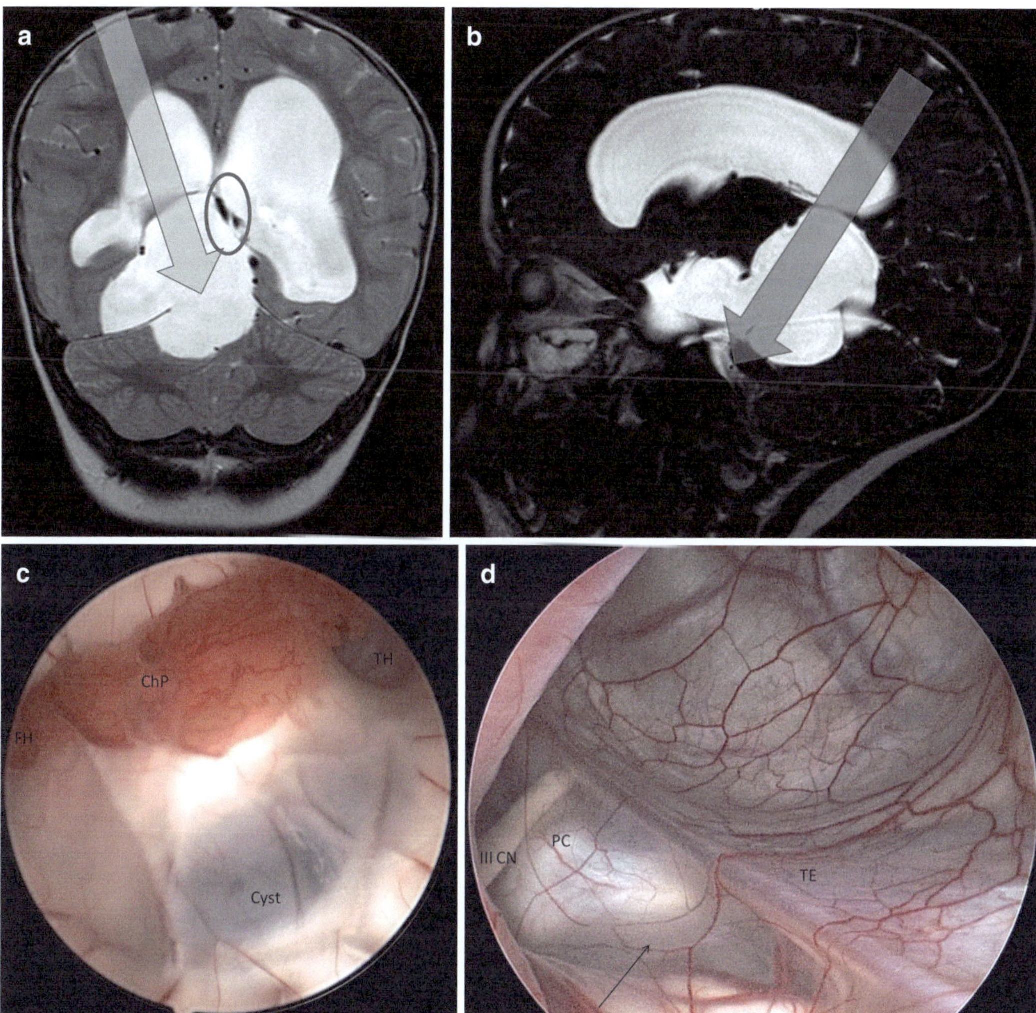

Fig. 16.8 Arachnoid cysts of the quadrigeminal cistern, type 3. Preoperative MRI showing surgical trajectory through a parietal burr hole on coronal (**a**) and sagittal (**b**) views to create a ventriculocystocisternostomy. Endoscopic vision of the cyst dome as seen through a right parietal approach (**c**), the head of the patient is in left lateral decubitus. The cyst wall is easily recognized as a dark layer visible through the attenuated ependyma medial to the choroid plexus. Endoscopic vision of the anterior pole of the cyst as seen after entrance into the cyst lumen (**d**). An area of perforation is identified behind the posterior clinoid (*arrow*). Basal cistern as seen endoscopically through the cyst-cisternostomy (**e**). Post operative MRI showing the flow artifact through the ventriculocystostomy (**f**) and through the cyst-cisternostomy (**g**). Both flow artifacts are visible on this sagittal T2 MRI (**h**). *Arrows* indicate the surgical trajectory, *Circle* indicates the internal cerebral veins

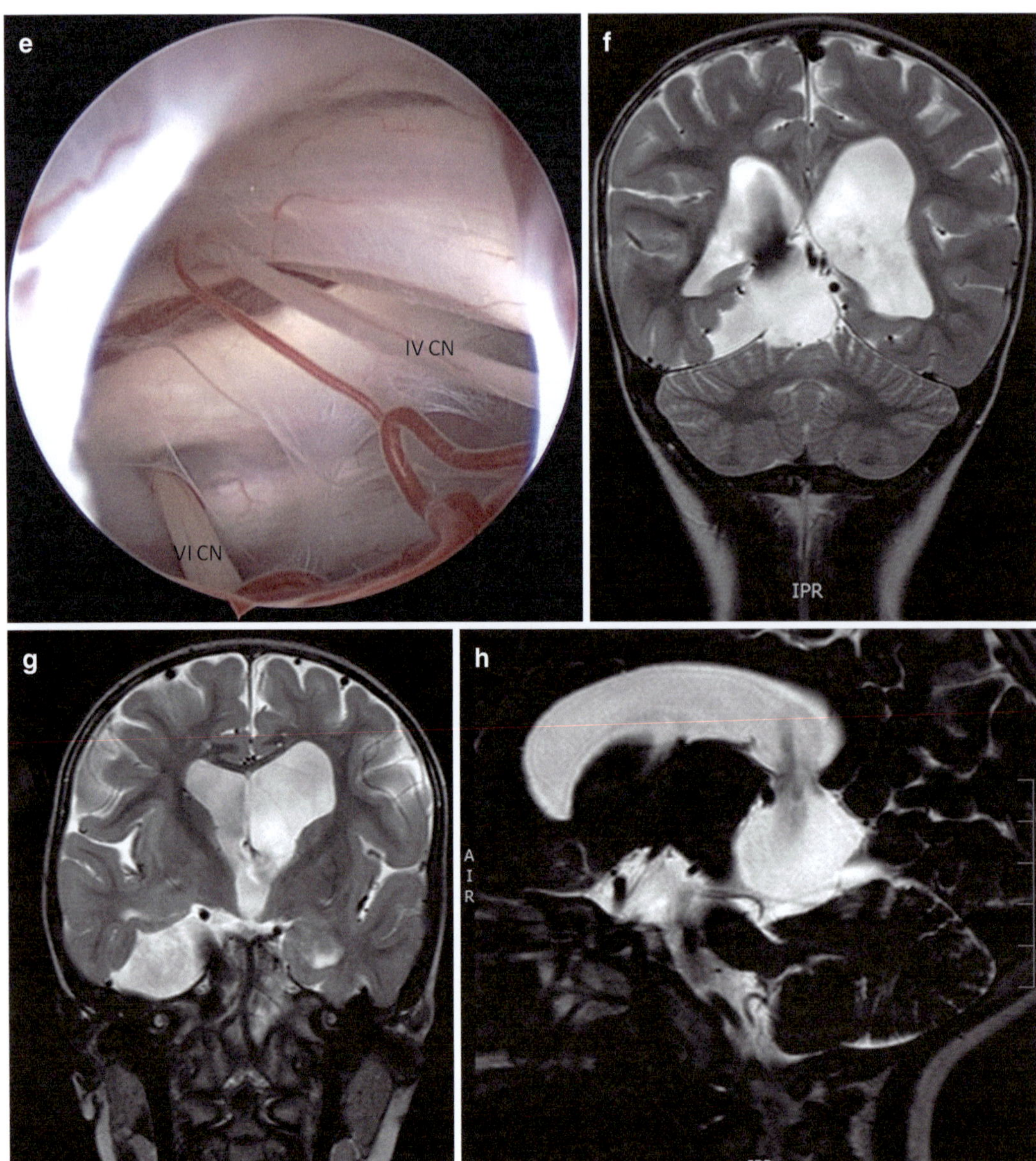

Fig. 16.8 (continued)

References

1. Abbott R (2004) The endoscopic management of arachnoidal cysts. Neurosurg Clin N Am 15:9–17
2. Artico M, Cervoni L, Salvati M, Fiorenza F, Caruso R (1995) Supratentorial arachnoid cysts: clinical and therapeutic remarks on 46 cases. Acta Neurochir 132:75–78
3. Galassi E, Gaist G, Giuliani G, Pozzati E (1988) Arachnoid cysts of the middle cranial fossa: experience with 77 cases treated surgically. Acta Neurochir Suppl 42:201–204
4. Cinalli G (1999) Alternatives to shunt. Childs Nerv Syst 15:718–731
5. Tirakotai W, Schulte DM, Bauer BL, Bertalanffy H, Hellwig D (2004) Neuroendoscopic surgery of intracranial cysts in adults. Childs Nerv Syst 20:842–851
6. Gaab MR, Schroeder HWS (1998) Neuroendoscopic approach to intraventricular lesions. J Neurosurg 88:496–505
7. Hopf NJ, Perneczky A (1998) Endoscopic neurosurgery and endoscope-assisted microneurosurgery for the treatment of intracranial cysts. Neurosurgery 43:1330–1337

8. Decq P, Brugieres P, Le Guerinel C, Djindjian M, Keravel Y, Nguyen JP (1996) Percutaneous endoscopic treatment of suprasellar arachnoid cysts: ventriculocystostomy or ventriculocystocisternostomy? Technical note. J Neurosurg 84:696–701
9. Caemaert J, Abdullah J, Calliauw L, Carton D, Dhooge C, van Foster R (1992) Endoscopic treatment of suprasellar arachnoid cyst. Acta Neurochir 119:68–73
10. Choudhri O, Feroze AH, Nathan J, Cheshier S, Guzman R (2014) Ventricular endoscopy in the pediatric population: review of indications. Childs Nerv Syst 30:1625–1643
11. Kirollos RW, Javadpour M, May P, Mallucci C (2001) Endoscopic treatment of suprasellar and third ventricle-related arachnoid cysts. Childs Nerv Syst 17:713–718
12. Spacca B, Kandasamy J, Mallucci CL, Genitori L (2010) Endoscopic treatment of middle fossa arachnoid cysts: a series of 40 patients treated endoscopically in two centres. Childs Nerv Syst 26:163–172
13. Di Rocco F, R James S, Roujeau T, Puget S, Sainte-Rose C, Zerah M (2010) Limits of endoscopic treatment of sylvian arachnoid cysts in children. Childs Nerv Syst 26:155–162
14. Galassi E, Tognetti F, Gaist G, Fagioli L, Frank F, Frank G (1982) CT scan and metrizamide CT cisternography in arachnoid cysts of the middle cranial fossa: classification and pathophysiological aspects. Surg Neurol 17(5):363–369
15. Choi JW, Lee JY, Phi JH, Kim SK, Wang KC (2015) Stricter indications are recommended for fenestration surgery in intracranial arachnoid cysts of children. Childs Nerv Syst 31:77–86
16. Cinalli G, Spennato P, Ruggiero C, Aliberti F, Trischitta V, Buonocore MC, Cianciulli E, Maggi G (2007) Complications following endoscopic intracranial procedures in children. Childs Nerv Syst 23(6):633–644
17. Tamburrini G, Caldarelli M, Massimi L, Santini P, Di Rocco C (2003) Subdural hygroma: an unwanted result of Sylvian arachnoid cyst marsupialization. Childs Nerv Syst 19(3):159–165
18. Levy ML, Wang M, Aryan HE, Yoo K, Meltzer H (2003) Microsurgical keyhole approach for middle fossa arachnoid cyst fenestration. Neurosurgery 53(5):1138–1144
19. Karabagli H, Etus V (2012) Success of pure neuroendoscopic technique in the treatment of Sylvian arachnoid cysts in children. Childs Nerv Syst 28(3):445–452
20. Elhammady MS, Bhatia S, Ragheb J (2007) Endoscopic fenestration of middle fossa arachnoid cysts: a technical description and case series. Pediatr Neurosurg 43(3):209–215
21. Karabatsu K, Hayhurst H, Buxton N, O'Brien DF, Mallucci CL (2007) Endoscopic management of arachnoid cysts: an advancing technique. J Neurosurg 106:455–462
22. El-Ghandour NM (2012) Endoscopic treatment of middle cranial fossa arachnoid cysts in children. J Neurosurg Pediatr 9:231–238
23. Miyajima M, Arai H, Okuda O, Hishii M, Nakanishi H, Sato K (2000) Possible origin of suprasellar arachnoid cysts: neuroimaging and neurosurgical observations in nine cases. J Neurosurg 93:62–67
24. Maher CO, Goumnerova L (2011) The effectiveness of ventriculocystocisternostomy for suprasellar arachnoid cysts. J Neurosurg Pediatr 7:64–72
25. Rizk E, Chern JJ, Tagayun C, Tubbs RS, Hankinson T, Rozzelle C, Oakes WJ, Blount JP, Wellons JC (2013) Institutional experience of endoscopic suprasellar arachnoid cyst fenestration. Childs Nerv Syst 29:1345–1347
26. Mori K (1992) Giant interhemispheric cysts associated with agenesis of the corpus callosum. J Neurosurg 76:224–230
27. Spennato P, Ruggiero C, Aliberti F, Buonocore MC, Trischitta V, Cinalli G (2013) Interhemispheric and quadrigeminal cysts. World Neurosurg 79(2 Suppl):S20.e1–S20.e7
28. Caldarelli M, Di Rocco C (1996) Surgical options in the treatment of interhemispheric arachnoid cysts. Surg Neurol 46:212–221
29. Ulu MO, Kafadar AM, Dashti R, Isler C, Uludağ S, Erdinçler P (2010) Treatment of symptomatic interhemispheric arachnoid cysts by cystoperitoneal shunting. J Clin Neurosci 17:700–705
30. Cinalli G, Peretta P, Spennato P, Savarese L, Varone A, Vedova P, Grimaldi G, Ragazzi P, Ruggiero C, Cianciulli E, Maggi G (2006) Neuroendoscopic management of interhemispheric cysts in children. J Neurosurg 105(Suppl):194–202
31. Giannetti AV, Fraga SM, Silva MC, Gurgel-Giannetti J (2012) Endoscopic treatment of interhemispheric arachnoid cysts. Pediatr Neurosurg 48:157–162
32. Cinalli G, Spennato P, Columbano L, Ruggiero C, Aliberti F, Trischitta V, Buonocore MC, Cianciulli E (2010) Neuroendoscopic treatment of arachnoid cysts of the quadrigeminal cistern: a series of 14 cases. J Neurosurg Pediatr 6:489–497
33. Ersahin Y, Kesikçi H (2009) Endoscopic management of quadrigeminal arachnoid cysts. Childs Nerv Syst 25:569–576
34. Tamburrini G, Di Rocco C, Caldarelli M, Massimi L (2005) Endoscopic management of supratentorial intra and paraventricular cysts. Childs Nerv Syst 21:500
35. Choi JU, Kim DS, Huh R (1999) Endoscopic approach to arachnoid cyst. Childs Nerv Syst 15:285–291
36. Gangemi M, Maiuri F, Colella G, Magro F (2005) Endoscopic treatment of quadrigeminal cistern arachnoid cysts. Minim Invasive Neurosurg 48:289–292
37. Schroeder HWS, Gaab MR, Niendore WR (1996) Neuroendoscopic approach to arachnoid cysts. J Neurosurg 85:293–298
38. Garg K, Tandon V, Sharma S, Suri A, Chandra PS, Kumar R, Mahapatra AK, Sharma BS (2015) Quadrigeminal cistern arachnoid cyst: a series of 18 patients and a review of literature. Br J Neurosurg 29(1):1–7
39. El-Ghandour NM (2013) Endoscopic treatment of quadrigeminal arachnoid cysts in children. J Neurosurg Pediatr 12:521–528

17 Transcranial Approaches

Francesco Maiuri

17.1 Classification and Anatomical Features

Arachnoid cysts of the midline skull base are located at the base of the brain in a region extending from the sella turcica to the foramen magnum. These cysts lie on the midline, foreword the third ventricle, diencephalon, and brainstem, in relationship to the cranial nerves and basilar artery and its branches.

According to the location and cisternal origin, midline basal arachnoid cysts may be classified as (Table 17.1 and Fig. 17.1):

1. Intrasellar
2. Suprasellar
3. Interpeduncular
4. Retroclival
5. Craniocervical

1. The *intrasellar cysts* lie within an enlarged sella turcica and may extend in the suprasellar cistern. They may show variable size and may become very large. Compression of the optic chiasm results in variable impairment of the visual function and bitemporal hemianopia [1]. Endocrinological disturbances from compression of the pituitary gland and stalk and hypothalamus often occur [2].
2. The *suprasellar cysts* arise from intra-arachnoid dilatation and upward herniation of the superior (or mesencephalic) layer of the Liliequist's membrane caused by cerebrospinal fluid (CSF) pulsation in the prepontine cistern [3]. Thus, they lie anterior to the interpeduncular cistern [4]. The third ventricle is compressed and displaced upwards, resulting in hydrocephalus, whereas the basilar bifurcation is pushed posteriorly against the brainstem. The suprasellar cysts may often be asymptomatic or may present with macrocephaly, intracranial hypertension syndrome, developmental delay, endocrine deficits, reduced visual field, and decreased visual acuity.
3. The *interpeduncular cysts* lie within the interpeduncular cistern, between the diencephalic and mesencephalic leaves of the Liliequist's membrane. Although these cysts have been considered a posterior variant of the suprasellar cysts [4], they are a peculiar, although rare, entity [5]. Interpeduncular cysts are small and tend to preserve the floor of the third ventricle, resulting in absence of hydrocephalus. Their limited expansion minimizes the effect on the neighboring structures (chiasm, CSF spaces). In the reported cases, the cyst was incidental or presented with third cranial nerve deficit [5–7]. Pure interpeduncular cysts tend to remain stable over time.

F. Maiuri, MD
Division of Neurosurgery,
Department of Neurosciences, Reproductive and Odontostomatological Sciences,
Università degli Studi di Napoli "Federico II",
Naples, Italy
e-mail: frmaiuri@unina.it

P. Cappabianca et al. (eds.), *Midline Skull Base Surgery*, DOI 10.1007/978-3-319-21533-4_17

Table 17.1 Location, indication to transcranial surgery, and approaches of skull base midline arachnoid cysts

Type of cyst	Location	Compression of the nervous structures	Hydrocephalus	Indication to transcranial surgery	Transcranial approaches	Site of fenestration and CSF drainage
Intrasellar	Sella turcica with suprasellar extension	None or slight chiasmal compression	No	Suprasellar extension, failed endoscopy	Supraorbital, subfrontal, pterional	Chiasmatic cistern
Suprasellar	Suprasellar cistern	Optic chiasm, hypothalamus, high brainstem, third ventricle	90 %	No hydrocephalus, failed endoscopy	Supraorbital, subfrontal, pterional, transcallosal	Basal cisterns
Interpeduncular	Interpeduncular cistern	Optic chiasm, hypothalamus, third cranial nerve	No or slight	No hydrocephalus, small cysts	Pterional	Chiasmatic and lamina terminalis cisterns
Retroclival	Prepontine cistern	Optic chiasm and tracts, pons and mesencephalon, fifth to eighth cranial nerves	Often present	Treatment of choice	Suboccipital retrosigmoid	Cerebellopontine angle and prepontine cisterns
Craniocervical	Anterior prebulbo-spinal Posterior retrobulbospinal	Medulla, high spinal cord, lower cranial nerves, C1–C2 roots	No	Treatment of choice	Midline suboccipital	Prebulbar cistern, cisterna magna, and spinal canal

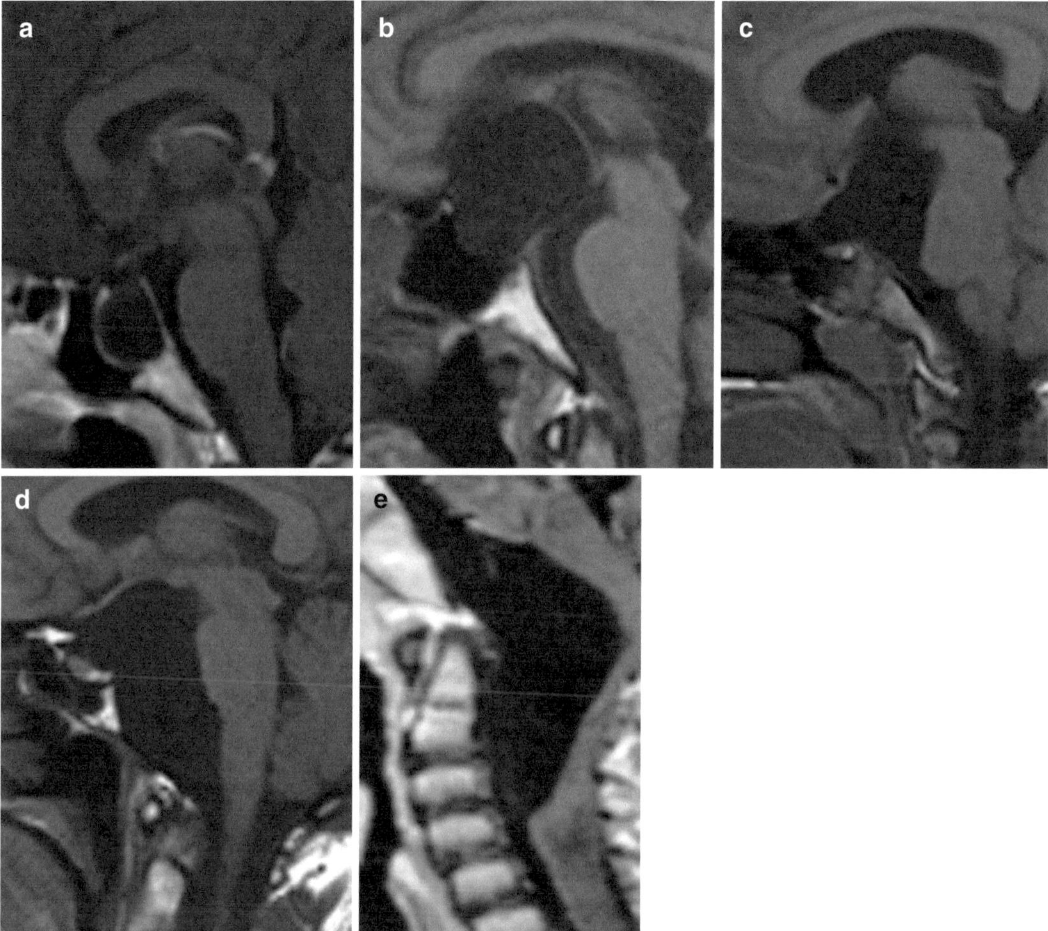

Fig. 17.1 Magnetic Resonance (MR), sagittal T1-sequences, of the various midline basal arachnoid cysts: (**a**) intrasellar; (**b**) suprasellar; (**c**) interpeduncular; (**d**) retroclival; (**e**) craniocervical (anterior)

4. The *retroclival cysts* arise posterior to the mesencephalic leaf of the Liliequist's membrane and lie in the prepontine cistern. They are exceptional, with only several reported cases [8–13]. They may extend upward in the interpeduncular cistern and laterally to the cerebellopontine angle. The typical magnetic resonance features of retroclival cysts are vertical displacement of the optic chiasm and tracts, upward deflection of the rostral mesencephalon and mammillary bodies, and effacement of the ventral pons.

   The retroclival cysts may present with signs of obstructive hydrocephalus, weakness on the limbs, and symptoms due to stretching of the cranial nerves [11, 12].

5. The *cysts of the craniovertebral junction* are rare and may lie posterior or anterior to the bulbo-medullary junction. Anterior cysts are exceptional, with only a few reported cases [14, 15]. They lie in relationship with the clivus and C1 to C3 bodies; they compress and displace backward the medulla and high spinal cord and may stretch the lower cranial nerves and C1 to C3 roots. There is no hydrocephalus. These cysts may be asymptomatic [15] or may present with lower limb weakness and gait disturbances [14].

   Dorsal cysts lie posterior to the medulla, within the cisterna magna, and variably extend downward into the spinal canal [14, 16–19]. Head and neck pain, ataxia, gait disturbances, and arm and leg numbness and paresis are the reported complaints.

17.2 Management Options

The management options for the skull base midline arachnoid cysts include observation, endoscopy, shunting, and transcranial surgery.

Factors involved in the management decision include patient age, size and location of the cyst, and neurological symptoms.

The *conservative management* with follow-up magnetic resonance studies is indicated for incidental cysts with no neurological symptoms. However, large asymptomatic cysts with mass effect should be treated, particularly in children [20], and if they show progressive enlargement on serial magnetic resonance studies.

The *endoscopic fenestration* into the ventricles and cisterns is the best option for midline cysts of middle or large size, mainly with hydrocephalus; in such cases it offers the best chances for definitive treatment and avoids the risk of the craniotomy and shunt dependence [20–22]. However, the endoscopic approach may be difficult for not large cysts without hydrocephalus [22].

The *cyst-peritoneal shunt* is an effective and not invasive procedure for the complete obliteration of large cysts. However, it may also present several complications, including shunt failure, malfunction and infection, hemorrhage, and lifelong shunt dependence [22–24]. Moreover, the shunt procedure may be difficult in cases of not large midline basal cysts [22].

The *microsurgical approach* by craniotomy allows to largely fenestrate the cyst into the subarachnoid spaces and leaves the patient shunt independent. However, it is considered too aggressive for a usually scarcely symptomatic cyst. Besides, it carries not negligible operative morbidity and the risk of complications, such as damage of the neural structures, infection, and hemorrhage [22, 25]. Thus, less invasive and even keyhole approaches should be preferred.

Large opening and partial excision of the cyst wall are the aim of the transcranial surgery; on the contrary, complete removal of the cyst is neither possible nor necessary. However, cyst recurrence even after large fenestrations has also been reported [22].

17.3 Indications to the Transcranial Surgery (Table 17.1)

17.3.1 Intrasellar Cysts

The intrasellar arachnoid cysts must be first treated by endoscopic endonasal transsphenoidal approach. The transcranial microsurgical fenestration is rarely required for large cysts with significant suprasellar extension and after failure of the endoscopic approach [1, 26, 27].

17.3.2 Suprasellar Cysts

The endoscopic fenestration by ventricle-cyst-cisternostomy is the treatment of first choice for suprasellar arachnoid cysts and results in clinical remission and decrease of the cyst size in most cases [20, 21, 26–28]. However, endoscopy is impractical in presence of tiny ventricles. Besides, even repeated endoscopic procedures may fail. In these instances, open microsurgical fenestration of the cyst into the basal cisterns is a safe and effective option, which should be preferred to shunt insertion [21, 29]. If the cyst is huge and causes severe intracranial hypertension, the open fenestration allows immediate relief of the pressure and reduces the cyst [22, 29].

When transcranial surgery is required, suprasellar arachnoid cysts may be treated by supraorbital, subfrontal, and pterional approaches or by transcallosal approach.

17.3.3 Interpeduncular Cysts

The choice of the best management for interpeduncular cysts depends upon the cyst size and the presence of hydrocephalus. Cysts with enlarged third ventricle may be treated by endoscopic ventricle-cyst-cisternostomy, as well as suprasellar cysts. In cases without hydrocephalus, the endoscopy is risky and may be realized with difficulty with the aid of the navigation. In these cases, the microsurgical fenestration and partial excision of the cyst wall through pterional craniotomy, eventually under endoscopic guidance, may be more advisable [5].

17.3.4 Retroclival Cysts

The retroclival arachnoid cysts are best treated by microsurgical fenestration through lateral suboccipital retrosigmoid approach [8–13]. The endoscopy is difficult to realize and not advisable, because of the risk of injuring the cranial nerves and arterial branches.

17.3.5 Cysts of the Craniovertebral Junction

The arachnoid cysts located at the craniovertebral region, anterior, or posterior to the bulbomedullary junction are treated through a midline posterior fossa approach [14]. If the cyst shows significant downward extension within the spinal canal, a posterior high cervical approach through laminectomy may be useful [15].

The endoscopy is more complex and difficult, because of the relationship of the cyst wall with the brainstem and lower cranial nerves.

17.4 Approaches and Techniques

17.4.1 Supraorbital Approach

The transcranial fenestration of arachnoid cysts of the sellar region may be easily performed by a less invasive supraorbital approach, first introduced by Perneczky [30].

This approach is realized by supraorbital skin incision along the eyebrow extended laterally for 2 cm and small frontal basal craniotomy. It allows to expose the suprasellar region through subfrontal route [31, 32]. The suprasellar cyst is well exposed and the cyst wall may be largely fenestrated and partially resected between the two optic nerves and between the homolateral optic nerve and carotid artery.

The classical subfrontal approach through coronal skin incision and frontal craniotomy may also be used. However, it is too invasive for a cyst fenestration.

17.4.2 Pterional Approach

The pterional frontotemporal approach may be realized through a small craniotomy. The large opening of the arachnoid of the sylvian cistern allows to well expose and fenestrate both the suprasellar and interpeduncular cysts. After opening and partial resection of the cyst wall, the lamina terminalis may also be opened posterior to the optic chiasm to drain the eventually enlarged third ventricle.

17.4.3 Transcallosal Approach

The transcallosal approach may be realized through a small or even keyhole craniotomy under endoscopic assistance [33]. A small sagittal section of the corpus callosum (1 cm) allows to reach the cyst. The dome of the cyst is opened into the lateral ventricle; the cyst wall is dissected with microsurgical technique and fenestrated in the basal cisterns. This procedure is helpful in cases of suprasellar cysts with difficult anatomical features (such as absence of hydrocephalus).

The transventricular approach requiring cortical incision to reach the lateral ventricle is too invasive and difficult in cases without hydrocephalus.

In our review of some series of transventricular and transcallosal interventions in the pre-endoscopic era, the success rate was 79 % [20]. The causes of failure included insufficient opening of the cyst wall, inability of the chiasmatic cistern to adapt itself to the CSF diversion from the cyst, and lack of communication between the cyst and the ventricular system [20, 34].

17.4.4 Retrosigmoid Approach

The lateral suboccipital retrosigmoid approach is the surgical technique of choice for retroclival arachnoid cysts. The approach should be realized on the side of the prevalent lateral expansion of the cyst or on the side of the eventual deficit of a cranial nerve (abducens [10] or facial [11]). The cyst is easily exposed; it displaces backward the pons and medulla and stretches the cranial nerves. Wide fenestration and partial wall resection may be performed both above and below the acoustic-facial complex, in order to ensure large communication between the cyst and the prepontine and cerebellopontine angle cisterns.

17.4.5 Suboccipital Midline Approach

A suboccipital midline approach may be used to treat arachnoid cysts located at the craniovertebral junction [14]. It is realized by suboccipital craniotomy and C1 laminectomy. Posterior cysts are immediately exposed after dural opening. The cyst wall may be easily resected, and communication of the cyst with posterior fossa cisterns and spinal canal may be established. Anterior cysts displace backward the brain stem and may have asymmetrical expansion. A surgical corridor is thus provided to reach the cyst. Fenestration and partial excision of the cyst wall are performed on both sides with minimal traction on the lower cranial nerves.

Conclusions

In spite of the widespread diffusion of the endoscopy, the transcranial surgery is still a useful option for selected patients harboring midline skull base arachnoid cysts. It must be considered when endoscopy fails (as for several intra- and suprasellar cysts) or cannot be performed for technical difficulties (as for interpeduncular, retroclival, or craniovertebral cysts without hydrocephalus). Small and less invasive craniotomies, such as supraorbital, mini-pterional, and small retrosigmoid, should be preferred to reduce the surgical morbidity. Large fenestrations into the cisternal spaces and partial resection of the cyst wall must be realized to ensure free CSF flow from the cyst.

References

1. Zielinski G, Podgorski JK, Koziarski A, Potakiewicz Z (2006) Intrasellar arachnoid cyst. A case report and review of the literature. Neurol Neurochir Pol 40:347–353
2. Yasuda K, Saitoh Y, Okita K, Morris S, Moriwaki M, Miyagawa J, Yoshimine T (2005) Giant intrasellar arachnoid cyst manifesting as adrenal insufficiency due to hypothalamic dysfunction, case report. Neurol Med Chir 45:164–167
3. Fox JL, Al-Mefty O (1980) Suprasellar arachnoid cysts: an extension of the membrane of Liliequist. Neurosurgery 7:615–618
4. Miyajima M, Arai H, Okuda O, Hishii M, Nakanishi H, Sato K (2000) Possible origin of suprasellar arachnoid cysts: neuroimaging and neurosurgical observation in nine cases. J Neurosurg 93:62–67
5. Paraskevopoulos D, Roth J, Beni-Adani L, Constantini S (2011) Interpeduncular arachnoid cyst in infants and children: insight into the entity based on a case series with long-term follow-up. Childs Nerv Syst 27:429–438
6. Ashker L, Weinstein JM, Dias M, Kanev P, Nguyen D, Bonsall DJ (2008) Arachnoid cyst causing third cranial nerve palsy manifesting as isolated internal ophthalmoplegia and iris cholinergic supersensitivity. J Neuroophthalmol 28:192–197
7. Dwarakamash S, Suri A, Mahapatra AK, Mehta VS, Gaikwad S, Sarkar C (2006) Endoscopic assisted excision of a retroclival arachnoid cyst presenting as hysterical breathlessness. Childs Nerv Syst 22:424–427
8. Boukeras EC, Raji MR, Dastur KJ, Francken GJ, Engle DJ, Nayak NT (1992) Retroclival arachnoid cyst. AJNR Am J Neuroradiol 13:353–354
9. Quint DJ (1992) Retroclival arachnoid cyst. AJNR Am J Neuroradiol 13:1503–1504
10. Ikeda H, Deinsberger W, Boker DK (2000) Retroclival arachnoid cyst presenting with spontaneous intracystic haemorrhage-case presentation. Acta Neurochir (Wien) 142:1317–1318
11. Bonde V, Muzumdar D, Goel A (2008) Retroclival arachnoid cyst with hemifacial spasm. Singapore Med J 49:e281–e282
12. Genc E, Ebru AD, Kocaogullar Y, Emlik D (2008) A case with prepontine (clival) arachnoid cyst manifested as trigeminal neuralgia. Headache 48:1525–1539
13. Akyuz M, Goksu E, Aralasmak A, Tuncer R (2010) Retroclival arachnoid cyst presenting with haemorrhage: a brief report of a special case. Acta Neurochir (Wien) 152:161–162
14. Mohindra S, Gupta S, Chhabra R, Gupta R, Kumar A, Radotra B (2007) Ventrally placed craniovertebral junction arachnoid cyst in children: a report of 2 cases and literature review. Surg Neurol 68:85–88
15. Lefranc M, Peltuer J, Fichten A, Desenclos C, Toussaint P, Le Gars D (2008) Giant prebulbomedullary arachnoid cyst. Case report and review of the literature. Neurochirurgie 54:89–92

16. Pego-Reigosa R, Branas-Fernandez F, Martinez-Vazquez F, Cortes-Laino JA (2000) Craniospinal intradural arachnoid cyst. Arch Neurol 57:128
17. Price SJ, David KM, O'Donovan DG, Aspoas AR (2001) Arachnoid cyst of the craniocervical junction: case report. Neurosurgery 49:212–215
18. Cakirer S (2004) Arachnoid cyst of the craniospinal junction: a case report and review of the literature. Acta Radiol 45:460–463
19. Panigrahi S, Mishra S, Das S, Patra S, Satpathy P (2012) Large intradural craniospinal arachnoid cyst: a case report and review of literature. J Craniovertebr Junction Spine 3:16–18
20. Gangemi M, Colella G, Magro F, Maiuri F (2007) Suprasellar arachnoid cysts: endoscopy versus microsurgical cyst excision and shunting. Br J Neurosurg 21:276–280
21. Crimmins DW, Pierre-Kahn A, Sainte-Rose C, Zerah M (2006) Treatment of suprasellar cysts and patient outcome. J Neurosurg 105:107–114
22. Shim KW, Lee YH, Park EK, Park YS, Choi JU, Kim DS (2009) Treatment option for arachnoid cysts. Childs Nerv Syst 25:1459–1466
23. Martìnez-Lage JF, Ruìz-Espejo AM, Almagro MJ, Alfaro R, Felipe-Murcia M, Lòpez-Guerrero AL (2009) CSF overdrainage in shunted intracranial arachnoid cysts: a series and review. Childs Nerv Syst 25:1061–1069
24. Maher C, Goumnerova L (2011) The effectiveness of ventriculocisternostomy for suprasellar arachnoid cyst. J Neurosurg Pediatr 7:64–72
25. Ciricillo SF, Cogen PH, Harsh GR, Edwards MS (1991) Intracranial arachnoid cysts in children. A comparison of the effects of fenestration and shunting. J Neurosurg 74:230–235
26. Iqbal J, Kanaan I, Al Homsi M (1999) Non neoplastic cystic lesions of the sellar region: presentation, diagnosis and management of eight cases and review of the literature. Acta Neurochir (Wien) 141: 389–398
27. Miyamoto T, Ebisubidani D, Kitamura K, Ohshima T, Horiguchi H, Nagahiro S (1999) Surgical management of symptomatic intrasellar arachnoid cyst – two case report. Neurol Med Chir (Tokyo) 39: 941–945
28. Gangemi M, Seneca V, Colella G, Cioffi V, Imperato A, Maiuri F (2011) Endoscopy versus microsurgical cyst excision and shunting for treating intracranial arachnoid cyst. J Neurosurg Pediatr 8: 158–164
29. Maiuri F, Gangemi M, Donati PA, Basile D (1999) Chronic hydrocephalus and suprasellar arachnoid cyst presenting with rhinorrhea. Minim Invasive Neurosurg 42:83–85
30. Perneczky A, Murrel Forell V, van Lindert E, Fries G (1999) Keyhole concept in neurosurgery: with endoscopic-assisted microneurosurgery and case studies. Thieme, New York
31. Joseph V, Chacko AG (2005) Suprabrow microcraniotomy for suprasellar tumors. Br J Neurosurg 19:33–37
32. Reisch R, Perneczky A (2005) Ten-year experience with the supraorbital subfrontal approach through an eyebrow skin incision. Neurosurgery 57:242–255
33. Charalampaki P, Filippi R, Welschehold S, Conrad J (2005) Endoscopic and endoscope-assisted neurosurgical treatment of suprasellar arachnoidal cysts (Mickey Mouse cysts). Minim Invasive Neurosurg 48:283–288
34. Di Rocco C, Caldarelli M, Ceddia A (1993) Incidence, anatomical distribution and classification of arachnoid cysts. In: Raimondi AJ, Choux M, Di Rocco C (eds) Intracranial cyst lesions. Springer, New York, pp 101–111

Part IV

Anterior Cranial Fossa Meningiomas

Introduction

18

Oreste de Divitiis, Carmela Chiaramonte, and Gianluigi Califano

The surgical treatment of meningiomas located at the base of the anterior cranial fossa continues to pose a big challenge to neurosurgeons despite that over the past century, many advances have taken place in both the treatment and the biological understanding of these lesions. The introduction of the microsurgical technique and the development of skull base approaches has allowed surgeons to achieve a better treatment, a big improvement in the outcome, and a higher cure rate of these tumors and was well founded in principle and proven beneficial in practice [1].

Once again in the history of modern neurosurgery, we must thank Harvey Cushing who made significant contribution in the understanding and treatment of meningiomas in general but particularly those involving the anterior cranial base, following early reports of prominent figures such as Sir William MacEwen and Francesco Durante, who were first to perform successful operations to treat these tumors [2–5].

Meningioma's cell of origin is supposed to be the arachnoid cap cell, and these tumors are listed under the heading "Tumors of the Meninges" and the subheading "Tumors of the Meningothelial Cells" in the *WHO classification* that are classified anaplastic, papillary, and rhabdoid as Grade III meningiomas; atypical, chondroid, and clear cell types as Grade II; and all the other variants as Grade I [6].

Today, it appears that cytogenetic analysis is a very important predictor of an aggressive meningioma. A normal karyotype is associated with a lower recurrence rate and slower growth being monosomy of chromosome 22 which is a frequent finding in benign meningiomas. The deletion of chromosome 1p or 14q has been definitively associated with a higher-grade meningioma and a more aggressive biology. One more prognostic factor could be the expression of TRF1 which is heterogeneously expressed in meningiomas [7–10]. Despite these considerations and because of their easy determination on fixed specimens, a high K_i-67 labeling index, or a lack of progesterone receptors, is considered a useful indicator in determining the aggressiveness of meningiomas.

Based on the site of dural attachment, even the most recent classifications, one above all of the *Al-Mefty classifications* of meningiomas is based on the following principles: convexity, parasagittal, falx, tentorial, peritorcular, falcotentorial, olfactory groove, tuberculum sellae, lateral and middle sphenoid wing, clinoidal, cavernous sinus, sphenoorbital, cerebellar convexity, cerebellopontine angle, clival and petroclival, temporal bone, foramen magnum, lateral and fourth

O. de Divitiis, MD (✉) • C. Chiaramonte, MD
G. Califano, MS
Division of Neurosurgery,
Department of Neurosciences, Reproductive and Odontostomatological Sciences,
Università degli Studi di Napoli "Federico II", Napoli, Italy
e-mail: oreste.dedivitiis@unina.it

P. Cappabianca et al. (eds.), *Midline Skull Base Surgery*, DOI 10.1007/978-3-319-21533-4_18

ventricles, third ventricle and pineal region, middle fossa floor [1].

Meningiomas of the anterior cranial fossa represent 12–20 % of all intracranial meningiomas. They are classified into *olfactory groove*, *planum sphenoidale*, *tuberculum sellae*, and *diaphragma sellae meningiomas*, according to the site of attachment, each of them with few distinct clinical features. However, despite that the original site of attachment may differ, we can consider this group of tumors as an unique entity that grows in an area where the brain has a high compliance, thus allowing these tumors to reach large sizes at the time of diagnosis and occupying a significant portion of the anterior cranial fossa [11, 12]. This characteristic, their slow growth, and subfrontal location give often to anterior cranial fossa meningiomas an insidious presentation. Especially for the olfactory groove and planum sphenoidale types, one of the most common symptoms is the change in personality, judgment, or motivation noted by family members or close contacts with headache, visual disturbance, or lack of smell occurring only late in the course of the disease. Working with prominent figures such as Sir William Gowers and Sir Victor Horsley at the National Hospital in Queen's Square in London, Dr. Robert Foster Kennedy made a significant contribution, recognizing a common clinical presentation of space-occupying lesions located in the frontal lobe known as "Foster Kennedy syndrome" (optic atrophy in the ipsilateral eye, papilledema in the contralateral eye, central scotoma in ipsilateral eye, anosmia, nausea and vomiting, memory loss, and emotional lability), during a time when imaging modalities were not widely available [13]. With earlier diagnosis achieved thanks to modern imaging, the Foster Kennedy syndrome is only seen in a minority of patients. Visual impairment is among the primary symptoms of patients with meningiomas of the anterior cranial fossa, especially those located in the tuberculum sellae and diaphragma. Because of the growth pattern of olfactory groove meningiomas and planum sphenoidale ones, these tumors may extend posteriorly and inferiorly compressing the optic nerves and causing an inferior visual field deficit. In contrast due to their location close to the visual pathways, tuberculum sellae meningiomas produce a bitemporal visual field defect caused by elevation and compression of the optic chiasm.

Historically, meningiomas were characterized by plain roentgenograms and conventional diagnostic angiography, but the introduction of computed tomography and the magnetic resonance imaging dramatically increased detection and accuracy of the diagnosis. Recent years have witnessed the development of advanced imaging techniques, such as MR spectroscopy, MR perfusion, indium-111-octreotide scintigraphy, and PET. Anyway, despite their usefulness in certain clinical scenarios, these newer tools remain peripheral at present and serve only as adjuncts to CT and routine MRI sequences [14].

Initially, large-sized unilateral or bilateral craniotomies were necessary to approach these deep-seated lesions. Technical advances such as the introduction of electrosurgery, the operating microscope, the cavitron ultrasound aspirator, and refined microsurgical instruments allowed neurosurgeons to perform less invasive surgical procedures with better results. Today, a wide variety of surgical strategies, including endoscopic surgery and radiosurgery, are used to treat these tumors [15].

Since the initial experience of the pioneering neurosurgeons, multiple advances have improved the safeness and the effectiveness of treatment of meningiomas. Starting with the unilateral frontal craniotomy performed by Cushing and evolved to a bifrontal craniotomy and a transbasal approach, due to the efforts of Dandy [16], we arrived to the Tonnis experience with the bifrontal approach preserving the brain tissue, which was followed later by multiple surgeons. The introduction of the operating microscope in the 1970s was a milestone in the removal of these neoplasms. The unilateral and bifrontal craniotomies have been further modified, and currently, some craniofacial approaches are used to treat tumors invading the nasal cavity and/or paranasal sinuses. The endoscope, which has been available for a long time for the treatment of other neurosurgical entities, was introduced recently in the treatment of anterior cranial fossa meningiomas and is acquiring more advocates as supporting evidence becomes available.

Nowadays, several approaches have been described to remove anterior cranial fossa meningiomas. Large tumors are often approached with a subfrontal approach with a bilateral or monolateral craniotomy [17, 18]. The pterional approach was popularized by Yasargil and since then largely used with his variations like the fronto-orbitozygomatic one [19, 20]. With the concept of minimally invasive neurosurgery and the development of modern neuroimaging techniques, neurosurgeons gained the possibility of a proper characterization of brain tumors and their relation to surrounding structures. This characterization is helpful in presurgical planning and in the intraoperative setting and makes it possible to approach deep-seated lesions through very small openings like the supraorbital "keyhole" craniotomy described by Perneczky and colleagues or the mini-pterional approach [21–23]. The introduction of the endoscope to the realm of neurosurgery led to successful treatment of deep-seated lesions without brain retraction. To gain access to the anterior skull base, the endoscope can be used via a low route, like in the extended endonasal approach, or via a high route using a small supraorbital craniotomy [24–28]. The extended endoscopic endonasal approach for the treatment of anterior cranial fossa meningiomas is relatively new and has been increasingly reported during the last decade, with significant contributions from different groups.

In its general principles, the ideal surgical approach should provide enough exposure of the tumor, including its dural attachment, to interrupt its blood supply early in the procedure. In addition, brain retraction and manipulation of critical neurovascular structures should be minimized as much as possible to avoid procedure-related morbidity. Sufficient access to the skull base is also desirable in cases in which bone resection and subsequent cranial base reconstruction are necessary. The selection of the most appropriate approach depends on multiple factors, including surgeon's preference and experience, tumor size and location, extent of dural attachment, and relation with the surrounding neurovascular structures [29].

Since 1957 when *Simpson* published his famous article correlating the extent of resection with the subsequent recurrence risk, neurosurgery gained a useful tool to predict the prognosis after the surgery of patients with meningiomas. His scale indicates *five grades of removal*: (I) macroscopically complete removal of tumor, with excision of its dural attachment, and of any abnormal bone including resection of venous sinus if involved; (II) macroscopically complete removal of tumor and its visible extensions with coagulation of its dural attachment; (III) macroscopically complete removal of the intradural tumor, without resection or coagulation of its dural attachment or its extradural extensions; (IV) partial removal, leaving intradural tumor in situ; and (V) simple decompression, with or without biopsy [30].

Nonsurgical therapies are used for recurrent or incompletely resected anterior cranial base meningiomas. Standard or stereotactic irradiation has been used.

According to Guthrie and associates conclusions, surgical excision is the treatment of choice, and radiotherapy should be considered after surgery (1) for a malignant meningioma, (2) following an incomplete resection of a meningioma whose risk of resection of an eventual recurrence is judged to be excessive, (3) for patients with multiple recurrent tumors for whom the surgeon judges repeat surgery to be too risky, and (4) as a sole therapy of a progressively symptomatic patient with a meningioma judged by the surgeon inoperable [31].

Bibliography

1. De Monte F, Mc Dermott MW, Al-Mefty O (2011) Al Mefty's meningiomas. Thieme, New York, pp 4–11
2. Cushing H (1938) Meningiomas, their classification, regional behaviour, life history and surgical end results. Charles C Thomas, Springfield
3. Durante F (1887) Contribution to endocranial surgery. Lancet 130:654–655
4. Durante F (1902) Observations on certain cerebral localizations. Br Med J 2:1822–1825
5. Macewen W (1881) Intra-cranial lesions: illustrating some points in connection with the localization of cerebral affections and the advantages of antiseptic trephining. Lancet 2:581–583

6. Louis DN, Ohgaki H, Wiestler OD et al (2007) WHO classification of tumors of the central nervous system. In: Bosman FT, Jaffe ES, Lakhani SR et al (eds) World Health Organization classification of tumors, 4th edn. International Agency for Research on Cancer, Lyon, p 309
7. Aragona M, De Divitiis O, La Torre D, Panetta S, D'Avella D, Pontoriero A, Morelli M, La Torre I, Tomasello F (2001) Immunohistochemical TRF1 expression in human primary intracranial tumors. Anticancer Res 21(3C):2135–2139
8. La Torre D, de Divitiis O, Conti A, Angileri FF, Cardali S, Aguennouz M, Aragona M, Panetta S, d'Avella D, Vita G, La Torre F, Tomasello F (2005) Expression of telomeric repeat binding factor-1 in astroglial brain tumors. Neurosurgery 56(4):802–810
9. Kane AJ, Sughrue ME, Rutkowski MJ, Shangari G, Fang S, McDermott MW, Berger MS, Parsa AT (2011) Anatomic location is a risk factor for atypical and malignant meningiomas. Cancer 117(6):1272–1278
10. Barbera S, San Miguel T, Gil-Benso R, Muñoz-Hidalgo L, Roldan P, Gonzalez-Darder J, Cerda-Nicolas M, Lopez-Gines C (2013) Genetic changes with prognostic value in histologically benign meningiomas. Clin Neuropathol 32(4):311–317
11. Rubin G, Ben David U, Gornish M, Rappaport ZH (1994) Meningiomas of the anterior cranial fossa floor. Review of 67 cases. Acta Neurochir (Wien) 129:26–30
12. Tuna H, Bozkurt M, Ayten M, Erdogan A, Deda H (2005) Olfactory groove meningiomas. J Clin Neurosci 12:664–668
13. Kennedy F (1911) Retrobulbar neuritis as an exact diagnostic sign of certain tumors and abscesses in the frontal lobes. Am J Med Sci 142:355–368
14. Okonkwo DO, Laws ER Jr (2008) Meningiomas: historical perspective. In: Lee JH (ed) Meningiomas: diagnostic treatment and outcome. Springer, London, pp 3–14
15. Pia HW (1972) The microscope in neurosurgery—technical improvements. Acta Neurochir (Wien) 26:251–255
16. Cushing H (1927) The meningiomas arising from the olfactory groove and their removal by the aid of electro-surgery. Jackson, Wylie & Co, Glasgow
17. Nakamura M, Struck M, Roser F, Vorkapic P, Samii M (2008) Olfactory groove meningiomas: clinical outcome and recurrence rates after tumor removal through the frontolateral and bifrontal approach. Neurosurgery 62(6 Suppl 3):1224–1232
18. Persing JA, Jane JA, Levine PA, Cantrell RW (1990) The versatile frontal sinus approach to the floor of the anterior cranial fossa. Technical note. J Neurosurg 72:513–516
19. Hassler W, Zentner J (1989) Pterional approach for surgical treatment of olfactory groove meningiomas. Neurosurgery 25:942–947
20. Tomasello F, Angileri FF, Grasso G, Granata F, De Ponte FS, Alafaci C (2011) Giant olfactory groove meningiomas: extent of frontal lobes damage and long-term outcome after the pterional approach. World Neurosurg 76:311–317
21. Perneczky A, Müller-Forell W, van Lindert E, Fries G (1999) Keyhole concept in neurosurgery. Thieme Medical Publishers, Stuttgart
22. Reisch R, Perneczky A (2005) Ten-year experience with the supra-orbital subfrontal approach through an eyebrow skin incision. Neurosurgery 57(4 Suppl):242–255
23. de Divitiis E, Esposito F, Cappabianca P, Cavallo LM, de Divitiis O (2008) Tuberculum sellae meningiomas: high route or low route? A series of 51 consecutive cases. Neurosurgery 62(3):556–563, discussion 556–63
24. Gardner PA, Kassam AB, Thomas A, Snyderman CH, Carrau RL, Mintz AH et al (2008) Endoscopic endonasal resection of anterior cranial base meningiomas. Neurosurgery 63:36–54
25. Schwartz TH, Fraser JF, Brown S, Tabaee A, Kacker A, Anand VK (2008) Endoscopic cranial base surgery: classification of operative approaches. Neurosurgery 62:991–1005
26. Van Gompel JJ, Frank G, Pasquini E, Zoli M, Hoover J, Lan-zino G (2011) Expanded endonasal endoscopic resection of anterior fossa meningiomas: report of 13 cases and meta-analysis of the literature. Neurosurg Focus 30(5):E15
27. Webb-Myers R, Wormald PJ, Brophy B (2008) An endoscopic endonasal technique for resection of olfactory groove meningioma. J Clin Neurosci 15:451–455
28. Spektor S, Valarezo J, Fliss DM, Gil Z, Cohen J, Goldman J et al (2005) Olfactory groove meningiomas from neurosurgical and ear, nose, and throat perspectives: approaches, techniques, and outcomes. Neurosurgery 57(4 Suppl):268–280
29. Rachinger W, Grau S, Tonn JC (2010) Different microsurgical approaches to meningiomas of the anterior cranial base. Acta Neurochir (Wien) 152:931–939
30. Simpson D (1957) The recurrence of intracranial meningiomas after surgical treatment. J Neurol Neurosurg Psychiatry 20(1):22–39
31. Couldwell WT, Cole CD, Al-Mefty O (2007) Patterns of Skull base meningioma progression after failed radiosurgery. J Neurosurg 106(1):30–35

19 The Expanded Endonasal Approach to Skull Base Meningiomas

Amin Kassam, Martin Corsten, and Richard Rovin

19.1 Introduction

Classic approaches to the skull base have involved either anterior, middle, or posterior fossa craniotomies, with retraction of the brain to expose the relevant intracranial anatomy, often with separate approaches from the mid-face or temporal bone to expose the relevant extracranial anatomy. The expanded endonasal approach (EEA) to skull base tumors was introduced as an alternative minimally invasive strategy for selected tumors in the late 1990s/early 2000s [3, 11, 12]. It offered some significant advantages in selected tumors, including the elimination of the need for skin incisions, the elimination of brain retraction, and the addition of excellent visualization of critical structures. In the early part of the experience with EEA, there was significant controversy about its safety, with critics of the approach citing the risk of infection and the possibility of cerebrospinal fluid leakage as a consequence of the procedure. However, early experience showed the safety of the procedure, especially relative to traditional skull base approaches, in selected tumors. We reported our experience in 800 consecutive patients performed by a single neurosurgeon over a decade and demonstrated the safety of the procedure for a broad range of pathologies [15]. Since then, the procedure has been adopted worldwide and has been made safer by advances in technology and reconstructive techniques. Since our original description of a modular anatomical classification system [25], expansion of the anatomic limits of the procedure has continued to increase the number of skull base tumors accessible by this approach. In this chapter, we will describe the use of EEA for skull base meningiomas, focusing on the anatomic limits of the use of EEA for these tumors, the advantages and disadvantages of EEA, and the technical nuances of the use of EEA for meningiomas.

19.2 The Expanded Endonasal Approach: Overview

EEA refers to a minimally invasive surgical approach to the skull base through the nares. Typically, the surgery is performed, as a two-surgeon, four-handed operation carried out by a neurosurgeon and an otolaryngologist – head and

A. Kassam, MD (✉) • R. Rovin
Department of Neurosurgery,
Aurora Health Care, Milwaukee, WI, USA
e-mail: kassamab@gmail.com; richard.rovin@aurora.org

M. Corsten
Department of Otolaryngology,
Aurora Health Care, Milwaukee, WI, USA
e-mail: martin.corsten@aurora.org

P. Cappabianca et al. (eds.), *Midline Skull Base Surgery*, DOI 10.1007/978-3-319-21533-4_19

neck surgeon. In our classical description of the approach, the right inferior turbinate is lateralized, and the right middle turbinate resected to gain space for the endoscope, which is brought in through the right nostril [3, 11, 12]. Nasoseptal flaps may be raised (see below), and a posterior septectomy is performed. The operating surgeon operates binarially, while his or her partner performs the endoscopy, with high-resolution views afforded to both surgeons from the endoscope displayed on monitors.

Several technological advances over the past 15 years have improved the safety and efficacy of EEA, with more technologies anticipated to improve the procedure even further. The development of high-definition television screens and advanced optics has allowed for views of anatomical structures with excellent levels of resolution and magnification. Image guidance has been an integral part of the development of EEA and its adoption by multiple centers around the world, by affording surgeons increased information about the proximity to critical structures such as the carotid arteries, optic nerves, and brain. Proponents of the procedure have partnered with equipment companies to create task-specific instrumentation designed for operating endoscopically in the ventral skull base. Some centers have been experimenting with 3-D optics platforms and "look-ahead" technologies to further enhance the operators' awareness of the anatomic environment of the operative field, in an attempt to make the procedure even safer [1, 5, 24].

It is key, however, to realize that image guidance techniques and enhanced endoscopic images are no replacement for surgical experience and a deep understanding of the anatomy. Identification of the location of the carotid artery, either unilaterally or bilaterally, through its six distinct segments (parapharyngeal, petrous, paraclival, parasellar, paraclinoid, and intradural) is usually a critical component of the dissection in EEA. We have recently published a detailed modular classification of EEA approaches using the carotid artery as a road map [16]. Other cranial nerves, including the optic nerve and chiasm, are often critical to the dissection as well.

Another critical advance that made EEA safer was not technological but surgical. In the early experience with EEA, reconstruction of the skull base was generally accomplished using non-vascularized tissue, along with tissue sealants. This was often successful, but high rates of cerebrospinal fluid leak were often observed. This problem was especially acute in high-flow situations such as craniopharyngiomas, with large dural openings, or with such patient risk factors as obesity or sleep apnea [26]. The introduction of the posteriorly based nasoseptal flap, popularized by Carrau [9], markedly reduced the incidence of CSF leaks and other intracranial complications. This flap, based on the posterior septal artery, is raised before the posterior septectomy and left pedicled posteriorly during the tumor resection. It allows reliable coverage of dural defects and encourages rapid remucosalization of the ventral skull base. This was in many ways the innovation that allowed for EEA to become a safe and reproducible surgical strategy. A later modification, described by Carrau, was the anteriorly based reverse flap [2]. This flap hastened the mucosalization of the denuded anterior septum left behind by the elevation of the NSF with an anteriorly based reverse flap, raised from the contralateral side.

There are other options for reconstruction after EEA; not all cases require a vascularized flap, and many centers continue to use non-vascularized reconstructions in simple cases at low risk for CSF leak. Some surgeons use a "rescue flap," also described by Carrau [23]. In these cases, the incisions for the NSF are created before the posterior septectomy, but the flap is not raised until the end of the procedure, when the decision is made that the case is of sufficiently high risk for CSF leak that a flap is necessary. Non-vascularized reconstruction can therefore be used in cases deemed to be low risk after the resection.

For cases in which vascularized reconstruction is deemed necessary but the NSF is unavailable, a large number of other flap options have been described, including a flap harvested from the lateral nasal wall [10, 22], pedicled pericranial [19, 28], buccinator [21] or temporoparietal flaps [6], turbinate flaps [7, 20], or even free flaps transferred into the skull base. While the details of reconstruction are beyond the scope of this chapter, this evolution of reconstruction options in EEA played a sentinel role in its development.

EEA is not the treatment of choice for all skull base lesions. The most critical issue in assessing whether EEA should be used for a particular lesion is the position of the tumor relative to cranial nerves. Nerves are significantly intolerant to manipulation and dissection, and EEA is largely a median and paramedian approach to the skull base. When skull base tumors are medial to critical nerve structures, EEA can often represent the preferred approach. Tumors that are lateral to cranial nerves are often better treated with lateral skull base approaches. As a central principle, we expressed the concept of avoiding crossing the plane of a cranial nerve. Tumors that cross cranial nerves may have their medial component treated with EEA, while the lateral component is addressed by an open approach, often at a second stage. In some cases, tumor debulking may be performed as part of a multidisciplinary approach utilizing radiation therapy.

19.3 Specific Considerations for the EEA in Meningiomas

Meningiomas represent the single largest subset of intracranial tumors, accounting for roughly 30 % of all primary brain tumors. Meningiomas are typically benign and cause symptoms through progressive growth and mass effect. These neurological symptoms can be quite dramatic, but these tumors rarely cause death; in fact, life expectancies may be quite long despite the presence of these meningiomas. The goal of surgical extirpation of meningiomas is to reduce or eliminate the neurological sequelae of this mass effect, ideally through complete resection of the tumor. Sometimes, however, a similar benefit for the patient can be obtained through subtotal tumor resection, especially if total tumor resection would result in the loss of neurological function. A careful assessment of the patient's life expectancy, current neurological disability, anatomic proximity to critical structures, and individual wishes must be made when weighing the optimal extent of resection of these tumors.

The surgical extirpation of meningiomas using EEA requires several important considerations. The first is the creation of tailored surgical working corridors to gain access to the tumor. Our modular approach to EEA has been described, with descriptions of the relevant working corridors to each area in the skull base [3, 11, 12]. The second consideration is the extent of bony dissection and drilling required for circumferential exposure of the meningioma. This bony exposure and removal should be completed before tumor removal is started. The third consideration is a circumferential devascularization of the tumor. Only after these three steps are performed should complete tumor removal and/or cytoreduction be attempted. Removal of tumor after devascularization can often be accomplished with powered, automated equipment such as the Myriad [17].

Preoperative evaluation of the tumor position, extent, and relationship with critical neurovascular structures is imperative. This evaluation certainly requires high-resolution imaging, usually with MRI. MRI imaging should be scrutinized to evaluate the relationship between the meningioma and cranial nerves, with special attention to whether the tumor is displacing nerves medially/laterally, or superiorly/inferiorly. The evaluation of whether EEA is a viable surgical approach to a meningioma depends entirely on the relationship between the tumor and cranial nerves. In addition to MRI, MRA or CTA is very useful to evaluate possible vascular invasion or encasement. Lastly, image guidance protocols will be necessary if the tumor is to be resected through EEA.

Physical examination and the assessment of preoperative cranial nerve function are likewise necessary. Neuro-ophthalmological exam and the evaluation of preoperative visual fields are imperative for any lesions centered around the optic apparatus. Papilledema should be identified; if present, this is often treated with CSF diversion. Evaluation of extraocular movements will give important information about the function of cranial nerves III, IV, and VI, while the presence or absence of facial pain or numbness will evaluate the function of cranial nerve V. Cranial nerves VII and VIII can be evaluated if necessary by facial nerve exam and audiometric studies. Lastly, lesions in the clivus or foramen magnum should have assessment of the lower cranial nerves, through evaluation of palatal movement, flexible laryngoscopy for assessment of vocal cord mobility, evaluation of shoulder function, and visualization of tongue mobility.

The identification of cranial nerve dysfunction and the duration of this dysfunction can be of paramount importance when evaluating the potential for using EEA for resection of meningiomas. Obviously, the absence of cranial nerve function does not rule out the possibility of restoration of function after tumor removal; however, long-standing cranial nerve dysfunction likely indicates permanent damage and allows for the possibility of transgressing those nerves as part of the resection.

19.3.1 Anterior Cranial Fossa (Cribriform Fossa, Planum Sphenoidale, Suprasellar, and Parasellar)

The working corridor and bone removal during EEA for olfactory groove meningiomas usually entail a wide opening of the frontal sinus (Draf 3) along with bilateral ethmoidectomies [8]. The posterior aspect of the frontal sinus and cribriform plate are removed; posterior extension of these tumors may require further removal of the planum sphenoidale as well. The position of the optic nerve (approximated by the midpoint of the orbit from medial to lateral) represents the lateral limit of resection using EEA. As mentioned earlier, olfactory groove meningiomas that have a component both medial and lateral to the optic nerve cannot be fully extirpated using EEA; a common approach is to resect the medial component with EEA and to return for the lateral component through a supralateral orbitotomy at a second stage.

Meningiomas more caudal along the ventral anterior cranial fossa can be addressed through a transplanum/transtuberculum approach [4]. In these cases, the working corridor is a wide bilateral sphenoidotomy and bilateral ethmoidectomies. Suprasellar meningiomas require a wide opening of the bone overlying the sella turcica and mobilization and displacement of the pituitary gland [13]. Further exposure of the suprasellar meningiomas may require resection of the tubercular strut and planum sphenoidale. The critical anatomic structures that need to be dissected and identified prior to the resection of a meningioma using EEA in this location are the carotid arteries and optic nerves. In a similar fashion to the evaluation of olfactory groove meningiomas, the relationship between the meningioma and the optic apparatus is critical to the decision-making process regarding the surgical approach to these lesions. Many meningiomas of the planum sphenoidale remain inferior to the optic chiasm and/or optic nerve and displace these structures superiorly; those are amenable to an endoscopic approach. If the tumor encases the optic chiasm or nerves, or is superolateral to these structures, a lateral approach will be necessary. A similar algorithm for resection applies to the anterior cerebral arteries.

Another option for the use of EEA for meningiomas superior and lateral to the optic nerves is for decompression of the optic apparatus prior to lateral resection. In many cases, the growth of the tumor causes significant compression of the optic chiasm or nerve, along with the possibility of ischemia of the vessels supplying these nerves. This may make the optic nerve or chiasm vulnerable to significant injury with even minimal manipulation. Bony decompression of the optic nerve and/or chiasm from an endonasal approach may minimize this ischemia and allow a corridor for the nerve to tolerate displacement when manipulated from the superior or lateral side. This may make it significantly safer to resect meningiomas that are superolateral to the optic apparatus or which encase the optic apparatus but have significant superior or lateral components.

19.3.2 Middle Cranial Fossa (Cavernous Sinus, Meckel's Cave, and Petrous Apex)

Meningiomas in Meckel's cave can be accessed through a well-described anteromedial corridor [14]. After a wide sphenoidotomy and medial maxillectomy, the pterygopalatine fossa is exposed. The vidian nerve is used as a landmark for the internal carotid artery, and V2 is exposed. Dissection through the "quadrangular space," bounded by the internal carotid artery inferomedially, the abducens nerve superiorly, and V2 laterally allows access to Meckel's cave for resection of tumors located within it.

Some cavernous sinus meningiomas can be resected through EEA. The major limitation of EEA access to the cavernous sinus is the potential of damage to the cranial nerves which traverse the sinus, including III, IV, V1, and VI. In the case of pre-existing nerve deficits, it may be reasonable to approach cavernous sinus lesions through EEA. Again, this would involve a wide sphenoidotomy and pterygopalatine fossa exposure. The internal carotid artery is widely exposed, and the cavernous sinus can be identified lateral to the ICA. Of course, compression of the cavernous sinus by the tumor may be relieved by tumor excision, and brisk bleeding may result and require control with hemostatic agents or packing.

Meningiomas of the medial petrous apex can likewise be approached with EEA. Three approaches to the medial petrous apex using EEA have been described by our group: (1) a medial approach, (2) a medial approach with lateralization of the internal carotid artery, and (3) a transpterygoid infrapetrous approach [27]. Of these, the transpterygoid infrapetrous approach would be the most common. In this approach, a wide sphenoidotomy and medial maxillectomy is performed, and the pterygoid wedge is identified and resected. The inferior portion of the carotid artery is identified, and using image guidance, access to the medial petrous apex is accomplished through directed drilling inferior to the petrous carotid.

19.3.3 Posterior Cranial Fossa (Clival, Petroclival, and Foramen Magnum)

Clival, petroclival, and foramen magnum meningiomas may be accessed through EEA. The corridor that can be accessed via EEA is limited laterally by the cranial nerves (as described below) and can be extended posteriorly into and through the clivus and through the dura of the anterior foramen magnum [3]. A wide sphenoidotomy is performed, and endoscopic resection of the nasopharyngeal mucosa and prevertebral musculature is performed. This allows access to the clivus below the vertebrobasilar junction (which can be approximated by the inferior limit of the sphenoid). The clivus can be drilled away; in the superior clivus, the nerve III is the lateral limit of bony resection, whereas in the lower clivus is the position of nerves IX, X, and in particular XII that limit lateral dissection. Bony dissection can be taken in a caudal direction through to the dura at the anterior margin of the foramen magnum, and this dura can be incised to gain access to meningiomas within the anterior portion of the foramen magnum. Bony dissection can also be carried more inferiorly to the craniocervical junction, or even further via a transodontoid approach to gain access to the C1–C2 junction.

The EEA approach can be expanded to lesions located more laterally in the clivus. A "far medial" approach recently described by our group uses dissection through the occipital condyle to increase the access to the lateral foramen magnum [18]. The inferolateral clivus can be divided into two compartments divided by the hypoglossal canal: the jugular tubercle (superior to the hypoglossal canal) and the condylar (inferior to the hypoglossal canal). Removal of the medial occipital condyle will increase exposure to lateral structures, including the vertebral artery. The hypoglossal canal is used as the posterior limit of the resection of the occipital condyle removal. Drilling above the hypoglossal canal in the medial aspect of the jugular tubercle can further increase the exposure to the lateral foramen magnum.

Conclusions

Meningiomas can occupy highly variable locations at the skull base. The expanded endonasal approach is a direct, low-morbidity approach to selected skull base tumors and can often be applied to meningiomas. EEA offers several advantages, including the absence of skin incisions, the elimination of the need for brain retraction, and direct, high-resolution visualization of critical structures. A substantial worldwide experience with EEA has been established, with low rates of morbidity, infection, and mortality. Advances in reconstruction have contributed significantly to the safety of this procedure. A series of modular approaches to the skull base using EEA have been described for tumors in various locations in the anterior, middle, and posterior cranial fossae. The determination of whether EEA is a viable surgical strategy for specific meningiomas depends on the location of the tumor and specifically the relationship between the tumor and cranial nerves. Resection of meningiomas through EEA may have as a goal complete resection, tumor debulking prior to radiation therapy, or resection of the medial component of the tumor prior to further resection through a lateral approach.

References

1. Beer-Furlan A, Evins AI, Rigante L, Anichini G, Stieg PE, Bernardo A (2014) Dual-port 2D and 3D endoscopy: expanding the limits of the endonasal approaches to midline skull base lesions with lateral extension. J Neurol Surg B Skull Base 75(3):187–197. doi:10.1055/s-0033-1364165
2. Caicedo-Granados E, Carrau R, Snyderman CH, Prevedello D, Fernandez-Miranda J, Gardner P, Kassam A (2010) Reverse rotation flap for reconstruction of donor site after vascular pedicled nasoseptal flap in skull base surgery. Laryngoscope 120(8):1550–1552. doi:10.1002/lary.20975
3. Cavallo LM, Messina A, Gardner P, Esposito F, Kassam AB, Cappabianca P, de Divitiis E, Tschabitscher M (2005) Extended endoscopic endonasal approach to the pterygopalatine fossa: anatomical study and clinical considerations. Neurosurg Focus 19(1), E5
4. de Lara D, Ditzel Filho LF, Muto J, Otto BA, Carrau RL, Prevedello DM (2013) Surgical management of craniopharyngioma with third ventricle involvement. Neurosurg Focus 34(1 Suppl): Video 5. doi:10.3171/2013.V1.FOCUS12330
5. Felisati G, Lenzi R, Pipolo C, Maccari A, Messina F, Revay M, Lania A, Cardia A, Lasio G (2013) Endoscopic expanded endonasal approach: preliminary experience with the new 3D endoscope. Acta Otorhinolaryngol Ital organo ufficiale della Societa italiana di otorinolaringologia e chirurgia cervico-facciale 33(2):102–106
6. Fortes FS, Carrau RL, Snyderman CH, Kassam A, Prevedello D, Vescan A, Mintz A, Gardner P (2007) Transpterygoid transposition of a temporoparietal fascia flap: a new method for skull base reconstruction after endoscopic expanded endonasal approaches. Laryngoscope 117(6):970–976. doi:10.1097/MLG.0b013e3180471482
7. Fortes FS, Carrau RL, Snyderman CH, Prevedello D, Vescan A, Mintz A, Gardner P, Kassam AB (2007) The posterior pedicle inferior turbinate flap: a new vascularized flap for skull base reconstruction. Laryngoscope 117(8):1329–1332. doi:10.1097/mlg.0b013e318062111f
8. Gardner PA, Kassam AB, Thomas A, Snyderman CH, Carrau RL, Mintz AH, Prevedello DM (2008) Endoscopic endonasal resection of anterior cranial base meningiomas. Neurosurgery 63(1):36–52; discussion 52–54. doi:10.1227/01.NEU.0000335069.30319.1E
9. Hadad G, Bassagasteguy L, Carrau RL, Mataza JC, Kassam A, Snyderman CH, Mintz A (2006) A novel reconstructive technique after endoscopic expanded endonasal approaches: vascular pedicle nasoseptal flap. Laryngoscope 116(10):1882–1886. doi:10.1097/01.mlg.0000234933.37779.e4
10. Hadad G, Rivera-Serrano CM, Bassagaisteguy LH, Carrau RL, Fernandez-Miranda J, Prevedello DM, Kassam AB (2011) Anterior pedicle lateral nasal wall flap: a novel technique for the reconstruction of anterior skull base defects. Laryngoscope 121(8):1606–1610. doi:10.1002/lary.21889
11. Kassam A, Snyderman CH, Mintz A, Gardner P, Carrau RL (2005) Expanded endonasal approach: the rostrocaudal axis. Part I. Crista galli to the sella turcica. Neurosurg Focus 19(1):E3
12. Kassam A, Snyderman CH, Mintz A, Gardner P, Carrau RL (2005) Expanded endonasal approach: the rostrocaudal axis. Part II. Posterior clinoids to the foramen magnum. Neurosurg Focus 19(1):E4
13. Kassam AB, Prevedello DM, Thomas A, Gardner P, Mintz A, Snyderman C, Carrau R (2008) Endoscopic endonasal pituitary transposition for a transdorsum sellae approach to the interpeduncular cistern. Neurosurgery 62(3 Suppl 1):57–72; discussion 72–54. doi:10.1227/01.neu.0000317374.30443.23
14. Kassam AB, Prevedello DM, Carrau RL, Snyderman CH, Gardner P, Osawa S, Seker A, Rhoton AL Jr (2009) The front door to Meckel's cave: an anteromedial corridor via expanded endoscopic endonasal approach- technical considerations and clinical series. Neurosurgery 64(3 Suppl):ons71–82; discussion ons82–83. doi:10.1227/01.NEU.0000335162.36862.54

15. Kassam AB, Prevedello DM, Carrau RL, Snyderman CH, Thomas A, Gardner P, Zanation A, Duz B, Stefko ST, Byers K, Horowitz MB (2011) Endoscopic endonasal skull base surgery: analysis of complications in the authors' initial 800 patients. J Neurosurg 114(6):1544–1568. doi:10.3171/2010.10.JNS09406
16. Labib MA, Prevedello DM, Carrau R, Kerr EE, Naudy C, Abou Al-Shaar H, Corsten M, Kassam A (2014) A road map to the internal carotid artery in expanded endoscopic endonasal approaches to the ventral cranial base. Neurosurgery 10(Suppl 3):448–471; discussion 471. doi:10.1227/NEU.0000000000000362
17. McLaughlin N, Ditzel Filho LF, Prevedello DM, Kelly DF, Carrau RL, Kassam AB (2012) Side-cutting aspiration device for endoscopic and microscopic tumor removal. J Neurol Surgery B Skull Base 73(1):11–20. doi:10.1055/s-0032-1304834
18. Morera VA, Fernandez-Miranda JC, Prevedello DM, Madhok R, Barges-Coll J, Gardner P, Carrau R, Snyderman CH, Rhoton AL Jr, Kassam AB (2010) "Far-medial" expanded endonasal approach to the inferior third of the clivus: the transcondylar and transjugular tubercle approaches. Neurosurgery 66(6 Suppl Operative):211–219; discussion 219–220. doi:10.1227/01.NEU.0000369926.01891.5D
19. Patel MR, Shah RN, Snyderman CH, Carrau RL, Germanwala AV, Kassam AB, Zanation AM (2010) Pericranial flap for endoscopic anterior skull-base reconstruction: clinical outcomes and radioanatomic analysis of preoperative planning. Neurosurgery 66(3):506–512; discussion 512. doi:10.1227/01.NEU.0000365620.59677.FF
20. Prevedello DM, Barges-Coll J, Fernandez-Miranda JC, Morera V, Jacobson D, Madhok R, dos Santos MC, Zanation A, Snyderman CH, Gardner P, Kassam AB, Carrau R (2009) Middle turbinate flap for skull base reconstruction: cadaveric feasibility study. Laryngoscope 119(11):2094–2098. doi:10.1002/lary.20226
21. Rivera-Serrano CM, Oliver C, Prevedello D, Gardner P, Snyderman C, Kassam A, Carrau RL (2010) Pedicled Facial Buccinator (FAB) flap: a new flap for reconstruction of skull base defects. The Laryngoscope 120(Suppl 4):S234. doi:10.1002/lary.21701
22. Rivera-Serrano CM, Bassagaisteguy LH, Hadad G, Carrau RL, Kelly D, Prevedello DM, Fernandez-Miranda J, Kassam AB (2011) Posterior pedicle lateral nasal wall flap: new reconstructive technique for large defects of the skull base. Am J Rhinol Allergy 25(6):e212–e216. doi:10.2500/ajra.2011.25.3693
23. Rivera-Serrano CM, Snyderman CH, Gardner P, Prevedello D, Wheless S, Kassam AB, Carrau RL, Germanwala A, Zanation A (2011) Nasoseptal "rescue" flap: a novel modification of the nasoseptal flap technique for pituitary surgery. Laryngoscope 121(5):990–993. doi:10.1002/lary.21419
24. Shah RN, Leight WD, Patel MR, Surowitz JB, Wong YT, Wheless SA, Germanwala AV, Zanation AM (2011) A controlled laboratory and clinical evaluation of a three-dimensional endoscope for endonasal sinus and skull base surgery. Am J Rhinol Allergy 25(3):141–144. doi:10.2500/ajra.2011.25.3593
25. Snyderman C, Kassam A, Carrau R, Mintz A, Gardner P, Prevedello DM (2007) Acquisition of surgical skills for endonasal skull base surgery: a training program. Laryngoscope 117(4):699–705. doi:10.1097/MLG.0b013e318031c817
26. Zanation AM, Carrau RL, Snyderman CH, Germanwala AV, Gardner PA, Prevedello DM, Kassam AB (2009) Nasoseptal flap reconstruction of high flow intraoperative cerebral spinal fluid leaks during endoscopic skull base surgery. Am J Rhinol Allergy 23(5):518–521. doi:10.2500/ajra.2009.23.3378
27. Zanation AM, Snyderman CH, Carrau RL, Gardner PA, Prevedello DM, Kassam AB (2009) Endoscopic endonasal surgery for petrous apex lesions. Laryngoscope 119(1):19–25. doi:10.1002/lary.20027
28. Zanation AM, Snyderman CH, Carrau RL, Kassam AB, Gardner PA, Prevedello DM (2009) Minimally invasive endoscopic pericranial flap: a new method for endonasal skull base reconstruction. Laryngoscope 119(1):13–18. doi:10.1002/lary.20022

Mini-Pterional Approach to Anterior Cranial Fossa Meningiomas

20

M. Yashar S. Kalani, Nicolas O. Koechlin, Hazem J. Abuhusain, and Charles Teo

20.1 Introduction

Anterior cranial fossa meningiomas include those involving the planum sphenoidale, the olfactory groove, the clinoid, the tuberculum sellae, the suprasellar region, and the sphenoorbital skull base. The majority of these tumors involve both anterior and middle fossae. Although some of these locations may be accessed via an endonasal endoscopic approach or an eyebrow craniotomy, the open mini-pterional approach remains a workhorse for access to these pathologies. In this chapter, we outline the indications, anatomical considerations, and techniques for the safe and effective extirpation of anterior cranial fossa meningiomas using this robust approach.

M.Y.S. Kalani, MD, PhD
Division of Neurological Surgery, Barrow Neurological Institute, Phoenix, AZ 85013, USA

Centre for Minimally Invasive Neurosurgery, Prince of Wales Private Hospital, Suite 3, Level 7, Barker Street, Randwick, NSW 2031, Australia

N.O. Koechlin, MD
Centre for Minimally Invasive Neurosurgery, Prince of Wales Private Hospital, Suite 3, Level 7, Barker Street, Randwick, NSW 2031, Australia

Neurosurgery Clinic, Lucerne Cantonal Hospital, Lucerne 6000, Switzerland

H.J. Abuhusain, MD, PhD • C. Teo, MBBS (✉)
Centre for Minimally Invasive Neurosurgery, Prince of Wales Private Hospital, Suite 3, Level 7, Barker Street, Randwick, NSW 2031, Australia
e-mail: Charlie@neuroendoscopy.info

20.2 Indications

Although a small, incidentally found meningioma can be followed with serial imaging and radiosurgery has been advocated for select patients, it is our policy to surgically treat all patients where comorbidities would not limit them undergoing general anesthesia.

The indication for the use of the mini-pterional approach as opposed to the endonasal endoscopic or the eyebrow approach (or other subfrontal variants) depends on several factors.

20.2.1 Location of the Optic Apparatus

Meningiomas of the anterior cranial fossa may displace the optic apparatus; therefore, the location of the optic apparatus can modify the choice of the approach. In most cases, the tumor displaces the optic apparatus superiorly and posteriorly. The lesion can be accessed safely via an endonasal corridor if the chosen is displaced superiorly. In contrast, a prefixed chiasm can limit the access to the suprasellar spaces and is therefore a relative contra-indication for an endonasal approach. Similarly, tumors with an

P. Cappabianca et al. (eds.), *Midline Skull Base Surgery*, DOI 10.1007/978-3-319-21533-4_20

extensive component above the optic chiasm benefit from a transcranial exposure.

20.2.2 Optic Canal Invasion

Anterior fossa meningiomas with extension into optic canal generally invade the canal in its medial aspect. The medial optic canal can be accessed endoscopically, but its full exposure can be arduous. Similarly, tumor invasion of the lateral optic canal is a contra-indication for an endoscopic approach.

20.2.3 Vascular Involvement

Significant vascular involvement and displacement is a contra-indication to endoscopic approaches. In most cases, both an eyebrow and mini-pterional approaches allow excellent vascular control.

20.2.4 Tumor with Significant Middle Fossa Component

Although tumors of the anterior cranial fossa with a small degree of overhang on the sphenoid wing can be approached via an eyebrow craniotomy with endoscopic assistance, most tumors with significant middle fossa components are best addressed from the anterolateral trajectory provided by a mini-pterional approach. Select tumors can be accessed endoscopically via a transmaxillary approach with good outcomes.

20.2.5 Surgeon Experience

Surgeon expertise and comfort strongly influences the choice of approach. For example, surgeons with extensive experience with the use of endoscopy may be able to tackle lesions that may not be appropriate for those without a broad experience with endoscopy. Other factors associated with experience including rates of CSF leak and experience with the repair of extensive skull base defects using vascularized flaps may alter the choice of approach.

20.3 Neuroimaging

Although in the current era of advanced imaging plain radiography is no longer used to diagnose anterior fossa meningiomas, historically, the sign of a "smoking pterion," reflected by thickening of the ala major in the sphenoid bone and pterion, was a highly specific sign for sphenoid meningiomas.

Adequate surgical planning relies on the correct interpretation of the meningioma and its dural attachment in relation to neighboring neurovascular structures. The soft tissue components of the tumor can generally be well depicted with a triplanar MRI including gadolinium-enhanced contrast sequences (Fig. 20.1a, b). However, the extent of dural invasion by the tumor cannot be judged reliably against adjoining neovascularization.

The T2-weighted sequences are especially useful to assess the course of the optic apparatus in cases of tumor proximity to the superior orbital fissure. Additionally, the passage of the intrasylvian MCA and any cortex edema adjacent to the tumor can be evaluated in these sequences.

For postoperative resection control and long-term follow-up, the multi-planar MRI has the greatest diagnostic value. As with all meningiomas, a correct evaluation of the resection grade according to Simpson (for grades I–III) is not possible [1].

MR angiography and MR venography can further elucidate the anatomical relations of the involved vasculature. Accordingly, in most cases, it is unnecessary to perform a digital subtraction angiography for diagnostic purposes alone.

On the other hand, there are authors who recommend embolization of tumors greater than 3 cm prior to surgery. Although historically particle and glue-based embolization was advocated for tumor devascularization, the advent of onyx has led to its broad use and replacement of prior embolysates [2, 3].

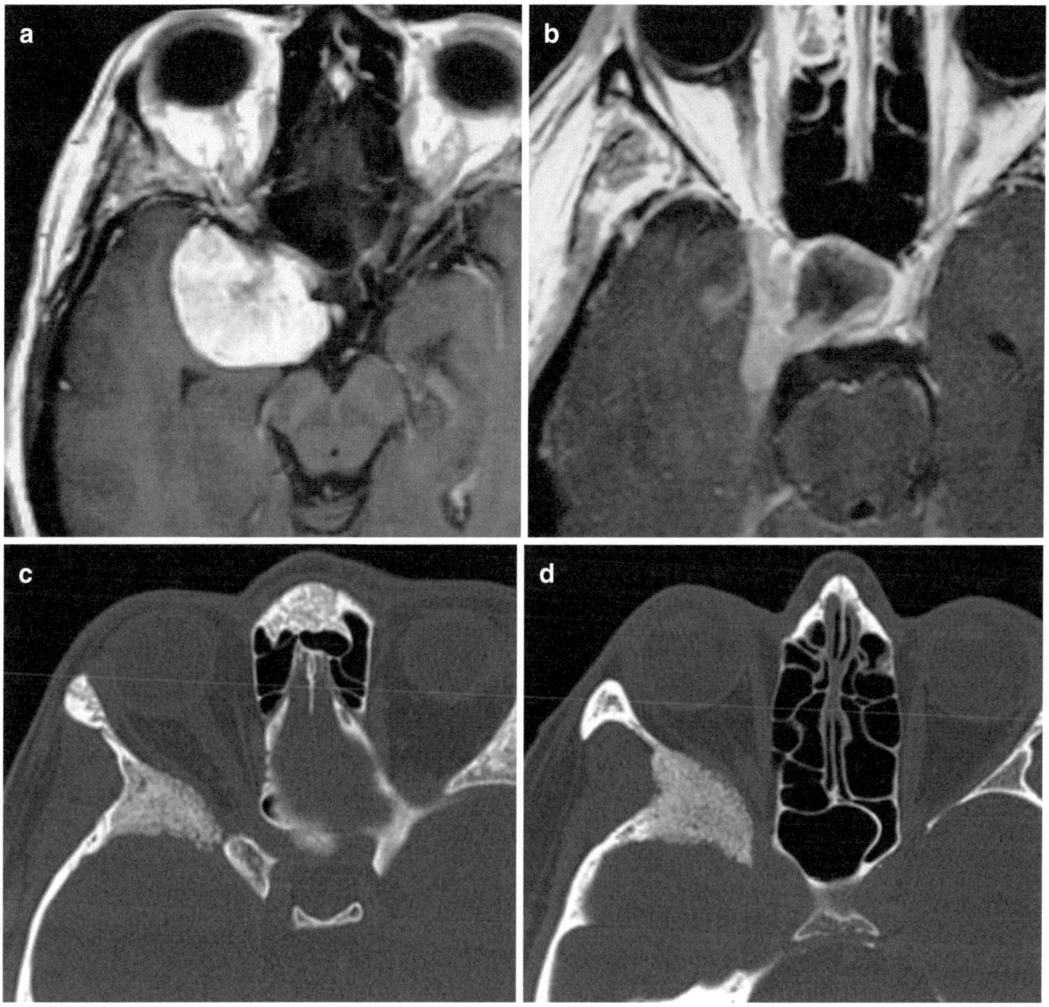

Fig. 20.1 Imaging modalities used in workup of meningiomas. (**a**) T1-weighted magnetic resonance imaging (MRI) with gadolinium-enhanced sequences provides anatomical detail about the location of tumors, as well as their dural tail, in relation to adjacent structures and is the most essential imaging modality in preparation of surgery. (**b**) Postoperative T1-weighted MRI with gadolinium enhancement depicts residual tumor in the cavernous sinus on the side. (**c**, **d**) Thin-sliced computed tomography (CT) of the skull demonstrates "en plaque" growth within the sphenoid wing and thickening of the clinoid process and lateral wall of the orbit with subsequent narrowing of the optic canal and proptosis

Computed tomography (CT), preferably thin sliced (1 mm), is essential to correctly estimate the degree of hyperostosis and width of optical canal and foramen, especially in cases where the tumor shows "en plaque" growth and involvement of the optic canal (Fig. 20.1c, d). In addition, the visualization of a possible pneumatization of the clinoid process is useful in preventing the occurrence of a postoperative CSF leak.

20.4 Anatomy

Most meningiomas of the anterior skull base, particularly the olfactory groove, tuberculum sellae, and clinoid, which were previously accessed through a classic pterional approach, are commonly accessed through transnasal endoscopic or subfrontal eyebrow approaches.

In our hands, the mini-pterional approach is reserved for lesions originating in the lateral and medial sphenoid ridge as well as some tumors of the cavernous sinus. This provides sufficient access to both the orbital roof and the base of the middle cranial and infratemporal fossae, if required.

20.4.1 The Pterion

The pterion is located in the temporal fossa and defines the point of junction of the parietal bone, squamous part of the temporal bone, greater wing of the sphenoid bone, and the frontal bone [4]. These bones are joined by the sphenoparietal, coronal, and squamous sutures which meet at the pterion. The anterior Sylvian point, an ideal starting point for the opening of the Sylvian fissure due to its cisternal enlargement, lies just behind the pterion. The inferior frontal gyrus is located between the pterion and the superior temporal line.

A recent study found the pterion to be located within a 1 cm diameter, 2.6 cm behind and 1.3 cm above the posterolateral margin of the frontozygomatic suture in most adults [5]. As it is easily palpable, the frontozygomatic suture serves as a practical external landmark to define the pterion. The thickness of the bone at the pterion as well as the relationship to the underlying middle meningeal artery is reported to be highly variable [5]. The most important structures to be aware of upon soft tissue dissection are the temporal branch of the facial nerve and the superficial temporal artery (STA).

20.4.2 The Temporal Branch of the Facial Nerve

Before exiting through the fascia of the parotid gland, the temporal branch of the facial nerve divides into an anterior, middle (frontal), and posterior ramus. The anterior ramus mainly innervates orbicularis oculi muscle, the frontal ramus innervates the ipsilateral frontalis muscle, and the posterior ramus innervates the tragus and anterior and superior auricular muscles. Of note, the number, usually between one and four, of rami and their pattern of innervation are highly variable.

In most cases, the temporal branch of the facial nerve runs in the superficial musculoaponeurotic system (SMAS) over the zygomatic arch, continuing initially in a superficial layer of fat between the temporoparietal and the deep temporal fascia. The deep temporal fascia consists of one layer at the level of the superior temporal line where it blends with the periosteum. However, at the orbital level, it consists of two layers separated by an intermediate fat pad. A recent study suggests that because of this fat pad, the point where the fascia splits differs at the anterior, middle, and posterior portions of the zygomatic arch. There is significant variability regarding the course of the temporal branch between these layers of fascia and fat, and the optimal method of dissection to avoid neural injury remains controversial. Finally, to reach their target muscles, the terminal twigs of the temporal branch penetrate the galea. Since the temporal branch of the frontal nerve usually has no anastomotic connections, spontaneous functional recovery after injury is generally poor.

20.4.3 The Superficial Temporal Artery

The STA originates from the external carotid artery (ECA) as a terminal branch. After its origin from the parotid gland, it courses superficially over the posterior root of the temporal bone zygomatic process and continues for 4–6 cm until it divides into a frontal and temporal branch. Injury to the STA can frequently lead to atrophy of the temporal muscle and in rare cases lead to the formation of an iatrogenic pseudoaneurysm.

20.4.4 Intracranial Anatomy of the Approach

The anterior part of the Sylvian fissure and the surrounding temporal and frontal lobes are the first relevant intracranial structures that are visualized after craniotomy and dural opening. The inferior frontal gyrus consists of the orbital, triangular, and opercular parts. In the dominant hemisphere, the opercular part is considered to be highly eloquent for it comprises Broca's area, a region involved in language-relevant semantic tasks. The superior temporal gyrus (STG) borders the Sylvian fissure inferiorly. In its opercular part, the STG harbors the transverse gyri with their primary auditory cortex. This region remains unexposed when a mini-pterional approach is fashioned as opposed to a classic large pterional craniotomy.

Great variability exists regarding the pattern of the venous drainage for the Sylvian fissure. The superficial middle cerebral vein (SMCV) drains typically anteriorly and caudally toward the skull base. After turning medially, it joins the anterior portion of the cavernous sinus. Alternatively, it may also join the superior petrosal sinus or the basal vein of Rosenthal. Anastomotic relations to the superior sagittal sinus through the plexus of Trolard and the transverse sinus through the vein of Labbé are common, but also hypoplastic SMCVs are seen not infrequently. Some authors suggest that an approach-related compromise of the SMCV might be the single most important factor contributing to morbidity in patients undergoing pterional craniotomies for aneurysmal repair [6]. The mini-pterional approach reduces the surface of potential venous injury compared to conventional craniotomies.

The arterial contents of the Sylvian fissure from lateral to medial are distal branches of the middle cerebral artery (MCA), the M1–2 bifurcation of the MCA, and the carotid bifurcation with the optic-carotid triangle and the carotid-oculomotor triangle as its neurovascular landmarks.

20.4.5 Anatomical Considerations Regarding Meningiomas of the Sphenoid Ridge

Meningiomas of the sphenoid ridge frequently show "en plaque" growth and prominent dural involvement. In some meningiomas, extensive bone invasion (hyperostosis) of the orbital roof, lateral orbital wall, and the orbit itself occurs. In these cases, loss of visual acuity and exophthalmos can be presenting symptoms.

Tumors located on the outer sphenoid ridge can for practical reasons be considered to behave essentially like meningiomas of the convexity. Their clinical presentation and surgical management does not differ from that of convexity meningiomas. In such cases, a mini-pterional craniotomy is usually not feasible as these tumors can grow quite large before they create symptoms, and a more extensive craniotomy is often required to completely resect the dural base of the tumor.

The vascular supply of lateral tumors mainly consists of feeding vessels arising from the STA and middle meningeal artery but sometimes includes anterior meningeal and branches of ethmoidal arteries.

Tumors located more medially on the sphenoid ridge may compress and encase the carotid artery and its branches, optic apparatus, or pituitary stalk. These tumors may also grow into the dural layers overlying the cavernous sinus and in the cavernous sinus itself and, therefore, typically become symptomatic at an earlier stage of the disease.

Neurologic compromise, especially cranial nerve deficits, after removal of intracavernous meningiomas is prohibitively high [7, 8]. There is growing agreement that these tumors should be resected less aggressively and any remnants that are left behind closely followed with serial imaging or treated with radiosurgery. These medially located meningiomas are mostly fed by direct branches of the ICA or ascending pharyngeal artery and sometimes by a recurrent branch of the ophthalmic artery through the superior orbital fissure.

20.4.6 Classification of Sphenoid Meningiomas

Any useful classification should help the surgeon in choosing an appropriate treatment strategy for the lesion. The most basic approach is to differentiate between globular tumors and en plaque (sphenoorbital) tumors.

Originally, the first classification of sphenoid meningiomas was proposed by Eisenhard and Cushing [9]. Later classifications reflected the involvement of the cavernous sinus, the extent of hyperostosis, and en plaque growth. The classification (Table 20.1) by Al-Mefty further categorizes medial tumors regarding their spatial

Table 20.1 Al-Mefty classifications of middle sphenoid meningiomas (clinoid meningiomas)

Group I	Tumor originating proximal to the end of the carotid cistern, directly enwrapping the ICA
Group II	Tumor with a superolateral point of origin on the clinoid process and an arachnoidal membrane interposed between tumor and ICA
Group III	Tumor originating medially in the region of the optic foramen

Table 20.2 Staged strategy to address meningiomas of the clinoid and sphenoid wing

Location of the lesion	Preferred strategy
Small lateral tumor	Mini-pterional centered over the tumor
Large lateral tumor	Pterional according to the dural base of the tumor +/– orbital, +/– temporal extension of the approach
Medial tumor without cavernous sinus involvement	Mini-pterional
Medial tumor with infiltration of the cavernous sinus	Mini-pterional conservative toward intracavernous tumor parts

relation toward the carotid cistern and their point of origin on the clinoid process [10]. This illustrates that a strict differentiation between medial sphenoid meningiomas, clinoid meningiomas, and meningiomas of the optic foramen and sheath is often not possible.

Our strategy regarding the choice of approach is guided by the size of the tumor, its location on the sphenoid ridge, arterial relations, bone invasion with or without orbital and middle fossae involvement, and finally involvement of the cavernous sinus beyond the infiltration of the outer wall (Table 20.2).

20.5 Technique

This section outlines the paradigm of keyhole surgery and technical nuances for performing the mini-pterional approach to the anterior cranial fossa. Our modification of the classic pterional approach makes use of the endoscope to provide robust access to the anterior and middle cranial fossae, the entire circle of Willis, and the top of the basilar artery.

20.5.1 The Keyhole Paradigm

Effective keyhole surgery depends on exquisite attention to details, meticulous microsurgical technique, and ample preoperative planning and evaluation of imaging to select the optimal approach. Keyhole surgery utilizes simple but maximally effective approaches that minimize extensive skull base resection and unnecessary static brain retraction while utilizing the endoscope to assist with improved visualization. Simplifying the steps associated with a procedure decreases the opportunities for mistake, saves operative time, facilitates closure, and provides the patient with a low-morbidity alternative to classic skull base approaches.

20.5.2 Mini-Pterional Craniotomy

The pterional craniotomy, championed by Yasargil [11, 12], is one of the classic approaches used for pathology involving the anterior and middle cranial fossae. Although the pterional craniotomy provides wide exposure to the skull base, the full exposure afforded by this approach is rarely needed or used. The approach involves a large C-shaped incision, temporalis muscle elevation (commonly resulting in devascularization, denervation, and subsequent atrophy of the muscle), extensive skull base drilling, and potential for injury to the frontal and temporal lobes [13–16].

In an effort to minimize the morbidity associated with the classical pterional approach, several authors have proposed modifications that limit morbidity while still providing the needed access to the anatomy of interest [17–19]. These approaches utilize smaller skin incisions, minimal temporalis dissection, reduced skull base drilling, and smaller craniotomies that avoid injury to the underlying brain while utilizing the critical operative corridor around the lesser sphenoid wing.

20.5.3 Key Steps of Opening

The incision used for the mini-pterional is a slightly curved 2–3 cm incision behind the temporal hairline (Fig. 20.2b). A line intersecting the sphenoid wing should bisect the incision. Once the incision is made, the scalp is gently elevated off of the temporalis fascia until the temporalis fat pad is visualized, while protecting the frontalis branch of the facial nerve using a subfascial approach (Fig. 20.2c, d). This is accomplished using a posterior C-shaped incision in the fascia, elevating the fascia off the muscle, and reflecting it anteriorly with the scalp using hooks. The temporalis muscle is incised parallel to its fibers from the posterior corner of the muscle toward the sphenoid wing (Fig. 20.2e). Retracting the elevated muscle with hooks minimizes the skin incision while providing the necessary angle to expose the sphenoid wing (Fig. 20.2f). In rare cases, where the tumor is adjacent to the brain surface, further exposure of the temporal squamosa may be necessary. A single burr hole is next used to garnish a submuscular bone flap. Upon elevation of the flap, the sphenoid wing is drilled flat (Fig. 20.2g). This approach should provide 270° of exposure to the meningoperiorbital band while flattening the orbit.

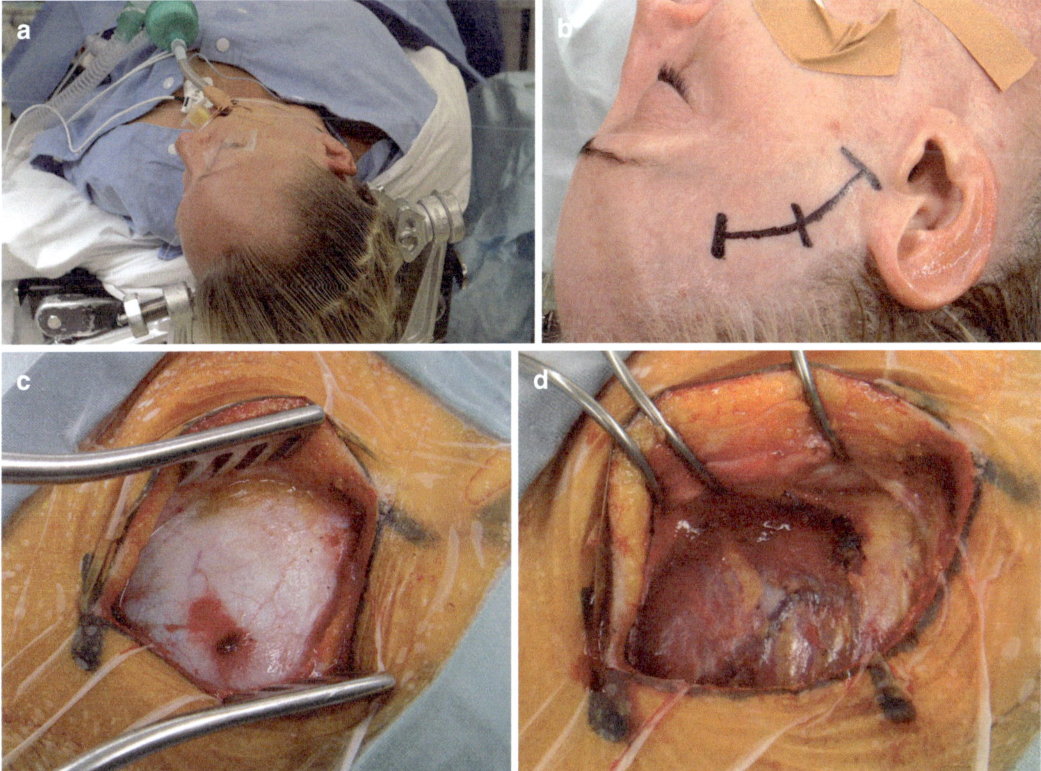

Fig. 20.2 The mini-pterional approach. (**a**) The head is positioned so that the malar eminence is the highest point in the operative field. (**b**) A 2–3 cm curved incision is garnished behind the temporal hairline. A *line* drawn perpendicularly from the sphenoid wing should bisect the incision. (**c**) The skin is elevated from the temporalis fascia until the superficial temporalis fat pad is identified. A subfascial dissection should be performed to protect the frontalis branch of the facial nerve. (**d**) The fascia is dissected away from the temporalis muscle and retracted anteriorly. (**e**) The temporalis muscle is split parallel to its fibers. (**f**) The pterion is exposed. The craniotomy is small and submuscular, minimizing cosmetic deformities. (**g**) Reduction of the sphenoid wing and orbital roof with a drill before the durotomy significantly increases the intradural space. (**h**) Closure should be performed in layers, ensuring meticulous approximation of tissues

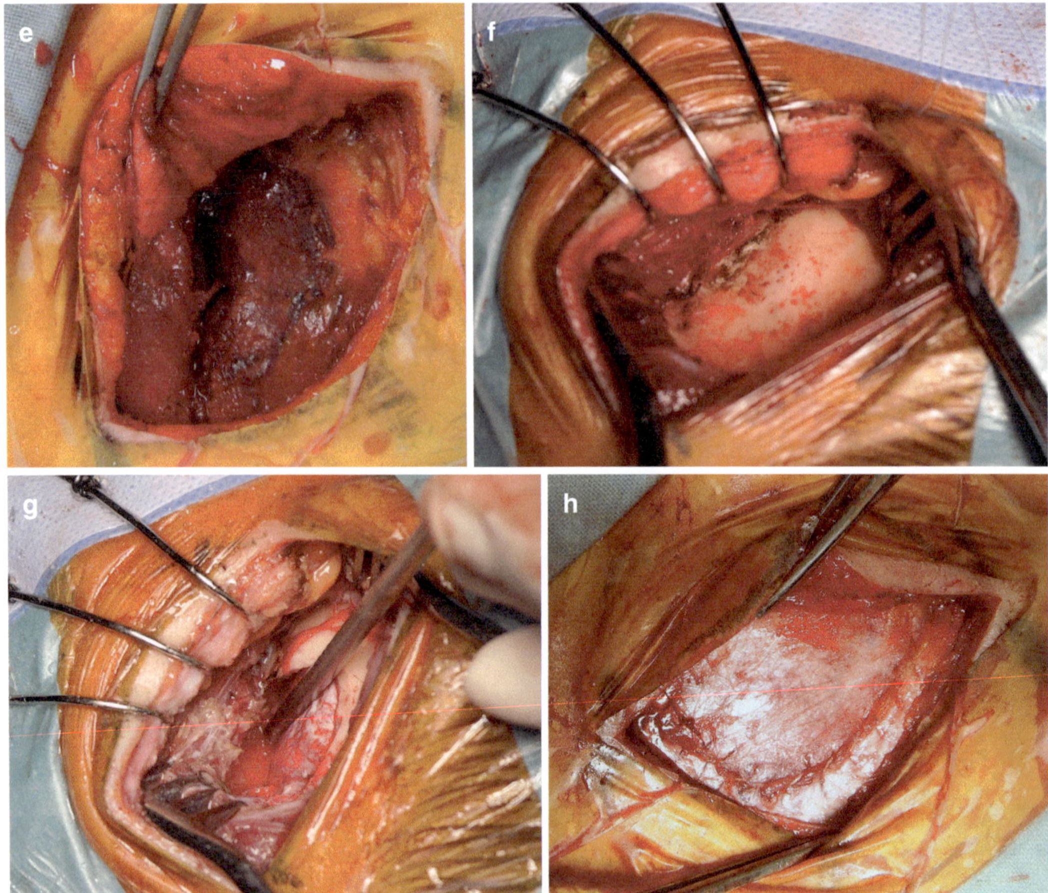

Fig. 20.3 (continued)

20.5.4 Key Steps of Approach and Tumor Resection

Although tumors involving the planum sphenoidale [20], lateral sphenoid wing [21], olfactory groove [22–24], clinoid [25], tuberculum sellae, and suprasellar region [20] can be accessed via a pterional or mini-pterional approaches, we generally approach the majority of these pathologies using an eyebrow craniotomy and reserve the mini-pterional approach for lesions with a significant middle fossa component that may not be readily accessible using a subfrontal approach via an eyebrow craniotomy or endoscopically via the transnasal corridor.

Once the craniotomy is complete, the dura is opened in a controlled fashion and retracted. A small amount of Sylvian fissure opening may be necessary to allow for release of cerebrospinal fluid (CSF) for brain relaxation and to allow a wider corridor down the barrel of the sphenoid wing. The Sylvian fissure split should be done carefully as to avoid sacrificing large Sylvian veins. Most Sylvian veins can be mobilized to the frontal or temporal lobes. If a Sylvian vein needs to be sacrificed, preference should be given to sacrificing small branches of the frontal lobe. Once CSF is released and adequate brain relaxation is obtained, the brain is covered with small patties to buttress it during periods of dynamic retraction. Fixed retractors are not used; instead, retraction is accomplished dynamically using the sucker, bipolar, or the shaft of other microsurgical instruments [26].

Technical considerations pertaining to meningiomas involving various surfaces of the anterior

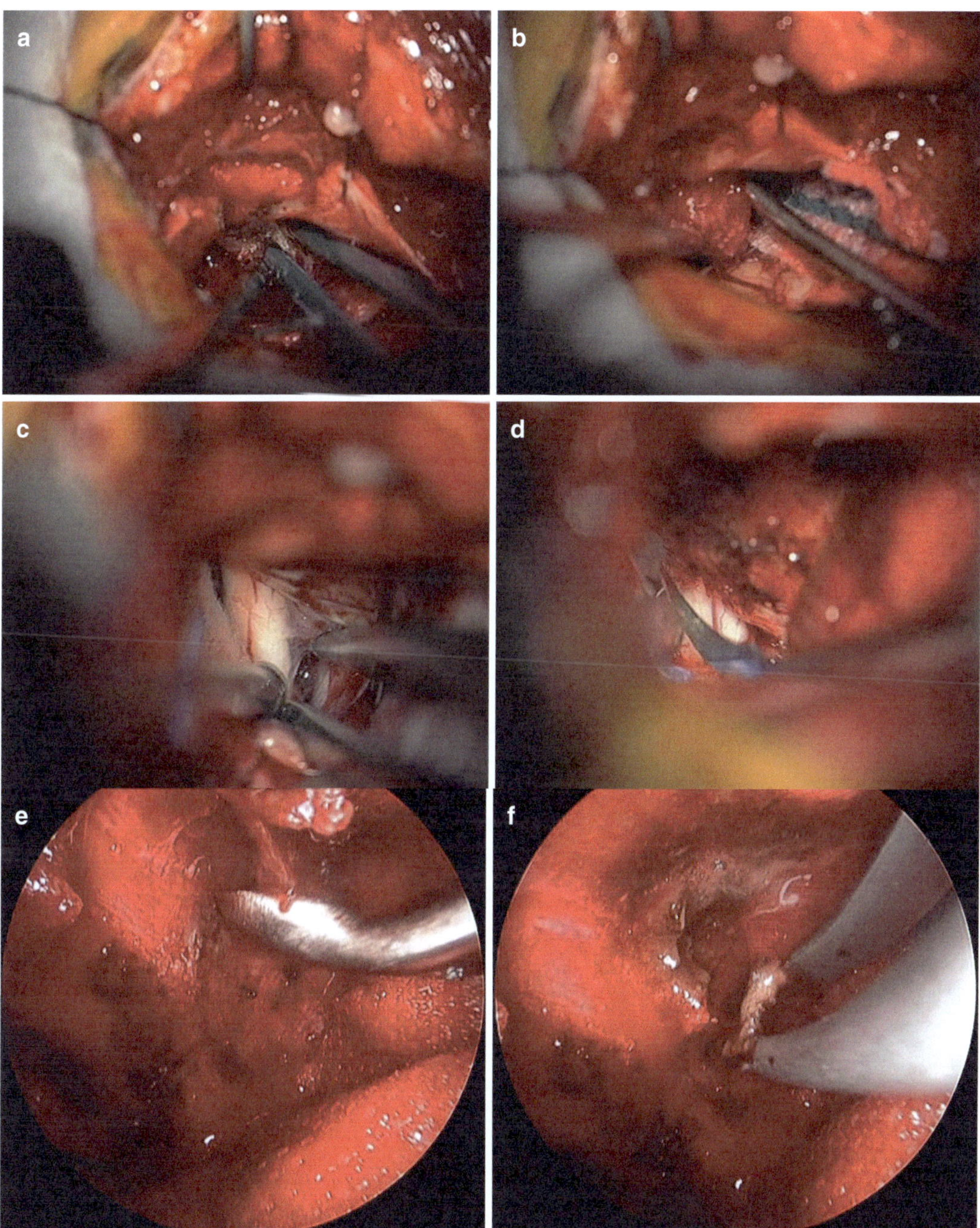

Fig. 20.3 Critical steps of tumor resection. (**a**) Coagulation and dissection of the tumor matrix deprive the tumor of most of its blood supply. (**b**) Piecemeal debulking of the tumor with suction and curettes. In some cases, an ultrasonic aspirator may be necessary. (**c**, **d**) The optic-carotid window and dura of the optic canal are opened to resect parts of the tumor that invade the cisternal spaces and bony foramina. (**e**, **f**) The endoscope and angled instruments are used to resect tumor and coagulate the dura in hidden corners of the surgical field

cranial fossa are discussed below. In approaching a meningioma, some common surgical pearls should be followed. Upon exposure of the tumor, the major blood supply to the lesion is identified and, when possible, interrupted early in the procedure (Fig. 20.3a). The tumor is internally debulked using mainly bipolar and suction as well as curettes allowing for it to be mobilized from adjacent critical neurovascular structures (Fig. 20.3b). Once the tumor is mobilized, it is sharply dissected from adjacent nerves and vessels. The difficulty of this is step is directly related to the intactness of arachnoid membranes between the tumor and the adjacent neurovascular structure (Fig. 20.3c, d). The endoscope can be a critical adjunct to improve visualization of residual tumor that may be obstructed by neurovascular structures, and angled instruments can be used to address these residual parts of the tumor (Fig. 20.3e, f). The dura involved by tumor should be resected to a normal margin or thoroughly coagulated in cases where this is not possible. The bone involved by the tumor should be thoroughly drilled to obtain the best chance of cure and minimize recurrence. At times this may result in significant defects in the skull base that need to be repaired. Skull base repairs are discussed elsewhere in this book, and the reader is referred to Part VI of this work for technical considerations. Once hemostasis is obtained, closure can commence.

20.5.5 Location-Specific Considerations

The initial steps of tumor exposure and resection are the same regardless of the specific location of the meningioma. Importantly, the surgeon should be cautious of the proximity of the internal carotid artery (ICA), anterior cerebral arteries (ACA), and anterior communicating artery (AComA) associated with tumors in this location. The pituitary gland and optic apparatus are other critical structures that must be visualized, decompressed, and preserved at all cost regardless of the approach. Specific surgical pearls pertaining to tumors involving various surfaces of the anterior cranial fossa are discussed below.

20.5.6 Planum Sphenoidale

Tumors involving the planum sphenoidale consist of those with predominantly a lateral base and those that are medial.

Lateral sphenoid tumors commonly involve the distal branches of the MCA. It is important to debulk the tumor and sharply dissect portions adherent to the arteries. Meningiomas may encase branches of the MCA, but true invasion is very rare. Regardless, one should be prepared to perform distal revascularization via an STA-to-MCA bypass or primary repair of the MCA should iatrogenic injury take place. Extensive dural resection is usually possible with these lesions and should be the goal.

Medial sphenoid tumors may involve the cavernous sinus complicating their gross resection. We do not favor entry into the cavernous sinus and resection of tumor from this compartment. The excessively high rate of cranial nerve palsies associated with surgery in the cavernous sinus must be weighed against the risks of radiation therapy in this patient population. In most cases, the residual tumor can be effectively controlled with radiosurgery obviating the need for surgical manipulation of cavernous sinus components. In select cases, medial tumors may involve the anterior clinoid and optic canal. Although some have advocated an extradural clinoidectomy and opening of the optic canal, we do not favor this approach given the risks associated with these maneuvers. Similar to lateral tumors, medial tumors may involve the branches of the MCA or the ICA bifurcation. Consequently, care should be taken to sharply dissect the tumor from adjacent vessels. Comfort with vascular reconstruction can assist in rare but catastrophic cases of vascular injury. Medial tumors may also compress the optic apparatus; therefore, care should be taken to avoid retraction or thermal injury to an already compromised optic apparatus.

20.5.7 Sphenoorbital

Careful removal of orbital bone involved by the tumor extradurally should be performed prior to commencing intradural work. The adequate management for most of these tumors requires removal of the clinoid and the lesser sphenoid wing. The foramen ovale and rotundum are commonly opened and the floor of the middle fossa is removed. Intraorbital tumor should be scrupulously removed; however, tumor extending into the cavernous sinus should be followed with serial imaging or treated with radiosurgery. In most cases, extraconal and extraperiorbital involvement is addressed by the removal of the lateral orbit. Invasion of the tumor into the orbital apex, the superior orbital fissure, and annulus of Zinn should not be surgically attempted, as the risk of cranial nerve injury is high. Entry into the sphenoid or ethmoid sinuses should be repaired to prevent CSF leak.

20.5.8 Olfactory Groove

Most olfactory groove meningiomas arise from the frontosphenoid suture and derive their blood supply from the anterior and posterior ethmoidal arteries. Olfactory meningiomas can be accessed usually by a lateral subfrontal trajectory. In most cases, extensive Sylvian fissure dissection is unnecessary, and simple fenestration of the subarachnoid cisterns via a subfrontal approach will provide adequate relaxation and access to the tumor. Care should be exercised to preserve the olfactory nerves. The olfactory nerve is usually displaced laterally and the optic apparatus interolaterally. The ACAs are generally adhered to the tumor capsule and displaced posteriorly and superiorly but should be preserved during tumor dissection. Like the subfrontal approach, the mini-pterional approach allows for early visualization of the optic apparatus and the ACA. Additionally, it avoids frontal sinus entry while providing a direct access to the cranial base. The major disadvantage with this approach is the narrow working corridor afforded by the anterolateral trajectory and the unnecessary exposure of the frontal lobe to approach related injury. Additional disadvantages include the difficulty with visualizing the upper portion of the tumor and the possibility of obstruction of the trajectory by a high-riding orbital roof.

20.5.9 Clinoid

These lesions can have high-riding components requiring an orbitotomy. In most cases, the removal of the orbital bar can be avoided with the judicious use of an angled endoscope. The initial steps of dissection include an extradural clinoidectomy. Since the majority of clinoidal tumors receive blood supply from the anterior dural branches of the middle meningeal, the posterior ethmoidal, and the meningioorbital arteries, the initial steps of extradural clinoidectomy lead to significant devascularization of the tumor. The clinoidectomy also exposes the clinoid segment of the ICA. This exposure, along with the exposure of the distal branches of the ACA and MCA, provides a route for the sharp dissection of the vessels displaced or engulfed by these tumors. The process of removing the clinoid usually results in orbital canal decompression by removal of the optic strut and optical roof. Small perforators to the optic apparatus, as well as the ophthalmic artery, should be preserved. The manipulation of these vessels may cause them to spasm, detrimentally affecting the visual outcome of the patient. Some tumors may extend into the cavernous sinus. Again one must weigh potential complications associated with entry into the cavernous sinus with the risk of tumor growth and radiation risks. We do not favor entry and resection of tumor from the cavernous sinus. For tumors with suprasellar or subchiasmatic extension, the dural rings should be dissected to widen the operative corridor between the ICA and the optic nerve to be able to access these domains. Again the use of the endoscope provides better visualization of possible residual tumor in these locations.

20.5.10 Tuberculum Sellae

Tumors involving the tuberculum sellae arise from the sellae proper, the chiasmatic sulcus, the diaphragm, or the limbus sphenoidale. Their major blood supply is from the posterior ethmoidal arteries. The olfactory nerves are commonly inferiorly displaced, while the optic apparatus is superolaterally displaced. The anterior cerebral arteries are displaced posteriorly and superiorly, similar to olfactory groove meningiomas. One of the most critical pearls associated with addressing tumors of the tuberculum sellae is the decision to unroof the optic canal or to remove the tumor without opening this canal. Although intuitively it makes good sense to open the optic canal to decompress the nerve, optic canal drilling is not without risks of injury to the nerve or the adjacent vasculature. In our practice, we expose the optic canal when there is clear compression of the optic apparatus.

20.5.11 Suprasellar

Tumors with suprasellar extension may require an orbitotomy for adequate visualization, but the endoscope obviates this in most cases. Care must be taken to minimize frontal lobe retraction via generous release of CSF and arachnoidal adhesions when approaching tumors in this location.

20.5.12 Key Steps of Closure

The closure is as important as any other step in the procedure, with the aim of an esthetically acceptable closure. Upon obtaining hemostasis, the dura is closed primarily in a watertight fashion. If the dura was sacrificed due to tumor involvement or shrunken, a dural substitute may be sown in place. Tack-up stitches are generally not necessary due to the small size of the craniotomy. The craniotomy is repaired using standard plating systems. The incision is closed in layers. The temporalis muscle should be re-approximated to minimize the chance of temporalis atrophy and to provide the best possible cosmetic outcome (Fig. 20.2h). The galea should be re-approximated using a 3-0 undyed Vicryl suture. The skin edges are re-approximated with a 3-0 nylon suture. Care should be taken to avoid strangulation of the muscle, galea, and skin edges as these delay wound healing and can jeopardize the cosmetic outcome.

Conclusions

The mini-pterional is a robust approach for resection of select anterior cranial fossa meningiomas. Although the majority of anterior fossa meningiomas, in our experience, can be accessed via endonasal endoscopic and eyebrow approaches, a select subset, notably those with significant middle fossa extension, requires the anterolateral approach afforded by the mini-pterional approach. A well-planned, meticulous operation can result in an excellent outcome in the majority of cases of anterior fossa meningiomas.

References

1. Simpson D (1957) The recurrence of intracranial meningiomas after surgical treatment. J Neurol Neurosurg Psychiatry 20(1):22–39
2. Borg A, Ekanayake J, Mair R, Smedley T, Brew S, Kitchen N et al (2013) Preoperative particle and glue embolization of meningiomas: indications, results, and lessons learned from 117 consecutive patients. Neurosurgery 73(2 Suppl Operative):244–251; discussion 252
3. Raper DM, Starke RM, Henderson F Jr, Ding D, Simon S, Evans AJ et al (2014) Preoperative embolization of intracranial meningiomas: efficacy, technical considerations, and complications. AJNR Am J Neuroradiol 35(9):1798–804
4. Rhoton AL Jr (2000) The temporal bone and transtemporal approaches. Neurosurgery 47(3 Suppl):S211–S265
5. Ma S, Baillie LJ, Stringer MD (2012) Reappraising the surface anatomy of the pterion and its relationship to the middle meningeal artery. Clin Anat 25(3):330–339. Epub 2011/07/30
6. Dean BL, Wallace RC, Zabramski JM, Pitt AM, Bird CR, Spetzler RF (2005) Incidence of superficial Sylvian vein compromise and postoperative effects on CT imaging after surgical clipping of middle cerebral artery aneurysms. AJNR Am J Neuroradiol 26(8):2019–2026
7. Sindou M, Wydh E, Jouanneau E, Nebbal M, Lieutaud T (2007) Long-term follow-up of meningiomas of the cavernous sinus after surgical treatment alone. J Neurosurg 107(5):937–944
8. Almefty R, Dunn IF, Pravdenkova S, Abolfotoh M, Al-Mefty O (2014) True petroclival meningiomas: results of surgical management. J Neurosurg 120(1):40–51
9. Cushing H (1938) Meningiomas of the sphenoid wing. In: Thomas CC (ed) Meningiomas: their classification, regional behavior, life history, and surgical end results. Charles C. Thomas, Springfield, pp 298–387
10. Al-Mefty O (1990) Clinoidal meningiomas. J Neurosurg 73(6):840–849
11. Krayenbuhl HA, Yasargil MG, Flamm ES, Tew JM Jr (1972) Microsurgical treatment of intracranial saccular aneurysms. J Neurosurg 37(6):678–686
12. Yasargil MG, Antic J, Laciga R, Jain KK, Hodosh RM, Smith RD (1976) Microsurgical pterional

approach to aneurysms of the basilar bifurcation. Surg Neurol 6(2):83–91
13. Bowles AP Jr (1999) Reconstruction of the temporalis muscle for pterional and cranio-orbital craniotomies. Surg Neurol 52(5):524–529
14. Patel RS, Yousem DM, Maldjian JA, Zager EL (2000) Incidence and clinical significance of frontal sinus or orbital entry during pterional (frontotemporal) craniotomy. AJNR Am J Neuroradiol 21(7):1327–1330
15. Bogaev CA (2002) Cosmetic considerations in cranial base surgery. Neurosurg Clin N Am 13(4): 421–441
16. Qing-Gong M, Si C, Xing L (2011) Conservative treatment of severe limited mouth opening after transtemporal craniotomy. J Craniofac Surg 22(5):1746–1750
17. Hernesniemi J, Ishii K, Niemela M, Smrcka M, Kivipelto L, Fujiki M et al (2005) Lateral supraorbital approach as an alternative to the classical pterional approach. Acta Neurochir Suppl 94:17–21. Epub 2005/08/03
18. Figueiredo EG, Deshmukh P, Nakaji P, Crusius MU, Crawford N, Spetzler RF et al (2007) The minipterional craniotomy: technical description and anatomic assessment. Neurosurgery 61(5 Suppl 2):256–264; discussion 264–265
19. Reisch R, Stadie A, Kockro R, Gawish I, Schwandt E, Hopf N (2009) The minimally invasive supraorbital subfrontal key-hole approach for surgical treatment of temporomesial lesions of the dominant hemisphere. Minim Invasive Neurosurg: MIN 52(4):163–169. Epub 2009/10/20
20. Fahlbusch R, Schott W (2002) Pterional surgery of meningiomas of the tuberculum sellae and planum sphenoidale: surgical results with special consideration of ophthalmological and endocrinological outcomes. J Neurosurg 96(2):235–243
21. Smith PG, Grubb RL, Kletzker GR, Leonetti JP (1990) Combined pterional-anterolateral approaches to cranial base tumors. Otolaryngol Head Neck Surg: Off J Am Acad Otolaryngol Head and Neck Surg 103(3):357–363
22. Hassler W, Zentner J (1989) Pterional approach for surgical treatment of olfactory groove meningiomas. Neurosurgery 25(6):942–945; discussion 945–947
23. Hassler W, Zentner J (1991) Surgical treatment of olfactory groove meningiomas using the pterional approach. Acta Neurochir Suppl 53:14–18
24. Turazzi S, Cristofori L, Gambin R, Bricolo A (1999) The pterional approach for the microsurgical removal of olfactory groove meningiomas. Neurosurgery 45(4):821–825; discussion 825–826
25. Puzzilli F, Ruggeri A, Mastronardi L, Agrillo A, Ferrante L (1999) Anterior clinoidal meningiomas: report of a series of 33 patients operated on through the pterional approach. Neuro Oncol 1(3):188–195
26. Spetzler RF, Sanai N (2012) The quiet revolution: retractorless surgery for complex vascular and skull base lesions. J Neurosurg 116(2):291–300

21 Subfrontal Approach

Giuseppe Catapano, Matteo de Notaris, Roberto Granata, Vincenzo Seneca, Giuseppe Di Nuzzo, Joaquim Enseñat, and Alberto Prats-Galino

21.1 Indications

Meningiomas arising in the midline of the anterior skull base (ASB) are generally separated in two main groups: (1) ventral ASB including the olfactory groove meningiomas and (2) dorsal ASB including the planum sphenoidale and tuberculum sellae meningiomas.

Among the different neurosurgical approaches commonly used for the management of ASB meningiomas, the subfrontal route, either in unilateral or bilateral fashion, is one of the most versatile and routinely performed. Indeed, using such route, it is possible to obtain an excellent midline orientation in order to expose the cribriform plate, the orbital roof, and the sellar, suprasellar, and parasellar areas.

The indications for a subfrontal approach to midline ASB meningiomas were firstly highlighted more the 100 years ago by Horsley [1] and Cushing [2]; afterward, Tönnies [3] described the first bifrontal craniotomy, with division of the anterior sagittal sinus and falx, with the aim of preserving the frontal brain tissue. Since then many advancements have been made in the development of this approach.

More recently, some other authors continue to use the bifrontal approach only for large meningiomas of the anterior cranial fossa, namely, Al-Mefty [4], Nakamura et al. [5], and Ransohoff [6]. The specific indications for a subfrontal bilateral approach are principally linked with the dimension of the tumor; as a matter of fact, this route is generally selected for large meningiomas involving the superior sagittal sinus due to the fact that this pathway gives direct access to both sides of the neoplasm. The direct access to the entire ASB and the opportunity to manage the sagittal sinus involvement and the possibility to create a large vascularized periosteal flap for reconstruction are key aspects to be considered when selecting a subfrontal bilateral approach. Moreover, retraction on the frontal lobes is usually minimal due to the ligation of the anterior aspect of the superior sagittal sinus.

On the other hand, the proposed surgical strategy for the unilateral subfrontal approach is quite

G. Catapano, MD (✉) • M. de Notaris, MD, PhD
V. Seneca, MD • G. Di Nuzzo, MD
Department of Neuroscience,
Neurosurgery Operative Unit,
'G. Rummo' Hospital, Benevento, Italy
e-mail: giuseppecatapano@libero.it

R. Granata, MD
Division of Neurosurgery, Department of Neurosciences and Reproductive and Odontostomatological Sciences,
Università degli Studi di Napoli "Federico II", Naples, Italy

J. Enseñat, MD, PhD
Department of Neurosurgery, Hospital Clinic, Faculty of Medicine, Universitat de Barcelona, Barcelona, Spain

A. Prats-Galino, MD, PhD
Laboratory of Surgical Neuroanatomy (LSNA), Faculty of Medicine, Universitat de Barcelona, Barcelona, Spain

P. Cappabianca et al. (eds.), *Midline Skull Base Surgery*, DOI 10.1007/978-3-319-21533-4_21

different from the bilateral one, and, actually, it represents the preferred route in many institutions, including our department. Historically, the unilateral subfrontal approach was firstly described in 1910, and, subsequently, Mc Arthur [7], Frazier [8], Krause [9], and, finally, Harvey Cushing [10] popularized this route. Regarding the specific indications, the unilateral subfrontal approach is preferred if the meningioma grows prominently on one side and does not possess an extensive basal dural attachment onto the contralateral side. However, this unilateral pathway can be safely performed also for wide ASB meningiomas after performing an extensive internal debulking of such neoplasm and if the contralateral olfactory nerve is expected to have a clear plane of dissection. This is an excellent, safe, and effective unilateral approach to midline structures; however, it allows a complex bilateral anatomical exposure. In some instances, retraction on the frontal lobe cannot be achieved safely or adequately without widely opening the sylvian fissure, increasing the temporal lobe, insula, draining veins, and middle cerebral artery dissection trauma. A simple frontal craniotomy, instead of extensive and time-consuming bilateral craniotomy that can be cosmetically disfiguring, offers some clear advantages.

In conclusion, subfrontal bilateral craniotomy is mostly used for large tumors and provides advantages such as wide symmetrical exposure that is useful when an extensive cranial base and vault reconstruction have to be performed. However, this strategy requires ligation of part of the superior sagittal sinus and exposes both frontal lobes to the risk of postoperative edema. Other disadvantages include the opening of the frontal sinuses and the possible late visualization of vital neurovascular structures such as the optic apparatus, the internal carotid arteries (ICAs), and the anterior cerebral-anterior communicating artery complex. Compared with the subfrontal bilateral approach, the unilateral frontal craniotomy allows sparing of the superior sagittal sinus and minimizes manipulation of the contralateral frontal lobe. The optic chiasm and ipsilateral carotid artery usually are identified early during the surgical procedure.

21.2 Neuroradiology

Several neuroradiological investigations may be performed in order to assess the main characteristic of anterior cranial base meningiomas [11].

Noncontrast computed tomography (CT) scans classically demonstrate a dural-based, homogeneous tumor of slightly increased density compared to the surrounding brain, with variable mass effect and surrounding edema. Hyperostosis of the adjacent skull base is a common feature, and it may be visualized also by means of simple radiography of the skull (Rx). Contrast agent administration determines an extensive homogeneous enhancement of the tumor in the majority of cases and often reveals the classical "dural tumor tail."

The gold standard diagnostic imaging for proper evaluation of anterior midline meningiomas is the magnetic resonance imaging (MRI). For preoperative and diagnostic evaluation, MRI is essential and provides very useful information to the surgeon (Fig. 21.1).

In T1-weighted scans, the tumor is of equivalent signal intensity compared to the surrounding brain, while in the T2-weighted scans, the meningioma usually shows a "sunburst" pattern with or without necrosis, cysts, hemorrhage, trapped hyperintense CSF clefts, and vascular flow voids. In FLAIR-weighted images, the hyperintense peritumoral edema can be identified, while T2-star gradient-echo sequences may detect calcifications. After the gadolinium injection, the tumor gains homogeneous and intense contrast enhancement; moreover, the possible presence of the "dural tail" (35–80 % of cases) can be detected.

Magnetic resonance angiography may provide essential information about blood supply and displaced arteries or even arteries embedded within the tumor.

Angiography, generally, has not been indicated unless preoperative embolization is planned. At any rate, the classic angiographic appearance of a meningioma is that of increasing hypervascular tumor blush throughout the arterial phase, persisting well into the late venous phase with slow washout.

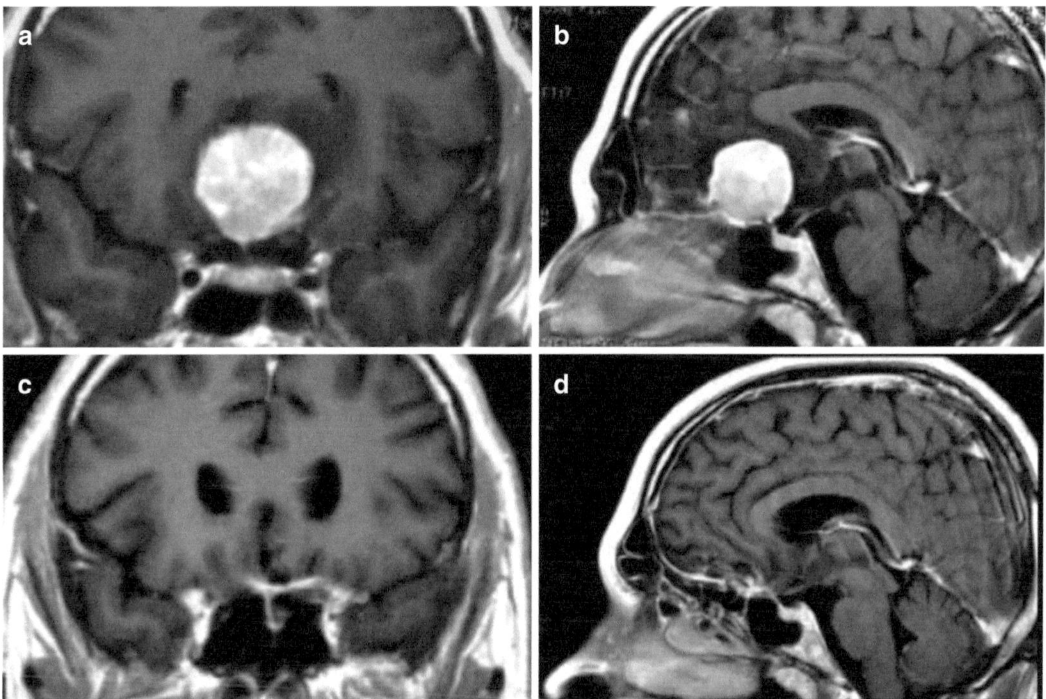

Fig. 21.1 T1-weighted MR images with gadolinium contrast enhancement showing a planum sphenoidale meningioma. Preoperative coronal (**a**) and sagittal (**b**) scans; postoperative coronal (**c**) and sagittal (**d**) scans

In conclusion, even if MRI has to be considered as the best diagnostic tool for the evaluation of a meningioma, cranial computed tomography (CT) and, in selected cases, angiography may be considered as important adjuncts to evaluate and characterize the involvement of the anterior skull base, the infiltration of the olfactory groove and ethmoid bone, the relationship of the major vessels, and the main vascular supply of the tumor, i.e., the ethmoidal arteries.

21.2.1 Surgical Planning

The knowledge of surgical anatomy is imperative for complex neurosurgical procedures in regions with vital structures nearby, as in skull base surgery.

In the field of neurosurgery, progress in neuroimaging studies, such as high-resolution CT scans, MRI studies, and digital subtraction angiography data, has certainly refined the visualization of the brain and skull base anatomy. On the other hand, the progress in computer technology and medical image processing techniques has enabled stereoscopic display of anatomical structures from computed imaging data. Indeed, three-dimensional (3D) imaging, which allows image manipulation and surgical simulation on-screen, has become an indispensable part of the neurosurgical planning and training.

Our surgical planning for skull base meningiomas generally provides two different methodologies: First of all, standard medical image data such as MRI and CT scan to obtain a general idea of the tumor and the surrounding structures is performed.

In a second step, a virtual preliminary exploration of patient's anatomy using the 3D reconstruction modules supported by the OsiriX software (Osirix®, advanced open-source PACS workstation DICOM viewer) in order to analyze the individual variability of the anatomy is performed. At the end of such step, the segmented objects (representing skin, tumor mass, vascular system, ventricular cavities) are displayed by a

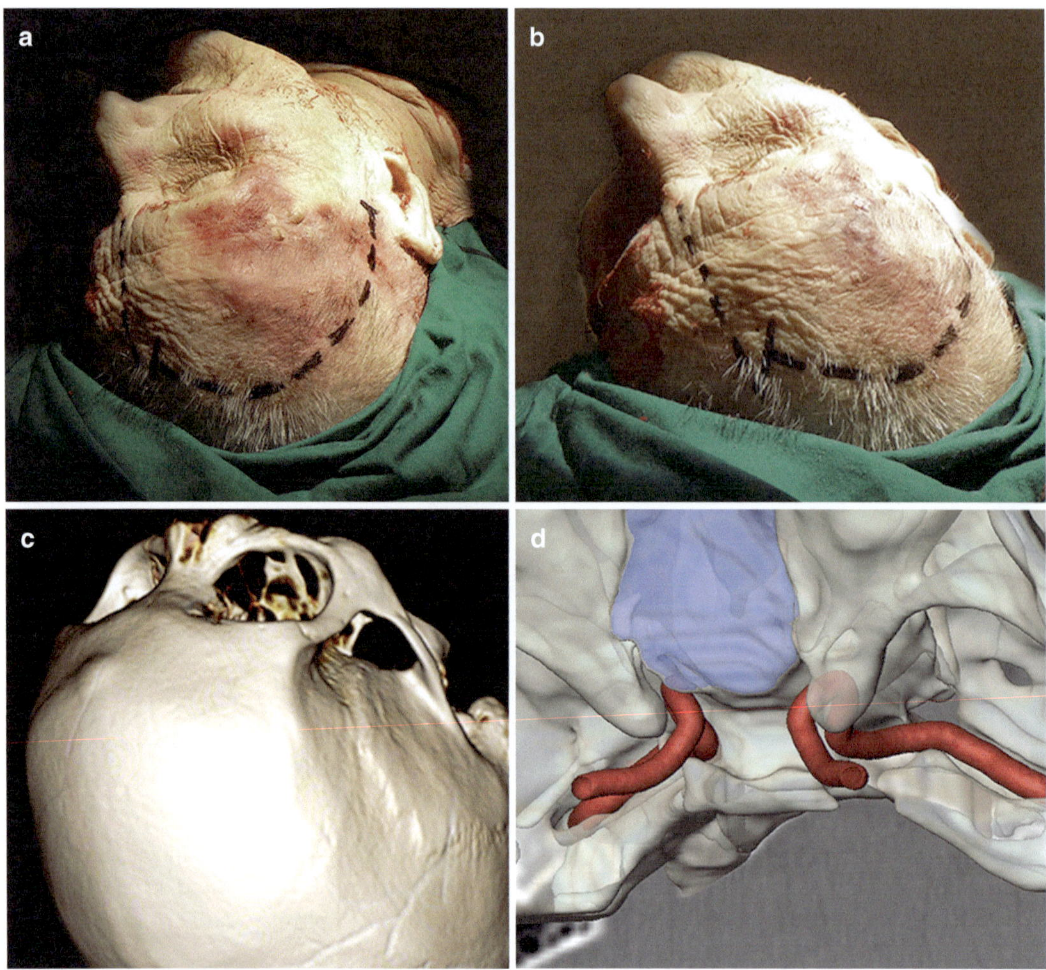

Fig. 21.2 Anatomical photographs (**a**, **b**) of a cadaveric dissection showing patient positioning and skin incision for a subfrontal unilateral approach. (**c**, **d**) Computed 3D virtual reality images showing CT reconstruction of the head (**c**) and the target area, i.e., anterior cranial fossa (**d**)

combination of volume rendering and polygonal iso-surfaces, ready to be manipulated.

Such types of 3D models have been previously utilized from recently published works of our group concerning the anatomy of microscopic and endoscopic skull base approaches [12–14] (Fig. 21.2).

21.3 Anatomy of the Approach

In order to perform a subfrontal approach, either uni- or bilateral, the anatomy of the anterior skull base and of the subfrontal pathway must be clearly understood.

First of all, it has to be remarked that frontal, parietal, temporal, zygomatic, and sphenoid bones, connected through their respective sutures, form the anterolateral region of the skull.

Moreover, the normal anatomy of the anterior cranial fossa should be deeply recognized. From the endocranial view, the anterior cranial base has a flat surface that comprises the anterior border of the sphenoid wings and the roof of the orbita, laterally, and the planum sphenoidale, medially. The anterior cranial fossa is principally formed by the orbital process of the frontal bone that is convex and has a variable number of orbital crests. A most anterior bony ridge, i.e., the frontal crest, is located in the midline and separates the two sides and gives attachment to the falx cerebri, which contains the origin of the superior and inferior sagittal sinuses. The central portion of the anterior fossa is deeper and is composed of the ethmoid bone, with the medial portion represented by the cribriform plate – that shows multiple perforations transmitting the olfactory nerve filaments – and the lateral one that is the fovea ethmoidalis, i.e., the roof of the ethmoid sinus. The crista galli is positioned at the center. The foramen cecum, crossed by an emissary anterior nasal vein, is located between the frontal crest and the crista galli. Lateral to the cribriform plate, the cribroethmoid foramina gives passage to the anterior and posterior ethmoidal arteries. On the other hand, the posterior portion of the anterior fossa is formed by the upper part of the sphenoid bone, namely, its body and lesser wings. Centrally, lies the planum or jugum sphenoidale, which constitutes the roof of the sphenoid sinus, bordered posteriorly by the anterior chiasmatic sulcus. Laterally, the lesser wing of the sphenoid roofs the optic canal, which contains the optic nerve and its dural sheath. The anterior clinoid process, i.e., the medial end of the lesser wings of the sphenoid, gives attachment to the tentorium cerebelli and covers the anteromedial portion of the cavernous sinus which contains the supraclinoid portion of the internal carotid artery (ICA). Other key neurovascular structures that can be exposed during the access to the anterior cranial fossa are the following: the olfactory bulb and tract, optic nerves, optic chiasm and lamina terminalis, the anterior cerebral arteries and the anterior communicating artery, the posterior communicating artery, the anterior choroidal artery, the third cranial nerve, the superior hypophyseal artery, the pituitary stalk and the diaphragma sellae, the ophthalmic arteries, and Heubner's recurrent arteries. Moreover, the opening of the Liliequist's membrane permits to get inside the interpeduncular cistern in order to expose the basilar artery, the posterior cerebral arteries, the superior cerebellar arteries, and the origin of the third cranial nerve.

It has to be reminded that before performing a subfrontal approach, unilateral or bilateral, a precise knowledge of the main frontal anatomic landmarks must be obtained (i.e., midline, orbital rim, supraorbital foramen, temporal line, and zygomatic arch). The orbital rim is the frontal bone part that forms the roof of the orbits, the zygomatic process of temporal bone, and the temporal process of the zygomatic bone form the zygomatic arch. The supraorbital foramen is situated along the supraorbital margin, which is entirely formed by the frontal bone and is crossed by the supraorbital nerve and vessels (supraorbital artery and supraorbital vein). Finally, the superior temporal line of the parietal bone gives attachment to the temporal fascia, indicating the origin of the temporalis muscle.

21.3.1 Brief Consideration of Surgical Neuroanatomy

As already said, meningiomas of the midline anterior cranial base are classified based on an anteroposterior direction: olfactory groove, planum sphenoidale, and tuberculum sellae meningiomas.

Olfactory groove meningiomas arise in the midline of the anterior cranial fossa over the cribriform plate and frontosphenoid suture. Those tumors generally grow in a symmetric fashion around the crista galli and, subsequently, may involve any part of the planum of the sphenoid bone and/or, less frequently, extend predominantly to one side. The anterior and posterior ethmoid arteries drive the primary blood supply to these tumors. However, these tumors may be also vascularized by the meningeal branches from the ophthalmic artery, anterior cerebral arteries, anterior communicating artery, pial collaterals, and external carotid circulation, such as anterior branches of the middle meningeal artery. Generally, in these cases, the olfactory nerves either are displaced laterally on the lower surface of the tumor or are adherent, compressed, or even not visible due to a diffuse spread within the tumor capsule. It has to be minded that in smaller tumors, the post-communicating segments of the anterior cerebral arteries usually are not involved in the tumor capsule. However, in large tumors, these and additional segments, i.e., the frontopolar or other small branches originating from the anterior cerebral arteries, may adhere to the tumor capsule.

Regarding the planum sphenoidal meningiomas, it has to be taken into consideration that planum sphenoidale and tuberculum sellae are part of the sphenoid bone. However, it is often difficult to clearly separate these tumors simply based on their bony covering. Rather, their relationship to the optic nerves and chiasm can distinguish these tumors as to their most likely origin. While planum sphenoidale meningiomas usually push the optic nerves dorsally and caudally, tuberculum sellae meningiomas lead to an upward and/or lateral bulging of these structures. At any rate, both entities might grow between, around, and beyond the optic nerves.

Tuberculum sellae meningiomas arise from the dura of the tuberculum sellae, chiasmatic sulcus, limbus sphenoidale, and diaphragma sellae. The tuberculum sellae is a bony elevation ridge that lines up the anterior aspect of the hypophyseal fossa, dividing it from the chiasmatic sulcus. The lateral end of this structure is just inferomedial to the intracranial outlet of the optic canal, through which the optic nerve runs to join the contralateral optic nerve at the chiasm. Behind the optic foramen, the anterior clinoid process is directed posteriorly and medially. The primary blood supply to these tumors is principally from the posterior ethmoid arteries. According to a recent proposed classification of suprasellar meningiomas, based on the origin and location of the tumor, Liu et al. [15] identified four groups: (a) tumor originating from the planum sphenoidale, rarely involves the optic pathway or pituitary stalk; (b) tumor located at the tuberculum sellae, mainly involves the optic pathway but rarely involves pituitary stalk; (c1) tumor located at the diaphragma sellae, which involves both the optic pathway and the pituitary stalk, pushing the chiasm anteriorly in to "prefixed chiasm" position, resulting in minimal pre-chiasmatic working area; (c2) tumor located at the diaphragma sellae but pushing the optic chiasm posteriorly, putting it in to "postfixed chiasm" position, resulting in expansion of the pre-chiasmatic area.

21.4 Technique

Generally, as the majority of meningiomas are benign tumors (WHO I), extra-axial and well-defined, complete surgical removal (Simpson Grade I) should be the primary goal in most cases. For anterior midline meningiomas, complete tumor excision even with resection of infiltrated dura or removal of hyperostotic bone might be achieved with low morbidity in most instances. However, when tumors are hardly adherent to the anterior brain circulation vessels, the optic apparatus, or within and near the pituitary gland and stalk, complete removal might represent a high-risk procedure for damage of those important neurovascular and endocrine structures [4, 16, 17].

21.4.1 Subfrontal Unilateral Approach

The patient is placed in the supine on the operating table with the head fixed in a three-pin Mayfield head holder. The positioning largely depends on the involvement of the midline structures, the displacement and orientation of the main vessels, and the optic nerves. As a general rule, the head has to be rotated toward the contralateral side of 20–40° and slightly extended posteriorly, as the frontal lobes follow gravity, thus making a natural exposure of the anterior cranial base and facilitates good venous drainage during surgery. In other words, the patient's neck has to be retroflexed, in order to form an angle of approximately 20° between the plane of the anterior cranial base and the vertical plane of the axis (Fig. 21.2). Fine adjustments of the patient's position can be obtained by tilting the operating table.

After a precise definition of the frontal anatomic landmarks, already described in the "anatomy of the approach section," the line of the incision is marked on the skin.

A curved frontal skin incision, beginning at the level of the top of the helix of the ear or slightly anterior to it on the side of the craniotomy and behind the hairline, is performed and extends until the midline in a curvilinear fashion above the superior temporal line. The skin incision is posterior to the superficial temporal artery, in order to include the artery in the skin flap. The incision should not be extended below the zygomatic arch to avoid injury of the frontal branch of the facial nerve (Fig. 21.3).

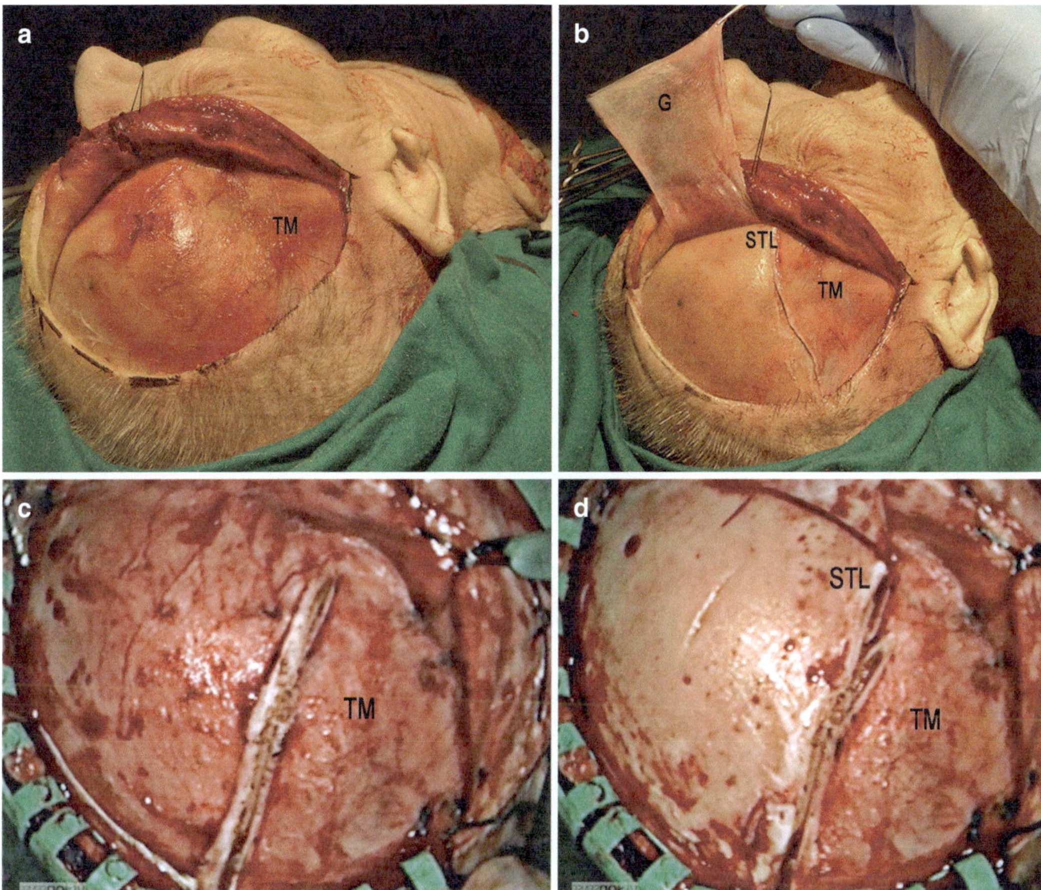

Fig. 21.3 Anatomical pictures of a cadaveric dissection showing the skin flap preparation; pericranium before (**a**) and after (**b**) its incision along the superior temporal line; corresponding intraoperative images (**c**, **d**). *TM* temporalis muscle, *G* galea capitis, *STL* superior temporal line

It is of utmost importance to preserve the pericranium for harvesting a potential flap that can be subsequently used in the reconstruction phase. As a matter of fact, a pericranial flap is usually prepared to cover potential dural tears or removed tumor matrix in case of anterior middle fossa involvement (Fig. 21.3).

The skin is reflected anteriorly along with the pericranium and retracted with temporary fishhooks. At the supraorbital ridge, care should be taken to identify and preserve the supraorbital nerve and the supraorbital artery passing along the medial third of the superior orbital rim.

Exposure and mobilization of the temporal muscle should be restricted to a minimum to avoid postoperative cosmetic and functional disabilities and chewing discomfort. Careful dissection of the temporal muscle from the superior temporal line should be sharply performed with the aim of exposing just the region of the keyhole (Dandy's keyhole) (Fig. 21.4). In other words, the temporalis muscle does not require elevation, although a small amount of dissection along the superior temporal line may be required to expose the keyhole for burr hole placement. Before starting the craniotomy, local hemostasis must be performed (Fig. 21.4).

The craniotomy is started using a high-speed drill, with the placement of a single frontobasal burr hole at Dandy's point, below the anterior aspect of the superior temporal line, just above the frontosphenoid suture.

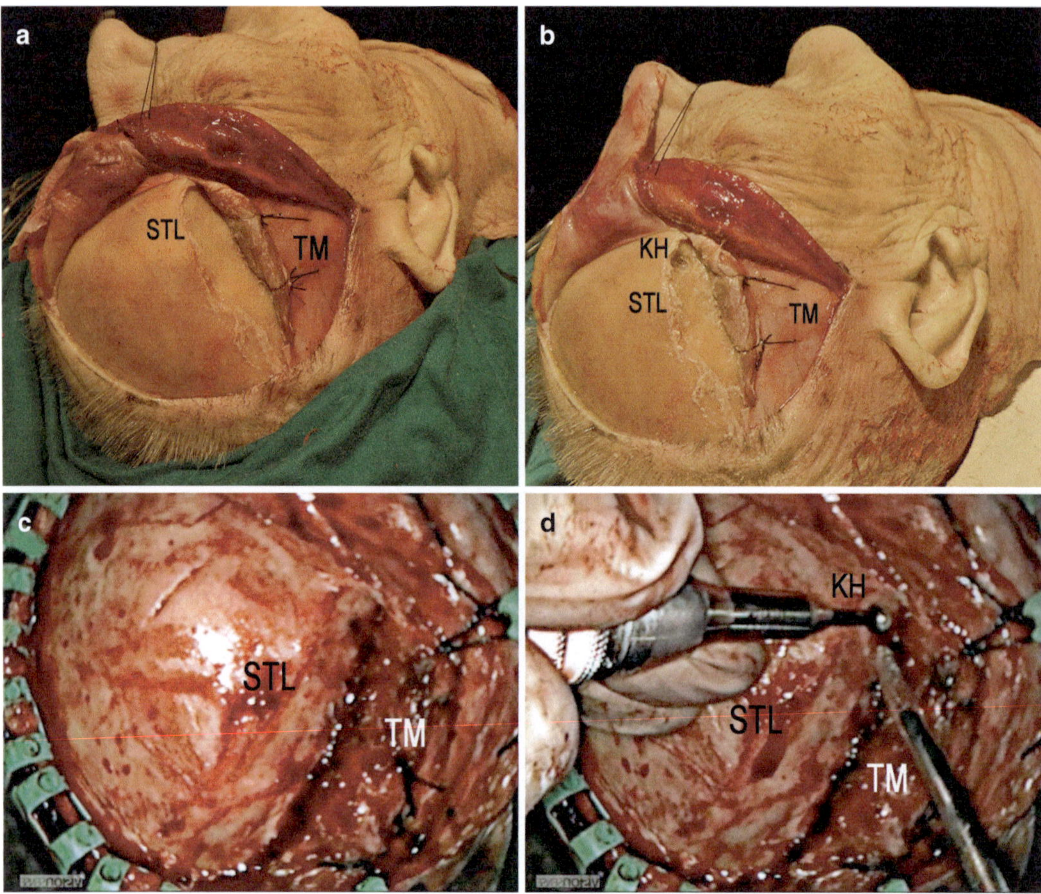

Fig. 21.4 Anatomical images of a cadaveric dissection. The temporalis muscle is slightly dissected from the superior temporal line in order to the site for the frontobasal burr hole; standard keyhole described by Dandy (**b**, *KH*); corresponding intraoperative images (**c**, **d**). *STL* superior temporal line, *TM* temporalis muscle, *KH* keyhole

A high-speed craniotome is then used to create the bone flap. The craniotome is directed anteriorly until the supraorbital foramen and it is then moved posteriorly to reach the superior temporal line (Fig. 21.5). Continuous irrigation during drilling avoids heat damage to the brain tissue and allows more precise bone cutting. It has to be stressed that the craniotomy should be shaped according to the expected irregularities of the frontal skull base.

Before removal of the bone flap, careful dissection of the dura from the inner surface of the bone using a blunt dissector avoids laceration of the dura mater. If the frontal sinus is accidentally entered, the posterior wall and all sinus mucosa are carefully removed away by cranialization. Subsequently, a galeaperiostal flap from the forehead sealed with fibrin glue can be used to cover the basal parts of the frontal sinus.

At this stage of the procedure, an important step is the drilling of the inner edge of the orbital roof protuberances with a high-speed drill (unroofing) in order to optimize the angle of attack of the approach and, accordingly, the exposure of the anterior cranial fossa (Fig. 21.5).

The dural opening is anticipated by positioning many sutures alongside the edges of the craniotomy. Typically, the dura is opened in a “X-” or “C-”shaped fashion, under the operating microscope, and anchored with stay sutures. Few millimeters should be left clear between the bone margin and the dural incision, to facilitate its

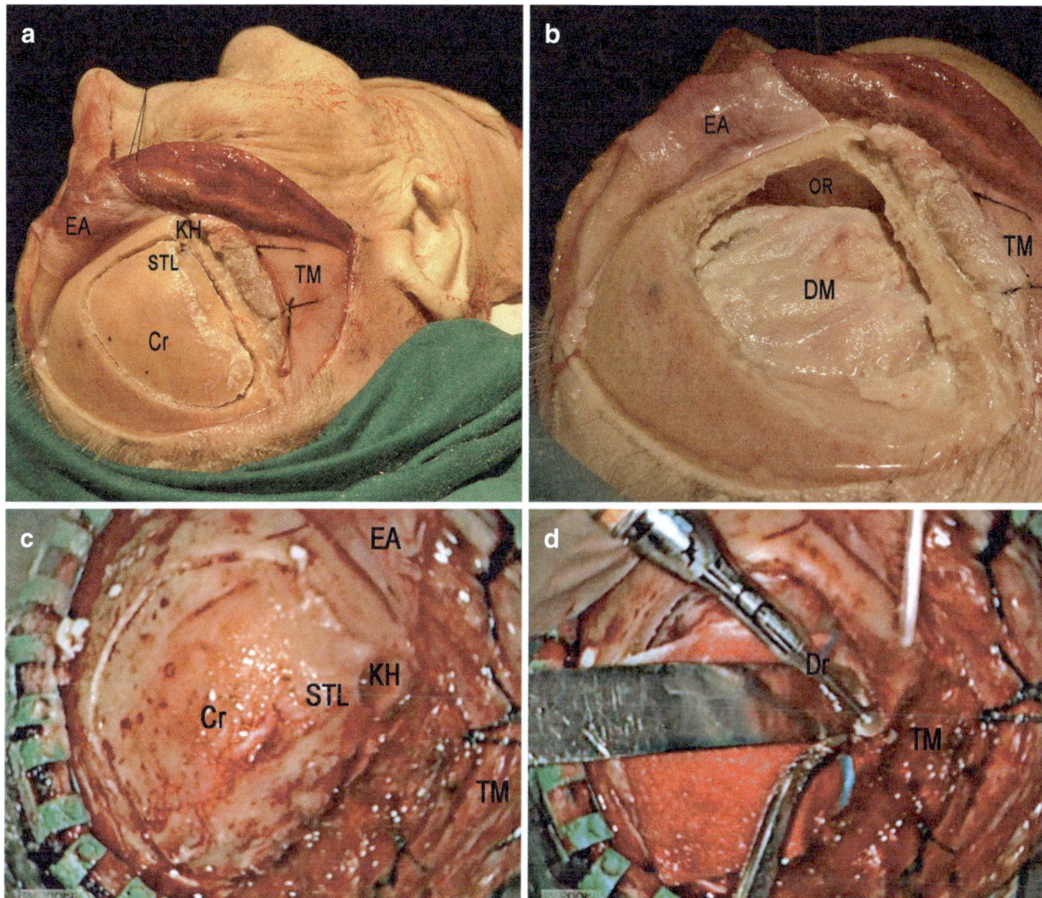

Fig. 21.5 Anatomical pictures of a cadaveric dissection demonstrating the frontal craniotomy (**a**, **b**). The unilateral subfrontal craniotomy extended anteriorly as close as possible to the supraorbital ridge and posteriorly along the convexity of the frontal bone; the removal of the bone flap shows the dura mater covering the frontal lobe; (**c**, **d**) intraoperative corresponding snapshots. *EA* epicranial aponeurosis, *KH* keyhole, *STL* superior temporal line, *Cr* craniotomy, *TM* temporalis muscle, *OR* orbital roof, *DM* dura mater, *Dr* drill

closure at the end of the procedure. Elevation and retraction of the frontal lobe pole will subsequently expose the target area at the frontal base of the skull.

Afterward, the sylvian fissure is dissected and opened in its most distal portion, exposing the first segment of the omolateral middle cerebral artery. As the release of cerebrospinal fluid (CSF) during sylvian dissection makes the brain relaxed, the frontal lobe starts to fall downward, following gravity. Further medial dissection of the arachnoid from the proximal sylvian fissure provides initial recognition of the tumor (Fig. 21.6). In this way, with the temporal lobe covered with cottonoids, only the ipsilateral frontal lobe is retracted.

The ipsilateral optic nerve should be compressed superiorly or superolaterally, angulated against the falciform ligament as it comes out of the optic foramen. The internal carotid artery is found lateral to the optic nerve (Figs. 21.6 and 21.7). When the optic nerve and the internal carotid artery are completely covered by the tumor, which occurs occasionally, dissection should first be carefully performed to identify the optic nerve and the carotid artery.

Devascularization of the tumor is then performed. This maneuver permits easier debulking

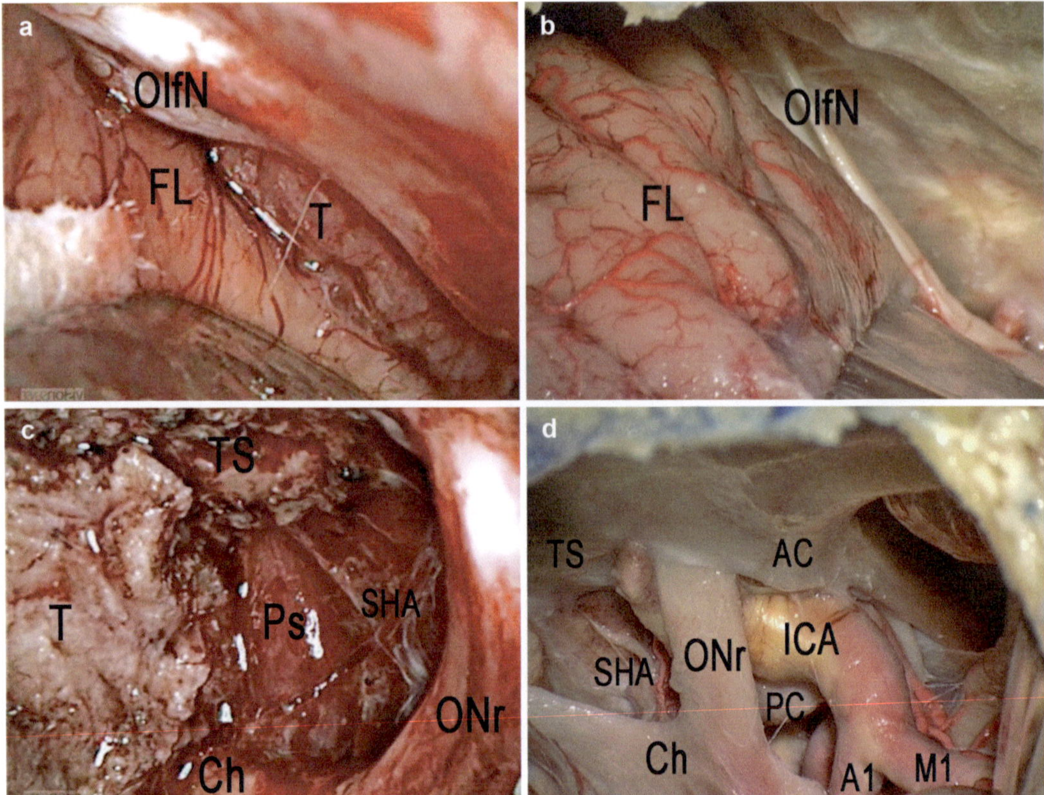

Fig. 21.6 Intraoperative microsurgical pictures showing the tumor (*T*) below the frontal lobe compressing the omolateral olfactory nerve (**a**) and adhering to the chiasm (**c**). Anatomical microsurgical images showing the key anatomical landmarks of the subfrontal unilateral approach (**b**, **d**). *OlfN* olfactory nerve, *FL* frontal lobe, *T* tumor, *TS* tuberculum sellae, *Ps* pituitary stalk, *SHA* superior hypophyseal artery, *Ch* chiasm, *ONr* right optic nerve, *AC* anterior clinoid, *PC* posterior clinoid, *ICA* internal carotid artery, *A1* pre-communicating segment of the anterior cerebral artery, *M1* pre-bifurcation segment of the middle cerebral artery

and further dissection of the tumor without bleeding (Fig. 21.7). Such maneuver starts from the most anterior part of the tumor, medial to the optic nerves, applying bipolar coagulation between the tumor and the underlying dura. Devascularization then proceeds posteriorly, with each devascularized part of the tumor detached and removed.

It has to be minded that the optic nerve is under significant tension, until enough decompression has been accomplished. Accordingly, it has to be protected with cottonoids, and frequent saline irrigation is recommended for cooling and cleaning during coagulation, thus avoiding thermal damage.

The tumor may be also debulked using an ultrasonic surgical aspirator or scissors.

After all these procedures have been carefully performed, the tumor capsule is meticulously spared from the surrounding neurovascular structure.

Special attention must be moved to the Heubner's artery or other perforating arteries. If these arteries are unintentionally injured, they should be repaired immediately by applying low-current bipolar cautery or by suturing the vessel wall. The medial aspect of the tumor is dissected from the contralateral optic nerve and the carotid artery by piecemeal removal. The contralateral optic nerve is usually displaced laterally. Finally, when sufficient decompression has been attained, the tumor is dissected and removed (Fig. 21.7).

Finally, after complete resection of the tumor, the involved dura around from which the tumor originated is excised, and the involved hyperostotic bone is also drilled, taking care not to enter the sphenoid or ethmoid sinuses.

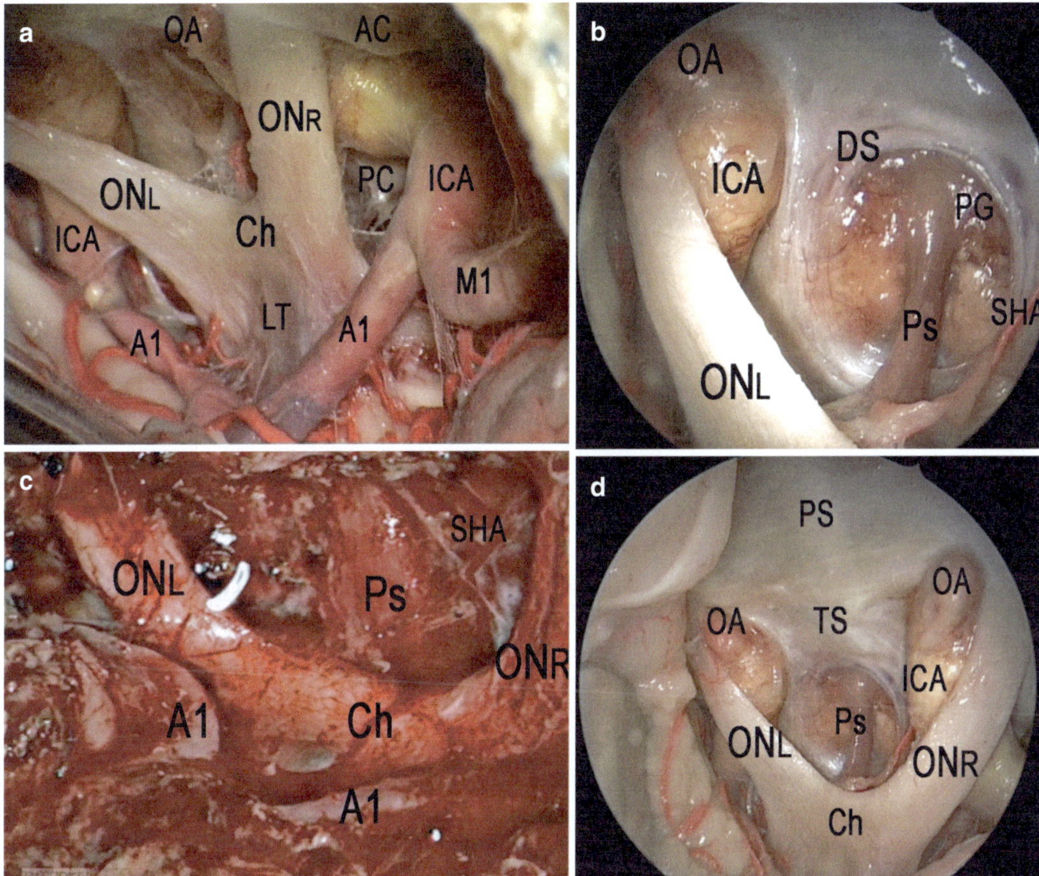

Fig. 21.7 Anatomical (**a**) and intraoperative (**c**) microsurgical images showing the exposure of the optic nerves, the chiasm, the carotid arteries, and the anterior communicating arteries complex; (**b**, **d**) endoscopic anatomical snapshots. *OA* ophthalmic artery, *AC* anterior clinoid, *PC* posterior clinoid, *ONr* right optic nerve, *ONl* left optic nerve, *Ch* chiasm, *ICA* internal carotid artery, *LT* lamina terminalis, *A1* pre-communicating segment of the anterior cerebral artery, *M1* pre-bifurcation segment of the middle cerebral artery, *PG* pituitary gland, *Ps* pituitary stalk, *SHA* superior hypophyseal artery, *DS* diaphragma sellae, *TS* tuberculum sellae, *PS* planum sphenoidale

In same cases, the unilateral subfrontal approach could be used for asymmetric midline lesions with the possibility of cutting the falx above the crista galli and saving the superior sagittal sinus, thus obtaining access to the contralateral side. In case of lesions such as meningiomas that involve the optic canal, a wider access could be gained by removal of the anterior clinoid that could be achieved via an extradural or intradural route.

After the lesion has been removed, the dural incision is sutured watertight using continuous sutures. The bone flap is positioned without significant bony distance to achieve the optimal cosmetic outcome and fixed with low-profile titanium plates and screws. After final verification of hemostasis, the galea and the subcutaneous layers are approximated with several interrupted absorbable sutures, and the skin is sutured as well. At the end of the procedure, the Mayfield is removed and general anesthesia is finished.

21.4.2 Endoscope-Assisted Technique

The endoscopic-assisted techniques have been developed to extirpate selected tumors that mainly involve the sphenoidal planum and tuberculum sellae areas. In the majority of cases, a 30- or 45-degree endoscope is used as an aid to excise tumor remnants in proximity of neurovascular structures such as the optic nerves, the pituitary stalk, and anterior cerebral arteries (Fig. 21.7). With the endoscope, a panoramic view of the sellar and suprasellar area is obtained. In selected cases, such as giant anterior skull base meningiomas or sinonasal tumors with large intracranial extension, a combined microscopic subfrontal and endoscopic endonasal transcribriform approach can be performed to optimize tumor resection. The main advantage of this approach is to combine the minimally invasive elements of the endonasal approach with the 3D view gained with the microscope. Moreover, a combined transcranial/endonasal procedure adds the significant advantage of a wide exposure of the intradural component of the lesion, especially over its lateral extension, together with a more accurate reconstruction of the bone and dural defects of the anterior skull base.

21.4.3 Subfrontal Bilateral Approach

The patient is placed supine with the head in the midline, slightly extended to bring the brows to the highest point of the surgical field. As already described for the subfrontal unilateral route, after a precise definition of the frontal anatomic landmarks, the line of the incision is marked on the skin.

A bicoronal skin incision, 13–15 cm from the orbital rim and 2 cm behind the coronal suture, is performed extending 1 cm anteriorly to the tragus on each side. Dissection continues in the immediate subgaleal plane taking care to preserve a thick and vascularized pericranial flap (Fig. 21.8).

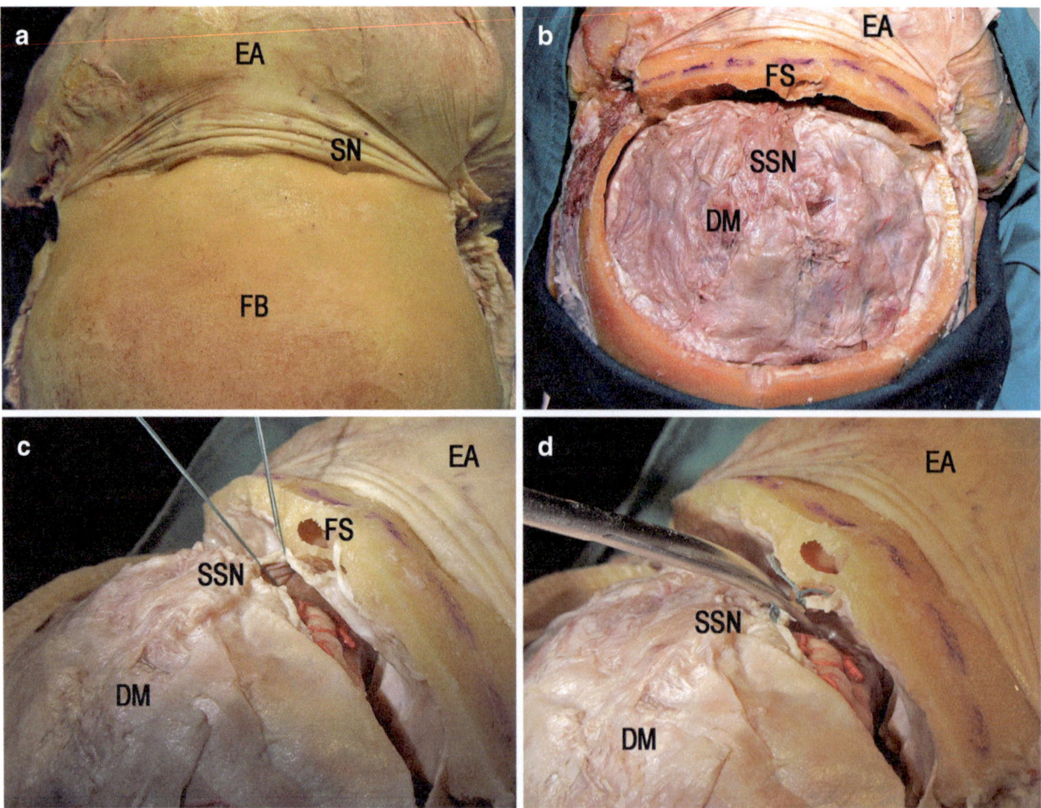

Fig. 21.8 Anatomical photographs of the subfrontal bilateral approach. The supraorbital nerve as it comes out from the supraorbital foramen (**a**), after the pericranium is taken up separately from the scalp flap; subfrontal bilateral craniotomy (**b**); (**c**, **d**) ligation and division of anterior third of superior sagittal sinus (*SSN*). *EA* epicranial aponeurosis, *SN* supraorbital nerve, *FB* frontal bone, *FS* frontal sinus, *SSN* superior sagittal sinus, *DM* dura mater

The skin of the posterior aspect of the incision is elevated, and the pericranial tissue is incised below the skin. The skin flap and underlying tissue, including the pericranial tissue, are then turned down together using fishhooks, taking care to preserve the supraorbital nerve as it comes out from the supraorbital foramen.

As already discussed, temporalis muscle does not require elevation, although a small amount of dissection along the superior temporal line may be required sometimes to expose the keyhole for burr hole placement.

The craniotomy is performed with two burr holes placed at the Dandy's keyhole bilaterally. After that, one or two additional burr holes are placed on the midline at the posterior aspect of the craniotomy straddling the superior sagittal sinus. After blunt dissection of the dura from the inner surface of the skull bone, particularly in the midline area, the bone flap is usually cut in one piece. The craniotomy is extended anteriorly as close as possible to the supraorbital ridge and posteriorly along the convexity of the frontal bone.

The frontal sinus is almost routinely encountered and requires cranialization if necessary as in the unilateral approach. The mucosa should be removed from the free flap, and cauterization is used to remove the accessible mucosa within the sinus. The sinuses are packed with bacitracin-soaked Gelfoam, and the pericranium is sewn in position over the open frontal sinuses.

A slightly curved dural incision is performed over each medial inferior frontal lobe adjacent to the anterior edge of the craniotomy opening but leaving a sufficient rim for safe and convenient closure of the dura. At this stage, attention should be moved toward the anterior portion of the superior sagittal sinus and the falx cerebri, and, generally, retraction on the mesial surface of each frontal lobe is needed for visualization of the falx cerebri below the sinus. The anterior portion of the superior sinus is then ligated between two silk sutures and then cut down together with the falx cerebri until its inferior margin as anteriorly as possible to disclose the operative field. As a rule, the inferior longitudinal sinus makes little or no bleeding, so that bipolar coagulation is enough (Fig. 21.9).

The frontal lobes are then gently retracted slightly laterally and posteriorly to open the view to the anterior and superior surface of the tumor, lying in the midline with attachments to the falx and crista galli.

The tumor is readily identifiable and often covered by a thick capsule. It is important to dissect within the arachnoid plane surrounding the tumor to avoid damage to the surrounding neurovascular structures. The capsule of the tumor is coagulated to shrink the lesion, and the process of devascularizing the tumor begins.

Small feeders along the skull base continue to supply the tumor; these can be divided as the dissection proceeds along the cranial base from anterior to posterior. Large tumors have usually displaced the frontal lobes superiorly and posteriorly, and brain retraction should be avoided as much as possible to prevent postoperative cerebral edema.

Internal tumor debulking with the ultrasonic aspirator may be useful. The olfactory nerves should be identified laterally to the tumor and can be preserved. As the tumor is debulked further, its superior, posterior, and inferior margins can be dissected in sequence with identification of the anterior cerebral artery and optic apparatus. Feeding vessels from the anterior cerebral circulation can be divided, but care must be taken not to mistake these vessels for perforating arteries that supply the optic chiasm and hypothalamus. The anterior cerebral vessels can become incorporated into very large tumors, and careful sharp dissection is required to free them from the tumor.

The blood supply typically enters from below the tumor. Thus, initial debulking of large tumors is necessary to expose the base of skull to interrupt the blood supply. Extensive internal decompression allows the surrounding structures to be identified and separated from the tumor capsule. Subsequentially, attention must be paid to the posterior aspect of the tumor. The surgeon must be vigilant to identify the anterior cerebral arteries and their respective branches. The capsule is followed posteriorly to expose the sphenoid wing. The edge of the sphenoid wing can be traced medially to the anterior clinoid process and optic apparatus. The posterior arachnoid

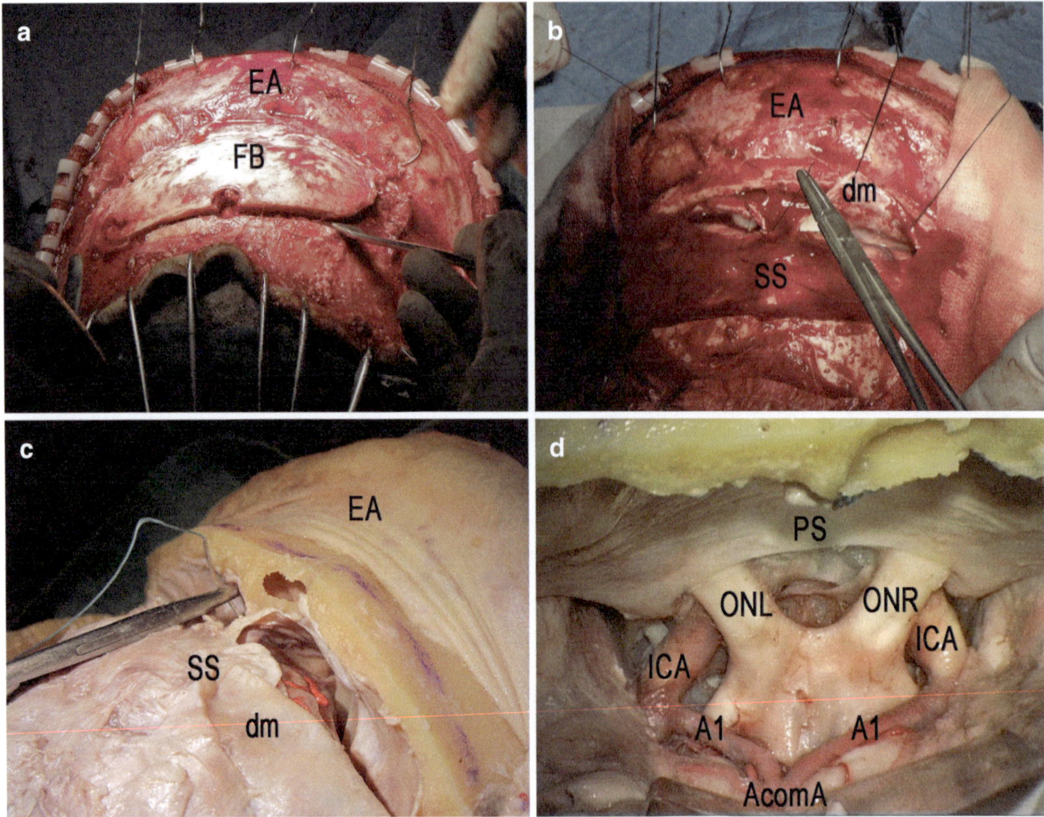

Fig. 21.9 Intraoperative images showing, respectively, bone flap removal (**a**) and superior sagittal sinus ligation (**b**) during a subfrontal bilateral approach; anatomical picture demonstrating the superior sagittal sinus ligation (**c**); anatomical pictures showing the wide and symmetrical anterior cranial fossa exposure of this approach (**d**). *EA* epicranial aponeurosis, *FB* frontal bone, *dm* dura mater, *SS* superior sagittal sinus, *PS* planum sphenoidale, *ONL* left optic nerve, *ONR* right optic nerve, *ICA* internal carotid artery, *A1* pre-communicating segment of the anterior cerebral artery, *AcomA* anterior communicating artery

plane must be preserved, allowing complete removal of the tumor after internal debulking.

After the bulk of the tumor has been removed, its dural attachment must be incised. Simple cauterization of the attachment is insufficient and is thought to leave the patient at high risk for a recurrence. Involved dura must be resected as completely as possible. After the tumor has been resected, attention should be turned toward the floor of the anterior cranial fossa. Any hyperostotic bone should be removed by drill curettage, and the dura of origin removed to reduce the risk of recurrence. Tumor extension into the ethmoid sinuses, nasal cavity, or orbits should be completely resected. A careful reconstruction of the anterior skull base with absorbable hemostatic gelatin sponge and fibrin glue can be necessary at this point. A large piece of vascularized pericranium that was preserved in the initial portion of the procedure is then brought down over the floor of the anterior cranial fossa and secured in place using holes drilled in the planum sphenoidale.

At the end of the procedure, the dural incision is sutured watertight using continuous sutures. The bone flap is positioned medially and frontally without bony distance to achieve the optimal cosmetic outcome and fixed with low-profile titanium plates and screws. After final verification of hemostasis, the galea and the subcutaneous layers are approximated with several interrupted absorbable sutures, and the skin is closed. At the end of the procedure, the Mayfield pin headrest is removed, and general anesthesia is reversed.

It has to be highlighted that for recurrent tumors where the pericranium has been previously utilized or disrupted, the galea can be harvested as a vascularized pedicled graft. Other methods of repair include use of fascia lata, dural substitutes, autologous fat, or fibrin glue. Rarely, in a multiply operated patient with no viable local options for reconstruction, free tissue transfer may be required.

References

1. Horsley V (1906) On the technique of operations on the central nervous system. Br Med J 2:411–423
2. Cushing H (1927) The meningiomas arising from the olfactory groove and their removal by the aid of electrosurgery. Lancet 1:1329–1339
3. Tonnies W (1938) Zur Operation der Meningeome der Siebbeinplatte. Zentralbl Neurochir 1:1–7
4. De Monte F, Mc Dermott M, Al-Mefty O (2011) Al-Mefty's meningiomas. Thieme, New York/Stuttgart
5. Nakamura M, Struck M, Roser F, Vorkapic P, Samii M (2008) Olfactory groove meningiomas: clinical outcome and recurrence rates after tumor removal through the frontolateral and bifrontal approach. Neurosurgery 62(6 Suppl 3):1224–1232. doi:10.1227/01.neu.0000333788.83349.1e
6. Ransohoff J, Nockels R (1993) Olfactory groove and planum meningiomas. In: Apuzzo MLJ (ed) Brain surgery complication avoidance and management. Churchill Livingstone, New York, pp 203–219
7. Mc Arthur L (1912) An aseptic surgical access to the pituitary body and its neighborhood. JAMA 58:2009–2011
8. Frazier CH (1913) An approach to the hypophysis through the anterior cranial fossa. Ann Surg 57:145–150
9. Krause F (1914) Freilegung der Hypophyse. In: Krause F (ed) Chirurgie der Gehirkrankheiten. Ferdinand Enke, Stuttgart, pp 465–470
10. Cushing H (1932) Intracranial tumors. Note upon a series of two thousands verified cases with surgical-mortality percentages pertaining thereto. Charles C. Thomas, Springfield
11. Osborn AG, Salzman KL, Barkovich AJ, Katzman GL, Provenzale JM (2009) Diagnostic imaging: brain. Amirsys Inc, Salt Lake City, Utah
12. de Notaris M, Prats-Galino A, Ensenat J, Topczewski T, Ferrer E, Cavallo LM, Cappabianca P, Solari D (2014) Quantitative analysis of progressive removal of nasal structures during endoscopic suprasellar approach. Laryngoscope. doi:10.1002/lary.24693
13. de Notaris M, Solari D, Cavallo LM, Ensenat J, Alobid I, Soria G, Gonzalez JB, Ferrer E, Prats-Galino A (2011) The use of a three-dimensional novel computer-based model for analysis of the endonasal endoscopic approach to the midline skull base. World Neurosurg 75(1):106–113. S1878-8750(10)00703-5 [pii]. doi:10.1016/j.wneu.2010.09.033
14. de Notaris M, Topczewski T, de Angelis M, Ensenat J, Alobid I, Gondolbleu AM, Soria G, Gonzalez JB, Ferrer E, Prats-Galino A (2013) Anatomic skull base education using advanced neuroimaging techniques. World Neurosurg 79(2 Suppl):S16 e19–13. doi:10.1016/j.wneu.2012.02.027
15. Liu Y, Chotai S, Ming C, Jin S, Pan J, Qi S (2014) Characteristics of midline suprasellar meningiomas based on their origin and growth pattern. Clin Neurol Neurosurg 125:173–181. doi:10.1016/j.clineuro.2014.08.002
16. Quinones-Hinojosa A (2012) Schmidek & Sweet operative neurosurgical techniques: indications, methods, and results. Elsevier Saunders, Philadelphia
17. Lee J (2007) Meningiomas: diagnosis, treatment, and outcome. Springer-Verlag, London

Supraorbital Approach

22

Henry W.S. Schroeder

Meningiomas of the anterior cranial fossa can be challenging lesions. They may spread extensively along the frontal skullbase and often involve olfactory tracts, optic nerves, pituitary stalk, carotid artery, and the anterior cerebral artery complex [1, 2]. Tumor resection via transcranial microsurgical approaches has been the standard of care for most of these lesions since more than 30 years. The surgical results have been improved significantly over the years because of refinement of the microsurgical instrumentation and dissection technique, better understanding of the surgical anatomy, and the availability of high-resolution MR imaging. After a period of extensive skullbase approaches which were mainly proposed in the late 1980s and 1990s [3–5], in the last decade, standard craniotomies have been recommended for skullbase tumors to reduce the approach-related morbidity and to improve the quality of life after surgery [1, 2]. A further step to reduce the approach-related trauma is the development of small craniotomies, also called mini-craniotomies or keyhole approaches [6]. For frontal skullbase meningiomas, the supraorbital craniotomy performed via an eyebrow incision is the most frequently used minimally invasive approach to that region. It is simply a smaller version of the standard frontolateral approach. Axel Perneczky was the main promoter of the eyebrow approach and used it for several lesions of the frontal skullbase [7–10]. Although the supraorbital approach provides a good overview over the anterior cranial base, there are some blind corners. Therefore, the additional use of endoscopes with various angles of view is sometimes advantageous to improve the visualization without the need for retraction [11]. The supraorbital craniotomy is a minimally invasive alternative to the endonasal approach, which has become popular recently in the treatment of anterior skullbase meningiomas [12–14].

22.1 Indications

Since the entire frontal skullbase can be explored via the supraorbital craniotomy, all kinds of anterior skullbase meningiomas can be treated via this surgical approach. However, because of the small height of the craniotomy of about 2 cm, there are some blind corners which require endoscope assistance to be visualized, for example, the olfactory groove. Additionally, because of the small width of about 2.5 cm, the angle of view cannot be changed significantly. There is always a blind corner under the ipsilateral optic nerve,

Electronic supplementary material The online version of this chapter (doi:10.1007/978-3-319-21533-4_22) contains supplementary material, which is available to authorized users.

H.W.S. Schroeder, MD, PhD
Department of Neurosurgery,
University Medicine Greifswald,
Sauerbruchstr., D-17487 Greifswald, Germany
e-mail: henry.schroeder@uni-greifswald.de

P. Cappabianca et al. (eds.), *Midline Skull Base Surgery*, DOI 10.1007/978-3-319-21533-4_22

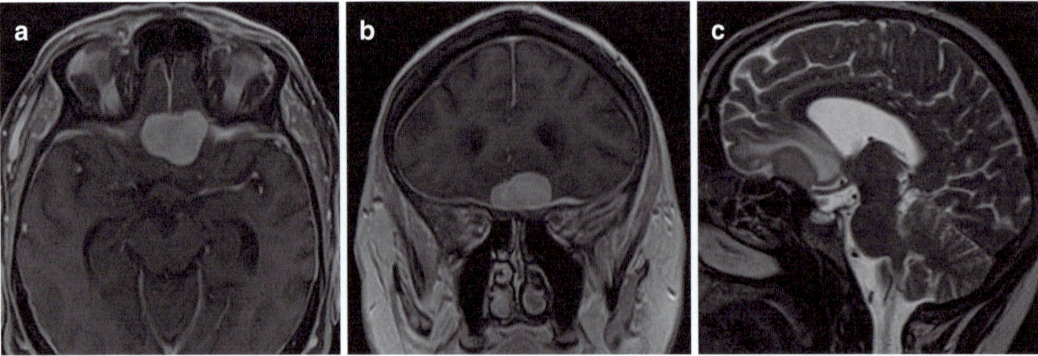

Fig. 22.1 MR imaging of a planum sphenoidale meningioma. (**a**) Axial T1-weighted contrast-enhanced image. (**b**) Coronal T1-weighted contrast-enhanced image. (**c**) Sagittal T2-weighted image showing perifocal edema (Created by H.W. Schroeder © Henry Schroeder 2015)

which requires endoscopic visualization as well. The major limitation of the eyebrow approach (at least for us) is the tumor size. If the tumor is 4 cm in size or larger, we prefer a standard frontolateral craniotomy (size 4×4 cm) via a frontotemporal skin incision behind the hairline because the access to the tumor is easier and the tumor resection is faster. Furthermore, in larger tumors, the amount of skullbase drilling required to remove the infiltrated skullbase is usually larger. Via a larger (higher) craniotomy, the entire skullbase can be drilled easily under microscopic visualization with standard straight high-speed drill handpieces. Via the small supraorbital craniotomy, the olfactory groove cannot be drill with standard straight high-speed drill handpieces but requires curved handpieces, sometimes even endoscopic visualization. Furthermore, harvesting of autologous material (usually pericranium) to cover the drilled skullbase is easy via the frontotemporal skin incision. In the eyebrow incision, harvesting of autologous material from the approach site is not recommended for cosmetic reasons. Since the skullbase defect is usually small, we take a collagen matrix or TachoSil® (Nycomed Austria GmbH, Linz, Austria).

Olfactory groove, planum sphenoidale, tuberculum sellae, and medial sphenoid wing meningiomas can be approached via the supraorbital craniotomy. In medial sphenoid wing meningiomas, lateral tumor extension going down to the floor of the middle cranial fossa represents a limitation of this approach. In these lesions, a pterional approach should be chosen. Although all tuberculum sellae meningiomas can be resected via a supraorbital approach, there are some tumors in which an endonasal approach is preferable. Especially smaller tumors, which are located under the chiasm or even behind the chiasm (prefixed chiasm), can be better reached via the endonasal approach avoiding undue manipulation of the optic apparatus. Rare tumors arising from the dorsum sellae are also better approached via the endonasal route. Other favorable factors for an endonasal approach include a very steep tuberculum sellae, involvement of the intrasellar space, and tumor invasion of the sphenoid sinus or nasal cavity.

22.2 Neuroradiology

Contrast-enhanced MR imaging is the preferred imaging modality to diagnose a skullbase meningioma. We routinely perform T1- and T2-weighted sequences followed by contrast-enhanced T1-weighted images in all three planes (Fig. 22.1). The degree of contrast enhancement provides some information about the vascularity of the lesion. A perifocal edema best shown in T2 or FLAIR images indicates brain invasion (Fig. 22.1c); however, sometimes brain invasion is even found during the tumor resection although no hyperintensity is seen around the tumor in the

T2 or FLAIR MR imaging. Calcifications can also be depicted with T2 images. Several other factors have to be considered for the surgery: encasement of carotid arteries or anterior cerebral artery complex, tumor extension into the optic canals, location of the tumor in relation to the optic chiasm, displacement of the pituitary stalk, intrasellar tumor extension, involvement of the paranasal sinus and nasal cavity, infiltration of the cribriform plate, and anatomy of the skullbase, i.e., steepness of the tuberculum sellae, size of the frontal sinus, and bony protuberances along the orbital roof.

CT scans were not performed routinely prior to surgery, but always the day after the surgery to rule out any complications. If a patient cannot have MR imaging because of a pacemaker or when some bony abnormalities need more accurate depiction, a high-resolution CT scan is carried out before surgery.

Three months after surgery, the first post-op contrast-enhanced MR imaging is performed to confirm gross total tumor resection or to show residual tumor. In all WHO grade 1 meningiomas, yearly MR images were taken to rule out recurrence or regrowth of residual tumor. Usually, radiation of residual tumor is not applied immediately, but only in the case of progression when surgical resection is not indicated.

22.3 Anatomy of the Approach

The eyebrow skin incision is located laterally from the supraorbital notch to avoid injury to the supraorbital branch of the frontal nerve (Fig. 22.2a, b). Since the incision is placed exactly within the eyebrow, the frontotemporal branch of the facial nerve is preserved additionally (Fig. 22.2a, b). After transection of the orbicularis oculi muscle, the temporal line is exposed, and the temporalis fascia and muscle are detached from the bone. Starting from a small burr hole behind the temporal line, a 2×2.5 cm craniotomy is performed close to the skullbase (Fig. 22.2c). The dura is incised in a curved fashion pediculated to the skullbase (Fig. 22.2d).

22.4 Technique

22.4.1 Patient Positioning and OR Setup

The patient is positioned supine with the body elevated 10–15° to reduce the venous cranial pressure. The head is fixed sharply in a Mayfield clamp with rotation to the contralateral side and hyperextension of the neck in a way that the zygoma is the highest point (Fig. 22.3a, b). Hyperextension is very important because it leads to frontal lobe retraction simply by gravity. The degree of head rotation depends on the target zone to be reached. Usually, we use 30° rotation in suprasellar lesions and 45° rotation for anteriorly located olfactory groove lesions. In midline tumors, we always come from the right side. In medial sphenoid wing meningiomas, we approach from the side of the lesion. After disinfection, the patient is draped. Microscope and endoscopes are draped as well and are ready to use. The microscope stands behind the surgeon in order to bring it easily out of the surgical field when the endoscopes are used for visualization. The video monitors displaying the MR data, and the endoscopic images are positioned in front of the surgeon to enable an ergonomic work (Fig. 22.4). A Gilsbach frame (Aesculap AG, Tuttlingen, Germany) is used for skin retraction and as a handrest (Fig. 22.5a). The endoscopes are used freehand for inspection, but are fixed to a mechanical holding arm (Karl Storz GmbH & Co. KG, Tuttlingen, Germany) when bimanual dissection and tumor removal are required (Fig. 22.5b).

22.4.2 Supraorbital Approach

At first, the skin incision is marked. It is placed exactly in the eyebrow and starts laterally to the supraorbital fissure avoiding injury to the supraorbital nerve (Fig. 22.6a). The incision follows the eyebrow to the lateral end, sometimes even a little bit longer (app. 4 cm). Then the orbicularis oculi muscle and the fat tissue overlying

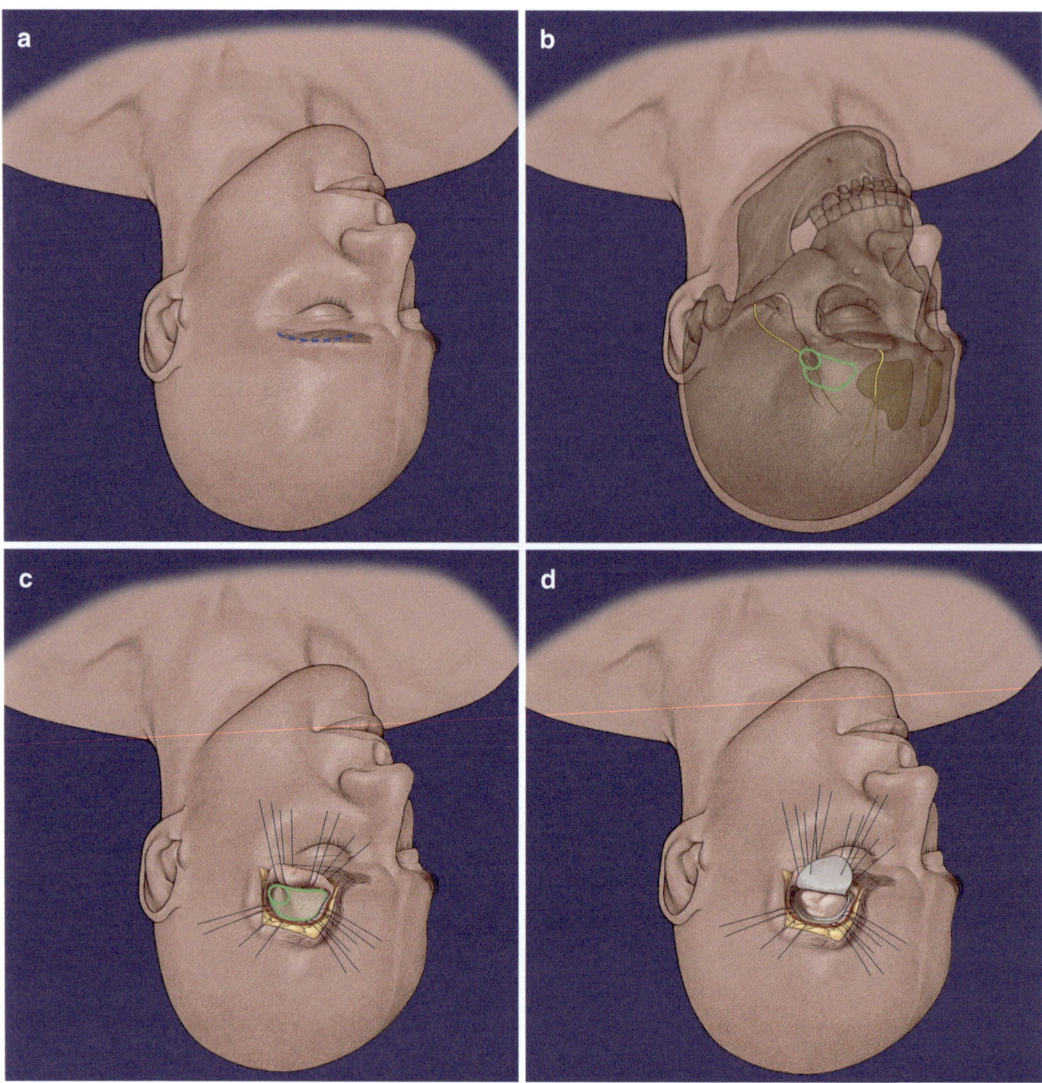

Fig. 22.2 Schematic drawing of the supraorbital eyebrow approach. (**a**) Skin incision. (**b**) Relation of the craniotomy to the supraorbital nerve and the frontotemporal branch of the facial nerve. (**c**) Position of the craniotomy after skin incision. (**d**) Approach with dural opening (Created by H.W. Schroeder © Henry Schroeder 2015)

the periosteum are incised. The skin is retracted upward away from the orbit. The superior temporal line indicating the attachment of the temporal fascia is identified (Fig. 22.6b). A periosteal flap based to the orbit is circumcised and elevated (Fig. 22.6c). The lateral incision follows the superior temporal line. Sometimes the supraorbital nerve can be identified at the medial end of the incision (Fig. 22.6d). The temporal fascia and the temporal muscle are detached from the temporal line and adjacent bone. They are retracted laterally with fish hooks (Fig. 22.6e). A small burr hole is placed as far as possible behind the temporal line for cosmetic reasons (Fig. 22.6f). It should be exactly made just over the frontal skullbase. If it is too deep, the orbit will be entered. Then a 2.5×2 cm craniotomy is made with the aid of a craniotome as close to the skullbase as feasible (Fig. 22.6g, h). The frontal sinus should be avoided whenever possible. The craniotomy should be approximately 2 cm in height (Fig. 22.6i). If it is too small, the microscopic

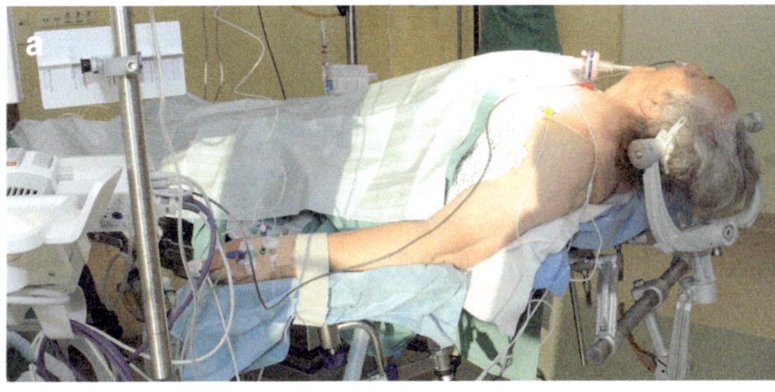

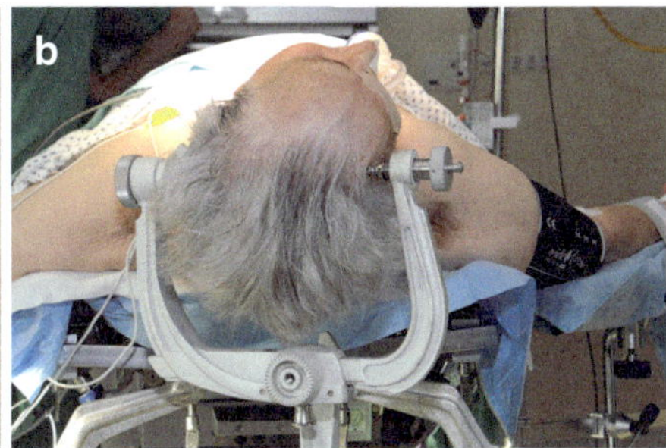

Fig. 22.3 Positioning of the patient. (**a**) Supine position with the body elevated 15°. (**b**) Sharp head fixation with rotation to the contralateral side and hyperextension of the neck (zygoma highest point) (Created by H.W. Schroeder © Henry Schroeder 2015)

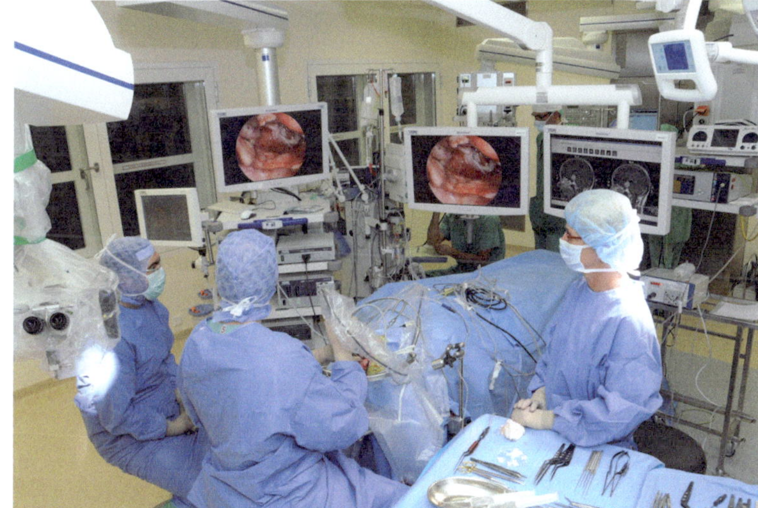

Fig. 22.4 Setup in the operating room for endoscope-assisted microsurgery (Created by H.W. Schroeder © Henry Schroeder 2015)

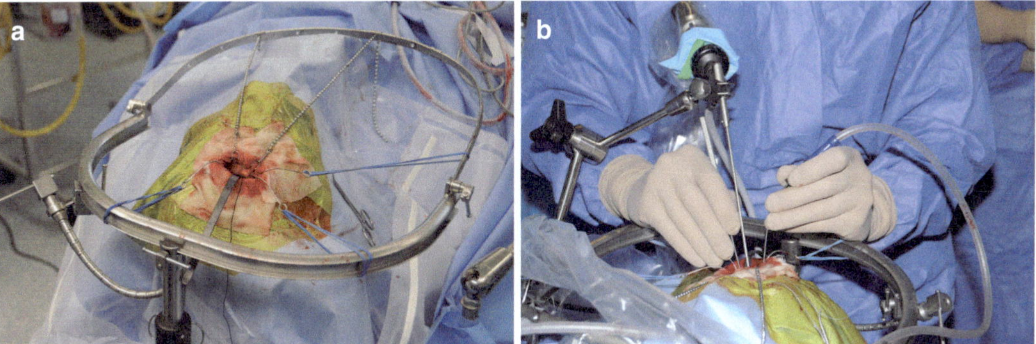

Fig. 22.5 (**a**) Gilsbach frame for skin and muscle retraction. (**b**) Bimanual endoscopic dissection with the endoscope fixed in a mechanical holding arm (Created by H.W. Schroeder © Henry Schroeder 2015)

visualization of the skullbase may be compromised, and the margins of the craniotomy may interfere with the bimanual dissection using the microinstruments. After elevation of the bone flap, the dura is detached from the frontal skullbase (Fig. 22.6j). The inner edge of the craniotomy and prominent protuberances of the orbital roof are drilled away to provide more space

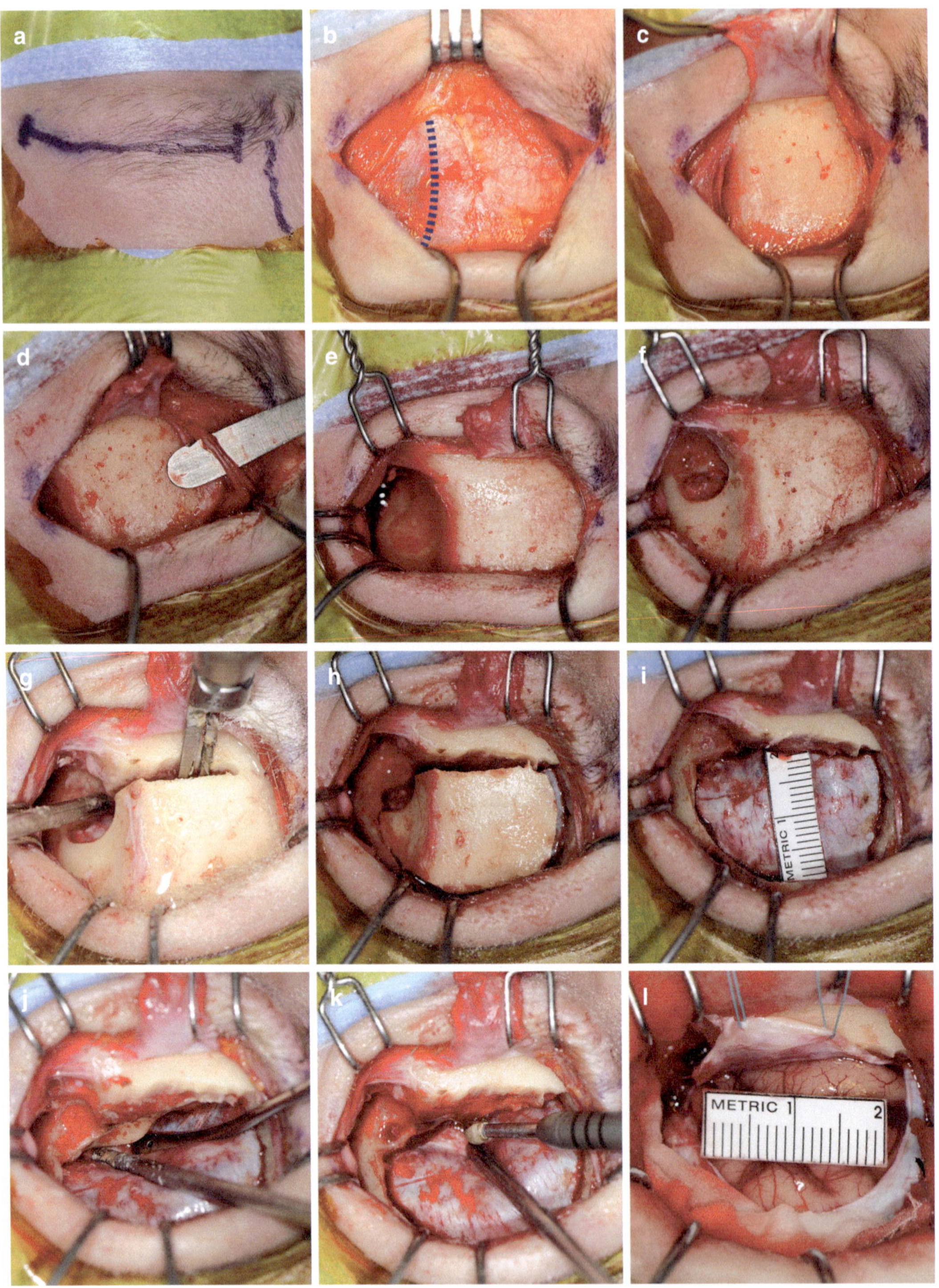

Fig. 22.6 Steps of the supraorbital approach. (**a**) Marking of the skin incision. (**b**) Exposed periosteum after skin and muscle incision with marked temporal line (*blue dots*). (**c**) Elevation of the periosteal flap. (**d**) Identification of the supraorbital nerve. (**e**) Retraction of the detached temporal muscle and fascia from the temporal line and adjacent bone. (**f**) Burr hole behind the temporal line. (**g**) Craniotomy with the craniotome. (**h**) Completed craniotomy. (**i**) Height of the craniotomy. (**j**) Detaching of the dura from the orbital roof. (**k**) Drilling of the inner edge of the craniotomy and prominent protuberances of the orbital roof. (**l**) Dural opening (Created by H.W. Schroeder © Henry Schroeder 2015)

for visualization and dissection (Fig. 22.6k). A curved dural incision based to the orbit is finally performed to complete the approach (Fig. 22.6l).

A cotton patty is placed on the frontobasal cortex, and the frontal lobe is carefully retracted from the skullbase with a suction and anatomical forceps. After olfactory tract and optic nerve have been identified, the optic cistern is opened, and CSF is released abundantly to relax the brain. Alternatively, the Sylvian fissure can be opened to drain CSF. If the head is positioned correctly, the frontal lobe falls back by gravity and provides space for the microsurgical manipulations (Fig. 22.7). Retractors should be avoided whenever possible. Sometimes, we use a retractor only to fix the patty which protects the frontal lobe. Excessive retraction of the frontal lobe has to be avoided because it can avulse the olfactory fibers at the cribriform plate.

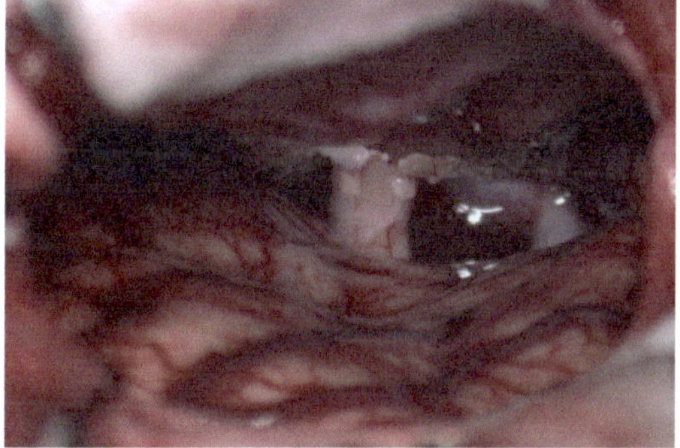

Fig. 22.7 Spontaneous brain retraction by gravity due to proper head positioning (Created by H.W. Schroeder © Henry Schroeder 2015)

After tumor resection, the dura is closed with a running suture (Fig. 22.8a). To achieve a watertight closure, TachoSil® (Nycomed Austria GmbH, Linz, Austria) can be placed on the suture line, if needed (Fig. 22.8b). This is especially helpful when the frontal sinus was opened during the craniotomy to avoid rhinorrhea. A piece of Gelfoam is placed in the craniotomy defect and the bone flap is fixed with mini plates (Fig. 22.8c). For cosmetic reasons, the bone flap has to be in close

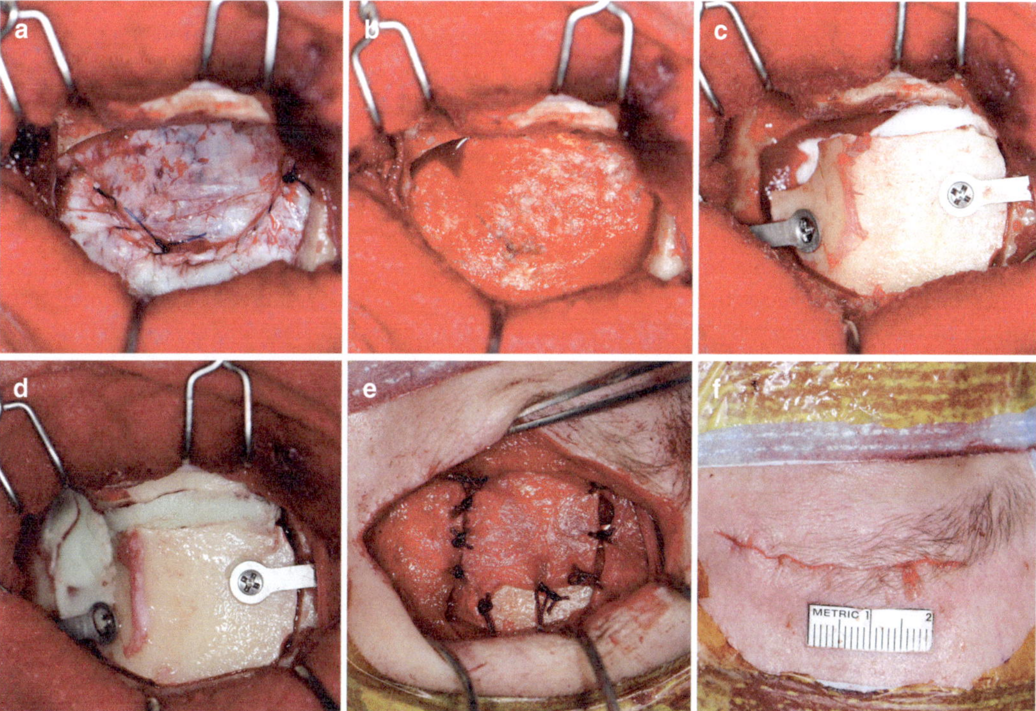

Fig. 22.8 Final steps of the supraorbital approach. (**a**) Watertight dural suture. (**b**) Covering of the suture line with TachoSil®. (**c**) Fixation of the bone flap with mini plates. (**d**) Filling of the burr hole and craniotome-related bony defects with bone cement. (**e**) Periosteal suture. (**f**) Intracutaneous skin suture (Created by H.W. Schroeder © Henry Schroeder 2015)

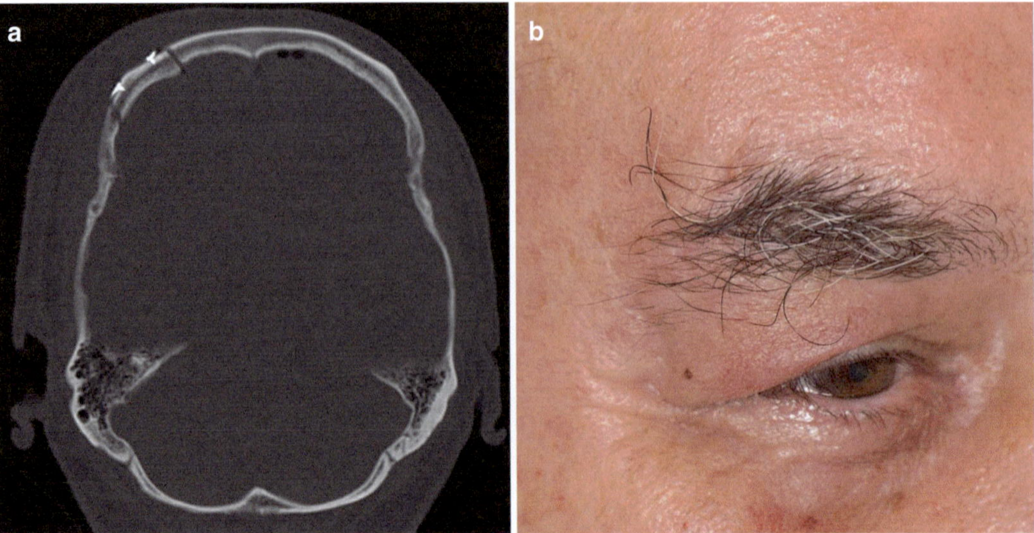

Fig. 22.9 (**a**) CT scan obtained 1 day after surgery showing the bone flap. (**b**) Eyebrow 3 months after surgery (Created by H.W. Schroeder © Henry Schroeder 2015)

contact to the upper margin of the craniotomy to avoid a visible indentation in the forehead later on. When the bony defect caused by the craniotome is at the lower aspect of the craniotomy hidden under the eyebrow, it usually remains invisible. When the temporal muscle and scalp are very thin, the initial burr hole and the lower craniotomy defect should be covered with a mini plate or filled with bone cement to avoid a visible indentation after scar formation (Fig. 22.8d). The wound is closed in layers – periost, muscle, subcutis, and skin. The periosteal suture is important to cover the bony defect caused by the craniotome (Fig. 22.8e). The periost is sutured additionally to the temporal fascia. For skin closure, we use running resorbable sutures (Fig. 22.8f). The patient is observed overnight in the intensive care unit. The day after surgery, a CT scan is performed to rule out any complication and to check the position of the bone flap (Fig. 22.9a). Usually, the cosmetic result after an eyebrow approach is excellent (Fig. 22.9b)

22.5 Olfactory Groove Meningiomas

The supraorbital craniotomy is our preferred approach for small olfactory groove meningiomas (<4 cm). However, because of the limited height of the craniotomy, there is usually a problem to visualize the olfactory groove with the microscope, especially when the groove is very steep. Therefore, 30° or 45° endoscopes are required to inspect the olfactory groove (Fig. 22.10). In larger tumors (>4 cm), we use a standard frontolateral craniotomy (4 × 4 cm) via a frontotemporal incision behind the hairline. With the standard frontolateral approach, there is no need to use the endoscope since all of the anterior skullbase can be seen with the microscope. Additionally, it is easy to harvest autologous periost for the skullbase reconstruction after drilling the base. In larger tumors, there is usually a large dural defect which should be covered to avoid a CSF fistula. Dural defects created via the eyebrow approach are smaller and usually covered with TachoSil®.

The most important point in olfactory groove meningiomas is the state of olfaction. Intact olfaction is an important factor in quality of life for enjoying food and drinks and sometimes even mandatory to stay employed, for example, as a cook or when working in livestock raising. When the sense of smell is still good, our intention is to preserve the olfaction, even when there is an infiltration of the cribriform plate. At least one olfactory tract should be preserved [15]. If the olfactory fibers are involved on both sides, we

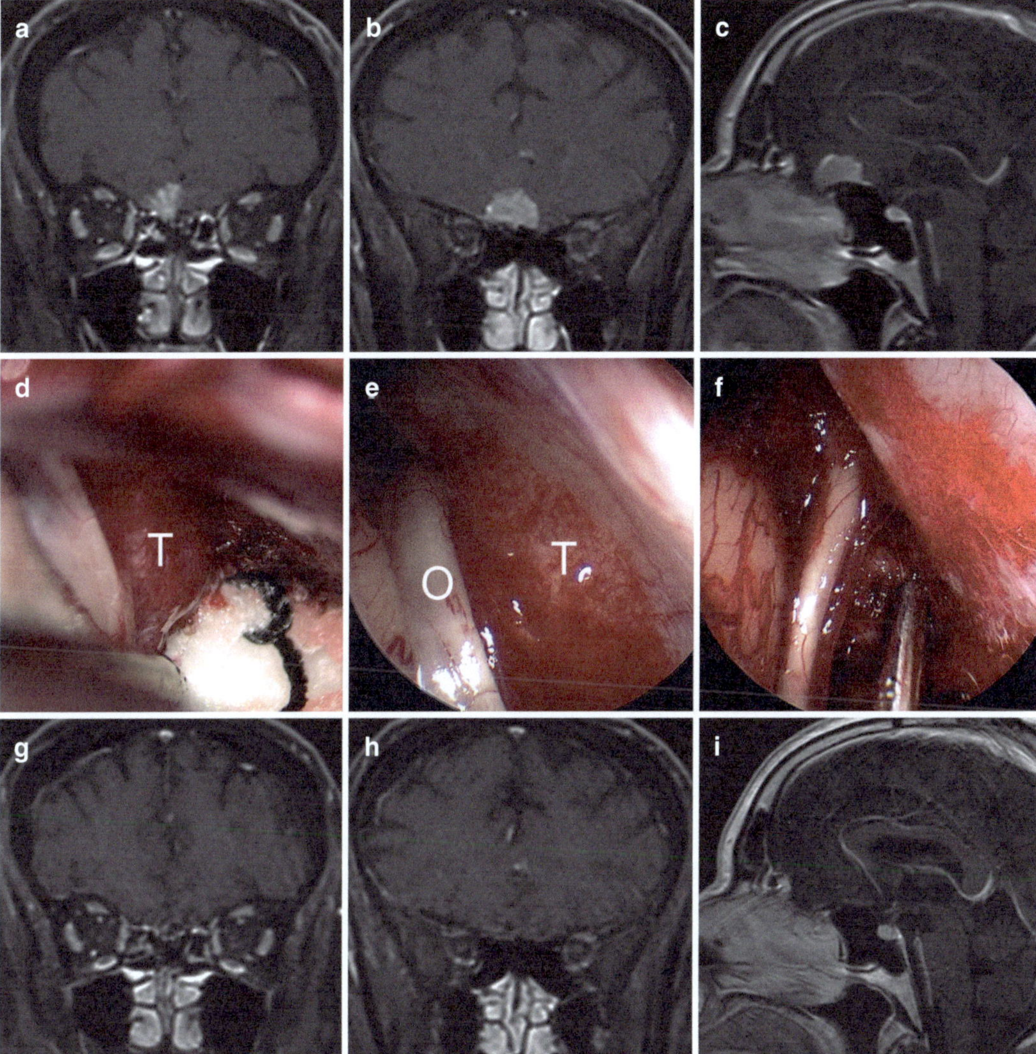

Fig. 22.10 Endoscope-assisted microsurgical resection of an olfactory groove meningioma. The 66-year-old male presented with headache. MR imaging revealed an olfactory groove meningioma which progressed within 2 years of follow-up. The patient had normal olfaction. (**a–c**) T1-weighted contrast-enhanced coronal (**a**, **b**) and sagittal (**c**) MR images showing an olfactory groove meningioma (note the unilateral tumor extension into the right olfactory groove). (**d**) The microscopic view showed that the anterior part of the tumor (*T*) within the olfactory groove could not be adequately visualized. (**e**) In contrast, the view with a 30° endoscope showed the entire tumor (*T*) located under the right olfactory tract (*O*). (**f**) The final endoscopic inspection confirmed the total tumor resection. (**g–i**) T1-weighted contrast-enhanced coronal (**g**, **h**) and sagittal (**i**) MR images obtained 5 years after surgery revealed gross total tumor resection without recurrence. The patient has a normal sense of smell (Created by H.W. Schroeder © Henry Schroeder 2015)

leave a small tumor remnant behind. However, smaller tumors can frequently be removed totally with bilateral preservation of the olfactory tracts and nerves. In larger tumors with bilateral infiltration of the cribriform plate, patients have mostly no useful olfaction, and the olfactory tracts and nerves can be sacrificed.

An indication to use the endonasal approach is a tumor with significant extension into the nasal cavity accompanied with loss of olfaction.

22.6 Planum Sphenoidale Meningiomas

Planum sphenoidale meningiomas can be easily approached via the supraorbital craniotomy. Because of the flat plateau of the planum, the tumors can usually be resected under microscopic visualization alone. However, if there are tumor extensions into the olfactory groove or to the tuberculum sellae, endoscope assistance can be helpful. Usually, olfactory tracts and olfaction can be preserved. The eyebrow approach is used for smaller tumor. Larger tumors (>4 cm) were removed via a standard frontolateral craniotomy.

22.7 Tuberculum Sellae Meningiomas

Most tuberculum sellae meningiomas are good indications for the supraorbital approach (Figs. 22.11 and 22.12). The tumors usually become early symptomatic because of optic nerve and/or chiasm compression with loss of visual acuity and visual field deficits. Therefore, they are mostly small (<3 cm) when diagnosed. They displace the chiasm backward (postfixed chiasm). This provides ample room for access to the tumor. The first step of the tumor resection is unroofing of the ipsilateral optic canal to release the optic nerve. The falciform ligament is cut and the intracanalicular dura is excised. The extent of the required unroofing depends on the extension of the tumor into the optic canal. Then the dural tumor base is coagulated to devascularize the tumor. Ideally, the vascular supply should be taken as much as possible before starting with debulking of the tumor. In soft tumors, the ultrasonic aspirator is very efficient in tumor debulking. However, when the tumor is very fibrous, the aspirator will fail, and bipolar coagulation is used to shrink the tumor down. Care has to be taken that no thermal damage occurs to the chiasm/optic nerve and the arachnoid plane with the supplying vessels. In fibrous tumors, sharp debulking with microscissors is required. The anterior part of the tumor is removed. As soon as the contralateral optic nerve can be visualized, the contralateral optic canal is unroofed too to release the optic nerve when it is compromised in the canal by the tumor. Then the most important step of the resection follows: the tumor is dissected within the arachnoid plane away from the chiasm in a bimanual dissection technique. The tumor is grasped with a tumor forceps, and the arachnoid overlying the tumor is peeled from the tumor surface with a sharp-pointed anatomical forceps. Utmost care has to be taken to preserve the small branches of the superior hypophyseal arteries supplying the chiasm. When the anterior cerebral artery complex is additionally involved in the tumor, it is dissected from the tumor too. Usually, the tuberculum sellae is drilled away to achieve a gross total tumor resection. Tumor extensions into the optic canals are removed after adequate unroofing of the optic canals. If the tuberculum is

Fig. 22.11 Endoscope-assisted microsurgical resection of a tuberculum sellae meningioma (Video 22.1). The 54-year-old female presented with decreased visual acuity and severe visual field deficits. (**a**, **b**) T1-weighted contrast-enhanced coronal (**a**) and sagittal (**b**) MR images showing a tuberculum sellae meningioma with intrasellar extension. (**c**) T2-weighted coronal MR image demonstrating the elevated and thinned chiasm (*arrows*) on top of the tumor. (**d**) Microscopic view showing tumor (*T*) and the right optic nerve (*ON*). (**e**, **f**) Bimanual dissection of the chiasm (*arrows*) and chiasm-supplying vessels within the arachnoid plane from the tumor surface (*T*). (**g**) Endoscopic inspection with a 30° endoscope revealed the right internal carotid artery (*C*) under the right optic nerve (*ON*). Blind corner under the microscope. (**h**) Endoscopic inspection with a 30° endoscope looking up showed the grooving (*arrows*) within the chiasm (*OC*) caused by compression of the chiasm against the anterior cerebral arteries by the tumor. Laterally, the left internal carotid artery (*C*) and the posterior communicating artery (*pcom*) are seen. (**i**) Incision after intracutaneous suture. (**j**, **k**) T1-weighted contrast-enhanced coronal (**j**) and sagittal (**k**) MR images obtained 2 years after surgery showing no tumor remnant or recurrence. (**l**) Photograph taken 3 months after surgery showing an excellent cosmetic result (Created by H.W. Schroeder © Henry Schroeder 2015)

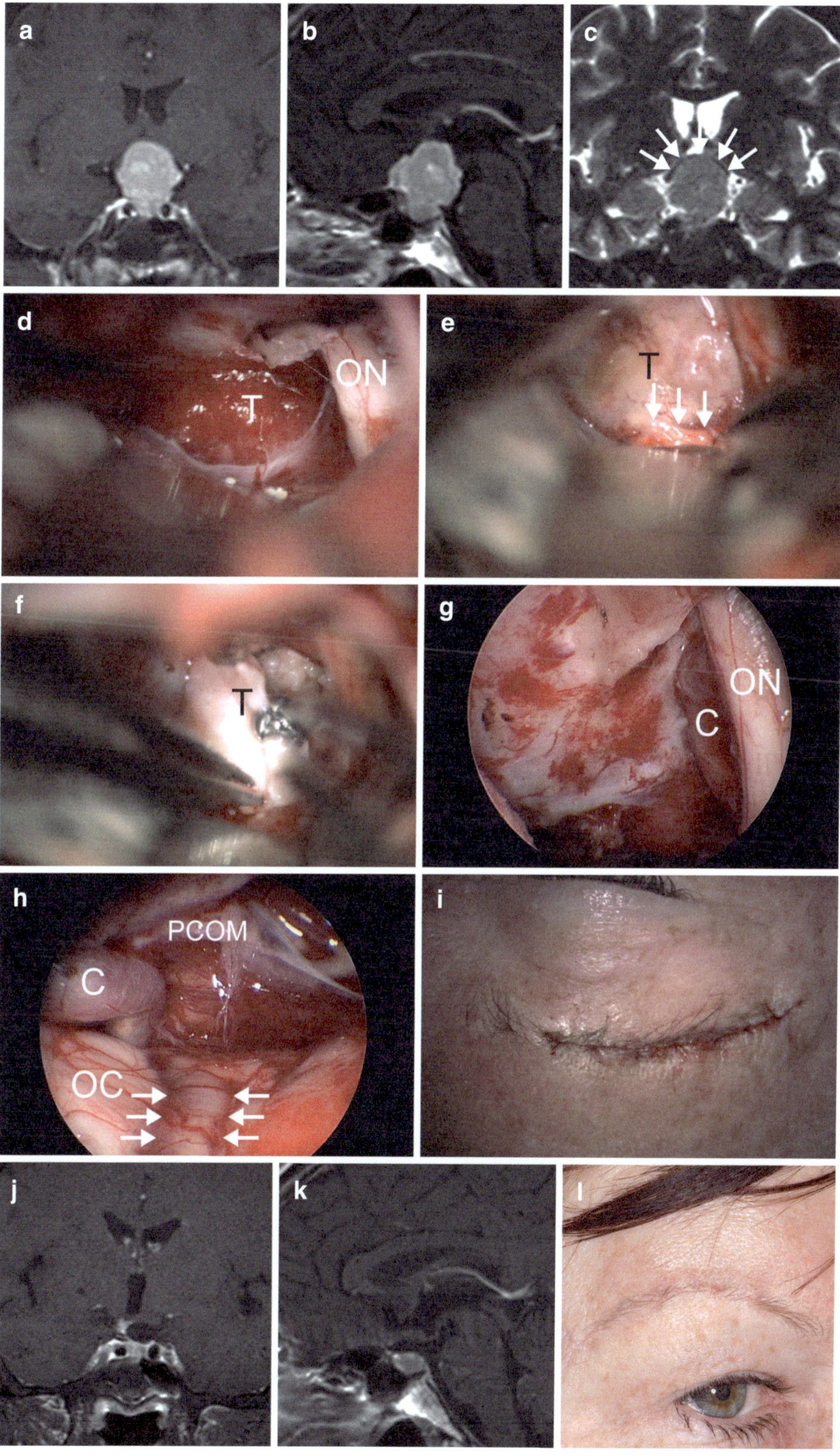
a
b
c
d
ON
T
e
T
f
T
g
ON
C
h
PCOM
C
OC
i
j
k
l

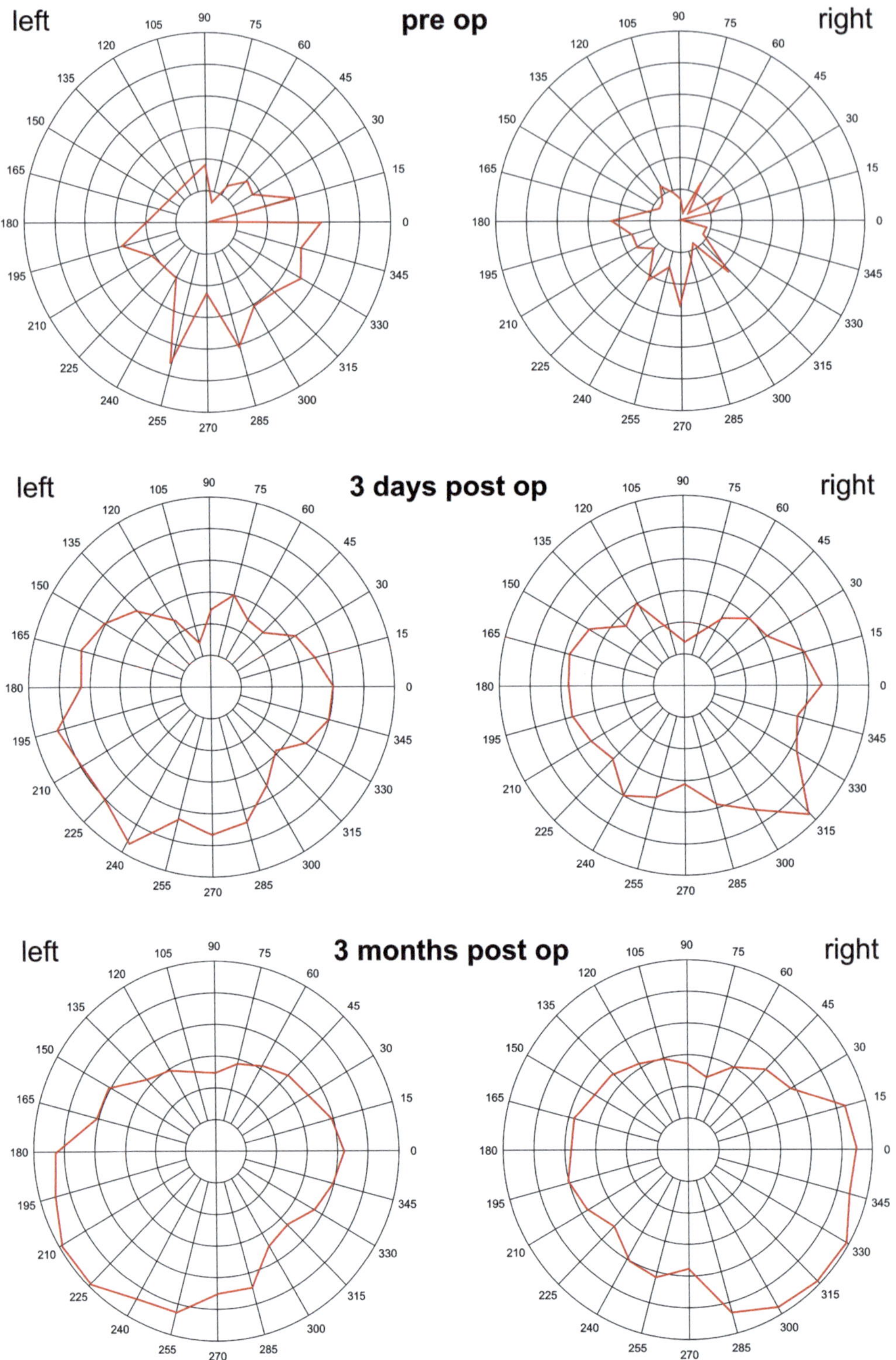

Fig. 22.12 Visual field of the patient with the tuberculum sellae meningioma shown in Fig. 22.11. *Upper*: visual field prior to surgery showed severe cuts (tunnel view). *Middle*: improved visual field 3 days after surgery. *Lower*: normalized visual field 3 months after surgery (Created by H.W. Schroeder © Henry Schroeder 2015)

steep, it cannot be visualized completely with the microscope as well as a deep-lying diaphragm. The space under the ipsilateral optic nerve is a blind corner too. Therefore, 30° or 45° endoscopes are used to inspect these regions and to remove residual tumor if still present. The final endoscopic inspection is carried out to confirm total tumor resection and to identify skullbase defects with communication to the sphenoid sinus caused by optic canal unroofing or drilling of the tuberculum. If such a defect is present, it is covered with muscle and/or TachoSil®. Larger tumors (>4 cm) are removed via a standard frontolateral craniotomy.

Although the endonasal approach is a valid alternative for many tuberculum sellae meningiomas, we usually prefer transcranial approaches. The main reasons are the following: in contrast to most craniopharyngiomas, tuberculum sellae meningiomas displace the chiasm backward and cause a postfixed chiasm. Therefore, there is usually a wide interoptic window for dissection. Furthermore, the dissection of the optic nerve and chiasm as well as the anterior cerebral arteries is easier and safer from above especially when the tumor is very adherent to these structures.

In my opinion, good indications for an endonasal approach are smaller tumors (<2 cm) under a prefixed chiasm, a very steep tuberculum sellae, and involvement of the intrasellar space. Additionally, tumors with invasion of the sphenoid sinus are good endonasal candidates too. Although there are advantages of the endonasal approach such as early optic canal decompression and tumor devascularization, the tumor resection is, at least in my hands, easier and faster via the supraorbital craniotomy.

22.8 Medial Sphenoid Wing Meningiomas

The supraorbital craniotomy is our preferred approach for smaller medial sphenoid wing meningiomas with little extension into the middle cranial fossa. For larger tumors (>3 cm), we use the standard frontolateral or pterional approach. If possible in smaller tumors, the location of the optic nerve and carotid artery is identified before starting with the tumor resection. At first, the main arterial feeders at the medial sphenoid wing are coagulated to devascularize the tumor. Then the tumor is debulked and resected. If an arachnoid plane is present, the tumor can totally be dissected from the carotid, anterior, and middle cerebral arteries although MR imaging shows complete encasement of the vessels. Tumor parts growing into the optic canal are removed after opening of the canal. 30° or 45° endoscopes are required to look under the ipsilateral optic nerve and around the medial sphenoid wing into the middle cranial fossa.

The endonasal approach should not be used for medial sphenoid wing meningiomas because these tumors grow above and lateral to the optic nerve and carotid artery.

22.9 Results

In our series of anterior skullbase meningiomas, we used the supraorbital eyebrow approach in 39 patients including 16 tuberculum sellae, 17 olfactory groove/planum sphenoidale, and 6 medial sphenoid wing meningiomas. In the 17 olfactory groove/planum sphenoidale meningiomas, we preserved the sense of smell in 14 patients (82 %). In the tuberculum sellae meningiomas, we had no permanent worsening of visual field or visual acuity after surgery. Eleven of thirteen (85 %) patients with visual symptoms improved. In the other three patients, the visual deficits did not change. Gross total tumor resection was achieved in 37 patients (95 %). In two patients with olfactory groove meningiomas, small tumor parts were left behind to preserve olfaction. The most frequent complications were CSF related. We observed two subgaleal CSF accumulations, which were treated with a lumbar drain. In one patient in whom the frontal sinus was opened by the craniotomy, a rhinoliquorrhoe occurred which required surgical revision. There was no mortality and no infection/meningitis.

22.10 Supraorbital Versus Endonasal Approach

The supraorbital craniotomy via eyebrow incision is a versatile, rapid, and minimally invasive surgical approach for meningiomas of the anterior cranial fossa. It provides a nice overview over the entire frontal skullbase. Thin en-plaque tumor growth around the meningioma which is not visible on MR imaging can easily be identified and removed. The supraorbital craniotomy allows the use of the operating microscope and endoscope, which is referred to as endoscope-assisted microsurgery. The surgeon can take advantage of both optical tools – high optical resolution and stereoscopic view of the microscope as well as panoramic view, high magnification, and large depth of field of the endoscope. Dissection of dense adhesion of the tumor to nerves and vessels is easier via a cranial craniotomy than via an endonasal approach. The argument that there is significant brain retraction in the transcranial approaches is not true: with proper head positioning and early release of CSF, the frontal lobe falls back by gravity without any retraction. And last but not least, usually the cosmetic result after the eyebrow skin incision is very satisfying.

Although successful endoscopic endonasal resection of skullbase meningiomas has been published recently [12, 13, 16–18], we are still convinced that in most meningiomas a transcranial approach is preferable to achieve a safe, rapid, and gross total tumor removal. To date, we have performed the endonasal approach for meningiomas in ten patients. We agree with the literature that rapid access to the vascular supply of the tumor and the avoidance of any brain retraction to expose the lesion are advantages. However, the creation of the approach takes longer and requires more skullbase drilling. Durations of surgery for olfactory groove meningiomas of 9 h have been reported [19]. The approach-related trauma to the nasal cavity and paranasal sinuses is significant. Frequently, one middle turbinate is resected, the sphenoid sinus is opened widely, the ethmoidal cells are removed, and depending on the location and size of the meningioma, the nasal septum and cranial base have to be resected. Furthermore, the frontal skullbase can only be explored in the midline. Therefore, the risk is higher to miss some lateral tumor parts hidden behind the margins of the created skullbase opening compared to the supraorbital craniotomy, which allows a good overview over the frontal skullbase. Early identification of nerves and major vessels is another advantage of the supraorbital approach. Although the nasoseptal flap has improved the leakage rate [20], CSF leaks are still a problem. CSF leak rates of up to 30 % have been reported [19]. Rhinoliquorrhoe after a supraorbital craniotomy is rare.

Additionally, the postoperative discomfort for the patient is clearly prolonged after the endonasal approach. Nasal discharge, smell and taste disturbances, sensory deficits, headaches, malodor, and serous otitis media have been described [21]. Nasal crusting and discharge have been reported for approximately 100 days after surgery [21]. The reverse flap, which covers the donor site of the septum from which the nasoseptal flap was harvested, has definitely reduced the crusting and discharge [22, 23], but still intensive rhinological care for about 2–3 months is necessary. After an eyebrow approach, we see usually a swollen eye, but at the latest 10 days after surgery, no additional care is necessary.

However, the most important reason why we prefer transcranial approaches is the unsatisfying rate of gross total resections, which should be the aim in most surgeries for anterior skullbase meningiomas. In olfactory groove meningiomas, a gross total resection rate of 67–75 % has been reported [19, 24]. The reason for incomplete resection was not preservation of olfaction, which is usually lost after an endonasal approach. In our series, the gross total resection rate in olfactory groove meningiomas was 88 %, but only because we left tumor to preserve the sense of smell. Otherwise, a 100 % gross total resection would have been achieved. Furthermore, a staged surgery (usually two surgeries) was required to remove olfactory groove meningiomas endonasally in 18 of 50 patients (36 %) which is inacceptable [19]. Even in giant tumors, a gross total tumor resection is usually accomplished in one surgery via a unilateral frontolateral craniotomy. In tuberculum sellae meningiomas, the reported gross total resection rate is 76–85 % [19, 24]. Improvement of visual complaints has been described in 82–86 % of the patients [19, 24] and is comparable with our series of the eyebrow approach. A recent literature review confirmed that open transcranial approaches for olfactory groove, tuberculum sellae, and planum sphenoidale meningiomas result in higher rates of gross total resection with lower postoperative CSF leak rates [25].

I agree that tumors with significant extension into the nasal cavity should be approached via the nose. I also agree that tumors located under a prefixed chiasm or arising from the dorsum sellae should be removed via an endonasal route to avoid retraction to the chiasm and optic nerves. Small midline tuberculum sellae meningiomas (<2 cm) are a good indication for an endonasal as well as supraorbital approach. In these lesions, the patient's preference is another important factor in the decision-making process. However, in most frontal skullbase meningiomas, the transcranial approach is easier, faster, and more convenient for the surgeon and the patient. Therefore, although I am very enthusiastic with the endoscopic endonasal approach for craniopharyngiomas, chordomas, and chondrosarcomas, in meningioma surgery, I still prefer the transcranial approach in most of the cases [15].

Acknowledgement I am very grateful to Marc Matthes, M.Sc., for helping with the creation of the figures and the video.

Disclosure HWSS is consultant for Karl Storz GmbH & Co. KG (Tuttlingen, Germany).

References

1. Nakamura M, Roser F, Struck M, Vorkapic P, Samii M (2006) Tuberculum sellae meningiomas: clinical outcome considering different surgical approaches. Neurosurgery 59(5):1019–1028. doi:10.1227/01.NEU.0000245600.92322.06; discussion 1028–1019
2. Nakamura M, Struck M, Roser F, Vorkapic P, Samii M (2007) Olfactory groove meningiomas: clinical outcome and recurrence rates after tumor removal through the frontolateral and bifrontal approach. Neurosurgery 60(5):844–852. doi:10.1227/01.NEU.0000255453.20602.80; discussion 844–852
3. Erkmen K, Pravdenkova S, Al-Mefty O (2005) Surgical management of petroclival meningiomas: factors determining the choice of approach. Neurosurg Focus 19(2), E7
4. Tatagiba M, Samii M, Matthies C, Vorkapic P (1996) Management of petroclival meningiomas: a critical analysis of surgical treatment. Acta Neurochir Suppl 65:92–94
5. Tuna H, Bozkurt M, Ayten M, Erdogan A, Deda H (2005) Olfactory groove meningiomas. J Clin Neurosci 12(6):664–668. doi:10.1016/j.jocn.2005.05.002
6. Fischer G, Stadie A, Reisch R, Hopf NJ, Fries G, Bocher-Schwarz H, van Lindert E, Ungersbock K, Knosp E, Oertel J, Perneczky A (2011) The keyhole concept in aneurysm surgery: results of the past 20 years. Neurosurgery 68(1 Suppl Operative):45–51. doi:10.1227/NEU.0b013e31820934ca; discussion 51
7. Fries G, Perneczky A (1998) Endoscope-assisted brain surgery: part 2 – analysis of 380 procedures. Neurosurgery 42(2):226–231; discussion 231–222
8. Perneczky A, Fries G (1998) Endoscope-assisted brain surgery: part 1 – evolution, basic concept, and current technique. Neurosurgery 42(2):219–224; discussion 224–215
9. Reisch R, Perneczky A (2005) Ten-year experience with the supraorbital subfrontal approach through an eyebrow skin incision. Neurosurgery 57(4 Suppl):242–255; discussion 242–255
10. van Lindert E, Perneczky A, Fries G, Pierangeli E (1998) The supraorbital keyhole approach to supratentorial aneurysms: concept and technique. Surg Neurol 49(5):481–489; discussion 489–490
11. Schroeder HW, Hickmann AK, Baldauf J (2011) Endoscope-assisted microsurgical resection of skull base meningiomas. Neurosurg Rev 34(4):441–455. doi:10.1007/s10143-011-0322-9
12. Fatemi N, Dusick JR, de Paiva Neto MA, Malkasian D, Kelly DF (2009) Endonasal versus supraorbital keyhole removal of craniopharyngiomas and tuberculum sellae meningiomas. Neurosurgery 64(5 Suppl 2):269–284. doi:10.1227/01.NEU.0000327857.22221.53; discussion 284–266
13. Gardner PA, Kassam AB, Thomas A, Snyderman CH, Carrau RL, Mintz AH, Prevedello DM (2008) Endoscopic endonasal resection of anterior cranial base meningiomas. Neurosurgery 63(1):36–52. doi:10.1227/01.NEU.0000335069.30319.1E; discussion 52–34
14. Laufer I, Anand VK, Schwartz TH (2007) Endoscopic, endonasal extended transsphenoidal, transplanum transtuberculum approach for resection of suprasellar lesions. J Neurosurg 106(3):400–406. doi:10.3171/jns.2007.106.3.400
15. Schroeder HW (2014) Indications and limitations of the endoscopic endonasal approach for anterior cranial base meningiomas. World Neurosurg 82(6 Suppl):S81–S85. doi:10.1016/j.wneu.2014.07.030

16. de Divitiis E, Cavallo LM, Cappabianca P, Esposito F (2007) Extended endoscopic endonasal transsphenoidal approach for the removal of suprasellar tumors: part 2. Neurosurgery 60(1):46–58. doi:10.1227/01.NEU.0000249211.89096.25; discussion 58–49
17. Fernandez-Miranda JC, Gardner PA, Prevedello DM, Kassam AB (2009) Expanded endonasal approach for olfactory groove meningioma. Acta Neurochir (Wien) 151(3):287–288. doi:10.1007/s00701-009-0201-0; author reply 289–290
18. Greenfield JP, Anand VK, Kacker A, Seibert MJ, Singh A, Brown SM, Schwartz TH (2010) Endoscopic endonasal transethmoidal transcribriform transfovea ethmoidalis approach to the anterior cranial fossa and skull base. Neurosurgery 66(5):883–892; discussion 892
19. Koutourousiou M, Fernandez-Miranda JC, Wang EW, Snyderman CH, Gardner PA (2014) Endoscopic endonasal surgery for olfactory groove meningiomas: outcomes and limitations in 50 patients. Neurosurg Focus 37(4), E8
20. Hadad G, Bassagasteguy L, Carrau RL, Mataza JC, Kassam A, Snyderman CH, Mintz A (2006) A novel reconstructive technique after endoscopic expanded endonasal approaches: vascular pedicle nasoseptal flap. Laryngoscope 116(10):1882–1886. doi:10.1097/01.mlg.0000234933.37779.e4
21. de Almeida JR, Snyderman CH, Gardner PA, Carrau RL, Vescan AD (2011) Nasal morbidity following endoscopic skull base surgery: a prospective cohort study. Head Neck 33(4):547–551. doi:10.1002/hed.21483
22. Caicedo-Granados E, Carrau R, Snyderman CH, Prevedello D, Fernandez-Miranda J, Gardner P, Kassam A (2010) Reverse rotation flap for reconstruction of donor site after vascular pedicled nasoseptal flap in skull base surgery. Laryngoscope 120(8):1550–1552. doi:10.1002/lary.20975
23. Kasemsiri P, Carrau RL, Otto BA, Tang IP, Prevedello DM, Muto J, Caicedo E (2013) Reconstruction of the pedicled nasoseptal flap donor site with a contralateral reverse rotation flap: technical modifications and outcomes. Laryngoscope 123(11):2601–2604. doi:10.1002/lary.24088
24. Khan OH, Anand VK, Schwartz TH (2014) Endoscopic endonasal resection of skull base meningiomas: the significance of a "cortical cuff" and brain edema compared with careful case selection and surgical experience in predicting morbidity and extent of resection. Neurosurg Focus 37(4), E7. doi:10.3171/2014.7.FOCUS14321
25. Komotar RJ, Starke RM, Raper DM, Anand VK, Schwartz TH (2012) Endoscopic endonasal versus open transcranial resection of anterior midline skull base meningiomas. World Neurosurg 77(5–6):713–724. doi:10.1016/j.wneu.2011.08.025

23 Radiotherapy and Radiosurgery

Alfredo Conti and Antonio Pontoriero

23.1 Introduction

Anterior skull base meningiomas are, in most instances, surgically accessible lesions, whose treatment of choice is the total resection of the tumor mass, ideally, together with the dural attachment. The total resection of benign meningiomas results in a tumor growth control rate averaging 95 % at 5 years, 90 % at 10 years, and 70 % at 15 years [1–3]. Nevertheless, there are a group of complex tumors, including those involving or encasing the optic apparatus and parasellar neurovascular structures, which could not be safely resected.

When a meningioma is subtotally resected and the surgical treatment is not followed by adjuvant radiotherapy (RT), progression rates range 37–47 % at 5 years, 55–63 % at 10 years, and >70 % after 15 years [4, 5].

In the 1980s, early studies demonstrated that external beam radiotherapy (EBRT) could provide durable local tumor control in incompletely resected benign meningiomas. Currently available advanced radio-oncology techniques, including fractionated stereotactic radiotherapy (FSRT), intensity-modulated radiotherapy (IMRT), and stereotactic radiosurgery (SRS), allow for a steeper dose gradient, meaning a more favorable dose distribution on target and surrounding normal tissue. This could improve the effects on the tumors reducing, at the same time, the risk of side effects.

Particularly, SRS has progressively emerged as the first-line treatment for both adjuvant treatment of residual tumors and an effective primary treatment of selected meningiomas. Radiosurgery is virtually noninvasive, but it does carry a risk of radiation-induced complications. For meningiomas, this risk ranges between 3 and 40 % [6]. Nevertheless, adverse effects induced by radiation appear to be more frequent in convexity or parasagittal meningiomas as compared to skull base tumors. In particular, brain edema is a fairly unpredictable consequence in parasagittal and convexity meningiomas, but it is less common in skull base meningiomas. In meningiomas of the anterior skull base, the main issue concerns the proximity of cranial nerves, including optic nerves and chiasm, that are extremely sensitive to radioinduced complications. We will provide an overview of therapeutic potential and risk of complications of different radiotherapy techniques. We also provide a more detailed analysis of issues related to optic nerve preservation.

A. Conti, MD, PhD (✉)
Division of Neurosurgery, Department of Biomedical Sciences, Dentistry, and Morphological and Functional Imaging, University of Messina, Messina, Italy
e-mail: alfredo.conti@unime.it

A. Pontoriero, MD
Radiation Oncology Unit, Department of Biomedical Sciences, Dentistry, and Morphological and Functional Imaging, University of Messina, Messina, Italy

P. Cappabianca et al. (eds.), *Midline Skull Base Surgery*, DOI 10.1007/978-3-319-21533-4_23

23.2 Conventionally Fractionated Radiotherapy

For a long time, EBRT has been the only available technique for adjuvant treatment of benign meningiomas. Using a dose of 50–55 Gy in 30–33 fractions, the 10-year and 20-year reported local control rates are 70–80 % [3, 7–17] (Table 23.1).

After the advent of CT planning, Goldsmith and coworkers [3] showed that local control using radiotherapy could rival that of surgical resection. They suggested that 5-year progression-free survival (PFS) in the post-1980 era with the aid of more modern techniques was 98 % compared with 77 % in patients treated before 1980 ($p=0.002$).

The first issue in the treatment of a benign meningioma, using a standard fractionation scheme (1.8–2 Gy/day), concerns the dose to be delivered. Most of published series showed no significant difference on tumor control with the use of doses ranging between 50 and 60 Gy with a 2 Gy daily fraction. However, a dose <50 Gy is associated with higher recurrence rates [14, 17]. Goldsmith et al. [3] reported that doses greater than 52 Gy resulted in a 10-year local control of 93 % compared with 65 % using lower doses, although the dose was not an independent predictor at multivariate analysis.

Size and tumor site have been suggested as a possible predictor of tumor control. Connell et al. [19] reported a 5-year control of 93 % for 54 patients with skull base meningiomas of <5 cm and 40 % for tumors >5 cm.

Late toxicity of EBRT is relatively low, ranging from 0 to 24 % (Table 23.1), and includes neurological deficits, especially optic neuropathy, cerebral radionecrosis, cognitive deficits, and pituitary function deficits.

Cerebral radionecrosis is a severe and potentially fatal complication of RT; however it remains exceptional when doses less than 60 Gy and 3-D planning system are used. Goldsmith et al. [3] identified complications in five out of 140 patients (3.6 %) attributable to EBRT. Authors described retinopathy in two patients, optic neuropathy in one patient, and cerebral necrosis in two patients [3]. Generally, optic complications are quite rare with doses lower than 54 Gy, particularly with fractional doses of 2.0 Gy or less [14, 38, 47]. Goldsmith et al. generated a radiobiology model to predict optic nerve tolerance and recommended a maximum dose of 890 optic ret (corresponding to 890 cGy in single fraction or 54 Gy in 30 fractions) to be delivered at the optic nerve [48].

Patients with parasellar meningiomas are at risk to develop late hypopituitarism and should be carefully assessed long life after RT. Neurocognitive dysfunction is a recognized consequence of large-volume RT for brain tumors [49] and has been occasionally reported in irradiated patients with meningiomas, especially impairment of short-term memory [11, 20, 21].

High-dose radiation may be associated with the development of a second brain tumor. In a large series of 426 patients with pituitary adenomas who received conventional RT at the Royal Marsden Hospital between 1962 and 1994, Minniti et al. reported that the risk of second brain tumors was 2.0 % at 10 years and 2.4 % at 20 years, measured from the date of RT [50].

23.3 Fractionated Stereotactic Conformal Radiotherapy (FSRT)

FSRT uses conventional fractionation schemes using modern high-precision image-guided radiotherapy (IGRT) approaches allowing for significantly improved precision over older radiotherapy paradigms. FSRT leads to a reduction in the volume of normal brain irradiated at high doses. Thus, the principal aims of radiosensitive structures sparing are to reduce the long-term toxicity of radiotherapy and to increase the precision of treatment maintaining or possibly increasing its effectiveness.

Toxicity is reported to be less than 0–12 % of patients in series reporting results on the use of FSRT in benign meningiomas (Table 23.1), including cranial deficits (leading especially to visual problems), hypopituitarism, and impairment of neurocognitive function. Reduced volume of normal brain receiving radiation doses may decrease the risk of radiation-induced tumors.

Table 23.1 Summary of results on main published studies on EBRT, FSRT, IMRT, and proton radiotherapy of skull base meningiomas

Authors	Year	No. of patients	Technique	Dose (Gy)	FU (months)	Tumor control (%)	Late toxicity (%)
Carella et al. [9]	1982	57	EBRT	55–60	NA	95	NA
Forbes and Goldberg [10]	1984	31	EBRT	53	45	72 at 4 years	13
Barbaro et al. [7]	1987	54	EBRT	52.5	78	68	0
Miralbell et al. [14]	1992	36	EBRT	45–64	88	84 at 8 years	16
Goldsmith et al. [3]	1994	117	EBRT	54	40	89 at 5 years; 77 at 10 years	3.6
Maire et al. [11]	1995	91	EBRT	52	40	94	6.5
Peele et al. [16]	1996	42	EBRT	55	48	100	5
Condra et al. [18]	1997	28	EBRT	53.3	98	87 at 15 years	24
Connell et al. [19]	1999	54	EBRT	54	55	76 at 5 years	19
Maguire et al. [20]	1999	26	EBRT	53	41	81 at 8 years	8
Nutting et al. [15]	1999	82	EBRT	55–60	41	92 at 5 and 83 at 10 years	14
Vendrely et al. [17]	1999	156	EBRT	50	40	79 at 5 years	11.5
Dufour et al. [21]	2001	21	EBRT	52	73	93 at 5 and 10 years	3.2
Pourel et al. [22]	2001	38	EBRT	56	30	95 at 5 years	4
Mendenhall et al. [23]	2003	101	EBRT	54	64	95 at 5, 92 at 10, and 15 years	8
Buglione et al. [24]	2014	18	EBRT	46–66	42	52.6 at 5 and 40 at 8 years	0
Debus et al. [25]	2001	189	FSRT	56.8	35	97 at 5 and 96 at 10 years	12
Jalali et al. [26]	2002	41	FSRT	55	21	100	12.1
Lo et al. [27]	2002	18	FSRT	54	30.5	93.3	5
Torres et al. [28]	2003	77	FSRT	48.4	24	97.2	5.2
Selch et al. [29]	2004	45	FSRT	56	36	100 at 3 years	0
Metellus et al. [12]	2005	38	FSRT	53	88.6	94.7	2.6
Milker-Zabel et al. [13]	2005	317	FSRT	57.6	67	90.5 at 5 and 89 at 10 years	8.2
Henzel et al. [30]	2006	84	FSRT	56	30	100	NA
Brell et al. [8]	2006	30	FSRT	52	50	93 at 4 years	6.6
Hamm et al. [31]	2008	183	FSRT	56	36	97 at 5 years	8.2
Minniti et al. [32]	2011	52	FSRT	50	42	93 at 5 years	5.5
Solda et al. [33]	2013	222	FSRT	50–55	43	93 at 5 years and 86 at 10 years	5
Fokas et al. [34]	2014	253	FSRT	50–55.8	50	92.9 at 5 years	3
Kaul et al. [35]	2014	179	FSRT	57	35	92.7 at 5 years and 85.8 at 10 years	0.7
Combs et al. [36]	2013	507	376 SRT/131 IMRT	57.6	107	91 at 10 years	NA
Uy et al. [37]	2002	40	IMRT	50.4	30	93 at 5 years	5
Pirzkall et al. [38]	2003	20	IMRT	57	36	100	0
Sajja et al. [39]	2005	35	IMRT	50.4	19.1	97 at 3 years	0
Milker-Zabel et al. [40]	2007	94	IMRT	57.6	52	93.6	4
Wenkel et al. [41]	2000	46	Prot/Phot	59	53	100 at 5 and 88 at 10 years	16
Vernimmen et al. [42]	2001	23	Protons	20.6	38	87	13
Weber et al. [43]	2004	16	Protons	56	34.1	91.7 at 3 years	24
Noel et al. [44]	2005	51	Prot/Phot	60.6	21	98 at 4 years	4
Slater et al. [45]	2012	72	Protons	59	74	99 at 5 years	8.3
Combs et al. [46]	2013	107	Protons	57.6	12	100 (grade I) and 33 (grades II–III) at 2 years	0

23.4 Intensity-Modulated Radiotherapy (IMRT)

Intensity-modulated radiotherapy (IMRT) is an advanced mode of 3D conformal radiotherapy that uses computer-controlled linear accelerators to deliver precise radiation doses to a malignant tumor or specific areas within the tumor. IMRT combines two advanced concepts to deliver 3D conformal radiotherapy: (A) inverse treatment planning with optimization by computer and (B) computer-controlled intensity modulation of the radiation beam during treatment. IMRT for meningiomas could result in greater conformality and better target coverage than 3D CRT [51].

Few series are available on the use of IMRT in patients with meningiomas [37–40] (Table 23.1). Milker-Zabel et al. [40] reported data of 94 patients with complex-shaped meningiomas treated with IMRT with a median follow-up of 4.4 years. Overall local control was 93.6 %. Sixty-nine patients had stable disease, whereas 19 had a tumor volume reduction after IMRT. In 39.8 % of the patients, preexisting neurological deficits improved. Transient side effects such as headache were seen in 7 patients. Treatment-induced loss of vision was seen in 1 of 53 with a grade 3 meningioma, 9 months after retreatment with IMRT.

Others have reported similar results in small series, with a reported local control of 93–97 % at median follow-up of 19–36 months and low toxicity [37–39], suggesting that IMRT is a feasible treatment modality for control of complexly shaped meningiomas.

23.5 Proton Radiotherapy

Proton therapy is a type of external beam radiotherapy using a cyclotron to generate beams of protons. Due to their relatively large mass, protons have little lateral side scatter in the living tissue. Therefore, the beams can be highly focused on the tumor and deliver only low dose to surrounding tissue with a potentially lower risk of side effect.

At the Centre de Protonthérapie d'Orsay (CPO), Noel et al. [52] treated, between December 1995 and December 1999, 17 patients using a 201-MeV proton beam combining high-energy photons and protons for approximately 2/3 and 1/3 of the total dose. The median total dose delivered within gross tumor volume was 61 cobalt gray equivalent (CGE) (25–69). The 4-year local control and overall survival rates were 87.5 ± 12 % and 88.9 ± 11 %, respectively. Authors recorded 11 stable diseases (65 %) and five partial responses (29 %).

Wenkel et al. [41] reported data of 46 patients with partially resected or recurrent meningiomas treated between 1981 and 1996 with combined photon and 160-MeV proton beam therapy at the Massachusetts General Hospital (MGH). Overall survival at 5 and 10 years was 93 and 77 %, respectively. At a median follow-up of 53 months, 8 (17 %) of patients developed severe long-term toxicity from RT, including ophthalmologic, neurological, and otologic complications.

At a median follow-up of 40 months, a tumor control of 89 % has been reported by Vernimmen et al. [42] in 27 patients with large skull base meningiomas treated with stereotactic proton beam therapy. Permanent neurological deficits were reported in three patients.

23.6 Stereotactic Radiosurgery (SRS)

Single-fraction stereotactic focused irradiation (stereotactic radiosurgery; SRS) has been extensively employed in the treatment of skull base meningiomas as alternative treatment for lesions not amenable to surgical removal. Since its introduction into clinical practice in 1985 by Colombo et al. [53], the procedure has proved to be safe and reliable. Reported results, in terms of clinical stabilization and tumor growth control, seem to be relatively independent of the device (GammaKnife or modified linear accelerator [LINAC]). Most studies describe 5-year tumor control rates of about 90–95 %, with a low or very low treatment-related complication rate [54] (Table 23.2).

In the largest single center series reported to date, Kondziolka et al. [61] described a series of

Table 23.2 Summary of results on main published studies on SRS of skull base meningiomas

	Year	System	No. of patients	FU (months)	5-year tumor control (%)	Late toxicity (%)
Roche et al. [55]	2000	GKS	92	30	94	2
Nicolato et al. [56]	2002	GKS	122	48	96	2.5
Kreil et al. [57]	2005	GKS	200	94	98.5	4.5
Malik et al. [58]	2005	GKS	309	96	87	3
Hasegawa et al. [59]	2007	GKS	115	62	94	5.5
Kollovà et al. [60]	2007	GKS	368	60	97.9	5.7
Kondziolka et al. [61]	2008	GKS	972	48	97	7.7
Villavicencio et al. [62]	2001	LINAC	56	60	95	9
Friedman et al. [63]	2005	LINAC	210	39	96	2.3
Patil et al. [64]	2009	CKS	102	20.9	–	14.7
Colombo et al. [54]	2009	CKS	199	30	93.5	0.5
Pollock et al. [65]	2012	GKS	416	60	96	11

972 patients, mostly with skull base meningiomas, who underwent GammaKnife SRS at the University of Pittsburgh. The median marginal dose was 13 Gy. Tumor control rates were 93 % at 5 years and 87 % at 10 and 15 years. Tumor volumes decreased in 34 %, remained stable in 60 %, and increased in 6 % of patients. No difference between 384 patients who underwent postoperative SRS and 488 patients treated with primary SRS was recorded [19].

In a meta-analysis published in 2010, Pannullo et al. [66] collected data of 2734 patients from ten series on GammaKnife and five on LINAC radiosurgery. The tumor volume ranged from 0.11 to 121.8 cm^3. The follow-up ranged 4–144 months. Radiosurgery was performed as first line in 0–78 % of cases and the proportion of benign meningiomas ranged from 77.5 to 100 %. Tumor control rates averaged 89 %. Authors did not find remarkable differences between the two techniques [66].

More recently the image-guided robotic radiosurgery system (CyberKnife; Accuray Inc., Sunnyvale, Ca, USA) has been employed for frameless SRS in patients with skull base meningiomas. The CyberKnife is a frameless 6 MV LINAC system [67–69]. Real-time image guidance is based on digitally reconstructed skull radiographs used to localize the patient head position during treatment. Two x-ray imaging devices positioned on either side of the patient's anatomy acquire real-time digital radiographs of the skull at repeated intervals during treatment.

The images acquired during the treatment are automatically registered to digitally reconstructed radiographs derived from the treatment planning CT scans. This registration process allows the position of the skull (and thus the treatment site) to be translated to the coordinate frame of the LINAC.

CyberKnife technology (Fig. 23.1) is basically designed to perform hypofractionated treatments (usually 2–5 fractions). Such strongly hypofractionated treatments allows the delivery of ablative, radiosurgical doses to the lesion in association with an enhanced protection of the adjacent tissues receiving lower doses and lower dose rates but also being allowed precious time to recover between fractions. Frameless hypofractionated radiosurgery of lesions affecting the cranial nerves including the optic nerves substantially enhances treatment safety and prevention of dreaded neurological complications [67]. Furthermore, frameless systems are not limited to delivering spherical dose distributions (i.e., treatment planning and delivery can be nonisocentric). Conventional radiosurgery systems use multiple spherical isocenters. Nonisocentric planning provides a straightforward approach for the treatment of irregularly shaped lesions.

Colombo et al. [70] in a series of 199 benign intracranial meningiomas (157 skull base meningiomas) reported a 5-year control of 93.5 %. Tumors larger than 8 ml and/or situated close to critical structures were treated with hypofractionated stereotactic RT (2–5 daily fractions).

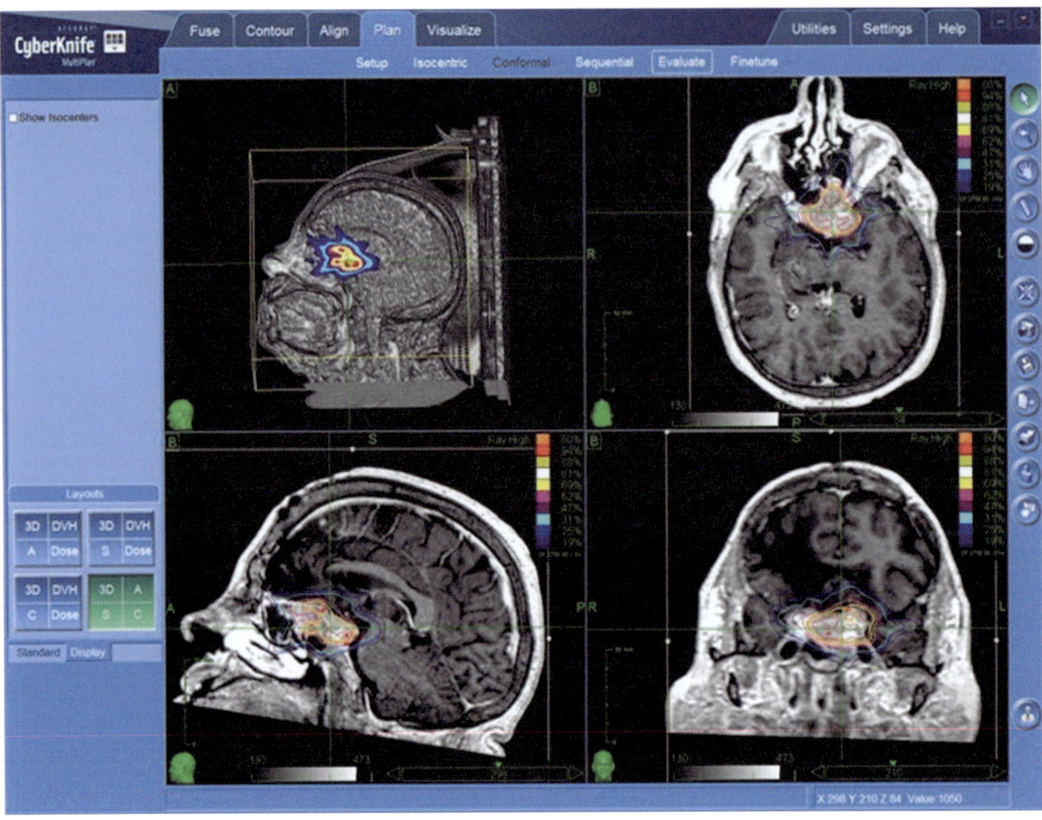

Fig. 23.1 CyberKnife hypofractionated radiosurgery treatment plan for a recurrent tuberculum sellae meningioma encasing the left optic nerve and the chiasm

The tumor volume decreased in 36 patients, was unchanged in 148 patients, and increased in 7 patients. Clinical symptoms improved in 30 patients. Tumor control in 63 patients with tumor volume up 65 ml treated with hypofractionated RT was similar to that obtained in smaller meningiomas treated with single-fraction SRS. Neurological deterioration was observed in 4 % of patients, represented mainly by visual deficits. Although the small numbers of fractions conventionally used with the CyberKnife, hypofractionated treatments seem safer than SRS for large parasellar meningiomas; further large series with appropriate follow-up should confirm the low risk of optic neuropathy in patients treated with hypofractionated regimens.

Few studies have compared the outcome of SRS and FSRT in skull base meningiomas [12, 27, 28]. Metellus et al. [12] found actuarial progression-free survival of 94.7 % in 38 patients treated by fractionated RT group and 94.4 % in 36 patients treated by SRS, with permanent morbidity of 2.6 % after FSRT and 0 % after SRS.

Torres et al. [28] reported on 77 patients treated with SRS and 51 patients treated with FSRT. Tumor control was achieved in 90 % of patients at a median follow-up of 40 months after SRS and in 97 % of patients at a median follow-up of 24 months following FSRT. Late complications were recorded in 5 % of patients treated with SRS and 5.2 % patients treated with FSRT.

Doses of radiations used to treat meningiomas ranged between 12 and 18 Gy. Nonetheless, over the last years, SRS doses have been progressively decreased. Ganz et al. [71] reported on 97 patients with meningiomas with median volume of 15.9 cm^3 treated with GammaKnife SRS using a dose of 12 Gy. At a median follow-up of 54 months, the 2-year progression-free survival was 100 %. Twenty-seven were smaller and 72 unchanged in volume. Three patients suffered adverse radiation effects. Overall, it seems that using 12–14 Gy, the rates of tumor control rate at 5 years remain in the range of 90–95 % as for higher doses [60, 71, 72].

Generally speaking, the concept of tumor control after irradiation of meningioma consists in the stabilization of its sizes. A proportion of cases may show a certain degree of shrinkage, ranging from 16 to 69 % in the different series, and tends to increase along with the time. A variable improvement of neurological functions has been shown in 10–60 % of patients, consisting in recovery of cranial nerve deficits, headache, and fatigue.

Analysis of factors predicting local tumor control in most series shows no significant differences between patients who underwent SRS as primary treatment and patients treated for incomplete resected or recurrent meningioma. Age, sex, site of meningioma, and neurological status did not affect significantly the outcome in most published series; however larger meningiomas are associated with worse long-term local control [61, 73]. DiBiase et al. [73] reported a significant higher 5-year tumor control in patients with meningiomas <10 ml than those with larger tumors (92 % vs 68 %, $p=0.038$). In the series by Kondziolka et al. [61], patients with meningioma poorer local control was correlated with increasing volume ($p=0.01$).

Complications of SRS are reported in 3–40 % of cases. Kondziolka et al. [61] reported permanent neurological deficits in 9 % of patients at 10 and 15 years in 972 patients treated with GK SRS for intracranial meningiomas. The morbidity rate for cavernous sinus meningiomas was 6.3 %, including visual deterioration, 6th nerve palsy, and trigeminal neuropathy. In the series by Nicolato et al. [56], late complications occurred in 4.5 % of patients, being transient in 80 % of them, and similar complication rates have been reported in main published series (Table 23.2). Other complications, as epilepsy, internal carotid occlusion, and hypopituitarism, have been rarely reported (less than 1–2 %).

A clear volume relationship for side effects has been reported, as well as a clear dose dependency; this holds true for toxicity to cranial nerves, as well as for the development of intracranial edema [65, 74, 75]. Based on these data, limitations can be seen for complex volumes adjacent to organs at risk and with increasing size, while fractionated treatments are associated with a comparable dose profile independent of tumor volume or diameter [25, 30, 31, 72, 76–78].

One main issue concerns whether "perioptic" meningiomas, tumors within 2 mm from the optic apparatus, can be managed by hypofractionated regimens, 2–5 fractions, as those typically delivered with the CyberKnife. Adler and coll. treated 49 patients with perioptic tumors, including 27 meningiomas, in 2–5 sessions with a cumulative average marginal dose of 2030 cGy [79]. At a follow-up of 49 months, vision was improved in eight patients (16 %), but worsened in three patients (6 %). In two cases the deterioration was attributed to tumor progression, but the use of 2100 cGy in 3 sessions was associated with loss of vision in one patient. Romanelli and coll. described four patients with optic nerve sheath meningiomas treated with 2000 cGy in 4 sessions with optimal preservation of vision after a follow-up of 37 months [80]. Colombo and coll. treated 29 perioptic meningiomas using up to 5 fractions and up to 2500 cGy [54]. Authors recorded visual worsening in two cases (1 % of the overall series); again this was ascribed to the tumor progression. In our series, 68 patients were treated for perioptic meningiomas and up to 500 cGy/fraction to the optic structures with no neuro-worsening neither tumor progression at 48 months [81].

Despite the very limited numbers of patients and follow-up, some considerations can be done on the basis of abovementioned data. The delivery of up to 500 cGy per fraction to the optic nerve, in a 5-session scheme, is commonly adopted and felt safe. Fundamentally, this is confirmed by midterm data, with no patient deteriorated with 22–25 Gy in 5 fractions. One patient deteriorated with 21 Gy in 3 fractions.

The issue visual deterioration due to tumor progression seems to be even more relevant than the radioinduced optic neuropathy at the currently used dose/fraction schemes. The loss of control of tumor progression in those meningiomas is not inconsequential and was the principal cause of functional deterioration in both the series of Adler et al. [79] and Colombo et al. [54].

Accordingly, it appears that the treatment of meningiomas in close proximity, or even encasing the optic nerves and chiasm, appears possible using hypofractionation paradigms. Definitive results on the safety in terms of tumor control/radioinduced neuropathy in the long term are still awaited.

Conclusions

The use of radiations to treat skull base benign meningiomas results in satisfactory results with local control rates that could rival those of surgical resection. Currently, 5-year progression-free survival with the aid of modern radiotherapy techniques averages 95 % and 10-year reaches 85–90 % in most series. Particularly, radiosurgery has progressively emerged as the first-line treatment for both adjuvant treatment of residual tumors and an effective primary treatment of difficult anterior skull base meningiomas. Radiosurgery is virtually noninvasive, but it does carry a risk of radiation-induced complications. The main issue, in such tumors, concerns the proximity of cranial nerves, including optic nerves and chiasm, that are extremely sensitive to radioinduced complications. Another possible complication is radioinduced hypopituitarism, for which patients should be checked for a long time after treatment. Oculomotor nerves and trigeminal nerves can be also involved by high dose of radiations, but stable deficits have been rarely reported. Hypofractionated radiosurgery has provided interesting results with very limited risks of optic neuropathy, even though longer-term results are still necessary to identify the best dose/fractionation schemes.

References

1. Cusimano M, Sekhar L, Sen C, Pomonis S, Wright D, Biglan A, Jannetta P (1995) The results of surgery for benign tumors of the cavernous sinus. Neurosurgery 37:1–9
2. Kallio M, Sankila R, Hakulinen T, Jaaskelainen J (1992) Factors affecting operative and excess long-term mortality in 935 patients with intracranial meningioma. Neurosurgery 31:2–12
3. Goldsmith B, Wara W, Wilson C, Larson D (1994) Postoperative irradiation for subtotally resected meningiomas. J Neurosurg 80:195–201
4. Mirimanoff RO, Dosoretz DE, Linggood RM, Ojemann RG, Martuza RL (1985) Meningioma: analysis of recurrence and progression following neurosurgical resection. J Neurosurg 62(1):18–24. doi:10.3171/jns.1985.62.1.0018
5. Stafford S, Pollock B, Foote R, Link M, Gorman D, Schomberg P, Leavitt J (2001) Meningioma radiosurgery: tumor control, outcomes, and complications among 190 consecutive patients. Neurosurgery 49:1029–1037
6. Conti A, Pontoriero A, Salamone I, Siragusa C, Midili F, La Torre D, Calisto A, Granata F, Romanelli P, De Renzis C, Tomasello F (2009) Protecting venous structures during radiosurgery for parasagittal meningiomas. Neurosurg Focus 27(5), E11. doi:10.3171/2009.8.FOCUS09-157
7. Barbaro N, Gutin P, Wilson C, Sheline G, Boldrey E, Wara W (1987) Radiation therapy in the treatment of partially resected meningiomas. Neurosurgery 20:525–528
8. Brell M, Villa S, Teixidor P, Lucas A, Ferran E, Marin S, Acebes J (2006) Fractionated stereotactic radiotherapy in the treatment of exclusive cavernous sinus meningioma: functional outcome, local control, and tolerance. Surg Neurol 65:28–33
9. Carella R, Ransohoff J, Newall J (1982) Role of radiation therapy in the management of meningioma. Neurosurgery 10:332–339
10. Forbes A, Goldberg I (1984) Radiation therapy in the treatment of meningioma: the Joint Center for Radiation Therapy experience 1970 to 1982. J Clin Oncol 2:1139–1143
11. Maire J, Caudry M, Guerin J, Celerier D, San Galli F, Causse N, Trouette R, Dautheribes M (1995) Fractionated radiation therapy in the treatment of intracranial meningiomas: local control, functional efficacy, and tolerance in 91 patients. Int J Radiat Oncol Biol Phys 33:315–321
12. Metellus P, Regis J, Muracciole X, Fuentes S, Dufour H, Nanni I, Chinot O, Martin P, Grisoli F (2005) Evaluation of fractionated radiotherapy and gamma knife radiosurgery in cavernous sinus meningiomas: treatment strategy. Neurosurgery 57:873–886
13. Milker-Zabel S, Zabel A, Schulz-Ertner D, Schlegel W, Wannenmacher M, Debus J (2005) Fractionated stereotactic radiotherapy in patients with benign or atypical intracranial meningioma: long-term experience and prognostic factors. Int J Radiat Oncol Biol Phys 61:809–816
14. Miralbell R, Linggood R, de la Monte S, Convery K, Munzenrider J, Mirimanoff R (1992) The role of radiotherapy in the treatment of subtotally resected benign meningiomas. J Neurooncol 13:157–164
15. Nutting C, Brada M, Brazil L, Sibtain A, Saran F, Westbury C, Moore A, Thomas D, Traish D, Ashley S (1999) Radiotherapy in the treatment of benign meningioma of the skull base. J Neurosurg 90:823–827

16. Peele K, Kennerdell J, Maroon J, Kalnicki S, Kazim M, Gardner T, Malton M, Goodglick T, Rosen C (1996) The role of postoperative irradiation in the management of sphenoid wing meningiomas. Ophthalmology 103:1761–1766
17. Vendrely V, Maire J, Darrouzet V, Bonichon N, San Galli F, Celerier D, Causse N, Demeaux H, Trouette R, Dahan O, Recaldini L, Guerin J, Caudry M (1999) Fractionated radiotherapy of intracranial meningiomas: 15 years' experience at the Bordeaux University Hospital Center. Cancer Radiother 3:311–317
18. Condra K, Buatti J, Mendenhall W, Friedman W, Marcus R, Rhoton A (1997) Benign meningiomas: primary treatment selection affects survival. Int J Radiat Oncol Biol Phys 39:427–436
19. Connell P, Macdonald R, Mansur D, Nicholas M, Mundt A (1999) Tumor size predicts control of benign meningiomas treated with radiotherapy. Neurosurgery 44:1194–1199
20. Maguire P, Clough R, Friedman A, Halperin E (1999) Fractionated external-beam radiation therapy for meningiomas of the cavernous sinus. Int J Radiat Oncol Biol Phys 44:75–79
21. Dufour H, Muracciole X, Metellus P, Regis J, Chinot O, Grisoli F (2001) Long-term tumor control and functional outcome in patients with cavernous sinus meningiomas treated by radiotherapy with or without previous surgery: is there an alternative to aggressive tumor removal? Neurosurgery 48:285–294
22. Pourel N, Auque J, Bracard S, Hoffstetter S, Luporsi E, Vignaud J, Bey P (2001) Efficacy of external fractionated radiation therapy in the treatment of meningiomas: a 20-year experience. Radiother Oncol 61:65–70
23. Mendenhall W, Morris C, Amdur R, Foote K, Friedman W (2003) Radiotherapy alone or after subtotal resection for benign skull base meningiomas. Cancer 98:1473–1482
24. Buglione M, De Bari B, Trevisan F, Ghirardelli P, Pedretti S, Triggiani L, Magrini SM (2014) Role of external beam radiotherapy in the treatment of relapsing meningioma. Med Oncol 31(3):866. doi:10.1007/s12032-014-0866-y
25. Debus J, Wuendrich M, Pirzkall A, Hoess A, Schlegel W, Zuna I, Engenhart-Cabillic R, Wannenmacher M (2001) High efficacy of fractionated stereotactic radiotherapy of large base-of-skull meningiomas: long-term results. J Clin Oncol 19:3547–3553
26. Jalali R, Loughrey C, Baumert B, Perks J, Warrington A, Traish D, Ashley S, Brada M (2002) High precision focused irradiation in the form of fractionated stereotactic conformal radiotherapy (SCRT) for benign meningiomas predominantly in the skull base location. Clin Oncol (R Coll Radiol) 14:103–109
27. Lo S, Cho K, Hall W, Kossow R, Hernandez W, McCollow K, Gerbi B, Higgins P, Lee C, Dusenbery K (2002) Single dose versus fractionated stereotactic radiotherapy for meningiomas. Can J Neurol Sci 29:240–248
28. Torres R, Frighetto L, De Salles A, Goss B, Medin P, Solberg T, Ford J, Selch M (2003) Radiosurgery and stereotactic radiotherapy for intracranial meningiomas. Neurosurg Focus 14, e5
29. Selch M, Ahn E, Laskari A, Lee S, Agazaryan N, Solberg T, Cabatan-Awang C, Frighetto L, Desalles A (2004) Stereotactic radiotherapy for treatment of cavernous sinus meningiomas. Int J Radiat Oncol Biol Phys 59:101–111
30. Henzel M, Gross M, Hamm K, Surber G, Kleinert G, Failing T, Strassman G, Engenhart-Cabillic R (2006) Significant tumor volume reduction of meningiomas after stereotactic radiotherapy: results of a prospective multicenter study. Neurosurgery 59:1188–1194
31. Hamm K, Henzel M, Gross M, Surber G, Kleinert G, Engenhart-Cabillic R (2008) Radiosurgery/stereotactic radiotherapy in the therapeutical concept for skull base meningiomas. Zentralbl Neurochir 69:14–21
32. Minniti G, Clarke E, Cavallo L, Osti MF, Esposito V, Cantore G, Cappabianca P, Enrici RM (2011) Fractionated stereotactic conformal radiotherapy for large benign skull base meningiomas. Radiat Oncol 6:36. doi:10.1186/1748-717X-6-36, 1748-717X-6-36 [pii]
33. Solda F, Wharram B, De Ieso PB, Bonner J, Ashley S, Brada M (2013) Long-term efficacy of fractionated radiotherapy for benign meningiomas. Radiother Oncol 109(2):330–334. doi:10.1016/j.radonc.2013.10.006, S0167-8140(13)00509-4 [pii]
34. Fokas E, Henzel M, Surber G, Hamm K, Engenhart-Cabillic R (2014) Stereotactic radiation therapy for benign meningioma: long-term outcome in 318 patients. Int J Radiat Oncol Biol Phys 89(3):569–575. doi:10.1016/j.ijrobp.2014.02.042, S0360-3016(14)00287-9 [pii]
35. Kaul D, Budach V, Wurm R, Gruen A, Graaf L, Habbel P, Badakhshi H (2014) Linac-based stereotactic radiotherapy and radiosurgery in patients with meningioma. Radiat Oncol 9:78. doi:10.1186/1748-717X-9-78, 1748-717X-9-78 [pii]
36. Combs SE, Adeberg S, Dittmar JO, Welzel T, Rieken S, Habermehl D, Huber PE, Debus J (2013) Skull base meningiomas: long-term results and patient self-reported outcome in 507 patients treated with fractionated stereotactic radiotherapy (FSRT) or intensity modulated radiotherapy (IMRT). Radiother Oncol 106(2):186–191. doi:10.1016/j.radonc.2012.07.008, S0167-8140(12)00324-6 [pii]
37. Uy N, Woo S, Teh B, Mai W, Carpenter L, Chiu J, Lu H, Gildenberg P, Trask T, Grant W, Butler E (2002) Intensity-modulated radiation therapy (IMRT) for meningioma. Int J Radiat Oncol Biol Phys 53:1265–1270
38. Pirzkall A, Debus J, Haering P, Rhein B, Grosser K, Hoss A, Wannenmacher M (2003) Intensity modulated radiotherapy (IMRT) for recurrent, residual, or untreated skull-base meningiomas: preliminary clinical experience. Int J Radiat Oncol Biol Phys 55:362–372
39. Sajja R, Barnett G, Lee S, Harnisch G, Stevens G, Lee J, Suh J (2005) Intensity-modulated radiation therapy (IMRT) for newly diagnosed and recurrent intracranial meningiomas: preliminary results. Technol Cancer Res Treat 4:675–682

40. Milker-Zabel S, Zabel-du Bois A, Huber P, Schlegel W, Debus J (2007) Intensity-modulated radiotherapy for complex-shaped meningioma of the skull base: long-term experience of a single institution. Int J Radiat Oncol Biol Phys 68:858–863
41. Wenkel E, Thornton A, Finkelstein D, Adams J, Lyons S, De La Monte S, Ojeman R, Munzenrider J (2000) Benign meningioma: partially resected, biopsied, and recurrent intracranial tumors treated with combined proton and photon radiotherapy. Int J Radiat Oncol Biol Phys 48:1363–1370
42. Vernimmen F, Harris J, Wilson J, Melvill R, Smit B, Slabbert J (2001) Stereotactic proton beam therapy of skull base meningiomas. Int J Radiat Oncol Biol Phys 49:99–105
43. Weber D, Lomax A, Rutz H, Stadelmann O, Egger E, Timmermann B, Pedroni E, Verwey J, Miralbell R, Goitein G, Group SPU (2004) Spot-scanning proton radiation therapy for recurrent, residual or untreated intracranial meningiomas. Radiother Oncol 71:251–258
44. Noel G, Bollet M, Calugaru V, Feuvret L, Haie-Meder C, Dhermain F, Ferrand R, Boisserie G, Beaudre A, Mazeron J, Habrand J (2005) Functional outcome of patients with benign meningioma treated by 3D conformal irradiation with a combination of photons and protons. Int J Radiat Oncol Biol Phys 62:1412–1422
45. Slater JD, Loredo LN, Chung A, Bush DA, Patyal B, Johnson WD, Hsu FP, Slater JM (2012) Fractionated proton radiotherapy for benign cavernous sinus meningiomas. Int J Radiat Oncol Biol Phys 83(5):e633–e637. doi:10.1016/j.ijrobp.2012.01.079, S0360-3016(12)00184-8 [pii]
46. Combs SE, Kessel K, Habermehl D, Haberer T, Jakel O, Debus J (2013) Proton and carbon ion radiotherapy for primary brain tumors and tumors of the skull base. Acta Oncol 52(7):1504–1509. doi:10.3109/0284186X.2013.818255
47. Glaholm J, Bloom HJ, Crow JH (1990) The role of radiotherapy in the management of intracranial meningiomas: the Royal Marsden Hospital experience with 186 patients. Int J Radiat Oncol Biol Phys 18(4):755–761. doi:0360-3016(90)90394-Y [pii]
48. Goldsmith BJ, Rosenthal SA, Wara WM, Larson DA (1992) Optic neuropathy after irradiation of meningioma. Radiology 185(1):71–76. doi:10.1148/radiology.185.1.1523337
49. Crossen J, Garwood D, Glatstein E, Neuwelt E (1994) Neurobehavioral sequelae of cranial irradiation in adults: a review of radiation-induced encephalopathy. J Clin Oncol 12:627–642
50. Minniti G, Traish D, Ashley S, Gonsalves A, Brada M (2005) Risk of second brain tumor after conservative surgery and radiotherapy for pituitary adenoma: update after an additional 10 years. J Clin Endocrinol Metab 90:800–804
51. Pirzkall A, Carol M, Lohr F, Hoss A, Wannenmacher M, Debus J (2000) Comparison of intensity-modulated radiotherapy with conventional conformal radiotherapy for complex-shaped tumors. Int J Radiat Oncol Biol Phys 48:1371–1380
52. Noel G, Bollet MA, Calugaru V, Feuvret L, Haie-Meder C, Dhermain F, Ferrand R, Boisserie G, Beaudre A, Mazeron JJ, Habrand JL (2005) Functional outcome of patients with benign meningioma treated by 3D conformal irradiation with a combination of photons and protons. Int J Radiat Oncol Biol Phys 62(5):1412–1422. doi:10.1016/j.ijrobp.2004.12.048, S0360-3016(04)03155-4 [pii]
53. Colombo F, Benedetti A, Pozza F, Zanardo A, Avanzo RC, Chierego G, Marchetti C (1985) Stereotactic radiosurgery utilizing a linear accelerator. Appl Neurophysiol 48(1–6):133–145
54. Colombo F, Casentini L, Cavedon C, Scalchi P, Cora S, Francescon P (2009) Cyberknife radiosurgery for benign meningiomas: short-term results in 199 patients. Neurosurgery 64(2 Suppl):A7–A13. doi:10.1227/01.NEU.0000338947.84636.A6, 00006123-200902001-00003 [pii]
55. Roche P, Regis J, Dufour H, Fournier H, Delsanti C, Pellet W, Grisoli F, Peragut J (2000) Gamma knife radiosurgery in the management of cavernous sinus meningiomas. J Neurosurg 3:68–73
56. Nicolato A, Foroni R, Alessandrini F, Maluta S, Bricolo A, Gerosa M (2002) The role of Gamma Knife radiosurgery in the management of cavernous sinus meningiomas. Int J Radiat Oncol Biol Phys 53:992–1000
57. Kreil W, Luggin J, Fuchs I, Weigl V, Eustacchio S, Papaefthymiou G (2005) Long term experience of gamma knife radiosurgery for benign skull base meningiomas. J Neurol Neurosurg Psychiatry 76:1425–1430
58. Malik I, Rowe JG, Walton L, Radatz MW, Kemeny AA (2005) The use of stereotactic radiosurgery in the management of meningiomas. Br J Neurosurg 19(1):13–20. doi:10.1080/02688690500080885, T60TT64L4540N119 [pii]
59. Hasegawa T, Kida Y, Yoshimoto M, Koike J, Iizuka H, Ishii D (2007) Long-term outcomes of Gamma Knife surgery for cavernous sinus meningioma. J Neurosurg 107:745–751
60. Kollova A, Liscak R, Novotny J, Vladyka V, Simonova G, Janouskova L (2007) Gamma Knife surgery for benign meningioma. J Neurosurg 107:325–336
61. Kondziolka D, Mathieu D, Lunsford L, Martin J, Madhok R, Niranjan A, Flickinger J (2008) Radiosurgery as definitive management of intracranial meningiomas. Neurosurgery 62:53–58
62. Villavicencio A, Black P, Shrieve D, Fallon M, Alexander E, Loeffler J (2001) Linac radiosurgery for skull base meningiomas. Acta Neurochir (Wien) 143:1141–1152
63. Friedman WA, Murad GJ, Bradshaw P, Amdur RJ, Mendenhall WM, Foote KD, Bova FJ (2005) Linear accelerator surgery for meningiomas. J Neurosurg 103(2):206–209. doi:10.3171/jns.2005.103.2.0206
64. Patil CG, Veeravagu A, Lad SP, Boakye M (2010) Craniotomy for resection of meningioma in the elderly: a multicentre, prospective analysis from the National Surgical Quality Improvement Program. J Neurol Neurosurg Psychiatry 81(5):502–505. doi:10.1136/jnnp.2009.185074, jnnp.2009.185074 [pii]

65. Pollock B, Stafford S, Link M, Garces Y, Foote R (2012) Single-fraction radiosurgery for presumed intracranial meningiomas: efficacy and complications from a 22-year experience. Int J Radiat Oncol Biol Phys 83:1414–1418
66. Pannullo SC, Fraser JF, Moliterno J, Cobb W, Stieg PE (2011) Stereotactic radiosurgery: a meta-analysis of current therapeutic applications in neuro-oncologic disease. J Neurooncol 103(1):1–17. doi:10.1007/s11060-010-0360-0
67. Romanelli P, Adler JR Jr (2008) Technology Insight: image-guided robotic radiosurgery – a new approach for noninvasive ablation of spinal lesions. Nat Clin Pract Oncol 5(7):405–414. doi:10.1038/ncponc1131, ncponc1131 [pii]
68. Romanelli P, Conti A, Pontoriero A, Ricciardi GK, Tomasello F, De Renzis C, Innocenzi G, Esposito V, Cantore G (2009) Role of stereotactic radiosurgery and fractionated stereotactic radiotherapy for the treatment of recurrent glioblastoma multiforme. Neurosurg Focus 27(6), E8. doi:10.3171/2009.9.FOCUS09187
69. Conti A, Pontoriero A, Arpa D, Siragusa C, Tomasello C, Romanelli P, Cardali S, Granata F, De Renzis C, Tomasello F (2012) Efficacy and toxicity of CyberKnife re-irradiation and "dose dense" temozolomide for recurrent gliomas. Acta Neurochir (Wien) 154(2):203–209. doi:10.1007/s00701-011-1184-1
70. Colombo F, Casentini L, Cavedon C, Scalchi P, Cora S, Francescon P (2009) Cyberknife radiosurgery for benign meningiomas: short-term results in 199 patients. Neurosurgery 64:A7–A13
71. Ganz J, Reda W, Abdelkarim K (2009) Gamma Knife surgery of large meningiomas: early response to treatment. Acta Neurochir (Wien) 151:1–8
72. Minniti G, Amichetti M, Enrici RM (2009) Radiotherapy and radiosurgery for benign skull base meningiomas. Radiat Oncol 4:42. doi:10.1186/1748-717X-4-42, 1748-717X-4-42 [pii]
73. DiBiase S, Kwok Y, Yovino S, Arena C, Naqvi S, Temple R, Regine W, Amin P, Guo C, Chin L (2004) Factors predicting local tumor control after gamma knife stereotactic radiosurgery for benign intracranial meningiomas. Int J Radiat Oncol Biol Phys 60:1515–1519
74. Morita A, Coffey R, Foote R, Schiff D, Gorman D (1999) Risk of injury to cranial nerves after gamma knife radiosurgery for skull base meningiomas: experience in 88 patients. J Neurosurg 90:42–49
75. Novotny J, Kollova A, Liscak R (2006) Prediction of intracranial edema after radiosurgery of meningiomas. J Neurosurg 105(Suppl):120–126
76. Combs S, Adeberg S, Dittmar J, Welzel T, Rieken S, Habermehl D (2013) Skull base meningiomas: long-term results and patient self-reported outcome in 507 patients treated with fractionated stereotactic radiotherapy (FSRT) or intensity modulated radiotherapy (IMRT). Radiother Oncol 106(2):186–191
77. Henzel M, Gross M, Hamm K, Surber G, Kleinert G, Failing T (2006) Stereotactic radiotherapy of meningiomas: symptomatology, acute and late toxicity. Strahlenther Onkol 182:382–388
78. Minniti G, Clarke E, Cavallo L, Osti M, Esposito V, Cantore G (2011) Fractionated stereotactic conformal radiotherapy for large benign skull base meningiomas. Radiat Oncol 6:36
79. Adler JR Jr, Gibbs IC, Puataweepong P, Chang SD (2006) Visual field preservation after multisession cyberknife radiosurgery for perioptic lesions. Neurosurgery 59(2):244–254. doi:10.1227/01.NEU.0000223512.09115.3E; discussion 244–254. 00006123-200608000-00005 [pii]
80. Romanelli P, Wowra B, Muacevic A (2007) Multisession CyberKnife radiosurgery for optic nerve sheath meningiomas. Neurosurg Focus 23(6), E11. doi:10.3171/FOC-07/12/E11
81. Conti A, Pontoriero A, Midili F, Iatì G, Siragusa C, Tomasello C, La Torre D, Cardali SM, Pergolizzi S, De Renzis C (2015) CyberKnife multisession stereotactic radiosurgery and hypofractionated stereotactic radiotherapy for perioptic meningiomas: intermediate-term results and radiobiological considerations. Springerplus. 4:37. doi:10.1186/s40064-015-0804-2

Part V

Clival Chordomas

24 Introduction

Paolo Cappabianca, Marialaura Del Basso De Caro, and Alessandra D'Amico

Chordomas are quite rare pathological entities occurring with an overall incidence rate of 0.08 per 100,000 [24, 26, 44, 47, 49]. They may occur at any age, although they are most commonly encountered in male patients during the third, fourth, and fifth decades of life and rarely appear in children (<5 %). Chordomas histologically derive from remnants of embryonic notochordal tissue a rodlike cord of cells from which the skull base and vertebral column develop [26, 32, 44, 46]; indeed, they can arise anywhere along the axial skeleton – nearly always within the bone – having a predilection for the sacrum, clivus, or cervical vertebrae [24, 26, 32, 44, 47, 57]. In rare cases (3–7 %), they arise from the cervical spine (cervical chordomas), presenting as a paravertebral or parapharyngeal mass [24, 26, 42, 44, 64].

P. Cappabianca, MD (✉)
Division of Neurosurgery,
Department of Neurosciences,
Reproductive and Odontostomatological Sciences,
Università degli Studi di Napoli "Federico II",
Naples, Italy
e-mail: paolo.cappabianca@unina.it

M. Del Basso De Caro, BS
Anatomopathology Unit,
Department of Advanced Biomedical Sciences,
University of Naples "Federico II", Naples, Italy

A. D'Amico, MD
Neuroradiology Unit,
Department of Advanced Biomedical Sciences,
Università degli Studi di Napoli "Federico II",
Naples, Italy

Almost a third of chordomas arise at the skull base (cranial chordomas) involving the clival area [26, 32, 46, 57]. These tumors are typically slow growing, with an indolent but progressive clinical course; they can be assumed as malignant but classified as tumors of low to intermediate malignancy with a propensity for locally aggressive behavior [14, 22, 26, 32, 49, 57].

Chordomas figure out as midline, usually extradural, masses originating within the bone and, grossly, appear as gelatinous, soft blue-gray multilobulated masses; sparse areas of hemorrhage, cystic and/or necrotic degeneration, or calcification may be encountered. If on one hand these lesions are often well circumscribed at surgical exploration, on the other hand they show a certain degree of local invasiveness with destruction of the adjacent bone and eventual dural invasion. Although there cannot be clearly identified features depicting lesion aggressiveness, several molecular markers could be associated with an aggressive biologic behavior [32, 44].

According to the *WHO classification*, there have been defined three histopathologic patterns of chordoma: classic or conventional, chondroid, and dedifferentiated [5, 26, 36, 44, 50, 51, 54, 64].

The *conventional chordoma* is the most frequent diagnosed lesion: this histotype accounts for islands and cords of eosinophilic and clear vacuolated cells immersed in a basophilic myxoid/mucoid background. Thin fibrous septa can be recognized dividing groups of cells into lobules.

P. Cappabianca et al. (eds.), *Midline Skull Base Surgery*, DOI 10.1007/978-3-319-21533-4_24

Above all, it should be said that this histotype is identified with the most representative microscopic aspect: the majority of cells are vacuolated, so it have been called "physaliphorous cells" (from the Greek word meaning bearer of bubbles). Eventual areas of necrosis seem to draw a more aggressive course, whereas scattered mitoses, nucleoli, vascular invasion, and nuclear pleomorphism seem to not affect the tumor's prognosis. Usually no chondroid or other mesenchymal tissue differentiations are observed [5, 26].

The second histologic pattern of chordomas is defined by the presence of clear chondroid differentiation, however to be not interpreted as evidence of cartilaginous differentiation. This so-called chondroid chordoma is usually related to a better prognosis, although several authors have advocated that this better outcome could be associated with patient age rather than with the histopathologic development. At microscopy there is a resemblance of this tumor with low-grade chondrosarcoma [36, 54].

Finally, the third histologic class of identifies *malignant chordomas*, which present a frank mesenchymal component. This aspect constitutes the basis for the diagnosis of dedifferentiated chordomas; the prognosis is very poor and this tumor leads to death within a year. Hematogenous metastases consisting entirely of sarcomatous elements are common; contrariwise, other patterns of chordomas rarely result in metastasis [14, 42, 50, 52].

Despite the distinctive appearance of most chordomas, there are several important considerations that could be drawn in terms of differential diagnosis: chordomas may be confused with skull base chondrosarcomas, chordoid meningiomas, extraskeletal myxoid chondrosarcomas, metastatic mucinous adenocarcinomas, and, a developmental lesion, ecchordosis physaliphora. Most of them present at direct pathological observation many characteristics similar to the chordomas that could mislead diagnosis. However, according to peculiar features, *chondrosarcomas* differ for negative cytokeratin, as well as extraskeletal myxoid chondrosarcomas. Metastatic mucinous adenocarcinomas are usually negative for S-100 protein and, finally, ecchordosis physaliphoras are easily distinguished by their inferior size, complete lack of osseous components, and benign clinical behavior [26, 32, 47, 50, 51, 57, 62, 64].

When considering radiological appearance, cranial base chordomas on high-resolution computed tomography and magnetic resonance imaging (MRI) can be identified as well-circumscribed, soft tissue masses arising from the clivus and are accompanied by lytic bone destruction. They are isointense on T1-weighted MRI scans and usually post GAD enhancement. On the T2-weighted MRI scans, a hyperintense signal, per bone erosion areas, is observed; chondroid chordomas eventually may present intratumoral calcification [14, 26, 32, 42, 44, 49].

Case history of chordomas is very insidious, with patients that complain of general symptoms as headache, dizziness, and lower limb paresthesia for months/years before medical attention is drawn; when cranial nerve involvement is present, especially the abducens nerve (cranial nerve VI), often it figures out as presenting sign. Seldom, cerebellar syndrome, local neck pain, brainstem syndrome, and/or lower cranial nerve palsies could be present, especially when lesion involves the lower aspect of the clivus [10, 26, 32, 42, 44, 46, 52, 53, 57].

Chordomas pose significant challenges for cranial base surgeons: their central location and their tendency to infiltrate the bone render total removal rarely possible; moreover such tumors are associated with a high incidence of recurrence [7, 14, 16, 22, 26, 42, 44, 49, 51, 55, 62, 64]. Indeed, the achievement of total resection at primary surgery determines a tremendous improvement in 5-year survival rate, whereas it fell down in case of partial removal [1, 17, 26, 32, 40, 57–59]. Besides, it has to be underlined that their proximity to vital neurovascular structures, including cranial nerves and the brainstem, carries significant potential for severe postoperative morbidities. It clearly stands though that the optimal operative approach should offer the best chance of radical removal while minimizing the potential for postoperative complications [1, 16, 17, 21, 23, 42, 55, 61].

Historically, different extensive and complex skull base approaches have been described for the resection of clival chordomas, thus providing neurosurgeons with a wide choice of surgical strategy of accomplishing radical removal [6, 17, 31, 49, 50, 55, 56, 62]. Because chordomas are mainly extradural and midline tumors that displace dorsally the neurovascular structures, ventral corridors have been preferred: indeed, in transfacial [3, 13, 20, 35, 45, 60], transsphenoidal [2, 15, 25, 30, 40, 42, 44, 46, 52, 57], and transoral [11, 19, 34] techniques, lesions have been defined and renewed along with the technological progress and surgical technique refinements.

Al-Mefty and Borba [1] introduced a surgical classification of skull base chordomas as related to their local extension: *type I* that includes lesions limited to one clival compartment, which are rare; *type II* that comprises two or more contiguous areas; and *type III*, in which the lesion extends into several compartments and more than one surgical procedure is necessary. Though, several factors – i.e., location, involvement of the bone and eventually of the occipital condyles, and craniocervical instability – have to be considered in detail when choosing the proper surgical management. Furthermore, it has to be said that in this era of minimally invasiveness, adjunctive proton beam treatment and maximum possible removal have been claimed as viable strategy to achieve a longer and better tumor control [4, 9, 16, 27, 33, 42, 44, 48, 61, 63].

In more recent times, the increasing use of the endoscope in transsphenoidal surgery has allowed the endonasal route to be considered for the management of lesions of the cranial base, thus unlocking new possibilities for skull base surgery [8, 12, 18, 37–39, 43]. This technique allows a wide and median exposure of the targeted area, with a more orientable and closeup view, while obviating brain retraction. The wider and panoramic view offered by the endoscope and the rapid growth of neuroradiological diagnostic techniques together with the intraoperative neuronavigation systems has expanded its applicability to the removal of skull base chordomas [10, 26, 28, 29, 40, 41, 59].

We herein present the surgical nuances – according to our experience – of the endoscopic endonasal approach in the treatment of chordomas, aiming to highlight the feasibility of this technique and evaluate its advantages and limitations.

References

1. Al-Mefty O, Borba LA (1997) Skull base chordomas: a management challenge. J Neurosurg 86(2):182–189. doi:10.3171/jns.1997.86.2.0182
2. Al-Mefty O, Kadri PA, Hasan DM, Isolan GR, Pravdenkova S (2008) Anterior clivectomy: surgical technique and clinical applications. J Neurosurg 109(5):783–793. doi:10.3171/JNS/2008/109/11/0783
3. Anand VK, Harkey HL, Al-Mefty O (1991) Open-door maxillotomy approach for lesions of the clivus. Skull Base Surg 1(4):217–225
4. Ares C, Hug EB, Lomax AJ, Bolsi A, Timmermann B, Rutz HP, Schuller JC, Pedroni E, Goitein G (2009) Effectiveness and safety of spot scanning proton radiation therapy for chordomas and chondrosarcomas of the skull base: first long-term report. Int J Radiat Oncol Biol Phys 75(4):1111–1118. doi:10.1016/j.ijrobp.2008.12.055
5. Barnes L, Kapadia SB (1994) The biology and pathology of selected skull base tumors. J Neurooncol 20(3):213–240
6. Bertalanffy H, Seeger W (1991) The dorsolateral, suboccipital, transcondylar approach to the lower clivus and anterior portion of the craniocervical junction. Neurosurgery 29(6):815–821
7. Borba LA, Al-Mefty O, Mrak RE, Suen J (1996) Cranial chordomas in children and adolescents. J Neurosurg 84(4):584–591. doi:10.3171/jns.1996.84.4.0584
8. Cappabianca P, Cavallo LM, Esposito F, de Divitiis O, Messina A, de Divitiis E (2008) Extended endoscopic endonasal approach to the midline skull base: the evolving role of transsphenoidal surgery. In: Pickard JD, Akalan N, Di Rocco C et al (eds) Advances and technical standards in neurosurgery. Springer, Wien/New York, pp 152–199
9. Catton C, O'Sullivan B, Bell R, Laperriere N, Cummings B, Fornasier V, Wunder J (1996) Chordoma: long-term follow-up after radical photon irradiation. Radiother Oncol 41(1):67–72
10. Chibbaro S, Cornelius JF, Froelich S, Tigan L, Kehrli P, Debry C, Romano A, Herman P, George B, Bresson D (2014) Endoscopic endonasal approach in the management of skull base chordomas – clinical experience on a large series, technique, outcome, and pitfalls. Neurosurg Rev 37(2):217–224; discussion 224–215. doi:10.1007/s10143-013-0503-9

11. Choi D, Crockard HA (2013) Evolution of transoral surgery: three decades of change in patients, pathologies, and indications. Neurosurgery 73(2):296–303; discussion 303–294. doi:10.1227/01.neu.0000430324.24623.10
12. Ciporen JN, Moe KS, Ramanathan D, Lopez S, Ledesma E, Rostomily R, Sekhar LN (2010) Multiportal endoscopic approaches to the central skull base: a cadaveric study. World Neurosurg 73(6):705–712. doi:10.1016/j.wneu.2010.03.033
13. Cocke EW Jr, Robertson JH, Robertson JT, Crook JP Jr (1990) The extended maxillotomy and subtotal maxillectomy for excision of skull base tumors. Arch Otolaryngol Head Neck Surg 116(1):92–104
14. Colli BO, Al-Mefty O (2001) Chordomas of the skull base: follow-up review and prognostic factors. Neurosurg Focus 10(3), E1. doi:10.3171/foc.2001.10.3.2
15. Couldwell WT, Weiss MH, Rabb C, Liu JK, Apfelbaum RI, Fukushima T (2004) Variations on the standard transsphenoidal approach to the sellar region, with emphasis on the extended approaches and parasellar approaches: surgical experience in 105 cases. Neurosurgery 55(3):539–550
16. Crockard HA, Steel T, Plowman N, Singh A, Crossman J, Revesz T, Holton JL, Cheeseman A (2001) A multidisciplinary team approach to skull base chordomas. J Neurosurg 95(2):175–183. doi:10.3171/jns.2001.95.2.0175
17. Crumley RL, Gutin PH (1989) Surgical access for clivus chordoma. The University of California, San Francisco, experience. Arch Otolaryngol Head Neck Surg 115(3):295–300
18. de Divitiis E, Cappabianca P, Cavallo LM (2002) Endoscopic transsphenoidal approach: adaptability of the procedure to different sellar lesions. Neurosurgery 51(3):699–705; discussion 705–707
19. Delgado TE, Garrido E, Harwick RD (1981) Labiomandibular, transoral approach to chordomas in the clivus and upper cervical spine. Neurosurgery 8(6):675–679
20. DeMonte F, Diaz E Jr, Callender D, Suk I (2001) Transmandibular, circumglossal, retropharyngeal approach for chordomas of the clivus and upper cervical spine. Technical note. Neurosurg Focus 10(3), E10
21. Diaz RJ, Cusimano MD (2011) The biological basis for modern treatment of chordoma. J Neurooncol 104(2):411–422. doi:10.1007/s11060-011-0559-8
22. Diaz RJ, Guduk M, Romagnuolo R, Smith CA, Northcott P, Shih D, Berisha F, Flanagan A, Munoz DG, Cusimano MD, Pamir MN, Rutka JT (2012) High-resolution whole-genome analysis of skull base chordomas implicates FHIT loss in chordoma pathogenesis. Neoplasia 14(9):788–798
23. Diaz RJ, Maggacis N, Zhang S, Cusimano MD (2014) Determinants of quality of life in patients with skull base chordoma. J Neurosurg 120(2):528–537. doi:10.3171/2013.9.JNS13671
24. Eriksson B, Gunterberg B, Kindblom LG (1981) Chordoma. A clinicopathologic and prognostic study of a Swedish national series. Acta Orthop Scand 52(1):49–58
25. Fatemi N, Dusick JR, Gorgulho AA, Mattozo CA, Moftakhar P, De Salles AA, Kelly DF (2008) Endonasal microscopic removal of clival chordomas. Surg Neurol 69(4):331–338. doi:10.1016/j.surneu.2007.08.035, S0090-3019(07)00985-8 [pii]
26. Fernandez-Miranda JC, Gardner PA, Snyderman CH, Devaney KO, Mendenhall WM, Suarez C, Rinaldo A, Ferlito A (2014) Clival chordomas: a pathological, surgical, and radiotherapeutic review. Head Neck 36(6):892–906. doi:10.1002/hed.23415
27. Feuvret L, Noel G, Weber DC, Pommier P, Ferrand R, De Marzi L, Dhermain F, Alapetite C, Mammar H, Boisserie G, Habrand JL, Mazeron JJ (2007) A treatment planning comparison of combined photon-proton beams versus proton beams-only for the treatment of skull base tumors. Int J Radiat Oncol Biol Phys 69(3):944–954. doi:10.1016/j.ijrobp.2007.07.2326
28. Frank G, Sciarretta V, Calbucci F, Farneti G, Mazzatenta D, Pasquini E (2006) The endoscopic transnasal transsphenoidal approach for the treatment of cranial base chordomas and chondrosarcomas. Neurosurgery 59(1 Suppl 1):ONS50–ONS57; discussion ONS50–57. doi:10.1227/01.NEU.0000219914.17221.55
29. Fraser JF, Nyquist GG, Moore N, Anand VK, Schwartz TH (2010) Endoscopic endonasal transclival resection of chordomas: operative technique, clinical outcome, and review of the literature. J Neurosurg 112(5):1061–1069. doi:10.3171/2009.7.JNS081504
30. Hardy J, Vezina JL (1976) Transsphenoidal neurosurgery of intracranial neoplasm. Adv Neurol 15:261–273
31. Harsh GR, Sekhar LN (1992) The subtemporal, transcavernous, anterior transpetrosal approach to the upper brain stem and clivus. J Neurosurg 77(5):709–717. doi:10.3171/jns.1992.77.5.0709
32. Hoch BL, Nielsen GP, Liebsch NJ, Rosenberg AE (2006) Base of skull chordomas in children and adolescents: a clinicopathologic study of 73 cases. Am J Surg Pathol 30(7):811–818. doi:10.1097/01.pas.0000209828.39477.ab
33. Igaki H, Tokuuye K, Okumura T, Sugahara S, Kagei K, Hata M, Ohara K, Hashimoto T, Tsuboi K, Takano S, Matsumura A, Akine Y (2004) Clinical results of proton beam therapy for skull base chordoma. Int J Radiat Oncol Biol Phys 60(4):1120–1126. doi:10.1016/j.ijrobp.2004.05.064
34. James D, Crockard HA (1991) Surgical access to the base of skull and upper cervical spine by extended maxillotomy. Neurosurgery 29(3):411–416
35. Janecka IP, Nuss DW, Sen CN (1991) Facial translocation approach to the cranial base. Acta Neurochir Suppl 53:193–198
36. Jeffrey PB, Biava CG, Davis RL (1995) Chondroid chordoma. A hyalinized chordoma without cartilaginous differentiation. Am J Clin Pathol 103(3):271–279

37. Kassam A, Snyderman CH, Mintz A, Gardner P, Carrau RL (2005) Expanded endonasal approach: the rostrocaudal axis. Part I. Crista galli to the sella turcica. Neurosurg Focus 19(1):E3, 1–12
38. Kassam A, Snyderman CH, Mintz A, Gardner P, Carrau RL (2005) Expanded endonasal approach: the rostrocaudal axis. Part II. Posterior clinoids to the foramen magnum. Neurosurg Focus 19(1), E4
39. Kassam AB, Prevedello DM, Carrau RL, Snyderman CH, Thomas A, Gardner P, Zanation A, Duz B, Stefko ST, Byers K, Horowitz MB (2011) Endoscopic endonasal skull base surgery: analysis of complications in the authors' initial 800 patients. J Neurosurg 114(6):1544–1568. doi:10.3171/2010.10.JNS09406
40. Komotar RJ, Starke RM, Raper DM, Anand VK, Schwartz TH (2011) The endoscope-assisted ventral approach compared with open microscope-assisted surgery for clival chordomas. World Neurosurg 76(3–4):318–327; discussion 259–362. doi:10.1016/j.wneu.2011.02.026. S1878-8750(11)00145-8 [pii]
41. Koutourousiou M, Gardner PA, Tormenti MJ, Henry SL, Stefko ST, Kassam AB, Fernandez-Miranda JC, Snyderman CH (2012) Endoscopic endonasal approach for resection of cranial base chordomas: outcomes and learning curve. Neurosurgery 71(3):614–624; discussion 624–615. doi:10.1227/NEU.0b013e31825ea3e0
42. Lanzino G, Dumont AS, Lopes MB, Laws ER Jr (2001) Skull base chordomas: overview of disease, management options, and outcome. Neurosurg Focus 10(3), E12
43. Laufer I, Anand VK, Schwartz TH (2007) Endoscopic, endonasal extended transsphenoidal, transplanum transtuberculum approach for resection of suprasellar lesions. J Neurosurg 106(3):400–406
44. Laws E (1993) Clivus chordomas. In: Sekhar LN, Janecka IP (eds) Surgery of cranial base tumors. Raven Press, New York, pp 679–685
45. Liu JK, Decker D, Schaefer SD, Moscatello AL, Orlandi RR, Weiss MH, Couldwell WT (2003) Zones of approach for craniofacial resection: minimizing facial incisions for resection of anterior cranial base and paranasal sinus tumors. Neurosurgery 53(5):1126–1135; discussion 1135–1127
46. Maira G, Pallini R, Anile C, Fernandez E, Salvinelli F, La Rocca LM, Rossi GF (1996) Surgical treatment of clival chordomas: the transsphenoidal approach revisited. J Neurosurg 85(5):784–792
47. McMaster ML, Goldstein AM, Bromley CM, Ishibe N, Parry DM (2001) Chordoma: incidence and survival patterns in the United States, 1973–1995. Cancer Causes Control 12(1):1–11
48. Mendenhall NP, Malyapa RS, Su Z, Yeung D, Mendenhall WM, Li Z (2011) Proton therapy for head and neck cancer: rationale, potential indications, practical considerations, and current clinical evidence. Acta Oncol 50(6):763–771. doi:10.3109/0284186X.2011.590147
49. Mendenhall WM, Mendenhall CM, Lewis SB, Villaret DB, Mendenhall NP (2005) Skull base chordoma. Head Neck 27(2):159–165. doi:10.1002/hed.20144
50. Mitchell A, Scheithauer BW, Unni KK, Forsyth PJ, Wold LE, McGivney DJ (1993) Chordoma and chondroid neoplasms of the spheno-occiput. An immunohistochemical study of 41 cases with prognostic and nosologic implications. Cancer 72(10):2943–2949
51. O'Connell JX, Renard LG, Liebsch NJ, Efird JT, Munzenrider JE, Rosenberg AE (1994) Base of skull chordoma. A correlative study of histologic and clinical features of 62 cases. Cancer 74(8):2261–2267
52. Pallini R, Maira G, Pierconti F, Falchetti ML, Alvino E, Cimino-Reale G, Fernandez E, D'Ambrosio E, Larocca LM (2003) Chordoma of the skull base: predictors of tumor recurrence. J Neurosurg 98(4):812–822. doi:10.3171/jns.2003.98.4.0812
53. Prevedello DM, Ditzel Filho LF, Solari D, Carrau RL, Kassam AB (2010) Expanded endonasal approaches to middle cranial fossa and posterior fossa tumors. Neurosurg Clin N Am 21(4):621–635. doi:10.1016/j.nec.2010.07.003, vi. S1042-3680(10)00059-8 [pii]
54. Rosenberg AE, Brown GA, Bhan AK, Lee JM (1994) Chondroid chordoma--a variant of chordoma. A morphologic and immunohistochemical study. Am J Clin Pathol 101(1):36–41
55. Samii A, Gerganov VM, Herold C, Hayashi N, Naka T, Mirzayan MJ, Ostertag H, Samii M (2007) Chordomas of the skull base: surgical management and outcome. J Neurosurg 107(2):319–324. doi:10.3171/JNS-07/08/0319
56. Sen C, Triana A (2001) Cranial chordomas: results of radical excision. Neurosurg Focus 10(3), E3
57. Sen C, Triana AI, Berglind N, Godbold J, Shrivastava RK (2010) Clival chordomas: clinical management, results, and complications in 71 patients. J Neurosurg 113(5):1059–1071. doi:10.3171/2009.9.JNS08596
58. Srivastava A, Vischioni B, Fiore MR, Vitolo V, Fossati P, Iannalfi A, Tuan JK, Orecchia R (2013) Quality of life in patients with chordomas/chondrosarcomas during treatment with proton beam therapy. J Radiat Res 54(Suppl 1):i43–i48. doi:10.1093/jrr/rrt057
59. Stippler M, Gardner PA, Snyderman CH, Carrau RL, Prevedello DM, Kassam AB (2009) Endoscopic endonasal approach for clival chordomas. Neurosurgery 64(2):268–277; discussion 277–268. doi:10.1227/01.NEU.0000338071.01241.E2. 00006123-200902000-00008 [pii]
60. Swearingen B, Joseph M, Cheney M, Ojemann RG (1995) A modified transfacial approach to the clivus. Neurosurgery 36(1):101–104; discussion 104–105
61. Tamaki N, Nagashima T, Ehara K, Motooka Y, Barua KK (2001) Surgical approaches and strategies for skull base chordomas. Neurosurg Focus 10(3), E9
62. Tzortzidis F, Elahi F, Wright D, Natarajan SK, Sekhar LN (2006) Patient outcome at long-term follow-up after aggressive microsurgical resection of cranial base chordomas. Neurosurgery

59(2):230–237; discussion 230–237. doi:10.1227/01.NEU.0000223441.51012.9D

63. Yasuda M, Bresson D, Chibbaro S, Cornelius JF, Polivka M, Feuvret L, Takayasu M, George B (2012) Chordomas of the skull base and cervical spine: clinical outcomes associated with a multimodal surgical resection combined with proton-beam radiation in 40 patients. Neurosurg Rev 35(2):171–182; discussion 182–173. doi:10.1007/s10143-011-0334-5
64. Yoneoka Y, Tsumanuma I, Fukuda M, Tamura T, Morii K, Tanaka R, Fujii Y (2008) Cranial base chordoma – long term outcome and review of the literature. Acta Neurochir (Wien) 150(8):773–778; discussion 778. doi:10.1007/s00701-008-1600-3

Endoscopic Endonasal Transsphenoidal Approach

25

Domenico Solari, Luigi Maria Cavallo, Enrico Tedeschi, Chiara Caggiano, Massimo Niola, Rosa Maria Gerardi, and Paolo Cappabianca

25.1 Indications

Clival chordomas are lesions located at the anterolateral aspect of the brainstem, involving the extradural and seldom the intradural spaces. These tumors have been historically accessed through posterolateral approaches, which offer a comfortable surgical corridor for this kind of lesions: indeed, the retrosigmoid approach is considered adequate for chordomas that involve mainly the cerebellomesencephalic and cerebellopontine cisterns [55], whereas in the far lateral approach, it is more suitable for those mainly interested in the cerebellomedullary cistern [45, 61].

Besides, it has been possible to expose chordomas via complex and often morbid procedures such as the presigmoid approach, anterior and posterior petrosectomies with or without labyrinthectomy [9], and the extreme lateral approach [4]. These approaches, however, provide narrow dissection corridors with limited working area and mandatory angle of attacks, above all, in between the cranial nerves. Hence, such surgical procedures have been burdened often by significant brain tissue and cranial nerve morbidity.

Because chordomas displace dorsally the neurovascular structures, ventral corridors have been preferred: indeed, in transfacial [2, 12, 18, 34, 46, 58], transsphenoidal [1, 13, 22, 30, 39, 42, 43, 47, 51, 56], and transoral [11, 17, 33] techniques, lesions have been adopted and refined along years.

In recent times, the endoscope brought in transsphenoidal surgery a wider and panoramic view, pushing the refinement of several routes targeted mainly to entire midline of the skull base from the anterior skull base to the craniovertebral junction and adjacent areas. These corridors represent a direct and minimally invasive approach to the suprasellar, retrosellar, and retroclival space, obviating brain retraction, visualizing safely and effectively the surgical field, and granting the lowest rates of morbidity and mortality in a safe and effective way. Hence, the

Electronic supplementary material The online version of this chapter (doi:10.1007/978-3-319-21533-4_25) contains supplementary material, which is available to authorized users.

D. Solari, MD, PhD (✉) • L.M. Cavallo, MD, PhD
C. Caggiano, MD • R.M. Gerardi, MD
P. Cappabianca, MD
Division of Neurosurgery,
Department of Neurosciences, Reproductive and Odontostomatological Sciences,
Università degli Studi di Napoli "Federico II",
Via Pansini 5, 80131 Naples, Italy
e-mail: d.solari.md@gmail.com

E. Tedeschi, MD
Neuroradiology Unit,
Department of Advanced Biomedical Sciences,
Università degli Studi di Napoli "Federico II",
Naples, Italy

M. Niola, MD, PhD
Division of Legal Medicine,
Department of Advanced Biomedical Sciences,
Università degli Studi di Napoli "Federico II",
Naples, Italy

P. Cappabianca et al. (eds.), *Midline Skull Base Surgery*, DOI 10.1007/978-3-319-21533-4_25

extended endoscopic approaches (EEAs) provided ideal surgical alternative options [5, 16, 29, 60] also for clival chordomas and, in particular, those with a major component ventral to the brainstem and/or to the lower cranial nerves [10, 26, 35, 57]. By using a direct anterior approach, the EEAs allow the surgeon to work in a large window and to work between and not cross the cranial nerves, achieving early devascularization of the tumor and microsurgical dissection under closeup view.

Chordoma surgery, as any other skull base procedure, requires careful and specific postoperative management and long-term patient follow-up, which can make the difference between a satisfactory result and a poor result.

Detailed anatomy, neuroimaging, pathophysiology, and natural history of the disease are knowledge prerequisite pillars to build up a multidisciplinary team, which becomes familiar with all the different therapeutic options and fully informed about current therapeutic possibilities in the interest of the patient and of the institution where the operation is done.

Indications for surgery have changed through time and refinements of the surgical techniques, as well as according to the evaluation of results and experience, to the development of knowledge about disease's molecular biology, and to the use of effective new pharmacological agents and radiation techniques [3, 6, 14, 24, 32, 42, 43, 48, 59, 62].

Whether an EEA represents an appropriate surgical management strategy for a clival chordoma, the epicenter and extent of the tumor's bony and/or dural relationships, as well as neurovascular structures involvement, should be carefully evaluated preoperatively.

Though, it is worth reminding that tumor to be resected should be ventral to the brainstem and medial to the cranial nerves, i.e., when extending into the interpeduncular cistern, the mass should not extend beyond the third cranial nerve; when involving the prepontine cistern, it should be medial to the sixth cranial nerve; or when in the premedullary cistern, it should be preferably enclosed within the hypoglossal nerves [10, 23, 25, 26, 39, 40, 52, 57].

Frequently, the nerves and perforating arteries are pushed away by the tumor, which allows direct visualization and safe tumor debulking. Hence, the possibility of running tumor removal with the vital structures located lateral and/or posterior to it and without any neural tissue retraction or dissection in between cranial nerves should be considered as a main advantage of the endonasal endoscopic approach.

Nevertheless, there are conditions that could limit and somehow hinder the choice of the endonasal route, either related to the anatomy of the surgical route or to the inner features of the lesion itself: the size and the pneumatization of the sphenoid sinus and/or carotid arteries position and shape, the caudal extension of the lesion, as well as the encasement of the main neurovascular structures and above all the lateral extension beyond the ascending tract of ICAs.

25.2 Radiology

Clivus chordoma originates at the spheno-occipital synchondrosis (35 % of all chordomas) and usually spreads as an expansile multilobulated mass from the midline toward the lateral neighboring regions. In fact, after eroding of the occipital bone, the neoplasm tends to invade anteriorly the sphenoid sinus and the rhinopharynx and, posterosuperiorly, the subarachnoid spaces of the brainstem. The brain parenchyma is seldom infiltrated, while the brainstem is compressed on the midline [50].

The first-choice imaging modality is contrast-enhanced magnetic resonance imaging, which demonstrates the different histological components of the mass [27]: typical chordomas show large areas with increased water content and prolonged relaxation times compared with the forms where chondroid tissue predominates. The lesion therefore usually appears isointense (75 %) or hypointense in T1-weighted images and markedly hyperintense in T2-weighted images, reflecting the high fluid content of vacuolated cellular components [20]. Often, within the mass it is possible to spot areas of signal void representing sequestered fragments of destroyed cortical bone (rather

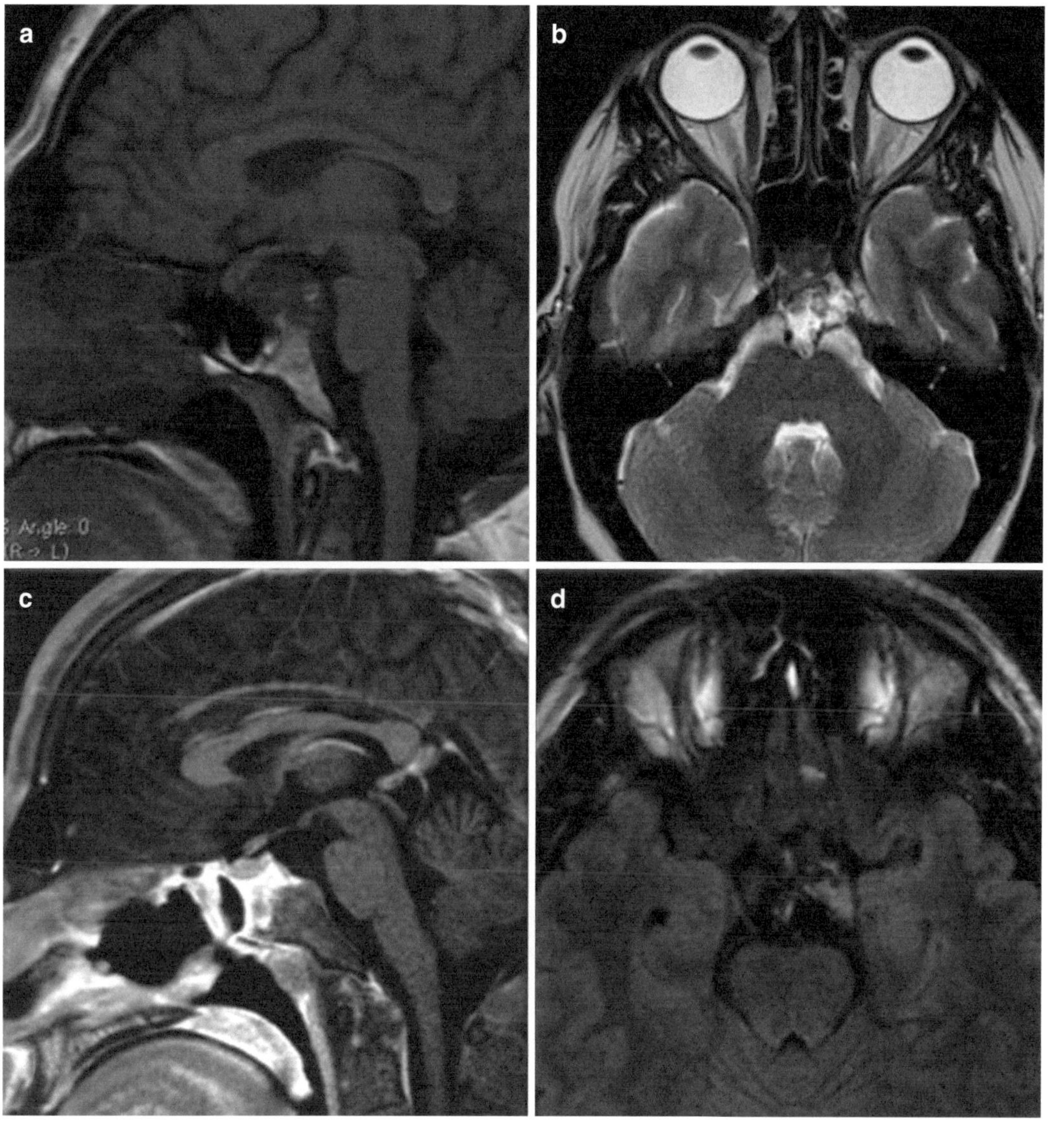

Fig. 25.1 (**a**) Sagittal and (**b**) axial preoperative MRI scans showing an invasive extradural sellar chordoma extending to the clivus. This latter T2-weighted image shows the typical inhomogeneous hyperintensity known as "thumb sign." (**c**) Axial and (**d**) sagittal postoperative scans showing complete tumor removal via an extended endoscopic endonasal approach

than calcific foci), fibrous connective septa, vessels or hemorrhage, or, conversely, areas with increased signal intensity in T1-weighted images that may reveal cyst-like mucoid material or hemorrhage (see Figs. 25.1 and 25.2).

Besides providing an optimal view on the sagittal plane, MRI permits the accurate definition of the intracranial extension of the tumor and its relationships with the brainstem – the impinging on the pons is typical and defined as "thumb sign" (see Fig. 25.1b) – the third ventricle, the sellar and hypothalamic structures, and the rhinopharynx [50].

Moreover, a better and earlier detection of the pathological substitution of the normal yellow marrow of the clivus can be obtained with MRI. Instead, the definition of intratumoral calcifications and osteolytic areas is more problematic compared to CT.

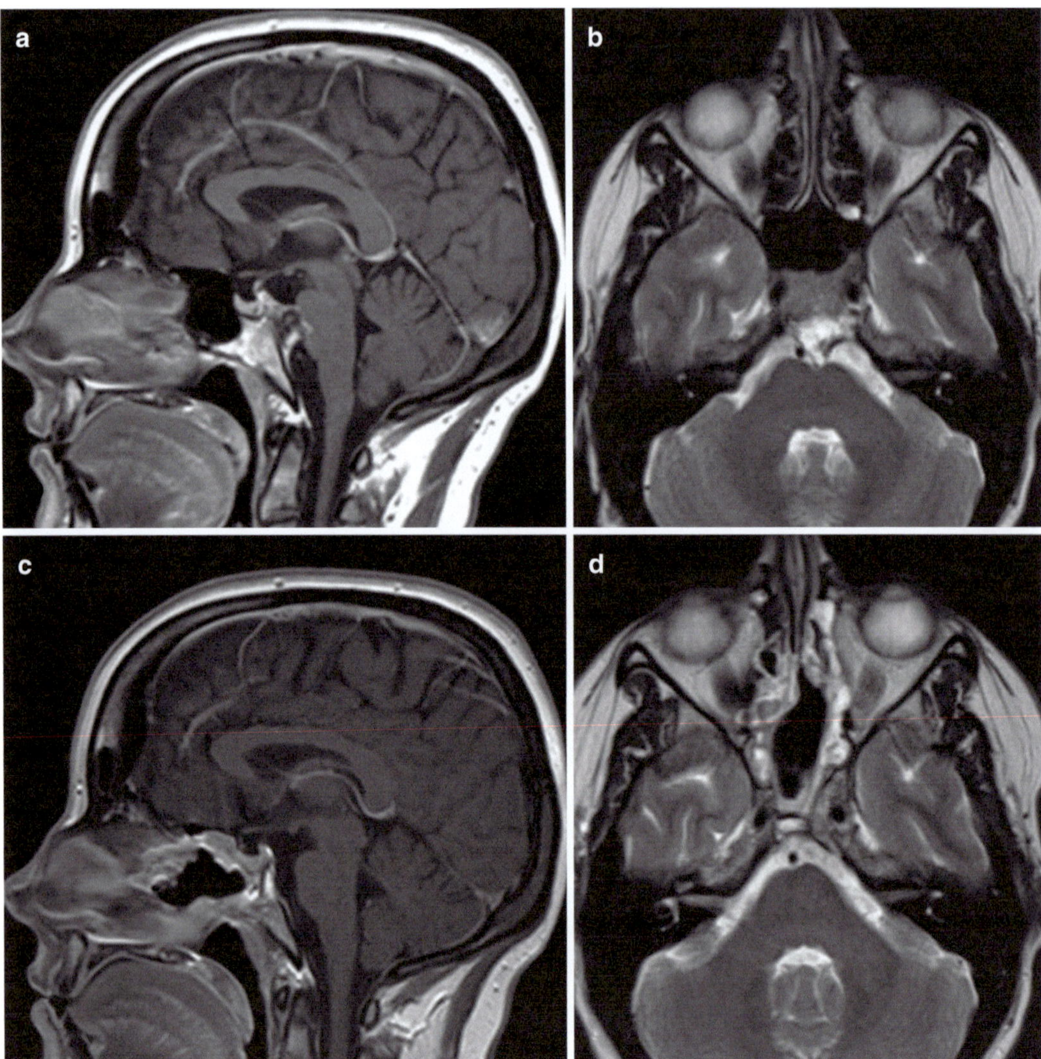

Fig. 25.2 (**a**) Sagittal and (**b**) axial preoperative MRI scans revealing an intradural clival chordoma; the lesion appears inhomogeneously enhancing post-GAD. (**c**) Axial and (**d**) sagittal postoperative scans showing complete tumor removal

The CT appearance of chordoma (see Fig. 25.3) is that of centrally located, well-circumscribed, inhomogeneous soft-tissue mass (hyperdense compared to the brain), with irregular intratumoral calcific spots and destructive osteolysis, sometimes with marginal sclerosis [27].

After contrast media administration, both on CT and MRI, the tumor shows variable areas of moderate to marked enhancement, creating a "honeycomb" appearance of the enhancement pattern [19].

As the usual clinical presentation is lined out by visual disturbances – i.e., oculomotor nerve palsies – and orbitofrontal headache, the diagnostic workup should start with contrast-enhanced MRI, with angiographic sequences to evaluate the encasement/displacement of carotid or vertebral arteries (80 %); then, unenhanced spiral CT may be used for the evaluation of the osseous skull base.

As for the differential diagnosis, chondroma and chondrosarcoma, clival meningioma, giant invasive pituitary macroadenoma, plasmacytoma, and nasopharyngeal carcinoma must be considered:

- Chondromas and chondrosarcomas, while similar in T1 and T2 signal intensity, tend to

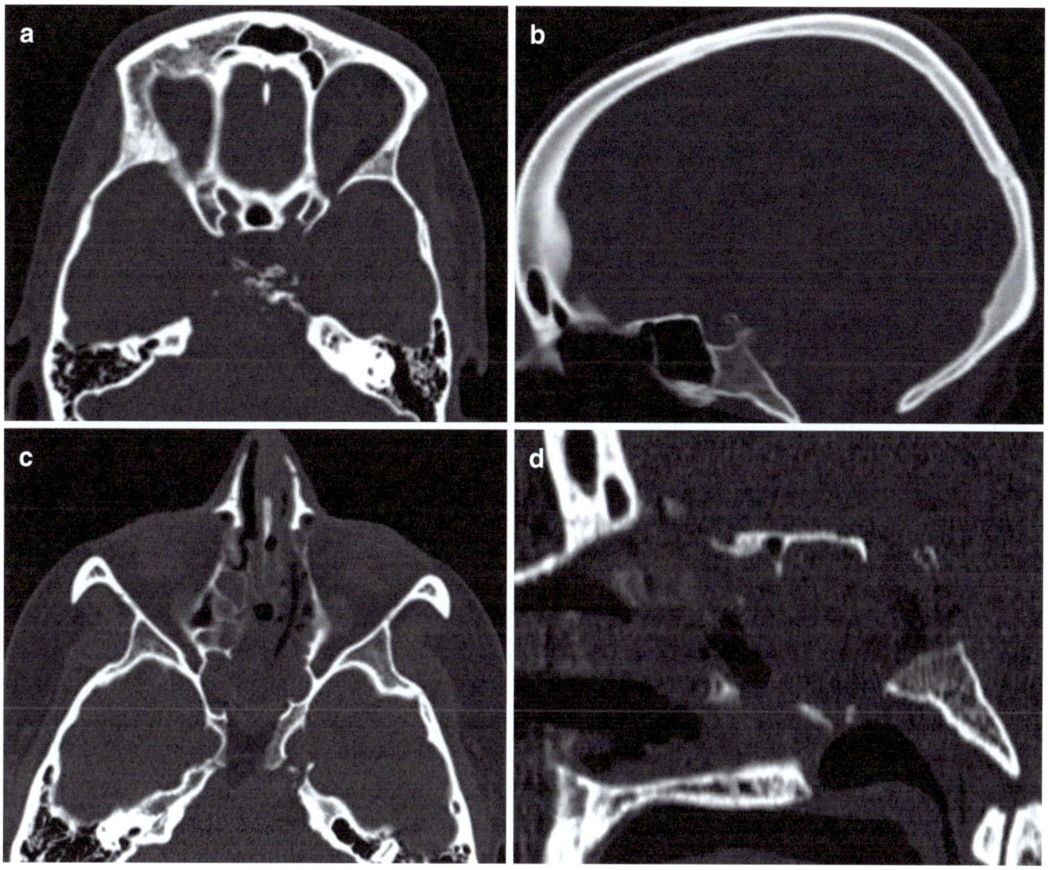

Fig. 25.3 (**a**) Axial and (**b**) sagittal preoperative CT scans showing a clival chordoma involving and partially destroying the dorsum sellae. Tumor calcifications are clearly seen. (**c**) Axial and (**d**) sagittal postoperative scans showing tumor removal

have a more lateral origin (the petro-occipital fissure) and show larger (archlike) calcifications compared to chordoma.

- In meningioma, the signs of bone destruction are usually less evident and a dural attachment may be seen.
- Macroadenomas of course cannot be separated by the pituitary gland, unlike chordomas, which usually displace but do not invade the gland.
- Plasmacytoma typically shows intermediate to low signal intensity in T2-weighted images.
- Nasopharyngeal malignancies usually extend more anteriorly and are associated with head and neck lymphadenopathy.

Chordomas very rarely metastatize, but they frequently recur, given also the difficulty in obtaining a radical resection in advanced cases. Therefore, radiation therapy is frequently employed and neuroradiological follow-up with MRI is warranted, to assess whether the residual disease is under control (i.e., if there is lack of progression) and also to evaluate the possible complications of radiation therapy, such as optic neuritis, edema, gliosis, or even necrosis in the temporal lobes [15].

25.3 Anatomy of the Approach

According to the anatomical classification introduced by Rhoton [53], the clivus can be divided into three segments in a cranio-caudal direction: the upper third extends from the level of dorsum sellae and posterior clinoids down to the sellar floor; the middle third limits are represented by the lower aspect of the sellar floor, superiorly, and the level of the sphenoid sinus floor, inferiorly; and finally, the lower segment goes from the sphenoid sinus floor to the foramen magnum. As described also in a recent publication by Prevedello et al. [52], this anatomical scheme could be adopted when exploring this area from endoscopic endonasal route (see Figs. 25.4 and 25.5)

25.3.1 Upper Third of the Clivus

The utmost superior aspect of the clivus is represented by the dorsum sellae and the posterior clinoids on both sides.

The anterior aspect of this area encloses posteriorly the sella: two layers of dura cover its bony surface. the periosteal and meningeal layers, the same two layers covering the sellar floor, between which run the superior, inferior, and posterior intercavernous sinuses (PIS) [54]. This latter venous channel is located behind the pituitary gland and could be seen upon elevation of the gland; the dorsum sellae could be identified posterior to the PIS. Upon bone removal, the clival dura harboring the basilar venous plexus is exposed (see Fig. 25.4): dural opening at this level gives access to the interpeduncular cistern encompassed laterally by Liliequist membrane and the posterior communicating arteries, the respective perforating arteries, and the third cranial nerves (see Figs. 25.5 and 25.6a, b). The mesencephalon, the basilar bifurcation, the posterior cerebral arteries, and the superior cerebellar arteries are noble neurovascular structure encountered in a deep level, being the epicenter of this area. The horizontal lamina of Liliequist membrane represents the inferior limit of this area [52, 53].

25.3.2 Middle Third of the Clivus

The bony aspect of this clival area is enclosed between the sellar floor superiorly and the sphenoid floor inferiorly; the protuberances of the ascending segments of ICAs, the so-called paraclival tract, represent the lateral limits of the area [41]. The identification of this region from a ventral endonasal route depends on the degree of pneumatization of the sphenoid sinus: it is well represented in sellar and presellar types, while it could be troublesome to recognize its boundaries in case of conchal sinuses (see Fig. 25.4).

Once the bone has been removed, the dura is exposed with the basilar venous plexus within: a

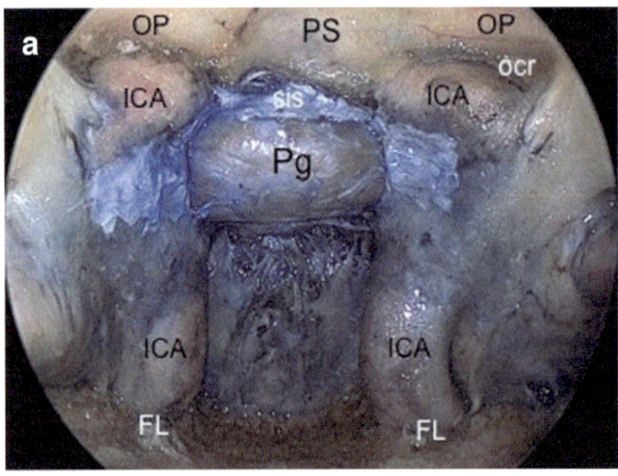

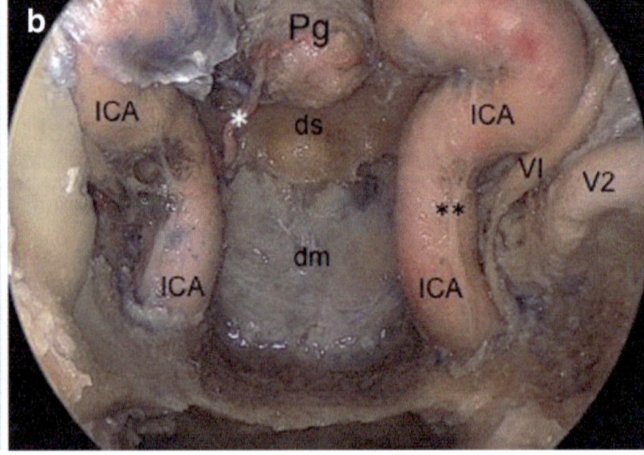

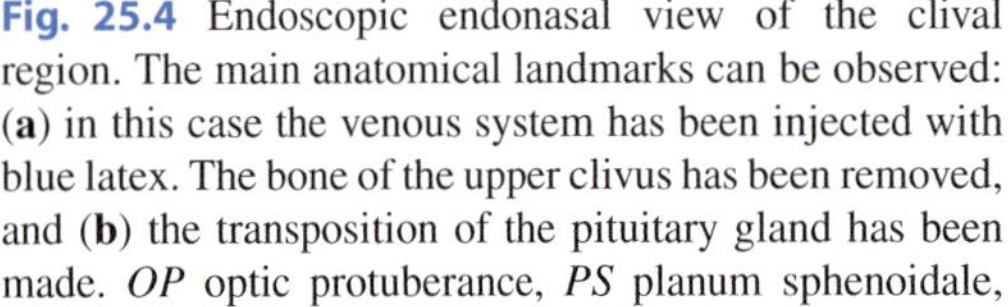
Fig. 25.4 Endoscopic endonasal view of the clival region. The main anatomical landmarks can be observed: (**a**) in this case the venous system has been injected with blue latex. The bone of the upper clivus has been removed, and (**b**) the transposition of the pituitary gland has been made. *OP* optic protuberance, *PS* planum sphenoidale, *ICA* internal carotid artery, *ocr* opto-carotid recess, *sis* superior intercavernous sinus, *Pg* pituitary gland, *FL* foramen lacerum, *ds* dorsum sellae, *VI* abducens nerve, *V2* maxillary branch of the trigeminal nerve, *dm* dura mater of the clivus, * inferior hypophyseal artery, ** pericarotid sympathetic plexus

segment of the sixth cranial nerve's root runs in between the two layers of clival dura just before piercing Dorello's canal [31]. The dural opening reveals the prepontine cistern with the sixth cranial nerves laterally; the pons with the basilar artery and its branches and the anteroinferior cerebellar arteries lie deeply (see Fig 25.6b). The pontomedullary junction and the vertebrobasilar junction (VBJ) are considered as the inferior edge of this region [7, 35].

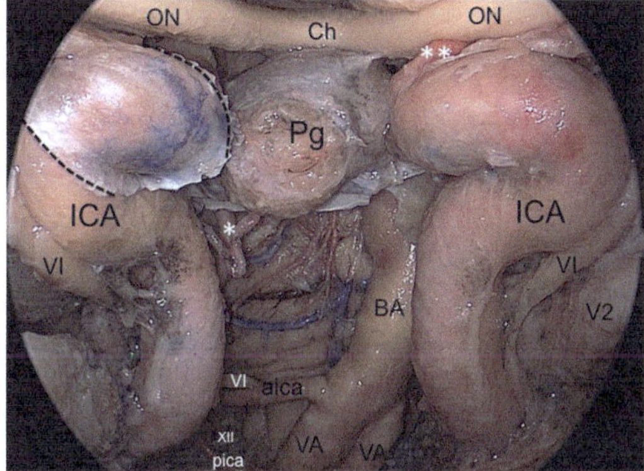

Fig. 25.5 Intradural exploration of the upper and middle clival area. The dura mater has been opened in order to show the main neurovascular structures. *ON* optic nerve, *Ch* optic chiasm, *Pg* pituitary gland, *ICA* internal carotid artery, *BA* basilar artery, *VI* abducens nerve, *V2* maxillary branch of the trigeminal nerve, *aica* anteroinferior cerebellar artery, *VA* vertebral artery, *XII* hypoglossal nerve, *pica*, postero-inferior cerebellar artery, * inferior hypophyseal artery, ** ophthalmic artery, *dotted lines* proximal and distal dural rings of the internal carotid artery

25.3.3 Inferior Third of Clivus

The inferior third has its superior border at the level of the floor of the sphenoid sinus and reaches down the foramen magnum; on both sides, the inferior third of the clivus is not limited directly by the ICA as in the middle third, so that dissection can be safely extended further laterally. Upon the lateral aspects of the clival bone, the petroclival synchondrosis can be identified and followed all the way to the jugular foramen (see Fig. 25.6c). The occipital condyles are found in the anterior portion of the foramen magnum: the lateral exposure can be increased by removing the condyles up to the hypoglossal canal, wherein the twelfth cranial nerve runs, this latter being fixed as the limit of maximum lateral extent [7, 35]. Once the dura has been opened, the premedullary cistern and the medulla oblongata are identified as the epicenter of this area. Whether a supracondylar approach is extended through the jugular tubercle, the ninth, tenth, and eleventh cranial nerves are exposed, in the lateral aspect of the cistern [49].

25.4 Surgical Technique

Surgical approach for a clival chordoma should be planned according to the location, dimension, and spread of the tumor. Clival lesions located predominantly in the midline are more fit to the endoscopic endonasal approach, which could

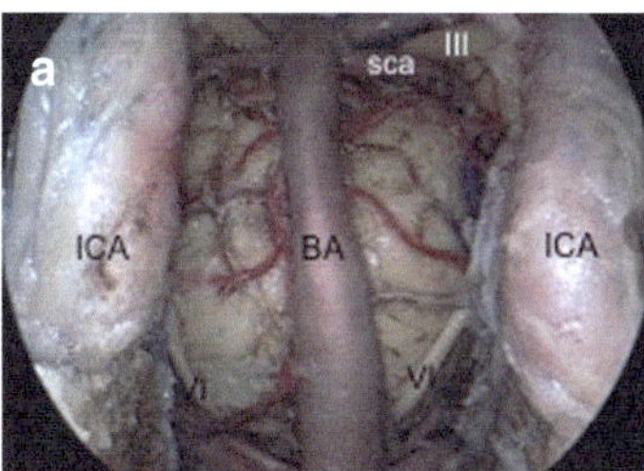

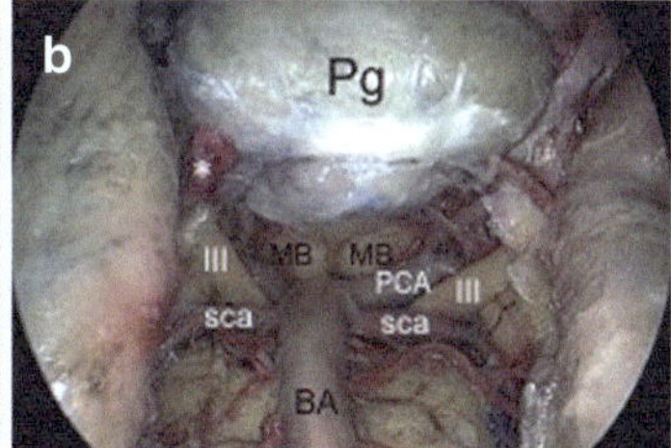

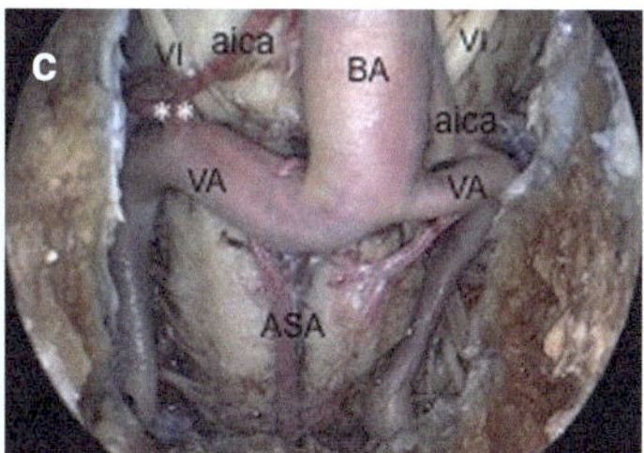

Fig. 25.6 Endoscopic endonasal panoramic view of the clival area with (**a**) the basilar trunk is clearly seen on the ventral side of the pons. (**b**) Closeup view of the upper clivus and (**c**) of the inferior third of the clivus. *Sca* superior cerebellar artery, *III* oculomotor nerve, *ICA* internal carotid artery, *BA* basilar artery, *VI* abducens nerve, *Pg* pituitary gland, *MB* mammillary bodies, * inferior hypophyseal artery, *PCA* posterior cerebral artery, *sca* superior cerebellar artery, *III* oculomotor nerve, *aica* anteroinferior cerebellar artery, *VI* abducens nerve, *VA* vertebral artery, *ASA* anterior spinal artery, ** postero-inferior cerebellar artery

offer a safer and more direct anatomical route. When tumor involves lateral aspects of the area, the endoscopic transclival approach can be implemented, gaining more exposure by the opening of bony surfaces around the different segments of the ICA. The concept behind this kind of surgery is to minimize the opening at the most superficial compartment while expanding the exposure in close proximity of the targeted area [25, 26, 39, 40, 52, 57].

The initial segments of the procedure are run according to the paradigm of Pittsburgh school for the expanded endoscopic endonasal approaches: middle turbinectomy in one nostril, accompanied by posterior ethmoidectomy, and a wider anterior sphenoidotomy are accomplished. At this time, whether reconstruction should rely on naso-septal flap [28, 37], it should be harvested and stored in the maxillary sinus or down into the choana. Upon sphenoid sinus opening, different steps are required to achieve a complete exposure of the clivus in each of the three portions as considered in the anatomical classification.

25.4.1 Superior Third

Once the main landmarks, i.e., clival indent, carotid protuberances, and sellar floor, have been identified, the bone removal can start at the level of the sellar floor: dura is exposed from the superior intercavernous sinus (SIS), down to inferior intercavernous sinus (IIS) and, posteriorly, at the sella-clival junction. Once circular sinuses have been managed, the dura is opened up to the supradiaphragmatic space to allow freeing the pituitary stalk. In order to gain a more comfortable corridor, Kassam et al. [36] introduced the so-called pituitary transposition/trans-dorsum sellae technique: the gland is mobilized superiorly after ligaments connecting the pituitary capsule to the medial cavernous sinus have been dissected. The posterior sellar dura is coagulated and transected so that the dorsum sellae and posterior clinoids are exposed; these are then drilled and carefully removed, minding attention to avoid injuries to the ICA and third and sixth cranial nerves. The retroclival dura harboring the basilar plexus is visualized: basilar plexus can determine intense venous bleeding, which can be controlled with hemostatic agents such as oxidized cellulose or thrombin/gelatin matrix.

Once the dura has been opened tumor, debulking is first performed and then the dissection from surrounding neurovascular structures completes the removal maneuvers. Chordomas in this location can be tightly attached to the branches of the superior hypophyseal artery, which should be preserved in order to avoid vascular damages to the pituitary stalk and the optic chiasm; as well, the basilar apex and its perforators are pushed posteriorly and attached to tumor capsule, while, laterally, the lesion can impinge the third cranial nerve and the posterior communicating artery from which it should be dissected carefully. Owing that, these maneuvers should be performed sharply under direct closeup view. Finally, it is useful to remark that when performing removal of the inferior aspects of tumor involving this area, the preservation of the inferior horizontal lamina of Liliequist membrane helps to decrease subarachnoid blood dissemination to other cisterns.

25.4.2 Middle Third (Clival Recess of Sphenoid Sinus)

In well-pneumatized sphenoid sinus, the middle third of the clivus is that thin bone, i.e., the clival recess, lying over the posterior wall of the sphenoid sinus, enclosed between the ascending tracts (paraclival) of the ICAs.

The bone is drilled away and the dura and the basilar plexus are exposed; laterally, the exposure is limited by the paraclival ICAs; particularly in cases of chordomas located immediately behind this vessel, removal maneuvers are hindered via this route. In such situations, to increase exposure and instruments maneuverability, the ICA bony canals should be opened and the periosteum exposed in order to allow ICA mobilization. It is important to identify the vidian nerve as referring landmark for this approach: indeed it points toward the anterior genu of the ICA, at the level of the foramen lacerum, thus helping the identification of the petrous ICA in non-pneumatized sphenoid sinuses and/or cases in which the anatomy is altered by the disease [38].

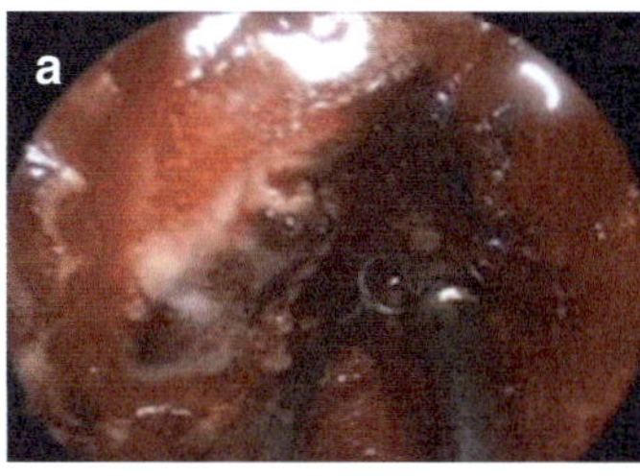

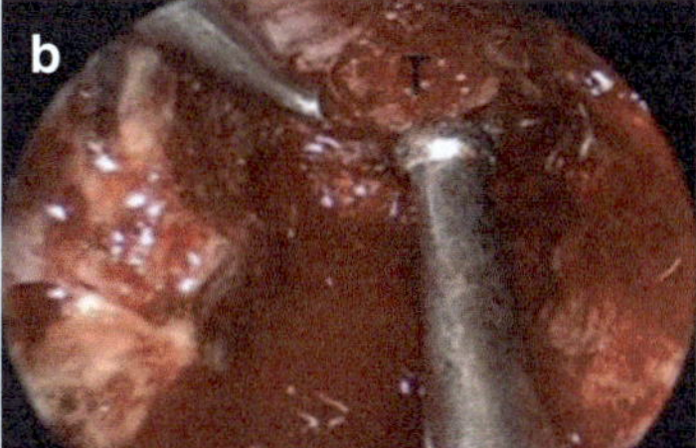

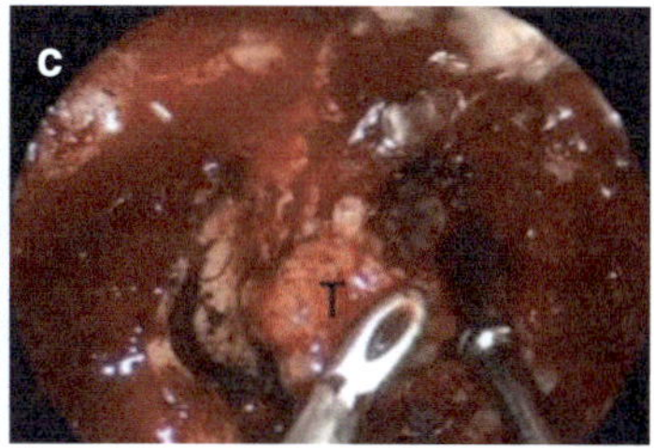

Fig. 25.7 Intraoperative picture showing the removal of a clival chordoma by means of the endoscopic endonasal technique. Dissection maneuvers are run with (**a**) ring curettes and (**b**) spoons. Thereafter, (**c**) the lesion is removed in piecemeal fashion. *T* tumor

In case of extradural chordomas, dissection maneuvers are run in a deep median plane according to bimanual microsurgical concept: this route offers a direct, safe corridor (see Fig. 25.7).

Whether chordomas have breached the dura, this is opened at the midline, under neurophysiology and nerve stimulation monitoring: it is of utmost importance to recognize at this level the sixth cranial nerve that could have been displaced medially by the tumor. Furthermore, image guidance system should also be used to determine the positioning of the vertebrobasilar junction (VBJ): dural opening should be performed below the VBJ, in order to ensure that the sixth cranial nerve origin remains above, at the brainstem.

When dissecting posterior aspects of the tumor, care should be taken to avoid injuries to the basilar artery and its perforator branches as well as their relationship with the pons.

25.4.3 Inferior Third

To properly expose this area, the nasal septum has to be detached from the anterior surface of the sphenoid bone, and the sphenoid sinus floor is completely drilled down to create a unique working room constituted of the sphenoid sinus and the nasopharynx; the basopharyngeal fascia is then stripped from the sphenoid rostrum and the clival bone.

Careful drilling of the anterior surface of the clivus down to the foramen magnum is carried out under image guidance; Kerrison rongeurs are used to bite off the bony speckles under endoscopic direct visual control. Dural exposure and whether or not the dura itself is opened depend on chordoma's features, each approach being tailored to the single patient. In case of intradural tumor, the vertebral arteries, VBJ superiorly, and medulla represent the posterior limit of the dissection.

According to Prevedello et al., the dissection can be refined in a coronal plane identifying three modules [52]:

1. Infrapetrous extension: in this module, the petrous bone below the ICA is removed and the area of the foramen lacerum exposed; the dense fibrous tissue attached to eustachian tube is transected.
2. Supracondylar or transjugular tubercle approach: the occipital bone medial to the petroclival synchondrosis and above the occipital condyle is removed; the dissection follows the petroclival synchondrosis inferiorly in order to expose ninth, tenth, and twelfth cranial nerves. In such module investigation of these inferior nerves with neurophysiology monitoring is mandatory.
3. Transcondylar route: a medial condylectomy is performed. The hypoglossal nerve represents the lateral limit of occipital condyles removal: this allows identification of the proximal aspect of the vertebral artery.

25.4.4 Reconstruction

This step of the procedure could tremendously affect the final surgical outcome. We usually adopt a multilayer technique that addresses all the single compartments of the osteodural defect

[8, 21, 44]. Initially, intradural closure, consisting of the obliteration of dead space, with fibrin glue and/or autologous fat is achieved. Thereafter, the extradural closure with positioning of one or multiple dural substitute layers, free mucosal flaps, and/or fascia lata in the extradural space and/or over the bony aperture is performed. Recently, we perform what we call “sandwich technique”: the surgical cavity is filled with fat sutured the inner layer of a three-layer foil of fascia lata or dural substitute; the first layer is positioned intradurally, the second between the dura and the bone, and the third outside to cover the bone. A vascular flap of septal mucosa harvested according to the Hadad-Bassagasteguy [28, 37] method is used to cover the skull base defect and a moderate inflated Foley balloon catheter is then placed in the sphenoid sinus to support the reconstruction.

References

1. Al-Mefty O, Kadri PA, Hasan DM, Isolan GR, Pravdenkova S (2008) Anterior clivectomy: surgical technique and clinical applications. J Neurosurg 109(5):783–793
2. Anand VK, Harkey HL, Al-Mefty O (1991) Open-door maxillotomy approach for lesions of the clivus. Skull Base Surg 1(4):217–225
3. Ares C, Hug EB, Lomax AJ, Bolsi A, Timmermann B, Rutz HP, Schuller JC, Pedroni E, Goitein G (2009) Effectiveness and safety of spot scanning proton radiation therapy for chordomas and chondrosarcomas of the skull base: first long-term report. Int J Radiat Oncol Biol Phys 75(4):1111–1118
4. Arnold H, Sepehrnia A (1995) Extreme lateral transcondylar approach. J Neurosurg 82(2):313–314
5. Cappabianca P, Cavallo LM, Esposito F, de Divitiis O, Messina A, de Divitiis E (2008) Extended endoscopic endonasal approach to the midline skull base: the evolving role of transsphenoidal surgery. In: Pickard JD, Akalan N, Di Rocco C, Dolenc VV, Lobo Antunes J, Mooij JJA, Schramm J, Sindou M (eds) Advances and technical standards in neurosurgery. Springer, Wien/New York, pp 152–199
6. Catton C, O'Sullivan B, Bell R, Laperriere N, Cummings B, Fornasier V, Wunder J (1996) Chordoma: long-term follow-up after radical photon irradiation. Radiother Oncol 41(1):67–72
7. Cavallo LM, Messina A, Cappabianca P, Esposito F, de Divitiis E, Gardner P, Tschabitscher M (2005) Endoscopic endonasal surgery of the midline skull base: anatomical study and clinical considerations. Neurosurg Focus 19(1), E2
8. Cavallo LM, Messina A, Esposito F, de Divitiis O, Dal Fabbro M, de Divitiis E, Cappabianca P (2007) Skull base reconstruction in the extended endoscopic transsphenoidal approach for suprasellar lesions. J Neurosurg 107(4):713–720
9. Chanda A, Nanda A (2002) Partial labyrinthectomy petrous apicectomy approach to the petroclival region: an anatomic and technical study. Neurosurgery 51(1):147–159; discussion 159–160
10. Chibbaro S, Cornelius JF, Froelich S, Tigan L, Kehrli P, Debry C, Romano A, Herman P, George B, Bresson D (2014) Endoscopic endonasal approach in the management of skull base chordomas--clinical experience on a large series, technique, outcome, and pitfalls. Neurosurg Rev 37(2):217–224; discussion 224–215
11. Choi D, Crockard HA (2013) Evolution of transoral surgery: three decades of change in patients, pathologies, and indications. Neurosurgery 73(2):296–303; discussion 303–304
12. Cocke EW Jr, Robertson JH, Robertson JT, Crook JP Jr (1990) The extended maxillotomy and subtotal maxillectomy for excision of skull base tumors. Arch Otolaryngol Head Neck Surg 116(1):92–104
13. Couldwell WT, Weiss MH, Rabb C, Liu JK, Apfelbaum RI, Fukushima T (2004) Variations on the standard transsphenoidal approach to the sellar region, with emphasis on the extended approaches and parasellar approaches: surgical experience in 105 cases. Neurosurgery 55(3):539–550
14. Crockard HA, Steel T, Plowman N, Singh A, Crossman J, Revesz T, Holton JL, Cheeseman A (2001) A multidisciplinary team approach to skull base chordomas. J Neurosurg 95(2):175–183
15. Curtin HD, Rabinov JD, Som PM (2003) Central skull base. In: Head and neck imaging. Mosby, Saint Louis
16. de Divitiis E, Cappabianca P, Cavallo LM (2002) Endoscopic transsphenoidal approach: adaptability of the procedure to different sellar lesions. Neurosurgery 51(3):699–705; discussion 705–707
17. Delgado TE, Garrido E, Harwick RD (1981) Labiomandibular, transoral approach to chordomas in the clivus and upper cervical spine. Neurosurgery 8(6):675–679
18. DeMonte F, Diaz E Jr, Callender D, Suk I (2001) Transmandibular, circumglossal, retropharyngeal approach for chordomas of the clivus and upper cervical spine. Technical note. Neurosurg Focus 10(3), E10
19. Doucet V, Peretti-Viton P, Figarella-Branger D, Manera L, Salamon G (1997) MRI of intracranial chordomas. Extent of tumour and contrast enhancement: criteria for differential diagnosis. Neuroradiology 39(8):571–576
20. Erdem E, Angtuaco EC, Van Hemert R, Park JS, Al-Mefty O (2003) Comprehensive review of intracranial chordoma. Radiographics 23(4):995–1009
21. Esposito F, Dusick JR, Fatemi N, Kelly DF (2007) Graded repair of cranial base defects and cerebrospinal fluid leaks in transsphenoidal surgery. Neurosurgery 60(4 Suppl 2):295–303; discussion 303–304

22. Fatemi N, Dusick JR, Gorgulho AA, Mattozo CA, Moftakhar P, De Salles AA, Kelly DF (2008) Endonasal microscopic removal of clival chordomas. Surg Neurol 69(4):331–338
23. Fernandez-Miranda JC, Gardner PA, Snyderman CH, Devaney KO, Mendenhall WM, Suarez C, Rinaldo A, Ferlito A (2014) Clival chordomas: a pathological, surgical, and radiotherapeutic review. Head Neck 36(6):892–906
24. Feuvret L, Noel G, Weber DC, Pommier P, Ferrand R, De Marzi L, Dhermain F, Alapetite C, Mammar H, Boisserie G, Habrand JL, Mazeron JJ (2007) A treatment planning comparison of combined photon-proton beams versus proton beams-only for the treatment of skull base tumors. Int J Radiat Oncol Biol Phys 69(3):944–954
25. Frank G, Sciarretta V, Calbucci F, Farneti G, Mazzatenta D, Pasquini E (2006) The endoscopic transnasal transsphenoidal approach for the treatment of cranial base chordomas and chondrosarcomas. Neurosurgery 59(1 Suppl 1):ONS50–ONS57; discussion ONS50–ONS57
26. Fraser JF, Nyquist GG, Moore N, Anand VK, Schwartz TH (2010) Endoscopic endonasal transclival resection of chordomas: operative technique, clinical outcome, and review of the literature. J Neurosurg 112(5):1061–1069
27. Gupta A, Harnsberger HR (2004) Chordoma, clivus. In: Diagnostic imaging. Head and neck. Amyrsis Inc, Salt Lake City
28. Hadad G, Bassagasteguy L, Carrau RL, Mataza JC, Kassam A, Snyderman CH, Mintz A (2006) A novel reconstructive technique after endoscopic expanded endonasal approaches: vascular pedicle nasoseptal flap. Laryngoscope 116(10): 1882–1886
29. Hardy J (2007) Transsphenoidal hypophysectomy. 1971. J Neurosurg 107(2):458–471
30. Hardy J, Vezina JL (1976) Transsphenoidal neurosurgery of intracranial neoplasm. Adv Neurol 15:261–273
31. Iaconetta G, Fusco M, Cavallo LM, Cappabianca P, Samii M, Tschabitscher M (2007) The abducens nerve: microanatomic and endoscopic study. Neurosurgery 61(3 Suppl):7–14; discussion 14
32. Igaki H, Tokuuye K, Okumura T, Sugahara S, Kagei K, Hata M, Ohara K, Hashimoto T, Tsuboi K, Takano S, Matsumura A, Akine Y (2004) Clinical results of proton beam therapy for skull base chordoma. Int J Radiat Oncol Biol Phys 60(4):1120–1126
33. James D, Crockard HA (1991) Surgical access to the base of skull and upper cervical spine by extended maxillotomy. Neurosurgery 29(3):411–416
34. Janecka IP, Nuss DW, Sen CN (1991) Facial translocation approach to the cranial base. Acta Neurochir Suppl 53:193–198
35. Kassam A, Snyderman CH, Mintz A, Gardner P, Carrau RL (2005) Expanded endonasal approach: the rostrocaudal axis. Part II. Posterior clinoids to the foramen magnum. Neurosurg Focus 19(1), E4
36. Kassam AB, Prevedello DM, Thomas A, Gardner P, Mintz A, Snyderman C, Carrau R (2008) Endoscopic endonasal pituitary transposition for a transdorsum sellae approach to the interpeduncular cistern. Neurosurgery 62(3 Suppl 1):57–72; discussion 72–74
37. Kassam AB, Thomas A, Carrau RL, Snyderman CH, Vescan A, Prevedello D, Mintz A, Gardner P (2008) Endoscopic reconstruction of the cranial base using a pedicled nasoseptal flap. Neurosurgery 63(1 Suppl 1):ONS44–ONS52; discussion ONS52–ONS53
38. Kassam AB, Vescan AD, Carrau RL, Prevedello DM, Gardner P, Mintz AH, Snyderman CH, Rhoton AL (2008) Expanded endonasal approach: vidian canal as a landmark to the petrous internal carotid artery. J Neurosurg 108(1):177–183
39. Komotar RJ, Starke RM, Raper DM, Anand VK, Schwartz TH (2011) The endoscope-assisted ventral approach compared with open microscope-assisted surgery for clival chordomas. World Neurosurg 76(3–4):318–327; discussion 259–362
40. Koutourousiou M, Gardner PA, Tormenti MJ, Henry SL, Stefko ST, Kassam AB, Fernandez-Miranda JC, Snyderman CH (2012) Endoscopic endonasal approach for resection of cranial base chordomas: outcomes and learning curve. Neurosurgery 71(3):614–624; discussion 624–625
41. Labib MA, Prevedello DM, Carrau R, Kerr EE, Naudy C, Abou Al-Shaar H, Corsten M, Kassam A (2014) A road map to the internal carotid artery in expanded endoscopic endonasal approaches to the ventral cranial base. Neurosurgery 10(Suppl 3):448–471; discussion 471
42. Lanzino G, Dumont AS, Lopes MB, Laws ER Jr (2001) Skull base chordomas: overview of disease, management options, and outcome. Neurosurg Focus 10(3), E12
43. Laws E (1993) Clivus chordomas. In: Sekhar LN, Janecka IP (eds) Surgery of cranial base tumors. Raven, New York, pp 679–685
44. Leng LZ, Brown S, Anand VK, Schwartz TH (2008) "Gasket-seal" watertight closure in minimal-access endoscopic cranial base surgery. Neurosurgery 62(5 Suppl 2):ONSE342–ONSE343; discussion ONSE343
45. Liu JK, Couldwell WT (2005) Far-lateral transcondylar approach: surgical technique and its application in neurenteric cysts of the cervicomedullary junction. Report of two cases. Neurosurg Focus 19(2), E9
46. Liu JK, Decker D, Schaefer SD, Moscatello AL, Orlandi RR, Weiss MH, Couldwell WT (2003) Zones of approach for craniofacial resection: minimizing facial incisions for resection of anterior cranial base and paranasal sinus tumors. Neurosurgery 53(5):1126–1135; discussion 1135–1137
47. Maira G, Pallini R, Anile C, Fernandez E, Salvinelli F, La Rocca LM, Rossi GF (1996) Surgical treatment of clival chordomas: the transsphenoidal approach revisited. J Neurosurg 85(5):784–792
48. Mendenhall NP, Malyapa RS, Su Z, Yeung D, Mendenhall WM, Li Z (2011) Proton therapy for head and neck cancer: rationale, potential indications,

practical considerations, and current clinical evidence. Acta Oncol 50(6):763–771
49. Morera VA, Fernandez-Miranda JC, Prevedello DM, Madhok R, Barges-Coll J, Gardner P, Carrau R, Snyderman CH, Rhoton AL Jr, Kassam AB (2010) "Far-medial" expanded endonasal approach to the inferior third of the clivus: the transcondylar and transjugular tubercle approaches. Neurosurgery 66(6):211–219; discussion 219–220
50. Osborn AG (2012) Clival chordomas. In: Osborn's brain: imaging, pathology and anatomy. Lippincott Williams & Wilkins, Philadelphia
51. Pallini R, Maira G, Pierconti F, Falchetti ML, Alvino E, Cimino-Reale G, Fernandez E, D'Ambrosio E, Larocca LM (2003) Chordoma of the skull base: predictors of tumor recurrence. J Neurosurg 98(4): 812–822
52. Prevedello DM, Ditzel Filho LF, Solari D, Carrau RL, Kassam AB (2010) Expanded endonasal approaches to middle cranial fossa and posterior fossa tumors. Neurosurg Clin N Am 21(4):621–635, vi
53. Rhoton AL Jr (2000) The cerebellar arteries. Neurosurgery 47(3 Suppl):S29–S68
54. Rhoton AL Jr (2002) The sellar region. Neurosurgery 51(4 Suppl):S335–S374
55. Samii A, Gerganov VM, Herold C, Hayashi N, Naka T, Mirzayan MJ, Ostertag H, Samii M (2007) Chordomas of the skull base: surgical management and outcome. J Neurosurg 107(2):319–324
56. Sen C, Triana AI, Berglind N, Godbold J, Shrivastava RK (2010) Clival chordomas: clinical management, results, and complications in 71 patients. J Neurosurg 113(5):1059–1071
57. Stippler M, Gardner PA, Snyderman CH, Carrau RL, Prevedello DM, Kassam AB (2009) Endoscopic endonasal approach for clival chordomas. Neurosurgery 64(2):268–277; discussion 277–288
58. Swearingen B, Joseph M, Cheney M, Ojemann RG (1995) A modified transfacial approach to the clivus. Neurosurgery 36(1):101–104; discussion 104–105
59. Tamaki N, Nagashima T, Ehara K, Motooka Y, Barua KK (2001) Surgical approaches and strategies for skull base chordomas. Neurosurg Focus 10(3), E9
60. Weiss MH (1987) The transnasal transsphenoidal approach. In: Apuzzo MLJ (ed) Surgery of the third ventricle. Williams & Wilkins, Baltimore, pp 476–494
61. Wen HT, Rhoton AL Jr, Katsuta T, de Oliveira E (1997) Microsurgical anatomy of the transcondylar, supracondylar, and paracondylar extensions of the far-lateral approach. J Neurosurg 87(4):555–585
62. Yasuda M, Bresson D, Chibbaro S, Cornelius JF, Polivka M, Feuvret L, Takayasu M, George B (2012) Chordomas of the skull base and cervical spine: clinical outcomes associated with a multimodal surgical resection combined with proton-beam radiation in 40 patients. Neurosurg Rev 35(2):171–182; discussion 182–183

Skull Base Approaches to Clival Chordomas

26

Salvatore Chibbaro, Damien Bresson, Philippe Herman, and Sebastien Froelich

26.1 Background

Chordoma is a rare neoplasm considered to be of low to intermediate malignancy and originating from the notochord cells. The incidence of chordoma is estimated around 0.51–0.80 cases per million [1, 2] accounting for 1–5.2 % of all malignant bone tumors [1–3]. Chordomas represent less than 0.1 % [4] of all skull base tumors. From the embryological point of view, the notochordal cells are distributed along the neural tube and play an important role in organizing and developing the axial spine and skeletal muscles [5]. The former start their regression at birth until complete disappearance by 6–10 years of age [6]. Few remnant tissues remain as the intervertebral disk nucleus pulposus and the ecchondrosis physaliphora in the clivus region [5–8]. Because of this topographical distribution of the notochord cells, chordoma usually occurs along the spinal column and/or in the midline skull base, especially into the clivus. According to previous reports, the sacrum represents the most common location of chordomas [1–3, 9–11]. Furthermore, 25–36 % of the tumors are found in the skull base and 15–34 % are located in the spine. From a pathological standpoint, chordoma is usually classified as a benign tumor due to the absence of malignant features although it has an aggressive local behavior with a high rate of recurrence. Metastasis may also occur and its long-term prognosis is poor. Some chemotherapy can be proposed in case of recurrences but have shown until now only limited results.

Several studies have emphasized the importance of radical resection and aggressive adjuvant radiotherapy [9, 12–21]. However, chordomas are usually located in complex anatomical region, and radical resection is challenging and not always achievable. Chordomas are usually refractory to an ordinary dose of radiotherapy [11, 19]. In the early 1980s, proton beam radiation was observed to be effective for the control of chordomas, and it has become a common treatment modality in the last decade [5, 22–27]. In the same period, new technologies, such as endoscopy, navigation systems, and microvascular ultrasound Doppler, have been introduced in the surgeon armamentarium opening new horizons; in fact nowadays the use of the natural nasal corridors to treat skull base chordomas has remarkably improved the quality of resection as well as the functional outcome.

S. Chibbaro, MD, PhD (✉)
Department of Neurosurgery,
Strasbourg University Hospital, Strasbourg, France
e-mail: schibbaro@hotmail.com

D. Bresson, MD • S. Froelich, MD, PhD (✉)
Department of Neurosurgery,
Lariboisiere University Hospital, Paris, France
e-mail: csebastien.froelich@chru-strasbourg.fr

P. Herman, MD
ENT Department,
Lariboisiere University Hospital, Paris, France

P. Cappabianca et al. (eds.), *Midline Skull Base Surgery*, DOI 10.1007/978-3-319-21533-4_26

Such an upward line of sight that uses the natural nasal and paranasal air cavities appears to be more logical than classic transcranial approach that requires a significant amount of soft tissue dissection, bone drilling, and brain retraction to reach a deeply located lesion such as clival chordomas.

26.2 Therapeutic Strategy

Our basic strategy is to try as much as possible to achieve maximal tumor resection combined with the preservation of neurological function and quality of life. Surgical procedure is tailored individually for conservation of important neurological structure and function. In those cases in which a radical resection is not achievable because of the extent of the lesion, the purpose of the surgery, while reducing the volume as much as possible, is to decompress the brain stem or the spinal cord and/or the optic apparatus in order to facilitate postoperative radiation therapy and enhance its efficacy. When the lesion surrounds the internal carotid artery (ICA), preoperative angiography with a BOT may be performed. However, the tumor, because of its soft consistency, can usually be separated from the ICA, and the sacrifice of a major vessel such as the ICA should be carefully considered and, as following a general principle, only performed if the goal of radical resection can be reached once the ICA is sacrificed.

Following surgery, all patients, whether or not radical resection has been achieved, receive a dose of at least 74 Gy proton-based radiation therapy, which most often consists of conventional fractionation (1.8–2 Gy) of mixed photon and proton therapy [28]. In case of a local recurrence, a new surgery in combination with additional radiation should be considered. In those cases because of the lack of initial landmark and scar tissue, the surgery is more technically challenging and the use of neuronavigation system and micro-Doppler is mandatory. Patients with a previous history of radiation may be able to receive additional radiation, according to their previous radiation plan.

26.3 Surgical Indications

The extended endoscopic endonasal approach is particularly indicated and a logical line of sight for midline-located chordomas although tumors extending laterally could also be reached by the same corridor bearing in mind that the ICA and the cranial nerves put the surgery at higher risk. In such approaches, the objectives, prior tumor resection, are (1) control of the ICA segments and (2) control of the cranial nerves using anatomical landmarks and neuromonitoring. As well as lateral tumor extension is more challenging than medially located chordomas, lesions located posteriorly, compressing the chiasma, fourth ventricle, and/or brain stem in the sagittal plane, are also more difficult to remove than anterior ones. However, if lower clivus and craniocervical junction (CCJ) lesions with extension to the occipital condyles, hypoglossal canal, jugular foramen, or lateral mass of C1 may have constituted a major theoretical limit of this surgical modality, recent advances allowed to consider this corridor as a valuable option. In our experience, lateral tumor extension around the ICA or, less frequently, around the vertebral arteries is not a formal contraindication to the endoscopic approach although such tumor locations are technically challenging to remove. Such chordomas extending very far laterally could also benefit of a combined EEA and transcranial approaches. A combination of an endoscopic endonasal approach for the medial part of the tumor with a transcranial approach for the lateral extension could result in lower approach-related morbidity than a single extensive approach.

26.4 Radiological Features

Chordomas are midline tumors lying in the bone. They are usually extradural and cause bone destruction. On CT scan, chordomas are osteolytic lesion destroying the bone trabeculation and the cortical bone. They are well limited without peripheral bone condensation (Fig. 26.1). They sometimes appear calcified; however, more often it is sequestered bone fragment rather than true calcification. On MRI scan, chordomas are well limited with hypo-signal on T1 sequences and a hyper-signal in T2 sequences and contrast enhancement (Fig. 26.2). It often shows signal heterogeneity, with some area of T2 hyposignal possibly due to a variety of components, including mucoid part, intratumoral hemorrhage, calcification, necrotic areas, and connective septa. Furthermore, it is worth noting that chondroid chordomas, which are mainly constituted by cartilaginous hyaline tissue, have shorter T1- and T2-weighted MRI signals because of low water content. MRI and CT scan have complementary roles in such lesion evaluation. CT is necessary to assess the degree of bone involvement or erosion and to identify calcification patterns within the tumor. It also allows identifying some reliable bony landmarks that will be used during the approach and the resection. MRI scan allows defining preoperatively the extension of the tumor in the cavernous sinus, sella, parapharyngeal space, and prevertebral space. It can also distinguish a true extension into subarachnoid space from an interdural or subdural extension of the tumor, and finally, it helps to define the relationship of the tumor with the cranial nerves (3D CISS or FIESTA sequences), the brain stem, and the major vessels (Fig. 26.3).

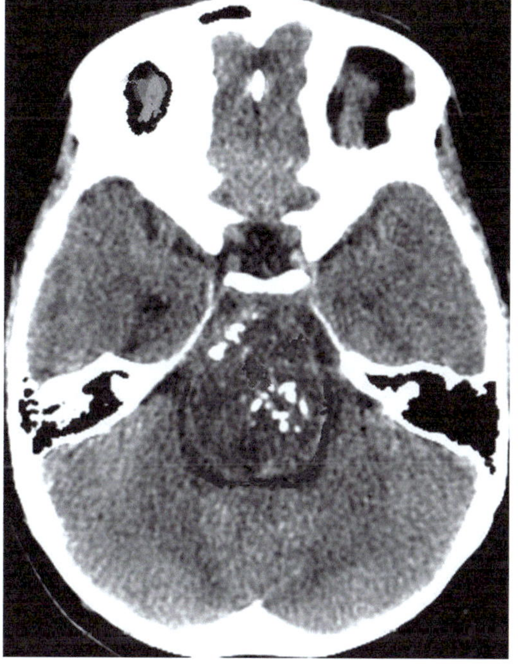

Fig. 26.1 Preoperative bony window sagittal CT scan

26.5 Anatomy of the Approach

A precise knowledge of the anatomy of the nose, paranasal sinuses, sellar and parasellar region, as well as clival, paraclival, and CCJ areas with all associated crucial neurovascular structure is

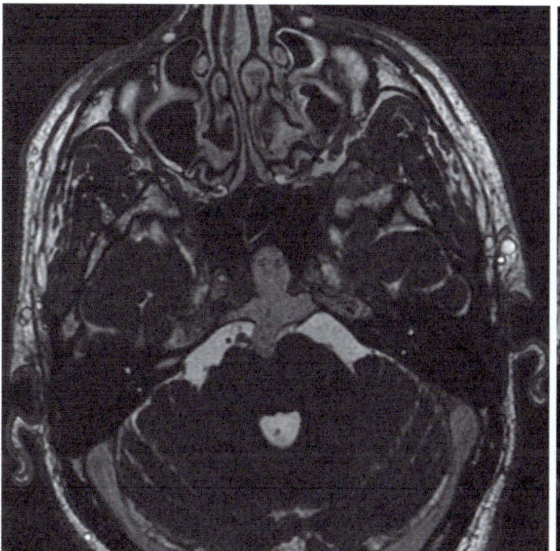

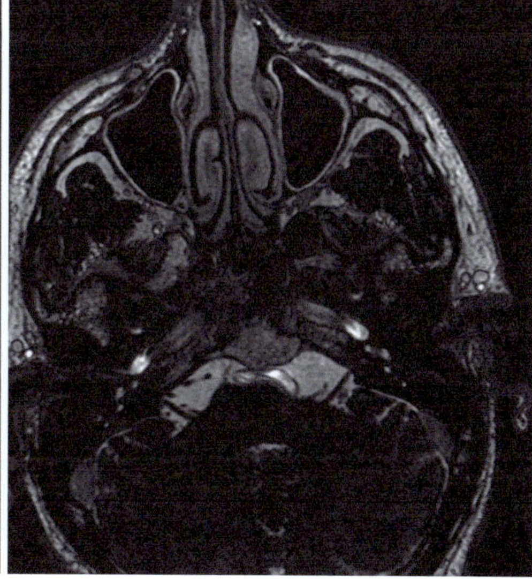

Figs. 26.2 and 26.3 Preoperative MRI scan

mandatory. Skull base neurosurgeons are used to the transcranial perspective of anatomical structures such as the ICA, but the endonasal view of it can be confusing for beginners. It definitely requires some effort, some practice in an anatomical laboratory, and the assistance of an ENT surgeon to safely identify crucial anatomical structures while performing such approaches. The use of neuronavigation system cannot replace a strong knowledge of the anatomy.

Landmarks are mandatory to navigate in the nasal cavities. One crucial landmark to begin with is the choanal arch. The choanal arch should be considered as a light in the dark for the beginners, and every time the surgeon get lost into the nasal cavities, going posteriorly, along the nasal fossa floor to the choanal arch, is particularly helpful to confirm that the line of sight of the approach is not too high toward the anterior skull base. The next major landmark is the middle turbinate. When the middle turbinate is mobilize medially, the uncinate process and, immediately behind, the bulla ethmoidalis come into view. One should keep in mind that the lateral wall of the bulla ethmoidalis is the thin medial wall of the orbit. The maxillary sinus will be reached behind and lateral to the inferior part of the uncinate process.

The sphenopalatine foramen (SPF) is a notch between the orbital and sphenoidal processes of the ascending process of the palatine bone. Following backward the ethmoid crest, which is a small spur of the bone of the medial surface of the ascending process of the palatine bone, the SPF with the sphenopalatine artery (SPA) running through is identified.

Following backward the nasal septum, the ostium of the sphenoid is located about 1.5 cm above the roof of the choanal arch. Below the level of the ostium runs the artery that vascularizes the mucosa of the nasal septum: the posterior septal artery (terminal branch of the sphenopalatine artery).

Once into the sphenoid sinus, some major landmarks may be recognized. Below the sella is the clival recess that is bordered laterally by the prominences created by the paraclival segment of the ICA. Those two prominences appear in case of a well pneumatized sphenoid sinus as two pillars on both side of the clival recess. The paraclival segment of the ICA corresponds to the posterior ascending segment of the cavernous segment of the ICA (C4 segment) that follows the lacerum segment of the ICA (C3 segment) [29]. The junction between the lacerum segment and the posterior segment of the ICA is also called the anterior or second genu of the ICA. The sellar floor limits superiorly the clival depression. On both sides of the anterior wall of the sella can be identified the slight prominence of the horizontal segment of the cavernous ICA followed by the recess formed by the middle clinoid process and, above it, the prominence of the clinoidal segment of the ICA. Above the prominence of the sella is the depression formed by the tuberculum sellae. Lateral to it is the medial opticocarotid recess that corresponds on the intracranial surface to the lateral tubercular crest. The opticocarotid recess that corresponds to the pneumatization of the optic strut (Inferior root of the anterior clinoid process) lies between the prominence of the clinoidal segment of the ICA and the prominence of the optic canal.

One should keep in mind that the shape of the posterior wall of the sphenoid sinus is highly variable from one patient to another. Two factors contribute to such variations: Firstly, the degree of pneumatization is variable, and in case of a conchal form of sphenoid sinus, none of those landmarks may be identified clearly. Secondly, the shape of the cavernous ICA is extremely variable [29], and the paraclival segment of the ICA can either run straightly vertical, slightly medially, or laterally or can be, rarely, tortuous. Those variations dictate the presence and shape of the clival depression and are important to consider preoperatively when planning an endoscopic transclival approach.

While resecting a tumor located into the clivus, the structure at high risk of damage is the abducens nerve (CN VI). From its emergence from the brain stem at the level of the bulbopontine sulcus (approximately at the level of the vertebral convergence which is a straightforward landmark after opening the dura mater in the midline), CN VI runs upward and slightly laterally. Following the same direction, it then runs

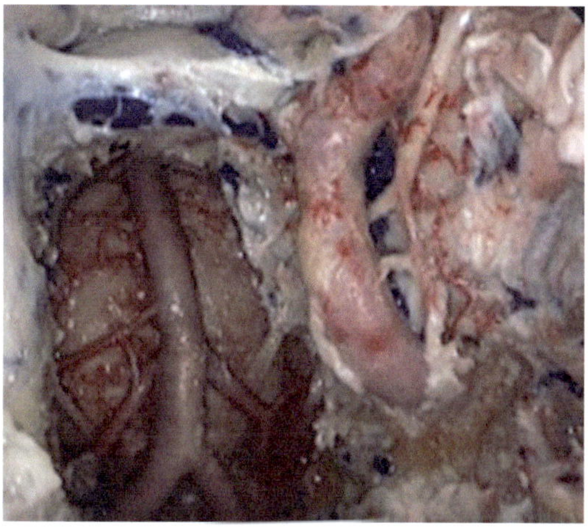

Fig. 26.4 Abducens nerve trajectory

into a dural canal in which CN VI is followed by a sleeve of arachnoid for a variable distance (abducens nerve cistern). Into Dorello's canal, below Gruber ligament, CN VI changes direction and became more horizontal and moves lateral to the posterior ascending segment of the ICA. Then, it courses slightly upward along the medial and inferior surface of the horizontal segment of the cavernous sinus ICA (Fig. 26.4). When looking at the CN VI from an endoscopic endonasal 2D perspective with a 0° scope, the CN VI in its cisternal segment is medial to the paraclival ICA until it reaches Dorello's canal. It then runs lateral to the paraclival segment of the ICA. The region at most risk for the CN VI nerve in case of clival chordomas is located immediately before and into Dorello's canal. CN VI nerve monitoring is therefore critical and helpful to identify CN VI. However, the efficiency of CN VI nerve monitoring is often diminished by a preoperative CN VI paresis, which is one of the most frequent presenting symptoms of clival chordomas.

26.6 Surgical Technique

26.6.1 Preoperative Planning

The approach should be carefully planned to achieve the three main goals of the surgery: (1) exposition, (2) resection, and (3) reconstruction. Considering those three steps, which are closely linked together, we have to consider several critical issues:

- If the patient had already prior surgery, the availability of vascularized flaps has to be evaluated: nasoseptal flap (NSF) in case of previous endonasal surgery and temporoparietal fascia flaps in case of previous craniotomy.

  A vascularized flap is mandatory in almost all cases because the procedure will often lead to at least a "naked" ICA or a dural defect. The vascularized flap serves as a remodeling tissue to reconstruct any dural defect and to prevent any secondary ICA rupture due to the inflammation and erosion of the wall of the ICA.

  The presence of scar tissue may also impede the tumor dissection as well as the identification of critical vascular and nervous structures.
- In case of previous radiotherapy, the issue of having a reliable vascularized flap is even more critical. Patients are at risk of radionecrosis, and the healing process is usually impaired with a higher risk of CSF leak. The identification and control of critical neurovascular structures such as the ICA surrounded by scar tissue is also at higher risk in case of previous irradiation.

Then, the side of the NSF harvest should be planned before the surgery, and it depends on several factors: its availability on both sides, the side of the main lateral extension, the presence of a septal deviation, and the size of the both nasal cavities.

The CT anatomy of the nasal cavities should be carefully reviewed, searching for septal deviation, Onodi cells, and bone defect over the ICA and studying the pneumatization of the sphenoid sinus. A CT angiography should be considered systematically as it offers a precise evaluation of the main intra- and extracranial vessel trajectories (ICA in all its segments, VA and BA, PCom) as well as their relationship with the tumor. The need of a proximal control of the ICA prior tumor resection must also be anticipated especially when the tumor is extending laterally and posteriorly to the paraclival ICA. In such

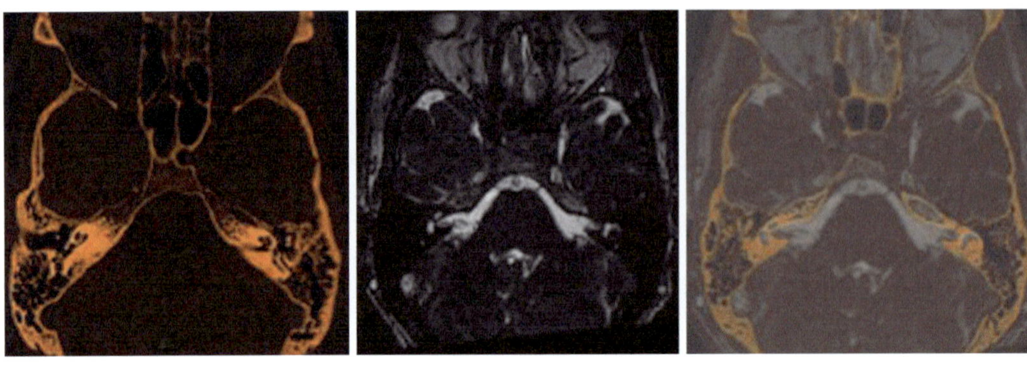

Fig. 26.5 Image-guided surgery (IGS) with MRI and CT imaging fusion

cases an additional transpterygoid approach, following the vidian nerve posteriorly toward the lacerum segment of the ICA, may be necessary before tumor resection.

Depending on the anatomy of the nasal cavities, the exact location and extent of the tumor, and the need of a NSF, one could consider a one nostril or binostril approach. In case of a small extradural chordomas, it may be possible to achieve a complete resection through only one nostril, keeping one nasal cavity intact and reducing the postoperative discomfort of the patient. In case of a large chordomas, with intradural extension, a binostril approach is almost unavoidable allowing a proper exposure of the tumor, enough space for the movement of the instruments, and a good control of the critical structures.

26.6.2 Surgical Technique and Pitfalls

26.6.2.1 Tools and Patient Preparation

The endonasal endoscopic approach is systematically performed using image-guided surgery (IGS) with MRI (contrast T1-weighted and T2-weighted) and CT imaging fusion (Fig. 26.5) as well as a microvascular ultrasound Doppler probe to accurately localize the internal carotid arteries. The precision of the navigation system should be confirmed regularly during the procedure. Before starting the surgery, we find very useful to test the accuracy of the neuronavigation using the groove between both superior incisive that are clearly visible on the properatice CT scan. Deeper, the accuracy is checked along the rail of the septum and using the bony septations into the sphenoid sinus. This is mandatory when working at high depth at the level of the lower clivus and CCJ.

Monitoring of the cranial nerve is also critical, especially the monitoring of CN VI that is most often involved in clival chordomas. In case of lower clivus chordomas with significant lateral extension toward the condyl and hypoglossal canal, monitoring of cranial nerve XII is also mandatory. It is even more important in case of unilateral cranial nerve palsy to avoid a bilateral XII nerve palsy that is a devastating complication for the patient. In case of brain stem compression or infitration, monitoring of motor evoked potential may also be helpful.

Standard 4 mm, 30° and inverted 30° scope is commonly used (KARL STORZ GmbH & Co., Tuttlingen, Germany). 70° scope may be very helpful for lesion located laterally, typically behind the horizontal segment of the ICA. Scope with variable direction of view from 0° to 120° might be also extremely useful to check the deep corners of the surgical field (KARL STORZ GmbH & Co., Tuttlingen, Germany). This ability to inspect such corners with multidirection scope may reduce the need of additional surgical steps required to expose those deep regions using regular 0° or 30° scopes.

Binostril approach is most commonly used. With experience and training, a one nostril approach can be considered in case of small well-defined lesion. However, the functional benefit for the patient of sparing one nasal cavity should not be overestimated and should not limit the ability to achieve a radical resection that is even more critical for the patient. The need for two, three, or four hands depends on the step of the surgery. The initial ENT steps of the approach most often require only two or three hands. The main surgeon is holding the scope while performing the approach with its other hand in a sequential use of the instruments. A third hand may be needed for suction of blood or smoke caused by the use of bipolar or monopolar coagulation. When drilling is required, the same combination can be used with one surgeon holding the scope and the drill and another one holding the suction. Another option is for the main surgeon to work with both hands with another surgeon holding the scope. Self-irrigating drills are mandatory. When working deep at the level of the CCJ, long instruments and an angled drill handpiece are most useful to navigate the curve of the palate.

In case of recurrence and reoperation, neuronavigation and Doppler are mandatory as most of the anatomical landmarks, and the initial bone protection over the ICA may not be present anymore. The main rule in such "redo procedure" is to spot the bony limits from the previous surgery. The Doppler is crucial and has to be used at early stage in the surgery if the ICA is proved to be "naked" on the preoperative CT angiography.

The nostrils are prepared by 2 ml of 10 % naphazoline with adrenaline, applied topically with patties. The septum and lateral nasal wall is injected with 2 ml of 2 % lidocaine with adrenaline. The thorax is slightly elevated and the head is slightly flexed, rotated, and tilted toward the surgeon and secured in a three-pin head holder. According to the navigation system that is used, the head has to be immobilized in a pin holder or could be moved freely. The pin holder headrest gives the advantage to freeze the position of the head. It's also important to adapt the flexion of the head according to the location of the tumor. The flexion needs to be accentuated for lesion located at the lower clivus and CCJ. If a temporoparietal flap is needed, a non-fixed head is more convenient to harvest the flap and tunnelize it.

Intraoperative elevation of the head and thorax should also be anticipated in order to diminish the venous pressure and the venous bleeding that may occur at the level of the cavernous sinus or basilar venous plexus if necessary. The abdomen or anterolateral thigh is prepared for harvesting a fat and/or fascia lata graft to repair the bone and dural defects.

26.6.3 Surgical Approach

26.6.3.1 Endonasal Steps

The approach is initiated doing a review of the anatomy of the nostril. To gain space inferiorly for the endoscope, inferior turbinate may be out fractured and lateralized. Then, a middle turbinectomy is performed in the right nostril to provide enough space for the endoscope and the suction. The resection of the left middle turbinate may not be necessary and can be only fractured laterally.

Following the resection of the middle turbinate, a posterior ethmoidectomy can be performed on the side of the NSF in order to facilitate the harvesting of the flap. This step is best performed by a microdebrider. Before starting the ethmoidectomy, the ostium of the sphenoid sinus as well as the posterior root of the middle turbinate must be identified in order to envision the position of the SPA and the pedicle of the NSF. The uncinate process is resected and the bulla ethmoidalis is removed exposing the lamina papyracea. Behind the inferior part of the uncinate process, the maxillary sinus is entered, and the medial wall of the maxillary sinus, above the inferior turbinate, is removed from front to back toward the angle between the medial and posterior wall of the maxillary sinus. The basal lamella of the middle turbinate is opened to enter the posterior ethmoid, and the subsequent ethmoid air cells are removed from front to back. Finally, the superior turbinate is removed and the sphenoid sinus is entered. Care must be taken to remain above the level of the ostium not to injure the SPA and the pedicle of the NSF. Another option to locate the SPF and SPA is to elevate the mucoperiosteum over the ascending process of the palatine bone and to follow backward the ethmoid crest.

It is not always necessary to open the maxillary sinus. The opening of the maxillary sinus is required for orientation purposes, when an ipsilateral transpterygoid approach is planned or in order to store the NSF during the surgery.

Then, the NSF is harvested from back to front starting with the inferior mucosal cut so that no blood trickle will obscure the surgical field [17]. Section of the mucosa is made with a monopolar diathermy needle at minimum effective power to spare the olfactory mucosa as much as possible.

The incision starts above the superior lip of the Eustachian tube and follows the inferior aspect of the choanal arch toward the septum. Then, the incision runs anteriorly along the angle between the septum and the floor of the nasal cavity. In case of an expected large dural defect, the size of the NSF can be increased with the adjunction of the mucosa of the floor of the nasal cavity and eventually the mucosa of the inferior meatus. The superior cut starts above the ostium of the sphenoid and runs anteriorly along the nasal septum, 1.5–2 cm below the roof of the nasal cavity in order to spare the olfactory fibers.

Then, a vertical anterior incision cut joins the superior and inferior cut.

The flap is elevated from anterior to posterior and placed either in the nasopharynx or into the maxillary sinus through a wider antrostomy, depending on the extent of the tumor. It can also be positioned in the sphenoid sinus in case of tumor located at the level of the CCJ. The flap can be hold in the maxillary sinus with the placement of large cottonoid into the maxillary sinus.

A crucial step consists in removing the posterior septum allowing an easy introduction of instruments from the contralateral nostril without contamination of the optic by the posterior septum itself. A rescue flap may be secondarily performed with the contralateral septal mucosa that is cut posteriorly and reversed anteriorly to cover the remaining denuded septum [30].

Whenever possible, the flap should be raised controlaterally to the side of the most lateral tumor extension site. The NSF flap makes a transpterygoid approach on the same side more difficult as it requires, in order to expose the pterygoid process, a more lateral mobilization of the NSF pedicle together with the lateral mobilization of the sphenopalatine fossa. Performing such a lateral mobilization of the NSF increases significantly the risk of injury to the SPA. It implies also the section of the palatine nerves.

The sphenoid sinus is then widely open until the lateral recess of the sphenoid sinus is exposed. The landmarks on the posterior surface of the sphenoid sinus are identified: the clival recess, the sella, the optic canal prominence, the opticocarotid recess, and the prominence of the paraclival segment of the ICA on both sides of the clival recess. The floor of the sphenoid sinus is drill down, as needed depending on the lower extension of the tumor. A wide opening of the sphenoid sinus also facilitates the transposition and adherence of the NSF. The mucosa of the sphenoid sinus is then completely removed.

The approach is then tailored depending on tumor location and extension, although generally a wide clival resection is performed [29].

26.6.3.2 Clival Resection

At this stage, the tumor is quite often visible in the posterior wall of the sphenoid sinus as it usually erodes the bone anteriorly. It therefore creates a door to get into the tumor. However, such tempting corridor toward the tumor should not eliminate the need to identify important landmarks and to envision the position of critical structure prior tumor resection. Moreover, it allows a wider opening, which is a critical step to perform a radical tumor resection.

The bone of the clivus is drilled out as far as needed and the underlying dura widely exposed. The structure at risk is the paraclival segment of the ICA. The bone covering the artery may be partially eroded by the tumor, and the tumor usually extends behind the paraclival segment. In such cases, it is strongly advocated to first identify the position of the paraclival segment of the ICA, before resecting the tumor. Complete unroofing of the carotid canal is not always necessary, but having a clear understanding of its position is necessary. Complete exposure of the ICA also allows to slightly mobilize the ICA laterally, which facilitates the resection of the tumor located behind it into the posterior cavernous sinus and upper petrous apex. Unroofing of the carotid canal should be performed with a diamond drill, and coarse diamond should be avoided when getting close to the ICA. Drilling of the floor of the sphenoid sinus inferiorly may be necessary depending on the lower extent of the tumor. One should remember that chordomas have a tendency to extend between the multiple connective tissue layers of the dura mater of the clivus sometimes beyond the limits of the tumor on the MRI. Therefore, to achieve a complete or subtotal resection, a sufficient and adequate drilling and resection of the bone is mandatory. For intradural exposure, if not already breached by the tumor, the dura mater needs to be incised. In extradural tumors with intradural extension, bleeding from the basilar plexus is usually not so intense as the venous channels are partially occluded by the tumor. The absence of venous bleeding from the dural margins usually means that there is still some tumor that has to be resected between the layers of the dura or between the dura and the bone.

26.6.4 Additional Steps

26.6.4.1 Upper Clivus, Dorsum Sellae

Tumor with an extension behind and above the level of the dorsum sellae and posterior clinoid may be difficult to reach even if the consistency of the tumor is soft and even if angled scopes are used. Situations exist where extradural approach along the dura mater of the sella is not sufficient. These are challenging lesions for two main reasons: (1) Firstly, the CN VI is at risk of damage at the level of the petrous apex. When the bone is not invaded by the tumor, the lateral drilling at the junction between the floor of the sella, the dorsum, and the petrous apex puts the CN VI at risk of damage by the heat from the drill. If the bone is totally invaded at the level of the petrous apex, the resection is easier because of the soft consistency of the tumor, but still care should be given not to damage the CN VI at the level of Dorello's canal with a strong suction used to remove the tumor as CN VI may be inside the tumor. (2) Secondly, the pituitary gland, which is usually embedded in its dura mater compartment, constitutes sometimes a barrier to reach the chordomas located behind it at the level of the dorsum sellae and posterior clinoids. In such cases, the transposition of the pituitary gland may be considered. In case of a lateral extension of the tumor, a lateral mobilization of the pituitary may be sufficient. This is done after sectioning the periosteal layer of the dura mater at the lateral margin of the sella that gives access to the dissection plane between the so-called medial wall of the cavernous sinus and the lateral border of the pituitary gland. The pituitary is gently and progressively mobilized medially with the tip of the suction (a small cottonoid is interposed between the suction and the gland), and a corridor is obtained by sectioning all connective tissue bridges between the gland and the medial wall of the CS. This step may be quite bloody, but a simple elevation of the thorax and head while reducing the venous pressure is often sufficient, together with the use of local hemostatic agents and cottonoids to rapidly control the bleeding. Then, the posterior clinoid comes into view. Dural covering is coagulated with the bipolar before drilling or biting the PCP with a small Kerrison rongeur. This step is facilitated, in our experience, by the section, from anterior to posterior, of the superior intercavernous sinus (cautiously coagulated or clipped) and the lateral insertion of the diaphragm sellae. The lateral mobilization of the gland provides full visualization of the lateral recess of the interpeduncular cistern containing the oculomotor nerve and the PCom and its perforators.

Another option is to sacrifice the pituitary gland. This situation is most often considered in case of previously operated and irradiated (at least 60–75 % of our series) patients that already have some degree of pituitary insufficiency and/or DI (diabetes insipidus). In those situations, when a retrosellar approach is considered, the resection of a nonfunctional pituitary gland seems reasonable if it guarantees a total resection. We have encountered few patients with a low pituitary stalk section that surprisingly had no postoperative DI or recovered from it. However, in case of pituitary gland resection, patient should be very carefully evaluated and supplemented postoperatively.

26.6.4.2 Lower Clivus

In case of tumor located into or arising from the lower clivus, the preclival tissue, the posterior nasopharyngeal mucosa, and the underlying soft tissue in front of the lower clivus must be removed or displaced in order to have access to the lower aspect of the tumor. In order to avoid profuse venous bleeding, one must perform the dissection staying against the bone with the monopolar coagulation or a laser-cutting tool. Two options may be encountered. If the chordoma is not only invading the clivus but also the soft tissue in front of the nasopharynx (muscle, fascia), the whole soft posterior nasopharyngeal wall must be resected. If there is no extension toward the soft tissue, a nasopharyngeal flap may be performed in order to improve postoperative healing. The lateral retraction of this structure allows the exposition of the inferior clivus, the atlantoaxial membrane, and the anterior arch of cervical vertebrae C1. During this step, it is necessary to strictly stay between the Eustachian tubes, as the ICAs run just laterally and posteriorly to them [24, 31, 32]. For this purpose, it is crucial to verify in the preoperative imaging ICA course to rule out any vascular loop that will be lying in front of the cervical spine.

26.6.4.3 Lateral Extension

In case of lateral extension of the tumor, into the petrous apex, care should be taken to identify the anterior genu between the horizontal petrous ICA and its vertical paraclival segment at the level of the foramen lacerum, which is best found by the vidian artery/nerve foramina [20, 33]. The former run in the pterygoid canal constituting a critical landmark when approaching a lateral tumor extension in the mid-clivus; thus, a transpterygoid approach should be performed. It starts with an antrostomy and SPA ligation. The posterior wall of the maxillary sinus is then resected allowing to access to the sphenopalatine fossa. The posterior wall of the maxillary sinus is removed inferiorly until the entrance of the pterygopalatine canal is exposed with the palatine nerves and descending palatine artery into it. The sphenopalatine fossa that is kept into its periosteal sac is then progressively transposed laterally, and the vidian bundle is sectioned as it exits from the vidian canal. Section of the palatine nerves is not necessary to transpose the sphenopalatine fossa laterally and to only expose the upper part of the pterygoid process. Then, following the vidian nerve posteriorly and drilling the root of the pterygoid process, the anterior ICA genu (C3 segment) is reached. In order to expose the inferior aspect of the petrous bone and once the position of the anterior or second genu of the ICA has been accurately controlled by the Doppler, the foramen lacerum is disconnected from the superior aspect of the ET cartilage.

26.6.4.4 Lateral Aspect of the Craniocervical Junction

The exposition of the CCJ in the midline doesn't raise any specific issues once a few rules are respected. Any abnormal loop of the cervical ICA should be evaluated with preoperative imaging. The lower clivus, the anterior arch of C1, and the odontoid are drilled once the thick posterior soft muscle-mucosal pharyngeal wall has been subperiosteally removed while performing an inferiorly pedicled flap. A lower trajectory is followed and middle turbinate resection is not necessary to access this region.

Gaining access laterally is trickier because vasculo-nervous structures may be encountered, i.e., the parapharyngeal ICA and the hypoglossal nerve. It requires the resection of the Eustachian tube. The medial pterygoid plate is drilled. The lateral plate is kept if possible because it acts as a barrier that limits the excursion of the instruments toward the ICA. The parapharyngeal carotid is usually located in the continuation of a line going through the anteroposterior axis of the lateral pterygoid plate. This can be confirmed preoperatively on the axial views of the CT angiography. Then, a transpterygoid approach is performed in order to expose the anterior or second genu of the ICA. The superior aspect of the Eustachian tube is dissected staying close to the cartilaginous portion. The Eustachian tube is then resected. The main cut is the superior one that is made below the level of the foramen lacerum. It should be done once the Doppler has accurately controlled the position of the anterior or second genu of the ICA. Cartilaginous and ligamentous structures of the foramen lacerum are sectioned, and the Eustachian tube is progressively lowered with the suction tube and cut laterally with strong scissors.

The lateral wall (hypoglossal nerve and parapharyngeal ICA) is then controlled working medial to lateral. The anterior arch of C1 is uncovered subperiosteally beginning at the midline and then moving laterally until the lateral mass of C1 and the capsule of the atlantooccipital joint are reached. The supracondylar groove located just above provides a reliable landmark for estimating the position of the hypoglossal canal and its exocranial orifice, which are located just posterior and lateral to the groove. Monitoring of CN XII in order to identify the nerve is particularly useful in this complex region. The ICA is situated lateral to the nerve and its proximity can be identified with a Doppler.

Once the exact position of all critical structures is identified, the drilling of the inferolateral clivus and condyle can be performed until the posterior aspect of the capsule of the atlantooccipital joint is reached. At this point, a Doppler probe can locate the VA.

Then, the resection of the tumor can be completed in a usual way. Postoperative CT scan is mandatory to evaluate the stability of the spine. If more than half condyle has been drilled off, an occipitocervical fixation should be performed in a second stage.

For large tumor, a two-stage procedure may be considered and planned especially for large and complex chordomas extending intradurally. Doing so the duration of the surgery is limited, and the closure that is a crucial step of the surgery is more easily performed. Moreover, a delay of few weeks between the approach and a second intradural step may greatly decrease/limit the amount of bleeding that is quite frequent in this region (basilar plexus, inferior petrosal sinus) [34].

Conclusions

Endoscopic approach to the clivus should nowadays be a part of the armamentarium of all modern skull base surgeons. The EEA is a valid alternative to transcranial or transoral ways when managing clival chordomas. Its main and largely accepted indication is for centrally sitting lesions. However, EEA approaches are not "minimally invasive" especially when they are performed for chordomas extending beyond the limit of clivus. This surgery is best performed by a combined team of ENT and neurosurgeon working closely together as real partners. Challenging and rare skull base tumor such as chordomas should be referred to skull base center in which all the skull base techniques and approaches are available in the surgeon's armamentarium, which enable to choose the best surgical strategy tailored to each specific tumor.

References

1. Eriksson B, Gunterberg B, Kindblom LG (1981) Chordoma. A clinicopathologic and prognostic study of a Swedish national series. Acta Orthop Scand 52(1):49–58
2. McMaster ML, Goldstein AM, Bromley CM, Ishibe N, Parry DM (2001) Chordoma: incidence and survival patterns in the United States, 1973–1995. Cancer Causes Control CCC 12(1):1–11
3. Mirra J, Nelson S, Della Rocca C, Mertens F (2002) Chordoma. In: Fletcher C, Unni K, Mertens F (eds) Pathology and genetics of tumours of soft tissue and bone. IARC Press, Lyon, pp 316–317
4. Tzortzidis F, Elahi F, Wright DC, Temkin N, Natarajan SK, Sekhar LN (2006) Patient outcome at long-term follow-up after aggressive microsurgical resection of cranial base chondrosarcomas. Neurosurgery 58(6):1090–1098. doi:10.1227/01.NEU.0000215892.65663.54; discussion 1090–1098
5. Munzenrider JE, Liebsch NJ (1999) Proton therapy for tumors of the skull base. Strahlenther Onkol Organ Dtsc Rontgengesellschaft [et al] 175 Suppl 2:57–63
6. Hunter CJ, Matyas JR, Duncan NA (2004) Cytomorphology of notochordal and chondrocytic cells from the nucleus pulposus: a species comparison. J Anat 205(5):357–362. doi:10.1111/j.0021-8782.2004.00352.x
7. Horten BC, Montague SR (1976) Human ecchordosis physaliphora and chick embryonic notochord. A comparative electron microscopic study. Virchows Arch A Pathol Anat Histol 371(4):295–303
8. Mehnert F, Beschorner R, Kuker W, Hahn U, Nagele T (2004) Retroclival ecchordosis physaliphora: MR imaging and review of the literature. AJNR Am J Neuroradiol 25(10):1851–1855
9. Chugh R, Tawbi H, Lucas DR, Biermann JS, Schuetze SM, Baker LH (2007) Chordoma: the nonsarcoma primary bone tumor. Oncologist 12(11):1344–1350. doi:10.1634/theoncologist.12-11-1344
10. Heffelfinger MJ, Dahlin DC, MacCarty CS, Beabout JW (1973) Chordomas and cartilaginous tumors at the skull base. Cancer 32(2):410–420
11. Rich TA, Schiller A, Suit HD, Mankin HJ (1985) Clinical and pathologic review of 48 cases of chordoma. Cancer 56(1):182–187

12. Carpentier A, Blanquet A, George B (2001) Suboccipital and cervical chordomas: radical resection with vertebral artery control. Neurosurg Focus 10(3), E4
13. al-Mefty O, Borba LA (1997) Skull base chordomas: a management challenge. J Neurosurg 86(2):182–189. doi:10.3171/jns.1997.86.2.0182
14. Almefty K, Pravdenkova S, Colli BO, Al-Mefty O, Gokden M (2007) Chordoma and chondrosarcoma: similar, but quite different, skull base tumors. Cancer 110(11):2457–2467. doi:10.1002/cncr.23073
15. Colli B, Al-Mefty O (2001) Chordomas of the craniocervical junction: follow-up review and prognostic factors. J Neurosurg 95(6):933–943. doi:10.3171/jns.2001.95.6.0933
16. Colli BO, Al-Mefty O (2001) Chordomas of the skull base: follow-up review and prognostic factors. Neurosurg Focus 10(3), E1. doi:10.3171/foc.2001.10.3.2
17. Gay E, Sekhar LN, Rubinstein E, Wright DC, Sen C, Janecka IP, Snyderman CH (1995) Chordomas and chondrosarcomas of the cranial base: results and follow-up of 60 patients. Neurosurgery 36(5):887–896; discussion 896–887
18. Pamir MN, Kilic T, Ture U, Ozek MM (2004) Multimodality management of 26 skull-base chordomas with 4-year mean follow-up: experience at a single institution. Acta Neurochir (Wien) 146(4):343–354. doi:10.1007/s00701-004-0218-3; discusion 354
19. Pearlman AW, Friedman M (1970) Radical radiation therapy of chordoma. Am J Roentgenol Radium Ther Nucl Med 108(2):332–341
20. Samii A, Gerganov VM, Herold C, Hayashi N, Naka T, Mirzayan MJ, Ostertag H, Samii M (2007) Chordomas of the skull base: surgical management and outcome. J Neurosurg 107(2):319–324. doi:10.3171/JNS-07/08/0319
21. Tamaki N, Nagashima T, Ehara K, Motooka Y, Barua KK (2001) Surgical approaches and strategies for skull base chordomas. Neurosurg Focus 10(3), E9
22. Austin-Seymour M, Munzenrider J, Goitein M, Verhey L, Urie M, Gentry R, Birnbaum S, Ruotolo D, McManus P, Skates S et al (1989) Fractionated proton radiation therapy of chordoma and low-grade chondrosarcoma of the base of the skull. J Neurosurg 70(1):13–17. doi:10.3171/jns.1989.70.1.0013
23. Hug EB, Loredo LN, Slater JD, DeVries A, Grove RI, Schaefer RA, Rosenberg AE, Slater JM (1999) Proton radiation therapy for chordomas and chondrosarcomas of the skull base. J Neurosurg 91(3):432–439. doi:10.3171/jns.1999.91.3.0432
24. Igaki H, Tokuuye K, Okumura T, Sugahara S, Kagei K, Hata M, Ohara K, Hashimoto T, Tsuboi K, Takano S, Matsumura A, Akine Y (2004) Clinical results of proton beam therapy for skull base chordoma. Int J Radiat Oncol Biol Phys 60(4):1120–1126. doi:10.1016/j.ijrobp.2004.05.064
25. Noel G, Feuvret L, Ferrand R, Boisserie G, Mazeron JJ, Habrand JL (2004) Radiotherapeutic factors in the management of cervical-basal chordomas and chondrosarcomas. Neurosurgery 55(6):1252–1260; discussion 1260–1252
26. Noel G, Habrand JL, Mammar H, Pontvert D, Haie-Meder C, Hasboun D, Moisson P, Ferrand R, Beaudre A, Boisserie G, Gaboriaud G, Mazal A, Kerody K, Schlienger M, Mazeron JJ (2001) Combination of photon and proton radiation therapy for chordomas and chondrosarcomas of the skull base: the Centre de Protontherapie D'Orsay experience. Int J Radiat Oncol Biol Phys 51(2):392–398
27. Suit HD, Goitein M, Munzenrider J, Verhey L, Davis KR, Koehler A, Linggood R, Ojemann RG (1982) Definitive radiation therapy for chordoma and chondrosarcoma of base of skull and cervical spine. J Neurosurg 56(3):377–385. doi:10.3171/jns.1982.56.3.0377
28. Feuvret L, Noel G, Weber DC, Pommier P, Ferrand R, De Marzi L, Dhermain F, Alapetite C, Mammar H, Boisserie G, Habrand JL, Mazeron JJ (2007) A treatment planning comparison of combined photon-proton beams versus proton beams-only for the treatment of skull base tumors. Int J Radiat Oncol Biol Phys 69(3):944–954. doi:10.1016/j.ijrobp.2007.07.2326
29. Cebula H, Kurbanov A, Zimmer LA, Poczos P, Leach JL, De Battista JC, Froelich S, Theodosopoulos PV, Keller JT (2014) Endoscopic, endonasal variability in the anatomy of the internal carotid artery. World Neurosurg 82(6):e759–e764. doi:10.1016/j.wneu.2014.09.021
30. Caicedo-Granados E, Carrau R, Snyderman CH, Prevedello D, Fernandez-Miranda J, Gardner P, Kassam A (2010) Reverse rotation flap for reconstruction of donor site after vascular pedicled nasoseptal flap in skull base surgery. Laryngoscope 120(8):1550–1552. doi:10.1002/lary.20975
31. Kassam AB, Snyderman C, Gardner P, Carrau R, Spiro R (2005) The expanded endonasal approach: a fully endoscopic transnasal approach and resection of the odontoid process: technical case report. Neurosurgery 57(1 Suppl):E213; discussion E213
32. Kassam AB, Thomas A, Carrau RL, Snyderman CH, Vescan A, Prevedello D, Mintz A, Gardner P (2008) Endoscopic reconstruction of the cranial base using a pedicled nasoseptal flap. Neurosurgery 63(1 Suppl 1):ONS44–ONS52. doi:10.1227/01.neu.0000335010.53122.75; discussion ONS52-43
33. Kassam AB, Prevedello DM, Thomas A, Gardner P, Mintz A, Snyderman C, Carrau R (2008) Endoscopic endonasal pituitary transposition for a transdorsum sellae approach to the interpeduncular cistern. Neurosurgery 62(3 Suppl 1):57–72. doi:10.1227/01.neu.0000317374.30443.23; discussion 72–54
34. Chibbaro S, Cornelius JF, Froelich S, Tigan L, Kehrli P, Debry C, Romano A, Herman P, George B, Bresson D (2014) Endoscopic endonasal approach in the management of skull base chordomas–clinical experience on a large series, technique, outcome, and pitfalls. Neurosurg Rev 37(2):217–224; discussion 224–225

Endoscopic Endonasal Odontoidectomy

27

Salvatore Chibbaro and Stephan Gaillard

27.1 Background

Removal of the peg is a procedure often required to manage basilar impression compressing the brain stem and/or spinal cord because of irreducible atlanto-axial dislocation. Various pathologies may cause atlanto-axial dislocation such as congenital malformation and especially Arnold–Chiari type II, genetic degenerative transformation such as in Down's syndrome, chronic inflammation related to rheumatoid arthritis and/or metabolic disorders, and finally trauma.

Until recently the transoral approach has been the most implemented and favored procedure to approach the craniocervical (CCJ) junction and largely used to manage either extradural or intradural disorders [1–14].

The former approaches although providing a direct access to the CCJ region present many disadvantages as follows:

1. The deepness of the surgical corridor.
2. Sometimes the splitting of the soft palate is needed.
3. The potential risk of tongue and teeth damage.
4. And finally, in case of dural opening, an important risk of CSF leak and meningitis.

Recently, based on the experience of endoscopic endonasal approaches [15, 16], several studies either anatomical and/or clinical have been reported showing the interest of approaching the CCJ through the nasal corridor. In fact, the availability of new technologies, such as endoscopy, navigation systems, and microvascular ultrasound Doppler coupled to dedicated devices, have opened new horizons to manage pathologies involving this complex region using the natural nasal corridors; this way/approach has demonstrated a remarkable improvement of the quality of disease resection as well as of the functional outcome with a lower morbidity.

This approach provides a direct access to the surgical field, minimizing the neurovascular manipulation passing through the oropharynx. The major limitation of this approach, in case of intradural disease, is the difficulty of dural closure with the related higher risk of CSF leakage and meningitis [17–26].

Thanking to the intrinsic features of the endoscope, the endonasal way provides a wider, panoramic, and multi-angled view of the region favoring also a closer-up view maximally reducing in this way the operating field deepness if comparing with the transoral microscopic approach. Furthermore,

Electronic supplementary material The online version of this chapter (doi:10.1007/978-3-319-21533-4_27) contains supplementary material, which is available to authorized users.

S. Chibbaro, MD, PhD (✉)
Department of Neurosurgery,
Strasbourg University Hospital, Strasbourg, France
e-mail: schibbaro@hotmail.com

S. Gaillard, MD (✉)
Department of Neurosurgery,
Foch Hospital, Sursenes, France
e-mail: s.gaillard@hopital-foch.org

P. Cappabianca et al. (eds.), *Midline Skull Base Surgery*, DOI 10.1007/978-3-319-21533-4_27

this way is less invasive reducing various morbidities associated to the transoral approach as follows:

1. There is no need of mouth retractors.
2. There is no need of neither prolonged tongue compression or split of the soft palate.

27.2 Indications

The indication for odontoid resection is irreducible atlanto-axial subluxation, associated with severe brain stem and/or spinal cord compression causing progressive neurological dysfunction. The possibility to perform an endonasal endoscopic odontoidectomy is necessarily related to the level of the C1–C2 junction. Practically, in the case of a quite low junction, generally far below the level of the hard palate, it is almost impossible to remove the peg by the endonasal way. On the contrary, in the presence of a higher junction position, the dens are more easily reachable and removed by the nasal route. Considering the complexity of the transoral approach to the CCJ, involving complicated maneuvers such as, sometimes, the splitting of the soft and even hard palate, we strongly believe that the former approach should nowadays be limited to selected case in which a very low C1–C2 junction is present. To summarize endonsal odontoidectomy could be performed in case of Arnold Chiari type II, genetic degenerative transformation as in Down's syndrome, chronic inflammation as in Rheumatoid arthritis, and very rarely in Trauma. Further it is very important to remember specific indication as in childrens (due to narrow mouth), in case of micrognathia and macroglossia (in which transoral way is very difficult) and finally this technique is also very suitable for achondroplasic and osteogenesis imperfecta patients.

27.3 Surgical Technique

The patient is positioned in a recumbent and slight Trendelenburg position (20°), the head is fixed in a Mayfield head-holder neuronavigation system based on CT, MRI image fusion is routinely used, and somatosensory evoked potential neuromonitoring is also suggestible (see also Figs. 27.1 and 27.2).

Preoperative antibiotic prophylaxis is routinely administered 20 min before the operation starts. The nose is routinely prepared by iodine 5 % and naphazoline.

A 0° and 30° angled endoscopes with an HDD camera (Storz, Germany) and dedicated endoscopic tools are used (Storz and Aesculap, Germany). The procedure could be usually dealt either by two-hand (coupled to an holder harm) or by four-hand technique; we strongly believe that the former choice is strictly related to the surgeon's skill and preference; for example, in the neurosurgical department of Foch Hospital in Paris, this procedure is ruled out using a two-hand technique by the senior author Dr. Stephan Gaillard; on the contrary, the same procedure in Strasbourg is realized using the four-hand technique by a combined neurosurgical and ENT team.

An endoscope, suction, and irrigation are typically introduced through the right nostril, while the dissecting instruments, the drill, and the navigation probes are entered through the left nostril. An inferior septectomy is performed, removing no more than 2 cm of vomer bone at its junction with the hard palate. We do not routinely perform a sphenoidotomy, and it is decided on a case by case basis depending on each patient's anatomical constitution if it is necessary to get enough room to maneuver in. Normally we use the clivus–nasal septum junction, as the most superior dissection limit. At this stage, few important anatomical landmarks should be identified as follows:

1. The clivus–septum junction superiorly.
2. The eustachian tubes laterally.
3. The nasal floor/soft palate inferiorly as marked by the hard and soft palate. The navigation is always utilized, before to proceed, to identify the midline and the upper and lower limits of the exposure.

Next step consists in creating an inverted U-shaped muco-pharyngeal flap using a diode laser or a monopolar electrocautery going from the level of the sphenoid floor to the level of the soft palate which is caudally reflected into the oropharynx during the bony removal and replaced back in its original site at the end of the procedure. Additional soft tissue is removed using a microdebrider to completely expose the body and arch of C1 and C2.

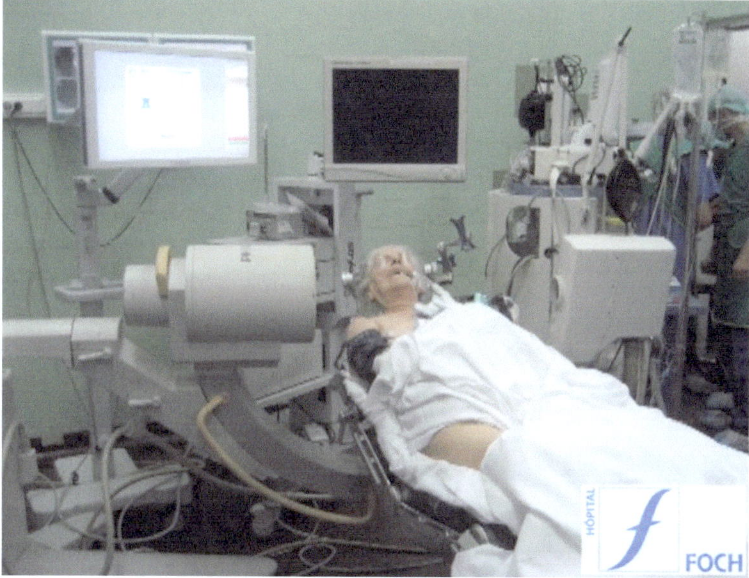

Fig. 27.1 Patient positioning in a recumbent and slight Trendelenburg position (20°), with the head fixed in a Mayfield head-holder

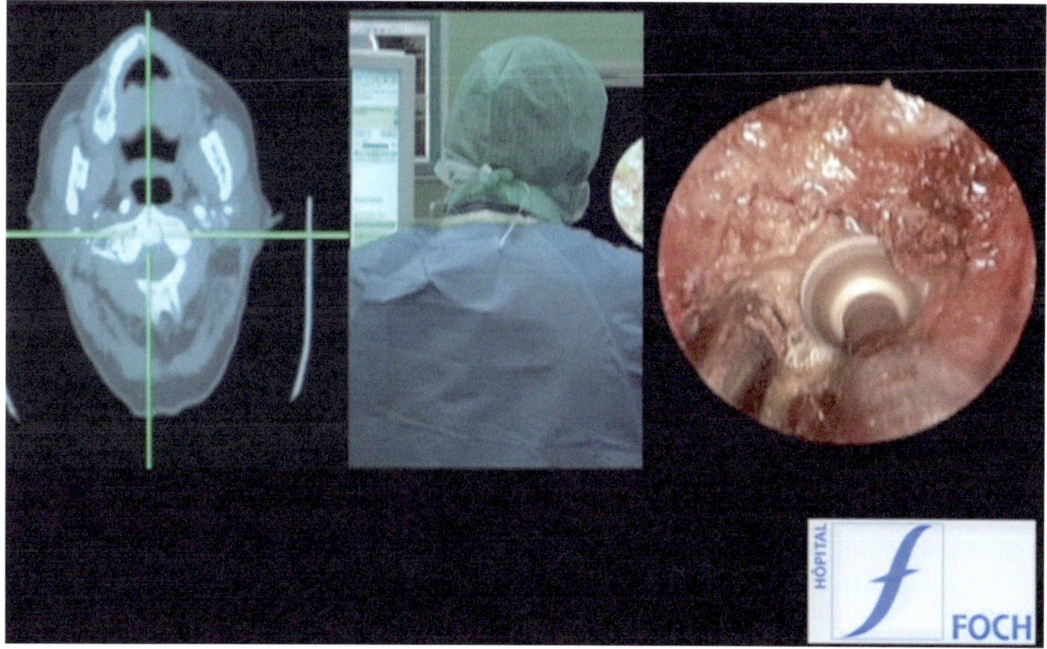

Fig. 27.2 Perioperative photos showing endoscopic view of peg drilling coupled to IGS on CT setting verification

At this stage, a 3–4 mm diamond drill bit coupled to Kerrison rongeurs is used to remove the anterior arch of C1 that allow to expose the dens, which is then drilled at its base to excise the tip and body of the dens from the remaining vertebral ring. Then removal could often be challenging due to dural and/or bony adhesion depending on specific pathology. The odontoid process could be adherent to the adjacent brain stem and/or spine dura with all associated connective tissue, and a CSF leak might occur. In some cases, instead of an "en-block" resection, an odontoid piecemeal removal may be required. Brain stem decompression is considered satisfactory when a wide dural pulsatile field is achieved (see also Figs. 27.3, 27.4, 27.5, and 27.6).

The reconstruction is completed by the placement of a multilayered Gelfoam/Surgicel and fibrin glue overlied by the pedicled regional paraspinal muscle and muco-pharyngeal flap which is also sealed by fibrin glue. If a CSF leak occurs, the multilayered closure is coupled to fascia lata and fat (for a better comprehension of the technique principal step, see also Video 27.1).

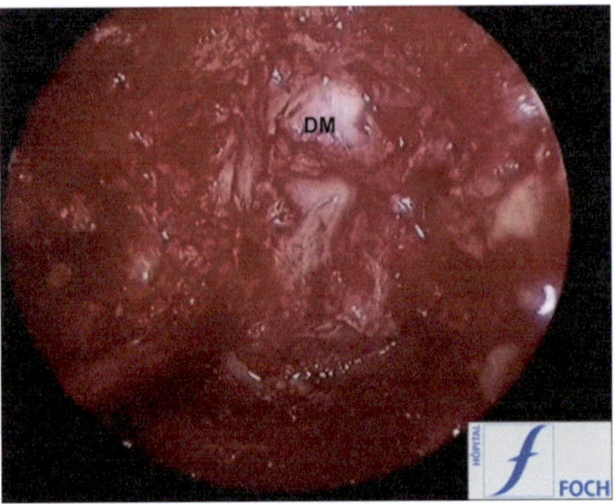

Fig. 27.3 Perioperative photos showing a wide dura mater freed area demonstrating a satisfactory brain stem decompression. *DM* dura mater

27.3.1 Technical Variation of Odontoidectomy Leaving Intact the Anterior Arch of C1

The technique and the approach is exactly the same until exposing the anterior arch of C1; after subperiosteal preparation of the anterior arch of C1, only its anteroinferior portion is drilled out in the midline to preserve the continuity of the atlas ring.

At this stage, the upper part and then the base of the peg is drilled off when it is still attached to the C2 body by working above and below the anterior arch of C1.

Once the odontoid base is completely drilled, its tip is freed from the ligaments and pushed down and removed together with any remaining

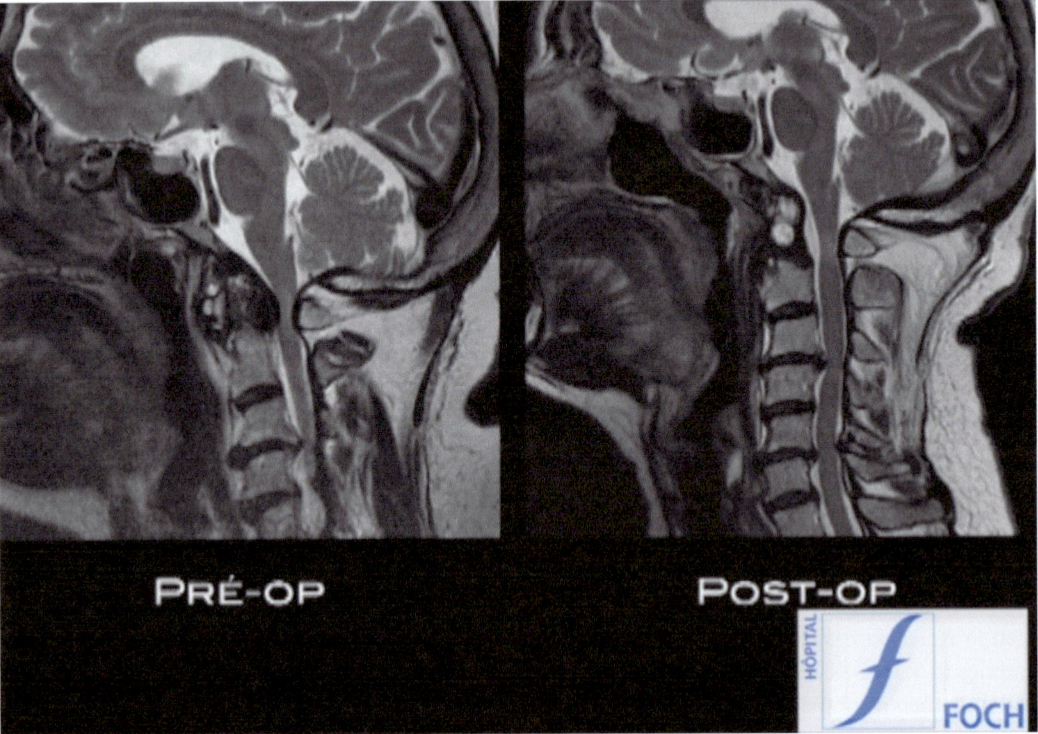

Fig. 27.4 Pre- and postoperative T2 sagittal MRI showing brain stem decompression

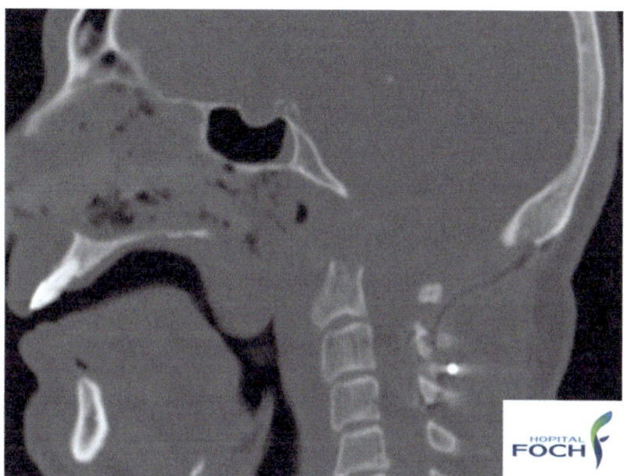

Fig. 27.5 Postoperative bony window sagittal CT scan showing optimal peg resection (same case of Fig. 27.4)

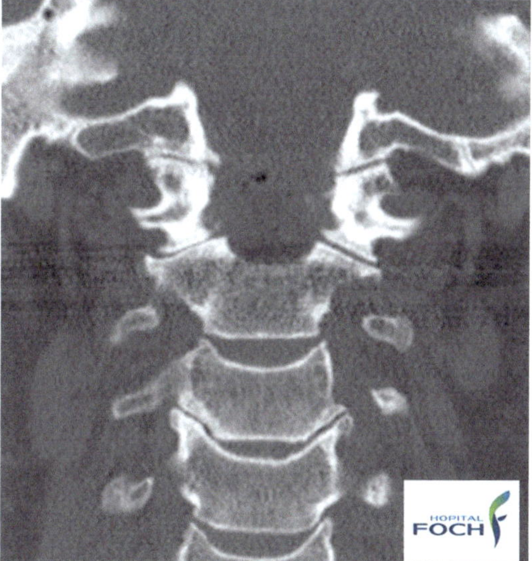

Fig. 27.6 Postoperative bony window coronal CT scan showing optimal peg resection (same case of Figs. 27.4 and 27.5)

compressive tissue. At the end, the residual surgical cavity should be inspected by angled endoscope to verify and ensure exact extension of resection which should also be confirmed by IGS. The final reconstruction is the same than standard technique. The former approach could be a nice option to treat odontoid inflammatory disease (i.e., rheumatoid arthritis) as it allows the preservation of the anterior arch of C1, reducing in this way the risk of a subaxial instability and above all avoiding a posterior fixation, thus preserving the rotational movement at C0–C2 [29].

27.4 Foch and Strasbourg Operative Series

In the neurosurgical department of Foch Hospital in Paris, a series of 10 endoscopic odontoidectomy procedures have been realized, as well as four cases have been operated in Strasbourg. Demographic, clinical, and management details are summarized in Tables 27.1 and 27.2.

27.5 Advantages, Disadvantages, and Pitfalls of Transoral Compared to EEA to the CCJ

Generally speaking, the standard transoral–transpalatal approach to the CCJ might be associated to various complications as follows:

1. Velopharyngeal incompetence (VPI)
2. Nasal speech and nasal reflux
3. Edema or tongue necrosis
4. Posterior pharyngeal wound dehiscence
5. Upper airway obstruction from retropharyngeal edema
6. Dysphagia and odynophagia
7. Pharyngeal cellulitis
8. Meningitis following CSF leakage
9. Dental injury [1–14, 27, 28]

On the other hand, the EEA has many advantages comparing to the open transoral as follows:

1. Better, wider, and angled views
2. Preservation of palatal function
3. Improved airway and swallowing morbidity, thus reduced frequency of tracheostomy
4. Decreased postoperative pain [25, 26]

The former features are possibly due to an upper placed incision of the nasopharynx comparing to the transoral way. It is a matter of fact that performing a nasopharyngeal incision above the level of the soft palate might preserve more the posterior pharyngeal muscles and mucosa which results in less tissue retraction and scarring. Furthermore, by the EEA, the patients have a lower rate of pharyngeal complications and VPI

Table 27.1 Operative series from Foch Hospital by Dr. Stephan Gaillard

No	Age/sex	Primary disease	Radiology	Preop C1–C2 shift (X-rays)	Management	Post-op shift (X-rays)	Frankel scale	Post-op external orthosis	F-U mths
1	20/M	Basilar impression	Brain stem compression	CCJ malformation	Endonasal endoscopic C0–C2 decompression with odontoidectomy *and occipitocervical stabilization at the same stage*	No	E5	No	15
2	36/M	Basilar impression	Brain stem compression	CCJ malformation	Endonasal endoscopic C0–C2 decompression with odontoidectomy *and occipitocervical stabilization at the same stage*	No	E5	No	12
3	48/M	Basilar impression	Brain stem compression	CCJ malformation	Endonasal endoscopic C0–C2 decompression with odontoidectomy *and occipitocervical stabilization at the same stage*	No	D4	No	30
4	56/M	Basilar impression	Brain stem compression	Large shift with brain stem compression and posterior deviation	Endonasal endoscopic C0–C2 decompression with odontoidectomy *and occipitocervical stabilization at the same stage*	No	E5	No	48
5	58/M	Basilar impression	Brain stem compression	Large shift with brain stem compression and posterior deviation	Endonasal endoscopic C0–C2 decompression with odontoidectomy *and occipitocervical stabilization at the same stage*	No	D4	No	30
6	67/F	Basilar impression	Brain stem compression	Large shift with brain stem compression and posterior deviation	Endonasal endoscopic C0–C2 decompression with odontoidectomy *and occipitocervical stabilization at the same stage*	No	E5	No	24
7	68/M	Degenerative disease	Brain stem compression	Large shift with brain stem compression and posterior deviation	Endonasal endoscopic C0–C2 decompression with odontoidectomy *and occipitocervical stabilization at the same stage*	No	E5	No	6
8	73/F	Degenerative disease	Brain stem compression	Large shift with brain stem compression and posterior deviation	Endonasal endoscopic C0–C2 decompression with odontoidectomy *and occipitocervical stabilization at the same stage*	No	E5	No	96
9	84/F	Degenerative disease	Brain stem compression	Large shift with brain stem compression and posterior deviation	Endonasal endoscopic C0–C2 decompression with odontoidectomy *and occipitocervical stabilization at the same stage*	No	E5	No	9
10	95/F	Degenerative disease	Brain stem compression	Large shift with brain stem compression and posterior deviation	Endonasal endoscopic C0–C2 decompression with odontoidectomy leaving C1 arch intact, no stabilization	No	E5	No	30

Table 27.2 Operative series from Strasbourg University Hospital by Dr. Salvatore Chibbaro

No	Age/sex	Primary disease	Radiology	Preop C1–C2 shift (X-rays)	Management	Post-op shift (X-rays)	Frankel scale	Post-op external orthosis	F-U mths
1	28/F	CVJ Skull base chordoma	Brain stem compression by tumor invasion of C0–C2	Brain stem compression, unstable on dynamic X-rays	Endonasal endoscopic C0–C2 decompression with odontoidectomy *and occipitocervical stabilization at the same stage*	No	E/5	No	48
2	59/F	Basilar impression	Extensive brain stem compression by C2 odontoid process	Large shift with brain stem compression and posterior deviation	Endonasal endoscopic C1 decompression with odontoidectomy *and occipitocervical stabilization at the same stage*	No	E/5	No	36
3	72/M	Degenerative compression	Extensive brain stem compression by hypertrophied "C2 odontoid process"	Large shift with brain stem compression and posterior deviation	Endonasal endoscopic C1 decompression with odontoidectomy *and occipitocervical stabilization at the same stage*	No	D/4	No	32
4	85/M	CVJ skull base chordoma	Brain stem compression	Large shift with brain stem compression and posterior deviation and instability	Endonasal endoscopic C1 decompression with odontoidectomy *and occipitocervical stabilization at the same stage*	No	E5	No	6

Pre- and Post-op preoperative, postoperative, *F-U mths* follow-up months avoiding the soft palate splitting. To date, the endonasal and transoral approaches have not been prospectively compared although in our experience, patients have less dysphagia being able to eat by the natural oral way immediately in the postoperative stage.

27.5.1 Pitfalls

27.5.1.1 CSF Leak and Meningitis

The goodness of the endoscope is its closer-up and multi-angled vision that could more easily detect the occurrence of a CSF leak, although it remains quite difficult to stitch up the dura and/or the overlying nasopharynx mucosa through the nose. For this purpose, care should be taken in creating a vascularized muscle-mucosal flap, including as much as possible of the muscular and mucosal tissue overlying the ventral CCJ. Also care should be taken to strip in the sphenoid inferior wall mucosa to favor the flap adhering, and finally, fibrin glue could be placed to seal the edges.

An endoscopic control should be performed 3 weeks later to verify the flap healing and integration.

27.5.1.2 CCJ Stability

The removals of the anterior arch of C1 as well as of the peg with its ligaments usually cause the CCJ destabilization obliging to realize an occipitocervical arthrodesis. A technical variation to avoid this problem might be performed in selected cases.

27.5.1.3 Hemostasis

The hemostasis during an EEA could constitute a major concern as it is always difficult to stop bleeding through the nose due to the deepness and narrowing of the corridor; for this purpose, dedicated bipolar forceps have been developed and are available in the market (Karl Storz GmbH, Tuttlingen, Germany) as well as various hemostatic products such as foam, matrix, etc. (and especially the activated thrombin).

Conclusions

Given our experience and up-to-date pertinent literature, we do believe that the EEA provides, similarly to the transoral way, a direct route to the CCJ being associated to lower morbidity. Analyzing the technique, the most common problem is a higher risk of CSF leakage and meningitis as well as a bleeding control. Performing a vascularized muscle-mucosal flap could represent a valid adjunct to the multilayered closure of the surgical field. Dedicated surgical instruments, IGS, and microvascular Doppler probe are necessary to perform safely such a procedure.

Finally, the EEA to CCJ represents a valid alternative to transoral and transcervical ways when managing CCJ disorders. Such approach is not "minimally invasive" although morbidity is limited compared to traditional open approaches. This technique has a steep learning curve, and it should be realized by a very experienced and skilled surgical team. Finally, the procedure could be realized using either the two- or four-hand technique as well as by a neurosurgeon alone or in cooperation with an ENT, and it is exclusively related to the surgeon's preference and habits; to date, we are not in the condition/position to affirm whether one technique is superior to the other, and the best way to perform it, we do believe, is the way each surgeon fell most comfortable to perform it.

References

1. Crockard H (1993) Transoral approach to intra/extradural tumors. In: Sekhar L, Janecka I (eds) Surgery of cranial base tumors. Raven, New York, pp 225–234
2. Crockard HA, Bradford R (1985) Transoral transclival removal of a schwannoma anterior to the craniocervical junction. Case report. J Neurosurg 62(2):293–295. doi:10.3171/jns.1985.62.2.0293
3. Crockard HA, Pozo JL, Ransford AO, Stevens JM, Kendall BE, Essigman WK (1986) Transoral decompression and posterior fusion for rheumatoid atlanto-axial subluxation. J Bone Joint Surg 68(3):350–356
4. Crockard HA, Sen CN (1991) The transoral approach for the management of intradural lesions

at the craniovertebral junction: review of 7 cases. Neurosurgery 28(1):88–97; discussion 97–88

5. Di Lorenzo N (1992) Craniocervical junction malformation treated by transoral approach. A survey of 25 cases with emphasis on postoperative instability and outcome. Acta Neurochir (Wien) 118(3–4):112–116
6. Dickman C, Spetzler R, Sonntag V (1998) Surgery of the craniovertebral junction. Thieme, New York
7. Donald P (1998) Transoral approach to the clivus and upper cervical spine. In: Donald P (ed) Surgery of the skull base. Lippincott-Raven, Philadelphia, pp 507–532
8. Hadley MN, Spetzler RF, Sonntag VK (1989) The transoral approach to the superior cervical spine. A review of 53 cases of extradural cervicomedullary compression. J Neurosurg 71(1):16–23. doi:10.3171/jns.1989.71.1.0016
9. Hayakawa T, Kamikawa K, Ohnishi T, Yoshimine T (1981) Prevention of postoperative complications after a transoral transclival approach to basilar aneurysms. Technical note. J Neurosurg 54(5):699–703. doi:10.3171/jns.1981.54.5.0699
10. Menezes AH, Graf CJ, Hibri N (1980) Abnormalities of the cranio-vertebral junction with cervico-medullary compression. A rational approach to surgical treatment in children. Childs Brain 7(1):15–30
11. Menezes AH, VanGilder JC (1988) Transoral-transpharyngeal approach to the anterior craniocervical junction. Ten-year experience with 72 patients. J Neurosurg 69(6):895–903. doi:10.3171/jns.1988.69.6.0895
12. Menezes AH, VanGilder JC, Clark CR, el-Khoury G (1985) Odontoid upward migration in rheumatoid arthritis. An analysis of 45 patients with "cranial settling". J Neurosurg 63(4):500–509. doi:10.3171/jns.1985.63.4.0500
13. Miller E, Crockard HA (1987) Transoral transclival removal of anteriorly placed meningiomas at the foramen magnum. Neurosurgery 20(6):966–968
14. Reisch R, Bettag M, Perneczky A (2001) Transoral transclival removal of anteriorly placed cavernous malformations of the brainstem. Surg Neurol 56(2):106–115; discussion 115–106
15. Cappabianca P, Alfieri A, de Divitiis E (1998) Endoscopic endonasal transsphenoidal approach to the sella: towards functional endoscopic pituitary surgery (FEPS). Minim Invasive Neurosurg 41:66–73
16. Jho HD, Carrau RL, Ko Y (1996) Endoscopic pituitary surgery. In: Wilkins H, Rengachary S (eds) Neurosurgical operative atlas. American Association of Neurological Surgeons, Park Ridge, pp 1–12
17. Alfieri A, Jho HD, Schettino R, Tschabitscher M (2003) Endoscopic endonasal approach to the pterygopalatine fossa: anatomic study. Neurosurgery 52(2):374–378; discussion 378–380
18. Alfieri A, Jho HD, Tschabitscher M (2002) Endoscopic endonasal approach to the ventral cranio-cervical junction: anatomical study. Acta Neurochir (Wien) 144(3):219–225. doi:10.1007/s007010200029; discussion 225
19. Cappabianca P, Frank G, Pasquini E, de Divitiis O, Calbucci F (2003) Extended endoscopic endonasal transsphenoidal approaches to the suprasellar region, planum sphenoidale and clivus. In: de Divitiis E, Cappabianca P (eds) Endoscopic endonasal transsphenoidal surgery. Springer, New York, pp 176–187
20. Cavallo LM, Messina A, Cappabianca P, Esposito F, de Divitiis E, Gardner P, Tschabitscher M (2005) Endoscopic endonasal surgery of the midline skull base: anatomical study and clinical considerations. Neurosurg Focus 19(1):E2
21. de Divitiis E, Cappabianca P, Cavallo LM (2002) Endoscopic transsphenoidal approach: adaptability of the procedure to different sellar lesions. Neurosurgery 51(3):699–705; discussion 705–697
22. Frank G, Pasquini E, Mazzatenta D (2001) Extended transsphenoidal approach. J Neurosurg 95(5):917–918
23. Jho HD, Carrau RL, McLaughlin MR, Somaza SC (1997) Endoscopic transsphenoidal resection of a large chordoma in the posterior fossa. Acta Neurochir (Wien) 139(4):343–347; discussion 347–348
24. Jho HD, Ha HG (2004) Endoscopic endonasal skull base surgery: part 3--the clivus and posterior fossa. Minim Invasive Neurosurg 47(1):16–23. doi:10.1055/s-2004-818347
25. Kassam A, Snyderman CH, Mintz A, Gardner P, Carrau RL (2005) Expanded endonasal approach: the rostrocaudal axis. Part II. Posterior clinoids to the foramen magnum. Neurosurg Focus 19(1), E4
26. Kassam AB, Snyderman C, Gardner P, Carrau R, Spiro R (2005) The expanded endonasal approach: a fully endoscopic transnasal approach and resection of the odontoid process: technical case report. Neurosurgery 57(1 Suppl):E213; discussion E213
27. Shaha AR, Johnson R, Miller J, Milhorat T (1993) Transoral-transpharyngeal approach to the upper cervical vertebrae. Am J Surg 166(4):336–340
28. Yang SY, Gao YZ (1999) Clinical results of the transoral operation for lesions of the craniovertebral junction and its abnormalities. Surg Neurol 51(1):16–20
29. Iacoangeli M, Gladi M, Alvaro L, Di Rienzo A, Specchia N, Scerrati M (2013) Endoscopic endonasal odontoidectomy with anterior C1 arch preservation in elderly patients affected by rheumatoid arthritis. Spine J. May;13(5):542–8.

Radiotherapy, Radiosurgery, and Proton Beam

28

Giuseppe Minniti and Claudia Scaringi

28.1 Introduction

Chordomas of the skull base are rare bone tumors with locally aggressive behavior. Surgery is the primary treatment of skull base chordomas, although long-term observation series have shown its limitation in achieving a complete removal of the lesion due to the critical location and the infiltrative patterns into the bone and neurovascular structures of the skull base.

External beam radiation therapy (RT) is usually recommended after surgery, even for patients with complete macroscopic resection. Chordomas respond to high radiation doses in the range of 70–74 Gy, although surrounding neurologic structures, including spinal cord, brainstem, and optic pathways, limit the safe delivery of high doses required for controlling the tumor [1–5]. Improvements in photon techniques are represented by intensity-modulated radiation therapy (IMRT) and stereotactic techniques, either fractionated stereotactic radiotherapy (FSRT) or stereotactic radiosurgery (SRS).

In light of the higher dose required, protons have been used in addition or instead of photons because of the superior dose distribution due to the rapid radiation falloff beyond the target [6]. Similar to proton beam therapy, carbon ions offer similar advantages relative to photon-based treatment; however, carbon ion therapy may have a number of biological differences in vivo, including a higher relative biological effectiveness and reduced oxygen-enhancement ratio in the tumor region.

28.2 Fractionated Radiotherapy

RT has been classically used in conjunction with surgery as a definitive treatment modality for unresectable or recurrent chordomas, although its efficacy is still matter of debate. At median doses of up to 50–60 Gy, the reported local control at 5 years with RT is in the range of 17–41 % (average 31 %) (Table 28.1) [4, 5, 7–17]. The optimum radiation dose is not yet well established, and no dose-response relationship has been clearly evidenced in the literature. A trend favoring highest doses has been suggested by some authors, with a better outcome for doses in the range of 60–75 Gy or even over 80 Gy as compared with

G. Minniti, MD (✉)
Radiation Oncology Unit, Department of Radiation Oncology, Sant' Andrea Hospital, University Sapienza, Via di Grottarossa 1035, Rome 00189, Italy

Department of Neuroscience, Neuromed Institute, Pozzilli, IS, Italy
e-mail: gminniti@ospedalesantandrea.it; giuseppe.minniti@ospedalesantandrea.it; giuseppeminniti@libero.it

C. Scaringi, MD
Radiation Oncology Unit, Department of Radiation Oncology, Sant' Andrea Hospital, University Sapienza, Via di Grottarossa 1035, Rome 00189, Italy

P. Cappabianca et al. (eds.), *Midline Skull Base Surgery*, DOI 10.1007/978-3-319-21533-4_28

Table 28.1 Summary of published studies on fractionated photon radiotherapy for chordoma

Authors	Patients no	Type of RT	Median dose Gy	Follow-up months	Tumor control (%)
Cummings et al. [7]	10	CRT	50	40	41 at 5 years
Chetiyawardana [8]	14	CRT	30–40	12–240	NA
Amendola et al. [9]	11	CRT	60	48	40 at 5 years
Fuller and Bloom [10]	13	CRT	55	31	23 at 5 years
Forsyth et al. [11]	39	CRT	50	99	39 at 5 years
Romero et al. [4]	18	CRT	50.1	3.1 years	17 at 5 years
Watkins et al. [12]	38	CRT	50–60	84	34 at 5 years
Catton et al. [5]	20	CRT	50	62	23 at 5 years
Zorlu et al. [13]	18	CRT	60	42	23 at 5 years
Cho et al. [14]	11	CRT/GK	59.4	55	40 at 5 years
Sahgal et al. [15]	24	IMRT	76	36	65.3 at 5 years
Debus et al. [16]	37	FSRT	66.6	27	50 at 5 years
Bugoci et al. [17]	12	FSRT	66.6	42	37.5 at 5 years

RT radiotherapy, *CRT* conventional radiotherapy, *NA* not assessed, *GK* Gamma Knife, *IMRT* intensity-modulated radiation therapy, *FSRT* fractionated stereotactic radiotherapy

doses of 55–65 Gy. Even though longer symptomatic control could be possible with higher doses, the intrinsic difficulty to achieve doses of at least 65–70 Gy without serious risks of long-term radiation-induced toxicity represents the main limitation of conventional radiotherapy.

Despite conventional RT does not appear to increase survival rates in all published studies, its role in the palliative setting in advanced, unresectable, or recurrent tumors is well established [11–19]. Tumor shrinkage and improvement of neurological function were reported in about 10 % and up to 60 % of patients; however, the criteria used to evaluate the neurological improvement are subjective or not available in most series. Complication rates following RT were reported in 0–5 % of patients, being represented especially by an impairment of preexisting neurologic symptoms due to cranial nerve deficits.

The use of new radiation techniques, including both IMRT and FSRT, which allow higher doses of radiation to the tumor while sparing more surrounding normal tissue, has been associated with better outcome (Table 28.1) [15–17]. In a series of 37 patients with skull base chordomas irradiated with FSRT using a median dose of 66.6 Gy, Debus et al. [16] observed 5-year overall survival and local control rates of 82 % and 50 %, respectively, at a median follow-up of 27 months. The reported rate of permanent complications was 2.2 %, including one case of hemiparesis. Using a similar dose and fractionation, at a median follow-up of 42 months, Bugoci et al. [17] reported an overall survival rate of 76.4 % at 5 years. Using IMRT with a median dose of 76 Gy given in 2 Gy per fraction in 24 patients, Sahgal et al. [15] reported a 5-year survival and local control rates of 85.6 % and 65.3 %, respectively, at a median follow-up of 36 months.

In conclusion, conformal photon RT is associated with longer progression-free survival in comparison to surgery alone, although without clear survival benefit. Certainly, it is difficult to draw a clear conclusion on the efficacy of RT from these data because all studies are retrospective and include a small number of patients treated over many years with different techniques or using different radiation doses. IMRT and FSRT allow for a better 5-year local control and survival; however, only large series and longer follow-up may allow for definitive conclusions regarding the efficacy of new radiation techniques.

28.3 Stereotactic Radiosurgery

SRS may represent a convenient approach for small skull base chordomas after surgery or at recurrence with a reported local control rates of 21–72 % at 5 years [18–32] (Table 28.2).

Table 28.2 Summary of published studies on SRS/HSRT for chordoma

Authors	Patients no	Type of RT	Median dose Gy	Follow-up months	Tumor control (%)
Miller et al. [18]	8	GK	15	2.3 years	100 at 2 years
Muthukumar et al. [19]	9	GK	18	48	NA
Crockard et al. [20]	26	GK[a]	15	51	NA
Krishnan et al. [23]	25	GK[a]	15	56	32 at 5 years
Hasegawa et al. [24]	30	GK[a]	14	59	72 at 5 years
Martin et al. [25]	18	GK	16.5	88	63 at 5 years
Liu et al. [26]	31	GK	12.7	30.2	21.4 at 5 years
Ito et al. [27]	19	GK	15	87.2	47.9 at 5 years
Kano et al. [28]	71	GK	15	60	66 at 5 years
Dassoulas et al. [29]	15	GK	12.7	88	50.3 at 5 years
Kondziolka et al. [30]	4	GK	20	22	100
Chang et al. [21]	10	CK[b]	19.4	4	80[c]
Gwak et al. [22]	4	CK	35–43.6	24	NA
Henderson et al. [31]	18	CK	35	46	59.1[c]
Zorlu et al. [32]	11	CK	30	42	73

SRS stereotactic radiosurgery, *HSRT* hypofractionated stereotactic radiotherapy, *RT* radiotherapy, *GK* Gamma Knife, *CK* CyberKnife, *NA* not assessed

[a]In conjunction with conventional radiotherapy

[b]Five patients treated with LINAC radiosurgery

[c]Series include both skull and cervical spine chordomas

In clinical practice, SRS is usually offered to patients with tumors smaller than 30 mm in diameter and not in close proximity of organs at risk, such as the optic apparatus and brainstem. Kano et al. [28] have recently reported the results of a multicenter study of the North American Gamma Knife Consortium including 71 patients with small-sized chordomas of the skull base treated with Gamma Knife (GK) SRS. The median SRS target volume was 7.1 cm^3 (range, 0.9–109 cm^3), and median margin dose was 15.0 Gy (range, 9–25 Gy). With a median follow-up of 5 years, the 5-year actuarial overall survival and local control rates after SRS were 80 % and 66 %, respectively. Overall survival rates were 43 % for patients who had prior RT and 93 % for those who had no prior RT, and respective 5-year tumor control rates were 62 and 69 %. Older age, recurrent group, prior RT, and larger tumor volume were significantly associated with worse tumor control. In a small series of 15 patients who had undergone GK SRS between 1990 and 2007 at the University of Virginia using a mean dose of 12.7 Gy, Dassoulas et al. [29] observed actuarial tumor control rates of 50.3 % at 5 and 10 years, and similar results have been observed in other few series [18–20, 26, 30]. A similar tumor control up to 60 % at 5 years has been reported when SRS has been used in combination with conventional RT [14, 20, 23, 24]. Complications are reported from 0 to 33 % (median 3 %), being represented mainly by brain radionecrosis and cranial nerve deficits; however, serious radiation-related complications are rarely reported.

Only a few series report on the use of hypofractionated stereotactic radiotherapy (HSRT) in patients with small-to-moderate-sized chordomas of skull base [21, 22, 31, 32]. In a small series of 11 patients with a chordoma of skull base treated with CyberKnife multi-fraction SRS (30 Gy in 5 daily fractions), Zorlu et al. [32] reported 2-year overall survival and tumor control rates of 91 % and 82 %, respectively, at a median follow-up time of 42 months. A similar tumor control has been observed in a few other small series using doses of 20–43.6 Gy delivered in 2 to 5 fractions [21, 22, 31], with a low incidence of serious radiation-induced complications. Although promising, available results on either photon-based single-fraction SRS or multi-fraction SRS are of difficult interpretation. The limited experience, the relatively small size of

Table 28.3 Summary of published studies on proton beam radiotherapy for chordomas

Authors	Patients no	Type of RT	Median dose CGE	Follow-up months	Tumor control (%)
Benk et al. [33]	18 (pediatric)	PhT/PBT	69	72	63 at 5 years[a]
Hug et al. [34]	33	PBT	71.9	33	76
Munzenrider and Liebsch [35]	169	PhT/PBT	66–83	41	73 at 5 years, 54 at 10 years
Terahara et al. [36]	115	PhT/PBT	68.9	41	59 at 5 years, 44 at 10 years
Hug et al. [37]	10 (pediatric)	PhT/PBT	73.7	30	60
Igaki et al. [38]	13	PhT/PBT	72	69.3	46 at 5 years
Noel et al. [39]	100	PhT/PBT	67	31	53.8 at 4 years[a]
Weber et al. [40]	18	PBT	74	29	87.5 at 3 years
Rutz et al. [41]	6	PBT	74	36	100
Ares et al. [42]	42	PBT	73.5	38	81 at 5 years
Fuji et al. [43]	8	PBT	63	42	100 at 3 years
Yasuda et al. [44]	40	PBT	68.9	56.5	70 at 5 years[a]
Rombi et al. [45]	19 (pediatric)	PBT	74	46	81 at 5 years[a]
Deraniyagala et al. [46]	33	PBT	77.4–79.4	21	86 at 2 years
Grosshans et al. [47]	10	PBT	69.8	27	88 at 3 years

RT radiotherapy, *CGE* cobalt gray equivalent, *PBT* proton beam radiotherapy, *PhT* photon beam radiotherapy
[a]Series included both skull and cervical spine chordomas

treated lesions, and the short follow-up periods do not allow for meaningful conclusions.

28.4 Proton Beam Radiotherapy

Protons represent a major advance in radiation therapy, because of their ability to concentrate dose in the tumor while simultaneously sparing surrounding healthy tissue. Surgery followed by proton beam RT has then considered the standard treatment for skull base chordomas. Several studies have reported the safety and efficacy using doses ranging between 63 and 83 CGE (Cobalt Gray Equivalent) at fractionation of 1.8–2.0 CGE for either adults or children with residual or recurrent chordomas of any size [33–47] (Table 28.3). Of these series, the largest one included 169 patients treated with proton beam RT at Massachusetts General Hospital [35]. At a median follow-up of 41 months, 5- and 10-year local control rates were 73 and 54 %, and respective overall survival rates were 80 and 54 %. Using a combination of FSRT and proton beam RT, Noël et al. [39] reported 2- and 4-year local control rates of 86.3 % and 53.8 %, respectively, in 100 patients with skull base and cervical spine chordomas. More recently, Deraniyagala et al. [46] found a 2-year local control rate of 86 % in 33 patients with skull base chordomas. Comparable results have been shown also by other authors, with reported 5-year tumor control and survival rates ranging from 46 % to 81 % and from 66.7 % to 89 %, respectively [33, 34, 36–38, 40–45, 47]. No differences have been observed in terms of local control and survival between children and adult patients.

Re-irradiation with protons for recurrent or progressive chordomas has been recently investigated by McDonald et al. [48] in a small series of 16 patients. At a median follow-up of 23 months, the 2-year local control and overall survival rates were 85 % and 80 %, respectively.

Proton beam RT for patients with chordoma may be associated with a potential risk of acute and late complications. Toxicity data are available for many of the reported series and are similar to that observed in patients treated with photon-based irradiation, although direct comparison is difficult due to differences in patient characteristics, dose, and treatment technique. Acute treatment toxicity is generally mild, including headache, loss of appetite, mucositis, fatigue, nausea, vomiting, and temporary epilation of the irradiated skin. Late complications have been reported in up to 45 % of patients, including visual deterioration [35, 39, 42, 49], pituitary deficits [33, 35, 39–41, 49–51], hearing loss [41, 52], and radiation necrosis at the temporal lobe [33, 52–56]. Factors potentially associated with an increased risk of complications include diabetes, smoking history, hypertension, and repeated surgical resection [48, 49]. Debus et al. [55] found that a dose of more than 60 CGE to a volume of brainstem of more than 0.9 cm^3 was the most significant factor related to a higher risk of brainstem damage. More recently, a dosimetric comparison study revealed improved high-dose conformality and better sparing of temporal lobes and brainstem with spot scanning compared to passive scattering proton therapy techniques [47].

Overall, data from literature provide evidence that proton beam RT is an effective and safe treatment option for chordomas, although it must be noted that long-term survival and local control data are reported only in a few studies [35, 36] and that local failure can occur even after 10 years of follow-up.

28.5 Carbon Ion Radiotherapy

Carbon ions are heavy particles that combine the physical advantage of protons of a highly conformal dose distribution to the tumor, to a higher relative biological effectiveness (RBE), which may allow for a greater tumor control when compared to protons. Currently, carbon ions are available only in eight particle therapy centers worldwide, and only a few studies have reported outcomes of carbon ion RT in patients with skull base chordomas [57–61]. Schulz-Ertner et al. [62] reported 5-year local control and overall survival rates of 70 % and 88.5 %, respectively, in 96 patients treated with carbon ions RT using a median dose of 60 CGE. Grade 3 optic nerve neuropathy was observed in 4.1 % of patients and grades 1–2 temporal lobe injury in 7.2 % of patients. Tsujii and Kamada [60] observed a 5-year local control rate of 88 % among 47 patients treated with a median dose of 60.8 CGE. In a recent series of 155 patients with skull base chordomas, Uhl et al. [61] reported 5-year local control and overall survival rates of 72 % and 85 %, respectively, at median follow-up of 72 months. A randomized phase III trial comparing proton with carbon ion RT is currently ongoing.

Conclusions

RT represents an essential part of the treatment of skull base chordomas. Both fractionated RT and SRS have been used in the management of skull base chordomas and published data indicate a tumor control in up to 50 % of patients 5 years after RT, with an acceptable incidence of long-term complications. Radiation therapy with charged particles may represent a treatment alternative to photon RT associated with a better clinical outcome, but prospective and methodologically rigorous studies need to clearly demonstrate its definitive superiority in terms of efficacy and toxicity in patients with skull base chordomas.

References

1. Tai PT, Craighead P, Bagdon F (1995) Optimization of radiotherapy for patients with cranial chordoma. A review of dose-response ratios for photon techniques. Cancer 75:749–756
2. Khairi S, Ewend MG (2002) Chordoma. Curr Treat Options Neurol 4:167–173
3. Mendenhall WM, Mendenhall CM, Lewis SB et al (2005) Skull base chordoma. Head Neck 27:159–165
4. Romero J, Cardenes H, la Torre A et al (1993) Chordoma: results of radiation therapy in eighteen patients. Radiother Oncol 29:27–32
5. Catton C, O'Sullivan B, Bell R et al (1996) Chordoma: long-term follow-up after radical photon irradiation. Radiother Oncol 41:67–72
6. Hug EB (2000) Proton radiation therapy for chordomas and chondrosarcomas of the skull base. Neurosurg Clin N Am 11:627–638
7. Cummings BJ, Hodson DI, Bush RS (1983) Chordoma: the results of megavoltage radiation therapy. Int J Radiat Oncol Biol Phys 9:633–642
8. Chetiyawardana AD (1984) Chordoma: results of treatment. Clin Radiol 35:159–161
9. Amendola BE, Amendola MA, Oliver E et al (1986) Chordoma: role of radiation therapy. Radiology 158:839–843

10. Fuller DB, Bloom JG (1988) Radiotherapy for chordoma. Int J Radiat Oncol Biol Phys 15:331–339
11. Forsyth PA, Cascino TL, Shaw EG et al (1993) Intracranial chordomas: a clinicopathological and prognostic study of 51 cases. J Neurosurg 78:741–747
12. Watkins L, Khudados ES, Kaleoglu M et al (1993) Skull base chordomas: a review of 38 patients, 1958–88. Br J Neurosurg 7:241–248
13. Zorlu F, Gürkaynak M, Yildiz F et al (2000) Conventional external radiotherapy in the management of clivus chordomas with overt residual disease. Neurol Sci 21:203–207
14. Cho YH, Kim JH, Khang SK et al (2008) Chordomas and chondrosarcomas of the skull base: comparative analysis of clinical results in 30 patients. Neurosurg Rev 31:35–43
15. Sahgal A, Chan MW, Atenafu EG et al (2015) Image-guided intensity modulated radiation therapy (IG-IMRT) for skull base chordoma and chondrosarcoma: preliminary outcomes. Neuro Oncol 17(6):889–894
16. Debus J, Schulz-Ertner D, Schad L et al (2000) Stereotactic fractionated radiotherapy for chordomas and chondrosarcomas of the skull base. Int J Radiat Oncol Biol Phys 47:591–596
17. Bugoci DM, Girvigian MR, Chen JC et al (2013) Photon-based fractionated stereotactic radiotherapy for postoperative treatment of skull base chordomas. Am J Clin Oncol 36:404–410
18. Miller RC, Foote RL, Coffey RJ et al (1997) The role of stereotactic radiosurgery in the treatment of malignant skull base tumors. Int J Radiat Oncol Biol Phys 39:977–981
19. Muthukumar N, Kondziolka D, Lunsford LD et al (1998) Stereotactic radiosurgery for chordoma and chondrosarcoma: further experiences. Int J Radiat Oncol Biol Phys 41:387–392
20. Crockard A, Macaulay E, Plowman PN (1999) Stereotactic radiosurgery. VI. Posterior displacement of the brainstem facilitates safer high dose radiosurgery for clival chordoma. Br J Neurosurg 13:65–70
21. Chang SD, Martin DP, Lee E et al (2001) Stereotactic radiosurgery and hypofractionated stereotactic radiotherapy for residual or recurrent cranial base and cervical chordomas. Neurosurg Focus 10, E5
22. Gwak HS, Yoo HJ, Youn SM et al (2005) Hypofractionated stereotactic radiation therapy for skull base and upper cervical chordoma and chondrosarcoma: preliminary results. Stereotact Funct Neurosurg 83:233–243
23. Krishnan S, Foote RL, Brown PD et al (2005) Radiosurgery for cranial base chordomas and chondrosarcomas. Neurosurgery 56:777–784
24. Hasegawa T, Ishii D, Kida Y et al (2007) Gamma Knife surgery for skull base chordomas and chondrosarcomas. J Neurosurg 107:752–757
25. Martin JJ, Niranjan A, Kondziolka D et al (2007) Radiosurgery for chordomas and chondrosarcomas of the skull base. J Neurosurg 107:758–764
26. Liu AL, Wang ZC, Sun SB et al (2008) Gamma knife radiosurgery for residual skull base chordomas. Neurol Res 30:557–561
27. Ito E, Saito K, Okada T et al (2010) Long-term control of clival chordoma with initial aggressive surgical resection and gamma knife radiosurgery for recurrence. Acta Neurochir (Wien) 152:57–67
28. Kano H, Iqbal FO, Sheehan J et al (2011) Stereotactic radiosurgery for chordoma: a report from the North American Gamma Knife Consortium. Neurosurgery 68:379–389
29. Dassoulas K, Schlesinger D, Yen CP et al (2009) The role of Gamma Knife surgery in the treatment of skull base chordomas. J Neurooncol 94:243–248
30. Kondziolka D, Lunsford LD, Flickinger JC (1991) The role of radiosurgery in the management of chordoma and chondrosarcoma of the cranial base. Neurosurgery 29:38–45
31. Henderson FC, McCool K, Seigle J et al (2009) Treatment of chordomas with CyberKnife: Georgetown University experience and treatment recommendations. Neurosurgery 64:A44–A53
32. Zorlu F, Gultekin M, Cengiz M et al (2014) Fractionated stereotactic radiosurgery treatment results for skull base chordomas. Technol Cancer Res Treat 13:11–19
33. Benk V, Liebsch NJ, Munzenrider JE et al (1995) Base of skull and cervical spine chordomas in children treated by high-dose irradiation. Int J Radiat Oncol Biol Phys 31:577–581
34. Hug E, Loredo LN, Slater JD et al (1999) Proton radiation therapy for chordomas and chondrosarcomas of the skull base. J Neurosurg 91:432–439
35. Munzenrider JE, Liebsch NJ (1999) Proton therapy for tumors of the skull base. Strahlenther Onkol 175:57–63
36. Terahara A, Niemierko A, Goitein M et al (1999) Analysis of the relationship between tumor dose inhomogeneity and local control in patients with skull base chordoma. Int J Radiat Oncol Biol Phys 45:351–358
37. Hug EB, Sweeney RA, Nurre PM et al (2002) Proton radiotherapy in management of pediatric base of skull tumors. Int J Radiat Oncol Biol Phys 52:1017–1024
38. Igaki H, Tokuuye K, Okumura T et al (2004) Clinical results of proton beam therapy for skull base chordoma. Int J Radiat Oncol Biol Phys 60:1120–1126
39. Noël G, Feuvret L, Calagaru V et al (2005) Chordomas of the spine and upper cervical spine. One hundred patient irradiated by a 3D conformal technique combining photon and proton beams. Acta Oncol 44:700–708
40. Weber DC, Rutz HP, Pedroni ES et al (2005) Results of spot-scanning proton radiation therapy for chordoma and chondrosarcoma of the skull base: the Paul Scherrer institute experience. Int J Radiat Oncol Biol Phys 63:401–409
41. Rutz HP, Weber DC, Goitein G et al (2008) Postoperative spot-scanning proton radiation therapy for chordoma and chondrosarcoma in children

and adolescents: initial experience at Paul Scherrer Institute. Int J Radiat Oncol Biol Phys 71:220–225
42. Ares C, Hug EB, Lomax AJ et al (2009) Effectiveness and safety of spot scanning proton radiation therapy for chordomas and chondrosarcomas of the skull base: first long-term report. Int J Radiat Oncol Biol Phys 75:1111–1118
43. Fuji H, Nakasu Y, Ishida Y et al (2011) Feasibility of proton beam therapy for chordoma and chondrosarcoma of the skull base. Skull Base 21:201–206
44. Yasuda M, Bresson D, Chibbaro S et al (2012) Chordomas of the skull base and cervical spine: clinical outcomes associated with a multimodal surgical resection combined with proton-beam radiation in 40 patients. Neurosurg Rev 35:171–183
45. Rombi B, Ares C, Hug EB et al (2013) Spot-scanning proton radiation therapy for pediatric chordoma and chondrosarcoma: clinical outcome of 26 patients treated at Paul Scherrer Institute. Int J Radiat Oncol Biol Phys 86:578–584
46. Deraniyagala RL, Yeung D, Mendenhall WM et al (2014) Proton therapy for skull base chordomas: an outcome study from the university of Florida proton therapy institute. J Neurol Surg B Skull Base 75:53–57
47. Grosshans DR, Zhu XR, Melancon A et al (2014) Spot scanning proton therapy for malignancies of the base of skull: treatment planning, acute toxicities, and preliminary clinical outcomes. Int J Radiat Oncol Biol Phys 90:540–546
48. McDonald MW, Linton OR, Shah MV (2013) Proton therapy for reirradiation of progressive or recurrent chordoma. Int J Radiat Oncol Biol Phys 87:1107–1114
49. Austin-Seymour M, Munzenrider J, Goitein M et al (1989) Fractionated proton radiation therapy of chordoma and low-grade chondrosarcoma of the base of the skull. J Neurosurg 70:13–17
50. Al-Mefty O, Borba LA (1997) Skull base chordomas: a management challenge. J Neurosurg 86:182–189
51. Pai HH, Thornton A, Katznelson L et al (2001) Hypothalamic/pituitary function following high-dose conformal radiotherapy to the base of skull: demonstration of a dose-effect relationship using dose-volume histogram analysis. Int J Radiat Oncol Biol Phys 49:1079–1092
52. Santoni R, Liebsch N, Finkelstein DM et al (1998) Temporal lobe (TL) damage following surgery and high-dose photon and proton irradiation in 96 patients affected by chordomas and chondrosarcomas of the base of the skull. Int J Radiat Oncol Biol Phys 41:59–68
53. Colli B, Al-Mefty O (2001) Chordomas of the skull base: follow-up review and prognostic factors. Neurosurg Focus 10:111
54. Slater JM (1995) Proton therapy for cranial base tumors. J Craniofac Surg 6:24–26
55. Debus J, Hug EB, Liebsch NJ et al (1997) Brainstem tolerance to conformal radiotherapy of skull base tumors. Int J Radiat Oncol Biol Phys 39:967–975
56. Tsujii H, Mizoe J, Kamada T et al (2007) Clinical results of carbon ion radiotherapy at NIRS. J Radiat Res 48 Suppl. 2:A1–A13
57. Mizoe JE, Hasegawa A, Takagi R et al (2009) Carbon ion radiotherapy for skull base chordoma. Skull Base 19:219–224
58. Takahashi S, Kawase T, Yoshida K et al (2009) Skull base chordomas: efficacy of surgery followed by carbon ion radiotherapy. Acta Neurochir (Wien) 151:759–769
59. Nikoghosyan AV, Karapanagiotou-Schenkel I, Münter MW et al (2010) Randomised trial of proton vs. carbon ion radiation therapy in patients with chordoma of the skull base, clinical phase III study HIT-1-Study. BMC Cancer 10:607
60. Tsujii H, Kamada T (2012) A review of update clinical results of carbon ion radiotherapy. Jpn J Clin Oncol 42:670–685
61. Uhl M, Mattke M, Welzel T et al (2014) Highly effective treatment of skull base chordoma with carbon ion irradiation using a raster scan technique in 155 patients: first long-term results. Cancer 120:3410–3417
62. Schulz-Ertner D, Karger CP, Feuerhake A et al (2007) Effectiveness of carbon ion radiotherapy in the treatment of skull-base chordomas. Int J Radiat Oncol Biol Phys 68:449–457

Part VI

Cranial Base Recontruction After Transcranial and Transnasal Skull Base Surgery

29 Cranial Base Reconstruction After Transcranial and Transnasal Skull Base Surgery for Median Lesions

Raewyn G. Campbell, Hafiz Patwa, Ing Ping Tang, Bradley A. Otto, Daniel M. Prevedello, and Ricardo L. Carrau

29.1 Introduction

Surgical approaches may be classified according to specific anatomic target areas, which in turn are associated with specific reconstructive idiosyncrasies. In addition, each approach creates a corridor with adjacent structures that may have different functions and significance. In the median skull base, EEAs can extend caudally to the level of C2 and anteriorly to the level of the posterior wall of the frontal sinus [1, 2]. Consequently, EEAs to the median skull base (i.e., sagittal plane) can be classified into six distinct corridors: transfrontal, transcribiform, transplanum, transsellar, transclival, and transodontoid [3]. Use of specific reconstructive techniques is contingent upon many factors aside from the corridor and target area: size and shape of the skull base defect, the condition of the surrounding bone and remaining dura, whether a CSF leak was encountered intraoperatively or not, the nature of the CSF leak encountered (high or low flow), extent of communication between the nasal and intracranial cavities, anticipated postoperative intracranial pressure (ICP), the nature of any lesion resected, patient comorbidities (e.g., diabetes mellitus, Cushing's disease, immunosuppression), prior sinonasal surgery, status of the nasal septum and lateral nasal wall, history of previous surgery or radiation therapy, and the anticipated need for adjuvant therapies (i.e., irradiation or chemotherapy).

A better understanding of the skull base anatomy, the development of appropriate instrumentation, and the evolution of vascularized flaps

Electronic supplementary material The online version of this chapter (doi:10.1007/978-3-319-21533-4_29) contains supplementary material, which is available to authorized users.

R.G. Campbell, MD • H. Patwa, MD
Department of Otolaryngology – Head and Neck Surgery, Wexner Medical Center, The Ohio State University, 320 West 10th Avenue, Starling-Loving Hall, B221, Columbus, OH 43210-1282, USA

I.P. Tang, MD
Department of Otolaryngology – Head and Neck Surgery, Wexner Medical Center, The Ohio State University, 320 West 10th Avenue, Starling-Loving Hall, B221, Columbus, OH 43210-1282, USA

Department of Otorhinolaryngology – Head and Neck Surgery, Faculty of Medicine, University Malaysia Sarawak, Kota Samarahan, Sarawak, Malaysia

B.A. Otto, MD • D.M. Prevedello, MD
R.L. Carrau, MD (✉)
Department of Otolaryngology – Head and Neck Surgery, Wexner Medical Center, The Ohio State University, 320 West 10th Avenue, Starling-Loving Hall, B221, Columbus, OH 43210-1282, USA

Department of Neurological Surgery, Wexner Medical Center, The Ohio State University, Columbus, OH, USA
e-mail: daniel.prevedello@osumc.edu; ricardo.carrau@osumc.edu

P. Cappabianca et al. (eds.), *Midline Skull Base Surgery*, DOI 10.1007/978-3-319-21533-4_29

have revolutionized the repair of the skull base following both open and endonasal approaches (EEA). Successful reconstruction of small skull base defects (generally <1 cm) appears to be independent of the reconstruction strategy [4–6], as these defects can be successfully repaired using a wide variety of free grafts and techniques; thus, these data suggest that their repair does not require a vascularized flap [5]. However, free tissue grafting is not as reliable when reconstructing large and complex skull base defects (>3 cm) [7–11, 5], which will be the focus of this chapter. Compared to small defects, large defects are characterized by a wide dural resection that frequently extends beyond the craniectomy defect, extensive dissection of the arachnoid membranes (opening of cisterns or ventricles), high-flow CSF leaks, and a large area to reconstruct. Currently, pedicled flaps offer the most reliable reconstruction of large skull base defects [9, 11], ensuring the successful isolation of the intracranial space from the sinonasal tract to prevent complications, such as meningitis, intracranial abscesses, encephaloceles, CSF leaks, and tension pneumocephalus.

One should note, however, that despite having their own vascularity, there are important differences between flaps with a random blood supply and those with an axial blood supply. Flaps with a random blood supply offer a limited surface area and require a broad-based pedicle. Length and width of a random flap may only be extended if accompanied by an increase in the dimensions of its base. A wide base consequently creates torsional forces that reduce the arc of rotation and reach of the flap, thus making it more difficult to mobilize into the defect and causing its retraction from defect [12].

Pedicled flaps, such as the posterior pedicle nasoseptal flap (i.e., Hadad-Bassagaisteguy flap), revolutionized the endoscopic repair of the skull base, as their axial blood supply can supply a large surface area with a small and relatively long pedicle. Therefore, a pedicled flap grants a superior arc of rotation, which facilitates its mobilization into the defect. In our experience, the adoption of pedicled flaps reduced our postoperative CSF leak rates from 33 % to less than 5 % [12]. One should note that open skull base surgery underwent a similar revolution with the adoption of the pericranial/galeopericranial flaps, and subsequently microvascular flaps, for the reconstruction of the anterior skull base [13].

29.2 General Principles

Upon the induction of the general anesthesia, the nasal cavity is decongested with cottonoids impregnated with a solution of 1:10,000 epinephrine. This aids with hemostasis throughout the surgery, including during flap harvesting. At the beginning of surgery, the lateral nasal wall is infiltrated with a solution of lidocaine 0.5–1 % with epinephrine 1/100,000–1/200,000. The sites corresponding to the incisions needed for flap harvesting may also be injected; however, we avoid injecting the area corresponding to the flap's vascular pedicle.

A multilayer technique is preferred for the reconstruction of any skull base defect. Prior to any repair, however, the site must be thoroughly prepared to receive the grafts and flaps. Any mucosa, bony spicule, or foreign body should be removed from the defect and immediate surroundings to allow the take of any free graft and healing of the pedicled flap. This is especially true for that area of the skull base framing the defect, as this is the surface that the flap will heal against, thus sealing the central defect. The fastest and most reliable reconstruction is furnished by bare vascularized tissue in full and unhindered contact with bare vascularized tissue (e.g., periosteal side of the flap against the bare bone of the skull base).

Multiple techniques (i.e., inlay, onlay, inlay/onlay) and materials have been reported to slow or stop the flow of CSF before the final flap or graft is placed. We prefer to use an inlay graft of collagen matrix (e.g., DuraGen Dural Regeneration Matrix, Integra Life Sciences Corporation, Plainsboro, NJ, USA) or fascia lata in the subdural or epidural space to stop the flow of CSF and, to some degree, obliterate the intracranial dead space. It is important to avoid any folding of the graft to prevent the formation of a channel leading to a CSF leak. One should also consider that inlay grafts require a blind insertion of the edges of the graft under the dura or bone; therefore, care must be taken to avoid injuring the vital structures in close proximity (i.e., ICA or optic chiasm). A subdural inlay graft can often be technically challenging due to the condition of the surrounding dura, the lack of a bony shelf to support the repair, or, as previously mentioned, the presence of critical structures around the defect. In this scenario, the graft may be placed between the dura and the bone (i.e., epidural), if a sufficient bony rim is present. Where an inlay graft is not possible, an onlay graft (i.e., extracranial) may be used. One should recognize, however, that an adequate bolster becomes more critical to maintain the position and avoid the migration or displacement of an onlay graft.

Free abdominal fat is a useful alternative or adjunct graft to fill a large bony cavity such as the bony tunnel created during a transclival or transodontoid approach or to obliterate the sphenoid sinus when appropriate (e.g., to complement a mucoperiosteal flap in supporting the intracranial contents following the sacrifice of significant areas of the skull base). If the length of the pedicled flap is inadequate, one may fill the sphenoid sinus with fat to reduce the surface area requiring coverage. This technique will also increase the reach of the flap by displacing the airspace anteriorly, therefore improving the ratio of the size of the defect to the flap length.

Free abdominal fat may also serve as a radiologic spacer to enable contrast between the soft tissue used in reconstruction and the tumor bed postoperatively. This improves the ability of the radiation oncologist to target any residual tumor and to minimize collateral radiation injury to adjacent vital structures. In addition, others have used free abdominal fat to obliterate intracranial dead space. However, free abdominal fat is best avoided if a second operation is planned or anticipated, as fat evolves into a strong scar and generates fibrosis that greatly compounds the approach and identification of neurovascular structures.

Defects with dimensions that approximate or surpass 2×2.5 cm may be considered for a gasket seal closure technique [14]. Using a piece of fascia lata or collagen matrix at least one third larger than the defect, the graft is inset into the defect and cartilage is then countersunk into the defect to ensure a tight closure and to anchor the graft. Although a Medpor prosthesis (Stryker Corporation, Kalamazoo, Michigan, USA) has been used to achieve the seal [14], we avoid using any alloplast due to the potential risk of infection, extrusion, and erosion into a critical structure. One concern with the gasket seal technique is the blind insertion of a hard graft into an intracranial space that may be in close proximity to critical structures. Several verbal communications have alluded to the formation of pseudoaneurysm or compression of the optic apparatus when using this technique.

Another similar technique involves an inlay and onlay technique without any hard material [15]. Using this technique, a piece of acellular dermal allograft or fascia lata is placed intracranially and then folded or wedged so that the margins of the graft then drape extracranially to overlay the denuded bony margins of the defect (Fig. 29.1). The graft is manipulated into place using ball probes and curved suction instruments. The graft is then further secured with pieces of gelatin foam or fat in the center of the wedged layers of the allograft (simulating a bath-plug technique). The intracranial portion of the graft is also held in place by the weight of the brain (i.e., this is only true for the anterior and middle cranial fossae) [15].

Relative contraindications when considering any pedicled flap include conditions that directly affect the vasculature (local or systemic) or predispose the patient to thrombotic phenomena. These include granulomatous diseases such as Wegener's granulomatosis, vasculitic diseases such as polyarteritis nodosa, or coagulopathies such as antithrombin III or protein C deficiency. Similarly, one must consider alternative reconstruction techniques in patients who have received high-dose irradiation in the area of the flap, its pedicle, or its terminal vessel.

29.3 Pedicled Flaps

An overview of mucoperiosteal and fascial vascularized flaps and their applications is provided in Table 29.1. These flaps can be further divided

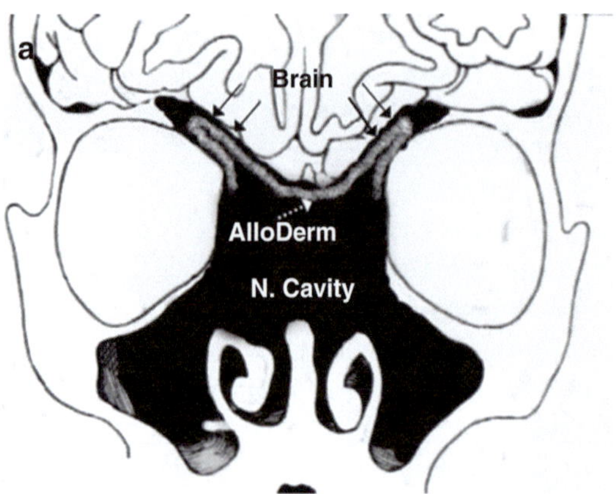

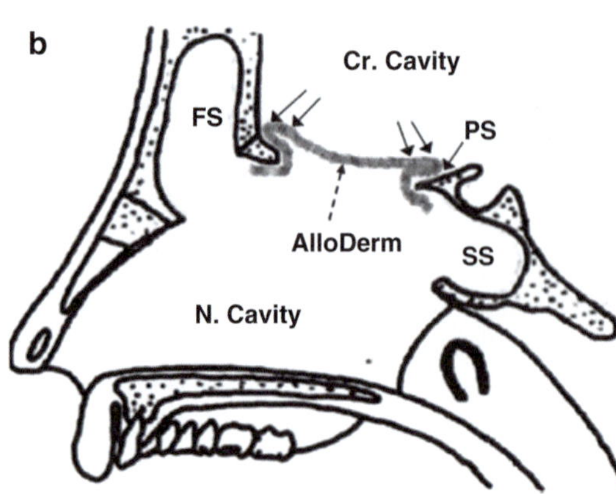

Fig. 29.1 Diagram showing inlay and onlay technique of synthetic dura placement. (**a**) Coronal view showing how the synthetic dura is introduced above the supraorbital walls in a double layer. *Arrows* demonstrate how the weight of the brain keeps the graft in position. (**b**) Sagittal view showing graft orientation in relation to planum sphenoidale and the frontal sinus. *FS* frontal sinus; *PS* planum sphenoidale; *SS* sphenoid sinus (Reproduced with permission: Germani et al. [16]. Oceanside Publications)

into intranasal and extranasal flaps. Intranasal flaps include the following:

- Pedicled nasoseptal flap
  - Reverse septal flap
  - Nasoseptal rescue flap
- Inferior turbinate flap
- Middle turbinate flap
- Anteriorly based lateral nasal wall flap
- Posteriorly based lateral nasal wall flap

Extranasal flaps include the following:

- Transfrontal pericranial flap
- Transpterygoid temporoparietal fascia flap
- Occipital galeopericranial flap
- Facial artery myomucosal (or mucosal) flap
- Oliver-modified pedicled palatal flap

A detailed discussion of the various myofascial or myocutaneous flaps used to reconstruct the skull base is beyond the scope of this chapter; however, a concise mention is appropriate. Briefly, these include flaps comprising the following muscles: temporalis, pectoralis major, sternocleidomastoid, trapezius, and latissimus dorsi. The temporalis myofascial flap is adequate for the most lateral aspect of the anterior cranial fossa and can be extended by harvesting the temporoparietal or pericranial fascia. However, the vascular pedicles of the remaining listed muscles originate below the clavicle; therefore, their reach to the skull base is limited. Free microvascular flaps overcome this limitation, allow flexibility in flap design, are not limited by the arc of rotation of their pedicle, and are ideal to fill large dead spaces. Free flaps suitable for skull base reconstruction include the anterolateral thigh, fibula, radial forearm, rectus abdominis, serratus, scapula, gracilis, and latissimus dorsi flaps [16, 13].

29.3.1 Intranasal Flaps

29.3.1.1 Posterior Pedicle Nasoseptal Flap

The posterior pedicle nasoseptal flap (NSF), also named the Hadad-Bassagaisteguy flap, was developed at the University of Rosario, Argentina, by Hadad and Bassagaisteguy et al. and modified by Carrau et al. in a quest to design a better intranasal vascular pedicled flap to reconstruct skull base defects [17, 12].

Indications

The posterior pedicle nasoseptal flap is a reliable flap, especially for the reconstruction of large skull base defects, as it provides an ample surface area with a superior arc of rotation. The

Table 29.1 Intranasal, extranasal, and free flaps available for skull base reconstruction

	Pedicled flaps										Free flaps
	Intranasal					Extranasal					
Defect location	Nasoseptal flap	Inferior turbinate flap	Lateral wall posteriorly based	Lateral wall anteriorly based	Middle turbinate flap	Palatal[a]	Transfrontal pericranial flap	Temporoparietal fascia flap	Occipital galeopericranial flap[a]	Facial artery myomucosal flap	
Anterior/ cribriform	X			X	X		X		X	X	X
Planum	X		X	X	X	X	X			X	X
Sella	X		X	X	X	X	X	X		X	X
Clivus	X	X	X			X		X	X		X
C1–C2	X					X					X

[a]Described in cadaveric studies only

length of the posterior pedicle nasoseptal flap is adequate to reconstruct cribriform, sella, planum sphenoidale, or clival defects [17]. The height of the septum provides enough width to cover the full width of any anterior skull base defect between the orbits. When considering posterior defects, the flap has sufficient length to cover all sellar defects and the roof or lateral walls of the sphenoid sinus, and it can cover a panclivectomy (i.e., from the posterior clinoids superiorly to the foramen magnum inferiorly) [18]. Anteriorly, the flap can cover the region extending from the posterior border of the frontal sinuses to the anterior wall of the sphenoid sinus. A single posterior pedicle nasoseptal flap, however, is not adequate to cover extensive defects involving multiple skull base locations, such as those extending from the posterior wall of the frontal sinus to the sella turcica or foramen magnum (i.e., more than two adjacent anatomical modules) [18]. Under these circumstances, bilateral posterior pedicle nasoseptal flap or a combination of different pedicled flaps or the use of free tissue grafts needs to be considered.

Contraindications

The posterior pedicle nasoseptal flap is not feasible in patients who have previously undergone procedures, which have compromised the vascular pedicle or the flap substance such as the following:

- Bilateral wide sphenoidotomies, sphenopalatine artery ligations, a previous septectomy, or in those with tumor involving the septum.
- A flap cannot be harvested on the side in which the tumor involves the sphenoid rostrum, lateral nasal wall, sphenopalatine foramen, or pterygopalatine fossa.

Careful consideration should be given to the use of this flap in children under 14 years of age as the impact of a posterior pedicle nasoseptal flap on facial skeletal growth in children is unknown [19]. Furthermore, the area of the septum in children under the age of 10 years may be insufficient relative to the area of the skull base; thus, a posterior pedicle nasoseptal flap in a child under this age may require supplementation with fascia or fat [19].

Anatomy

The flap consists of the mucoperiosteum and mucoperichondrium of the nasal septum and is pedicled on the posterior septal artery, a branch of the sphenopalatine artery. The posterior septal artery arises from the sphenopalatine artery in the pterygopalatine fossa, and its course is divided into three segments: the pterygopalatine, sphenoidal, and septal [20]. The posterior septal artery bifurcates into a superior and inferior branch in the sphenoidal segment, and the inferior branch is typically the larger/dominant branch [20]. The mean distance between the sphenoid ostium and the superior branch is 9.3 mm (range 5–15 mm) [21]. The branches of the posterior septal artery then form a dense network along the septum to supply the inferior two thirds of the septum and a large portion of the nasal floor [20]. The posterosuperior portion of the septum is supplied by the posterior ethmoid artery. The inferior branch of the posterior septal artery sends a branch to the incisive canal, which supplies the hard palate and anastomoses with the anterior branch of the greater palatine artery.

Technique

Several factors influence the laterality of the flap being harvested. First, tumors that invade the rostrum of the sphenoid, nasal septum, lateral pterygoid recess, or pterygopalatine fossa preclude the harvesting of the ipsilateral flap; thus, one should elevate the flap on the contralateral side. Second, when both sides of the nasal septum are available for flap harvesting, we generally prefer the right side, as it is usually easier to dissect for a right-handed surgeon, especially if a right middle turbinectomy is completed as part of the EEA. Last, the presence of nasal septal spurs or severe septal deviation increases the technical difficulty and the risk of perforation during the harvesting the flap. Thus, the contralateral side may be preferred in this instance, or a septoplasty should be performed first. If a patient has had prior sphenoidal sinus surgery, then the viability of the posterior pedicle nasoseptal flap vascular pedicle may be confirmed using an acoustic Doppler sonography with an endoscopic probe.

The posterior pedicle nasoseptal flap requires prior planning as one of its limitations is that this flap, or at least its pedicle, must be harvested at the beginning of surgery (i.e., prior to the posterior septectomy) and before the size of the skull base defect is known. Therefore, the flap dimensions must be overestimated, and the flap may require trimming to ensure it lies square against the bony rim of the resultant defect.

One advantage of the posterior pedicle nasoseptal flap is that it may be reused in cases of benign pathology such as a recurrent craniopharyngioma, incomplete pituitary adenoma resection, or in staged procedures. The flap tends to retain the shape of the defect, and, therefore, any defect that is enlarged may require additional tissue to supplement the repair.

Surgical steps to harvest the posterior pedicle nasoseptal flap are described below:

1. A posterior pedicle nasoseptal flap may be designed based on the anticipated size and shape of the defect. In our practice, however, we harvest its maximum surface area, which spans from the vomer posteriorly to the mucocutaneous junction of the columella anteriorly and from the floor of the nasal cavity to 1–2 cm below the olfactory cleft (to preserve the olfactory epithelium). Anterior to the anterior head of the middle turbinate, where there is no significant olfactory epithelium, we harvest the entire height of the nasal septum.
2. First, the nasal cavity is decongested and prepared as previously described.
3. To facilitate the visualization of the nasal septum and surgical field, and, therefore, the harvesting of the flap, the inferior turbinates and the left middle turbinate are out-fractured bilaterally and the right middle turbinate is removed.
4. The inferior third of the right superior turbinate is removed using a microdebrider or the straight tru-cut forceps, and the sphenoid ostium is identified.
5. To harvest the posterior pedicle nasoseptal flap, we incise the mucosa with a monopolar electrocautery equipped with an extended insulated needle tip bent at 90° (Arthroscopic hook electrode; Valley Lab, Boulder, CO) set at 15 W.
6. Two posterior incisions encompass the pedicle. The superior incision begins at the level of the natural ostium of the sphenoid sinus. The inferior incision starts at the junction of the superior border of the choana and lateral nasal wall, anterior to the torus tubarius.
7. The inferior incision of the pedicle is extended along the posterior choana toward the nasal septum medially. This incision is then continued anteroinferiorly following the free edge of the posterior nasal septum toward the junction of the nasal crest of the palatine bone and the vomer. At this point it continues as a sagittally oriented incision along the junction between the nasal crest of the palatine bone/maxilla and the vomer/nasal cartilage. The incision continues toward the columella and ceases at its mucocutaneous junction.
8. The superior incision extends from the superior aspect of the sphenoid ostium (incorporating the ostium into the incision) and crosses the rostrum of the sphenoid toward the septum. This incision continues sagittally following an imaginary line drawn to spare the olfactory epithelium. The olfactory epithelium can be identified as a raised, yellowish area with vertical striations over the most cephalic 1–2 cm of the nasal septum in the region posterior to the head of the middle turbinate.
9. At the level of the head of the middle turbinate, the incision is extended vertically to the most superior aspect of the septum. This incision is then carried anteriorly toward the mucocutaneous junction of the columella.
10. These two sagittally oriented incisions traverse the entire length of the septum and are connected at their most anterior aspect by a vertical incision that follows the mucocutaneous junction of the columella (Fig. 29.2).
11. These incisions can be modified to suit specific areas and needs of the reconstruction or

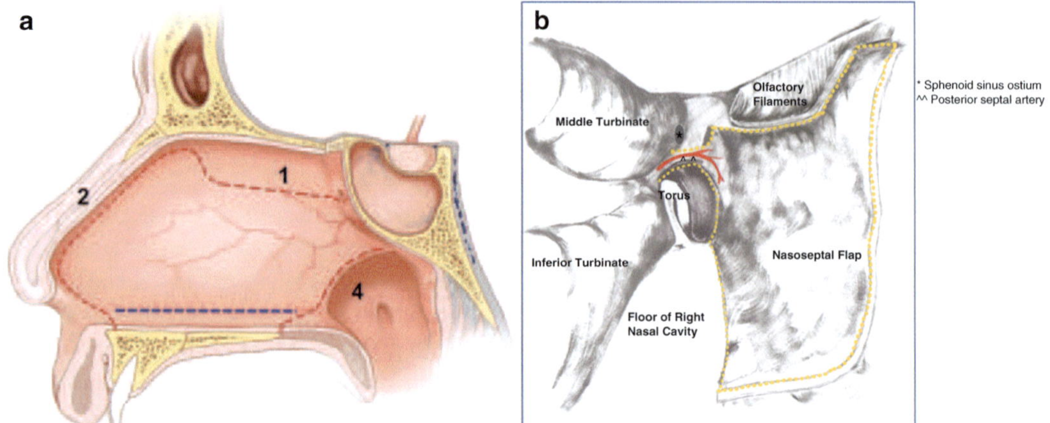

Fig. 29.2 Outline of incisions for a posterior pedicle nasoseptal flap. *1*. Superior incision parallel to the skull base and below the olfactory epithelium. *2*. Vertical anterior incision from the nasal dorsum to meet the inferior incision on the floor of the nose. *4*. Posterior incision along the posterior septum to the junction of the palatine crest and vomer (Reproduced with permission: Peris-Celda et al. [22]. Thieme Publishers)

to ensure a complete resection with adequate oncologic margins. The flap may be extended laterally onto the floor of the nose and into the inferior meatus. This adds 20 mm and 774 mm^2 of surface area to the posterior pedicle nasoseptal flap [22].

12. A Cottle dissector is used to elevate the mucoperichondrium and mucoperiosteum of the flap from anterior to posterior. If the flap has been extended onto the nasal floor, care must be taken during elevation of the mucoperichondrium and mucoperiosteum along the nasal floor as a strong matrix of collagenous fibers (Sharpey's fibers) connecting the periosteum and bone exists in this location. Sharp dissection reduces the risk of tearing the flap during its elevation in this location.
13. Once harvested, the nasoseptal flap may be stored in the nasopharynx, or inside the maxillary sinus, or against the lateral nasal wall to avoid injury during the extirpative surgery. During any clival or nasopharyngeal surgery pathology, we often prefer to place the posterior pedicle nasoseptal flap along the lateral nasal wall after placing a suture through its anterior border. This avoids congestion of the flap. The suture is brought out through the nostril and clamped with a hemostat, which is allowed to hang freely from the nostril. The hemostat provides a counterweight that maintains the flap in an extended position along the lateral nasal wall and, thus, out of the way of any instrumentation. If the flap is on the right lateral nasal wall, then the endoscope shaft will displace it and keep it out of the way. If the flap is on the left, the endoscope should be used to guide any instrumentation into the nasal cavity to avoid injury to the flap.
14. Prior to placement of the posterior pedicle nasoseptal flap over the defect, the mucosa of the surrounding bone is removed to ensure no mucosa is buried beneath the flap. This prevents the development of a mucocele. Subsequently, the nasoseptal flap is positioned over the defect ensuring its full contact against the surrounding denuded bone. It must overlap the bone to allow for any retraction of the flap (potentially up to 20 %). One should note that if the periosteal side of the pedicle is exposed to air, it would heal by secondary intention leading to contraction. Abdominal free fat maybe used to obliterate any dead space, a bony tunnel (e.g., after a transclival or transodontoid approach), or the sphenoid sinus when appropriate so that the periosteal side is against fat and not exposed to air.
15. Others apply a biologic glue to further fix the flap (optional). However, we have abandoned this practice as we feel its value is

questionable. Subsequently, nonadherent nasal packing materials, such as Nasopore (Polyganics, Groningen, the Netherlands), and expandable sponges (Merocel, Medtronic Corporation; Jacksonville, Florida) are inserted under direct endoscopic visualization to bolster the flap against the defect.

16. If a perforation is accidentally made in the flap at any stage during the surgery, the surgeon may align the flap so that the perforation does not directly overlay the defect. If this is not possible, then the hole may be sutured, bolstered with collagen matrix, or plugged with fat [23].

29.3.1.2 Reverse Flap

Indications

This flap was described by Caicedo et al. in 2010 and is also known as the Caicedo reverse rotation flap [24]. The reverse flap is harvested as part of the posterior pedicle nasoseptal flap to avoid crusting on the exposed cartilage of the denuded anterior septum donor site, which can persist for 3–6 months postoperatively [12]. Nasal crusting leads to nasal obstruction, an offensive smell, halitosis, and olfactory dysfunction. The reverse flap has been shown to reduce crusting of the donor site to 1–2 weeks [25]. Any crusting after the reverse flap most commonly occurs at the site of the sutures, and patients should be warned about this to avoid any attempts to digitally remove the crusts.

Contraindications

See Sect. 29.3.1.1.

Anatomy

This flap is based on branches of the anterior ethmoid artery (a branch of the ophthalmic artery), the greater palatine artery (a branch of the internal maxillary artery), and alar branches of the facial artery.

Technique [24, 25]

1. After the posterior pedicle nasoseptal flap is harvested and placed in the nasopharynx, along the lateral nasal wall, or in the maxillary sinus, the contralateral septal mucoperichondrium and mucoperiosteum is elevated. A posterior septectomy, removing the posterior septal cartilage and portions of the vomer and perpendicular plate of the ethmoid bone, creates a single cavity that can be approached through either nostril. Intraoperative image guidance may be used to ensure that the septectomy does not include the structural support of the nasal septum (that portion inferior to the nasal bones and resting over the premaxilla), thus avoiding a saddle nose deformity.
2. An extended, insulated needle tip electrocautery is used to make the three incisions. Prior to making these incisions, cottonoids are placed in the left nostril between the septum and the inferior and middle turbinates to protect them from any injury due to the cautery.
3. Superior and inferior incisions are made in a similar fashion to those of the posterior pedicle nasoseptal flap except that the inferior incision is made approximately 1 cm above the level of the floor of the nose. They are brought to the level of the remaining cartilaginous septum anteriorly.
4. A posterior vertical incision is made at the level of the rostrum of the sphenoid, joining the superior and inferior incisions and completing the anteriorly based flap (Fig. 29.3).
5. The posterior edge of the flap is then grasped with a Blakesley forceps and brought anteriorly to cover the denuded septal cartilage (Fig. 29.4).
6. The flap can then be trimmed to size and is sutured to the columella with a 4-0 absorbable suture such as chromic.
7. Quilting transmural absorbable 3-0 or 4-0 sutures are then used to appose the flap against the septum.
8. The remaining inferior mucosa is incised vertically at its posterior and anterior borders, extending the incisions down to the floor of the nose. This creates an inferiorly based flap that can be placed/folded over the maxillary crest to avoid further crusting in this region.
9. Silicone splints are then cut to size and sutured to the remnant septum using a nonabsorbable suture, i.e., 3-0 Nylon. These splints protect the flap from the trauma caused by the repeated passage of instruments during surgery.

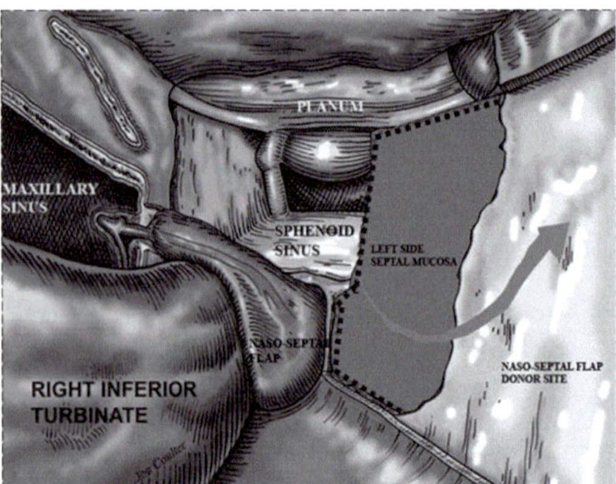

Fig. 29.3 Right nasal cavity after endoscopic endonasal approach shows right maxillary antrostomy, vascular pedicled nasoseptal flap positioned in the nasopharynx, posterior septectomy with preservation of opposite nasal septal mucosa (reverse rotation flap). *Black dotted line* demonstrates incisions for the reverse flap on opposite nasal septal mucosa. *Gray arrow* indicates the direction of flap transposition (Reproduced with permission: Caicedo-Granados et al. [24]. Wiley and Sons)

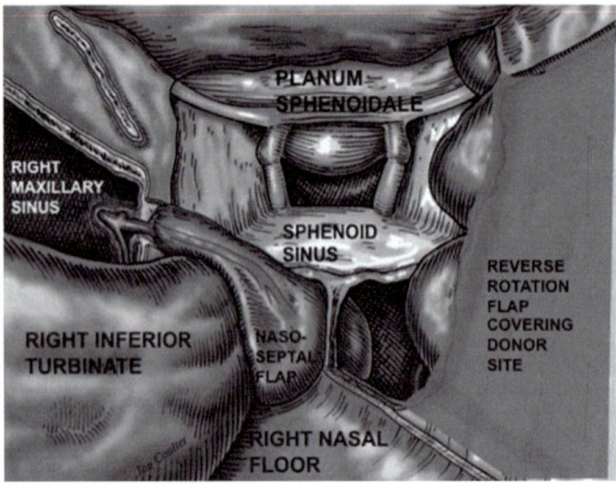

Fig. 29.4 Right nasal cavity after reverse rotation flap is positioned against the contralateral septum (Reproduced with permission: Caicedo-Granados et al. [24]. Wiley and Sons)

29.3.1.3 Rescue Flap

Indications

This technique is a modification of the original posterior pedicle nasoseptal flap that involves the elevation and preservation of its pedicle, while the flap paddle remains attached anteriorly. This flap is indicated when a CSF leak is not anticipated in any expanded endonasal approach, such as in routine pituitary surgery.

Contraindications

See Sect. 29.3.1.1.

Anatomy

See Sect. 29.3.1.1.

Technique

1. First, the nasal cavity is decongested and prepared as previously described (see Reconstruction technique).
2. Superior and inferior incisions are made with the needle tip electrocautery as described in the posterior pedicle nasoseptal flap. However, unlike the posterior pedicle nasoseptal flap, these incisions are not extended anteriorly to the mucocutaneous junction. Instead, the superior and inferior incisions are brought to a level that is just anterior to the head of the middle turbinate.
3. Using a Cottle dissector and a ball-tipped seeker probe, the mucoperiosteum is elevated from the septum toward the pedicle. This creates a bi-pedicled flap with attachments at the lateral nasal wall and nasal septum.
4. The bi-pedicled flap is then pushed inferiorly enough to allow a Frazier suction tip to sit under the choana without compromising the flap.
5. Dissection of the sphenoid sinus can then proceed without risk to the flap. However, surgeons must be wary of the flap during dissection as an unprotected drill shaft may inadvertently injure the flap and/or pedicle.
6. At the end of the procedure, if a posterior pedicle nasoseptal flap was not required, the rescue flaps are transposed posteriorly to cover the denuded floor of the sphenoid sinus. Silicone splints are placed along the septum and sutured with a nonabsorbable suture. These are generally removed at 1–2 weeks postoperatively.

29.3.1.4 Inferior Turbinate Flap

Indications

An inferior turbinate flap will cover small clival and sellar defects and may require combining it with free abdominal fat due to its limited reach [9]. Flap donor site crusting is a consequence of the inferior turbinate flap and lasts for up to 4 weeks until remucosalization is complete [9].

Contraindications

An inferior turbinate flap is contraindicated in any patient who has undergone an ipsilateral sphenopalatine artery ligation. Prior inferior turbinectomy or turbinate surgery may reduce the surface area and pliability of the flap, limit its ability to mold to the shape of the defect, and may also compromise its blood supply.

Anatomy

The inferior turbinate flap is based on the inferior turbinate arterial branch of the posterior lateral nasal artery, a branch of the sphenopalatine artery. The posterior lateral nasal artery branches from the sphenopalatine artery and runs in an inferolateral direction along the perpendicular plate of the ascending process of the palatine bone and sends a branch to the middle turbinate medially. The inferior turbinate branch enters the inferior turbinate on the anterior aspect of its lateral attachment, 1.0–1.5 cm from its posterior border [26]. It runs inside the bone 50 % of the time, through soft tissue in 14 % and in a mixed pattern in 36 % [27]. The artery runs through the soft tissue on the medial aspect of the bone for a mean of 1.2 cm before piercing the soft tissue and bone and dividing into up to six branches [27]. Of note, the artery increases in size as it moves anteriorly, possibly due to contributions from the angular artery, a branch of the facial artery, which could be considered the anterior vascular pedicle to the inferior turbinate [28]. The dominant blood supply to the inferior turbinate is the inferior turbinate artery, however [29]. The inferior turbinate flap provides a surface area of approximately 4.97 cm^2 [28]. To enlarge this surface area, bilateral flaps may be harvested for larger defects.

Technique [9, 30]

1. First, the nasal cavity is decongested and prepared as previously described (see Reconstruction technique).
2. It is important to avoid disruption to the nasolacrimal duct by sharply dissecting its attachment during flap harvest.
3. Next the inferior turbinate is medialized in such a way that the medial surface of the inferior turbinate is well visualized. Steps 4–6 are performed to identify the pedicle of the inferior turbinate flap.
4. The natural ostium of the ipsilateral maxillary sinus is identified after performing an uncinectomy.
5. The maxillary sinus ostium is enlarged posteriorly toward the posterior maxillary sinus (antral) wall.
6. Submucoperiosteal elevation from the ascending process of the palatine bone allows the identification of the crista ethmoidalis and the sphenopalatine foramen, thus identifying the sphenopalatine artery and its terminal branches. There is significant anatomical variation of the sphenopalatine artery branches, and the posterolateral nasal artery may be anterior to the posterior wall of the maxillary antrum [31, 32]. It is important to recognize this anatomic variation during the maxillary antrostomy and mucoperiosteal elevation so as not to injure the vascular pedicle.
7. Once the vascular pedicle is well defined, two sagittal incisions are made to define the superior and inferior limits of the flap (Fig. 29.5).
8. A posterior to anterior incision is made along the superior sagittal plane of the inferior turbinate.
9. An inferior sagittal incision is made along the caudal margin of the inferior turbinate.
10. A vertical incision is made at the head of the inferior turbinate at its attachment at the pyriform aperture joining the two sagittal incisions.
11. A periosteal elevator (Freer dissector or Cottle elevator) is used to raise the mucoperiosteum off the inferior turbinate in an anterior to posterior direction both medially and laterally to the inferior turbinate bone. Elevation has to be done in a submucoperiosteal plane to prevent injury to the vascular supply.
12. Care is taken not to injure the vascular pedicle as it enters the turbinate at the superior aspect of its lateral attachment, 1–1.5 cm from its posterior aspect.

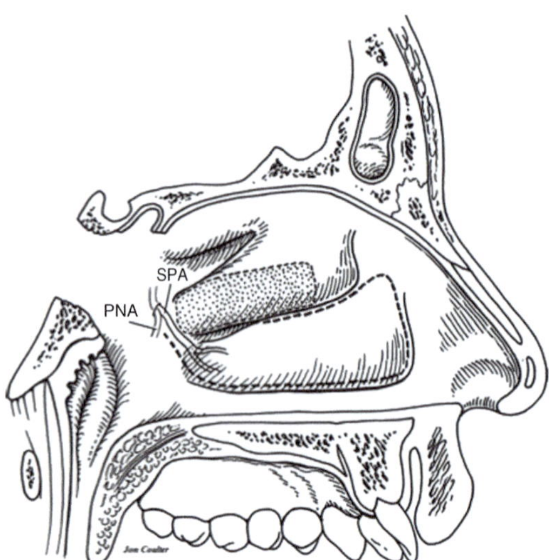

Fig. 29.5 Left lateral inferior turbinate flap incisions. *Shaded area* nasoantral window opened to facilitate identification of the sphenopalatine artery (*SPA*) and the posterior lateral nasal artery (*PLNA*) (Reproduced with permission: Fortes et al. [9]. Wiley and Sons)

13. The inferior turbinate bone is kept in situ until the flap is elevated. The bone is then taken down once the flap is elevated using true-cutting forceps.
14. The flap is then rotated into the skull base defect and secured in place.

29.3.1.5 Middle Turbinate Flap

Indications

This is a small intranasal flap which may be used for reconstruction of anterior cranial fossa, fovea ethmoidalis, planum sphenoidale, and limited sellar defects less than 1 cm [33, 34]. The flap has a mean surface area of 5.6 cm^2 [34].

Contraindications

This is a technically difficult flap to elevate due to its thin mucoperiosteum that is firmly attached to the multiple pits and crevices of the middle turbinate bone. In addition there is some risk to avulse the bony attachments of the middle turbinate to the cribriform plate, resulting in a CSF leak. This flap is especially difficult to harvest in any patient who has a destabilized middle turbinate, concha bullosa, paradoxical middle turbinate, and unilateral hypoplasia of the middle turbinate or in patients who have undergone previous surgery involving the middle turbinate. The middle turbinate flap is contraindicated in any patient who has undergone a sphenopalatine artery ligation on the involved side.

Anatomy

The middle turbinate flap comprises the mucoperiosteum of the middle turbinate and is based on the middle turbinate branch of the posterior lateral nasal artery, a branch of the sphenopalatine artery. This artery is located inferiorly in the middle turbinate and has anterior and posterior branches, which supply the lateral and medial mucosa of the turbinate, respectively [35]. See Sect. 29.3.1.4 for a further description of the vascular anatomy.

Technique [34]

1. First, the nasal cavity is decongested and prepared as previously described.
2. A vertical incision is made along the anterior face of the middle turbinate head using a 15 blade scalpel (Fig. 29.6a), a straight Beaver blade (Beaver-Visitec International Inc., Waltham, MA, USA), or monopolar electrocautery equipped with an extended insulated needle tip bent at 90° (Arthroscopic hook electrode; Valley Lab, Boulder, CO). Care must be taken not to injure the pedicle during this incision.
3. A periosteal elevator is used to raise the mucoperiosteum of the middle turbinate in a superior to inferior direction both medially and laterally to the middle turbinate bone. Care must be taken not to destabilize the middle turbinate during dissection or to fracture the ethmoid sinus cells resulting in a CSF leak.
4. The thin bone of the middle turbinate is removed from the inner aspect of the flap in a piecemeal fashion using true-cutting forceps (Fig. 29.6b).
5. Once the middle turbinate bone has been removed, the middle turbinate mucoperiosteum is detached from the lateral nasal wall and the skull base. This is done by making a horizontal cut through the axilla (Fig. 29.7) and following it posteriorly in a sagittal plane

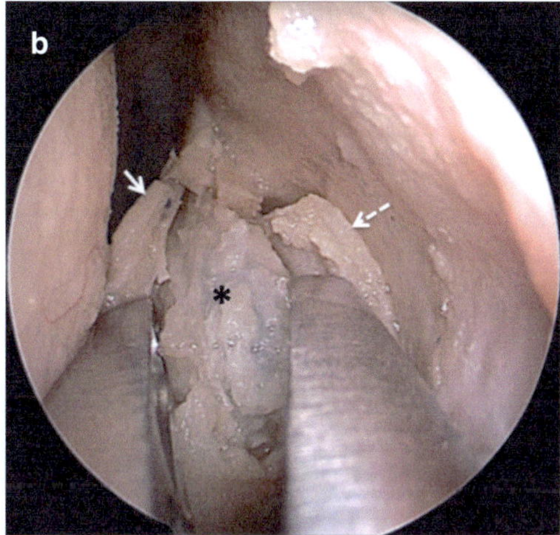

Fig. 29.6 (**a**) Endoscopic photograph of a cadaveric dissection demonstrating the anterior vertical incision of the middle turbinate flap. *Asterisk* septum; *dashed arrow* inferior turbinate; *white arrow* middle turbinate. (**b**) Endoscopic photograph of a cadaveric dissection demonstrating the removal of the middle turbinate bone. *White arrow* medial limb of flap; *white dashed arrow* lateral limb of flap; *asterisk* middle turbinate bone with concha bullosa. (Reproduced with permission: Prevedello et al. [34]. Wiley and Sons)

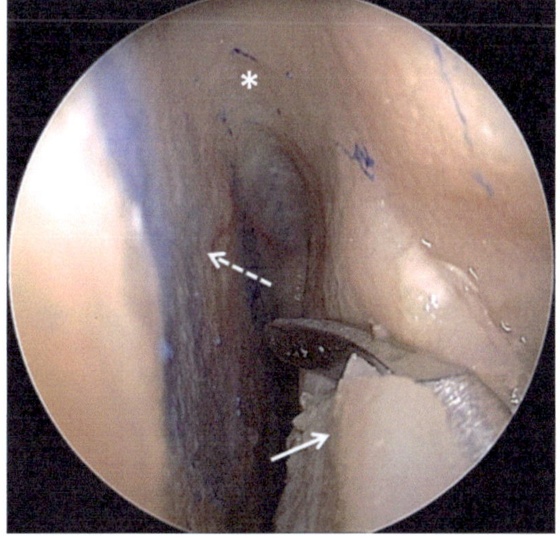

Fig. 29.7 Endoscopic photograph of a cadaveric dissection demonstrating the medial horizontal incision of the middle turbinate flap. Scissors are angled to avoid injury to the septum or skull base. *White arrow* medial limb of flap; *white asterisk* skull base; *white dashed arrow* septum

to the posterior pedicle yielding a posterior pedicle flap. Caution must be taken not to enter the skull base.

6. Identification of the pedicle is key, and following it to the sphenopalatine foramen allows for an increased length and a better arc of rotation.
7. The flap is then rotated into the skull base defect and secured in place.

29.3.1.6 Anteriorly Based Lateral Nasal Wall Flap

Indications

This flap, also known as the Hadad-Bassagaisteguy 2 or HB2 flap, is amenable to cover defects in the region from the frontal sinus to the tuberculum sella and from orbit to orbit [36]. An HB2 flap is designed based on the anticipated size and shape of the defect. The width of the flap can be extended to the nasal septum as required or can be combined with a nasoseptal flap to reconstruct very large skull base defects. Unfortunately, this flap tends to have "memory" for the original shape of the inferior turbinate [36].

Contraindications

Any patient who has undergone surgery that may compromise the blood supply or the tissue comprising the flap such as an anterior ethmoid artery ligation, previous facial fractures (particularly those involving the frontal, maxillary, ethmoid, or nasal bones) or orbital fractures, neck dissections, excision of the submandibular gland, or inferior turbinate surgery. It is also uncertain if the pedicle of this flap can withstand postoperative radiotherapy. Vascularity of the flap can be assessed preoperatively using contrast imaging or a Doppler.

Anatomy

The inferior turbinate receives a dual blood supply, from the inferior turbinate branch of the posterolateral nasal artery posteriorly, and the angular artery branch of the facial artery anteriorly [36]. The anteriorly based lateral nasal wall flap, also known as the Haddad-Bassagaisteguy (HB2) flap, is based on the facial (angular and lateral nasal branches) and anterior ethmoidal arteries.

Technique [36]

1. First, the nasal cavity is decongested and prepared as previously described (see Reconstruction technique).
2. To facilitate the visualization of the surgical field and harvesting of the flap, the middle turbinate ipsilateral to the flap is usually removed.
3. A monopolar electrocautery equipped with an extended insulated needle tip bent at 90° (Arthroscopic hook electrode; Valley Lab, Boulder, CO) is used to harvest the flap.
4. The pedicle of the flap is aligned vertically in the sagittal plane and extends from the roof of the nasal cavity, just anterior to the middle turbinate, to the head of the inferior turbinate. Its anterior incision follows the anterior border of the ascending maxillary process. Its posterior incision follows the uncinate process and extends over the superior aspect of the inferior turbinate. Although technically difficult, this incision can be extended superiorly to incorporate the fontanelle of the maxillary sinus (to increase the width of the flap) (Fig. 29.8).
5. The sphenopalatine neurovascular bundle will be encountered at the most posterior aspect of the incision and needs to be controlled either by clipping or cauterization.
6. A perpendicular incision starting at the most posterior aspect of the incision over the lateral nasal wall travels medially to cross the floor of the nose and to reach the inferior border of the septum.
7. Another perpendicular incision is made anteriorly from the head of the inferior turbinate to cross the floor of the nose and reach the inferior border of the septum.
8. Two horizontal incisions at the floor of the nose are joined by another incision that follows the maxillary crest at the junction of the floor of the nose with nasal septum. This incision can be extended to the nasal septum superiorly depending on the size of the defect.

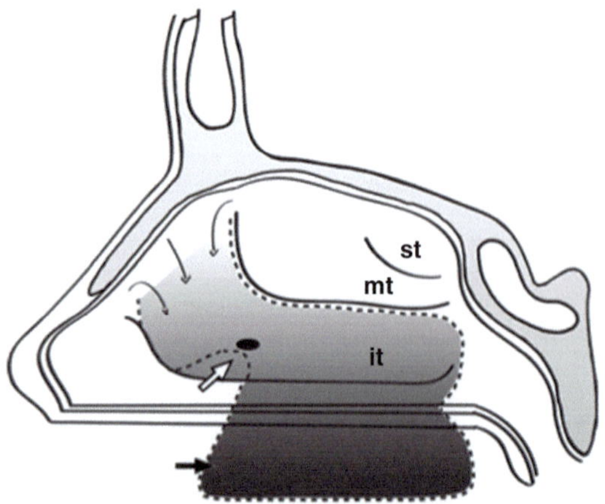

Fig. 29.8 Incisions for a right anterior pedicle lateral nasal wall flap. *IT* inferior turbinate, *MT* middle turbinate, *ST* superior turbinate. *Curved arrows* demonstrate the pedicle base and blood flow. *White arrow* points to the incision over the head of the middle turbinate. *Black arrow* extension of the incision over the nasal floor (Reproduced with permission: Hadad et al. [36]. Wiley and Sons)

9. A separate vertical incision is performed over the head of the inferior turbinate and extended laterally to intersect the pedicle's anterior incision. This latter incision is critical to allow the elevation of the mucoperiosteal lining of the nasal and meatal sides of the inferior turbinate. The dissection continues along the medial aspect of the inferior turbinate.
10. The opening of the nasolacrimal duct is spared by curving the anterior horizontal incision around it or by performing an elliptical incision around the opening.
11. Then, the inferior turbinate is fractured medially, and the mucoperiosteum together with the inferior turbinate bone is elevated from the lateral nasal wall. Later, the turbinate bone is removed with Kerrison rongeurs or true-cutting instruments.
12. The nasal floor mucosa is subsequently elevated, and the flap is freed posteriorly.
13. The placement of the HB2 flap over the defect requires rotation of its pedicle from the sagittal to the axial plane; thus, it needs to be bolstered in place with packing.

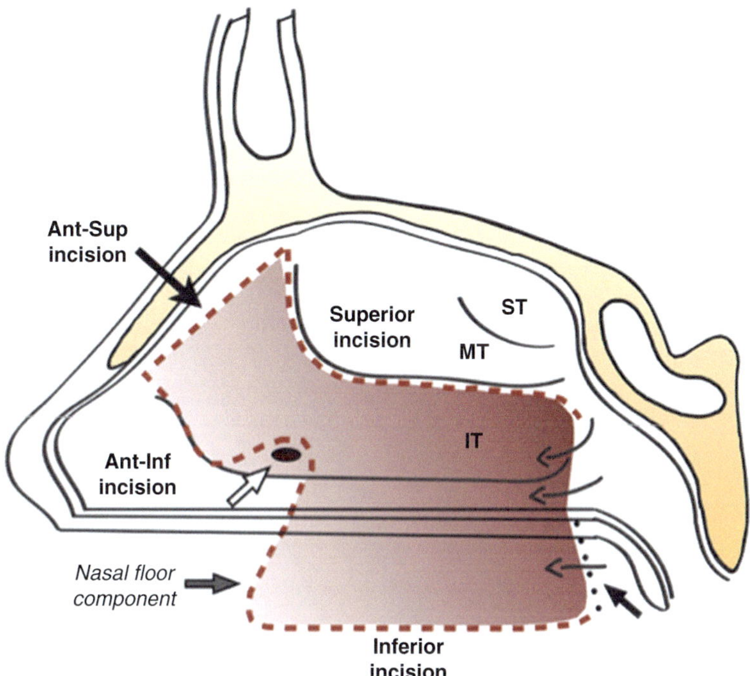

Fig. 29.9 Incisions for the posterior-based lateral nasal wall flap. *Dashed lines* incisions, *Ant-Sup incision (large black arrow)* anterosuperior incision, *Ant-Inf incision* anteroinferior incision, *IT* inferior turbinate, *MT* middle turbinate, *ST* superior turbinate, *small curved black arrows* blood supply of the flap, *white arrow* nasolacrimal duct opening, *dashed black (circles) line* and *small black arrow* an incision can be made at the nasal floor to increase the arc of rotation of the flap (Reproduced with permission: Rivera-Serrano et al. [37]. Oceanside Publications)

29.3.1.7 Posteriorly Based Lateral Nasal Wall Flap

Indications

The posterior pedicle lateral nasal wall flap, also named as Carrau-Hadad (C-H) flap, was designed by Carrau and Hadad et al. in 2011 [37]. It provides a large surface area that is adequate for the reconstruction of skull base defects that extend from the planum sphenoidale to the nasopharynx anteroposteriorly and from orbital apex to orbital apex or internal carotid artery canal to internal carotid artery canal, laterolaterally [37].

Contraindications

Careful consideration should be given to any patient who has had a sphenopalatine artery ligation on the involved side, surgery of the sphenoid sinuses, or inferior turbinate surgery.

Anatomy

The posteriorly based lateral nasal wall flap encompasses the mucoperiosteum of the inferolateral wall and floor of the nasal cavity. The pedicle is based on branches of sphenopalatine artery.

Technique [37]

1. First, the nasal cavity is decongested and prepared as previously described.
2. Resecting the middle turbinate greatly improves visualization of this flap.
3. Using a needle tip monopolar cautery (ValleyLab, Boulder, CO), the anterior mucoperiosteal incision is made along the anterior border of the ascending maxillary process. This starts at the level of the caudal aspect of the nasal bone and extends inferiorly to the level of the head of the inferior turbinate (Fig. 29.9).
4. The anterior incision extends onto the lateral nasal wall and then onto the nasal floor if a larger flap is required, preserving the nasolacrimal duct.
5. The anterior incision then continues posteriorly along the lateral nasal wall or along the nasal floor to a point that is level with the sphenopalatine foramen. This incision is then continued in a coronal plane toward the sphenopalatine foramen.
6. The posterior incision starts at a level that is superior to the anterior incision (axilla of the middle turbinate) and extends along the posterior aspect of the lacrimal bone and

along the superior aspect of the inferior turbinate to reach the level of the sphenopalatine foramen.
7. An incision is made connecting the superior aspects of both incisions.
8. The head of the inferior turbinate is incised vertically, and this incision is extended to connect with the anterior incision.
9. The mucoperiosteum of the inferior turbinate is then elevated using a Cottle dissector or Freer periosteal elevator.
10. The inferior turbinate bone is then removed using true-cutting instruments and Kerrison rongeurs.
11. The mucoperiosteum is elevated further along the lateral nasal wall and floor of nose. As the elevation continues posteriorly, care must be taken not to injure branches of the sphenopalatine artery.
12. Once elevated, the flap is rotated with a pivot point at the sphenopalatine foramen. The pedicle of the sphenopalatine artery may be freed from the foramen to facilitate its rotation (up to 180°).

29.3.2 Extranasal Flaps

29.3.2.1 Indications

Extranasal pedicled flaps may be used in instances where the vascular supply to the nasoseptal flap or local regional intranasal flaps has been compromised or when multiple flaps are needed for the reconstruction. Other potential scenarios when these flaps may be necessary include neoplastic involvement of intranasal tissue that would otherwise be used as a flap or previous use of flaps (e.g., recurrent tumor).

29.3.2.2 Anatomy of the Frontal and Temporal Scalp

Elevation of the pericranial flap, temporoparietal flap, and the galeofrontalis flap requires a thorough understanding of the anatomy of the scalp. The scalp is divided into five layers, from superficial to deep:

1. Skin.
2. Subcutaneous layer.
3. Aponeurotic layer – this includes the galea and frontalis muscle anteriorly, occipitalis muscle posteriorly, and the temporoparietal fascia laterally.
4. Subaponeurotic layer which is made up of loose areolar tissue.
5. Periosteal layer – the periosteal layer on the frontal scalp is contiguous with the deep temporalis fascia, which overlies the temporalis muscle. The pericranium is often described as a combination of the periosteal layer and the subaponeurotic layer (i.e., areolar tissue).

29.3.2.3 Transfrontal Pericranial Flap

Indications

The transfrontal pericranial flap is a regional vascular pedicled flap comprising the anterior pericranium. The pericranial flap has a long pedicle and may be utilized to cover defects from the frontal sinus to the sella and from orbit to orbit [33]. It is extremely useful for large anterior skull base defects when intranasal pedicled flaps are not available or when the extent of the defect may require the use of multiple flaps. Multiple reports have addressed excellent outcomes associated with the use of a pericranial flap for the reconstruction of skull base defects resulting from anterior craniofacial resection [38–40].

Contraindications

Careful consideration should be given to any patient who has undergone open cranial surgery, particularly via a subfrontal approach, a brow lift, or one who has suffered orbital rim fractures. Consideration should also be given to placement of the coronal incision in younger men due to the possibility of future hairline recession. Postoperatively, a compressive cranial dressing should be avoided to preserve the vascular pedicle.

Anatomy

The pericranial flap is based on the supraorbital and supratrochlear neurovascular bundles and, therefore, may be harvested as two separate flaps. The supratrochlear and supraorbital nerves are cutaneous branches of the ophthalmic division of the trigeminal nerve. The supraorbital nerve supplies the forehead and scalp back to the vertex, and the supratrochlear nerve supplies the midline forehead to the hairline [41]. The supraorbital and supratrochlear arteries are branches of the ophthalmic artery, a branch of the supraclinoid segment of the internal carotid artery (ICA). The ophthalmic artery branches from the ICA as it emerges from the roof of the cavernous sinus [41]. The supratrochlear artery is one of the two terminal branches of the ophthalmic artery and emerges as part of the neurovascular pedicle through the frontal notch or foramen. The supratrochlear notch or foramen is medial to the supraorbital notch or foramen, which lies approximately 22.2 mm from the midline [42]. A supraorbital notch is found approximately 70 % of the time, and a foramen is found approximately 30 % of the time [42]. The arteries ascend in the galea-frontalis muscle layer and then provide branches which supply the pericranium [40]. When elevating this flap, the frontalis layer should not be separated from the pericranium within 10 mm of the orbital rim in order to preserve the neurovascular pedicle [40]. Both arteries anastomose with each other and the superficial temporal artery, a terminal branch of the external carotid artery, thereby providing an anastomosis between the internal and external carotid arterial systems.

Technique [43]

1. First, the nasal cavity is decongested and prepared as previously described.
2. Prior to elevation of the pericranial flap, a Draf III frontal sinus resection is performed to maintain frontal sinus drainage and to prevent a frontal sinus mucocele postoperatively.
3. A coronal incision is marked at the vertex of the scalp extending from one ear to the other. Depending on the goals of resection, the marked incision may be carried down and forward in the preauricular region to allow increased mobility of the flap. Advantages of placing the incision at the vertex are that it allows for optimal cosmesis from potential hair loss at the incision site and also prevents transection of anterior branches of the superficial temporal artery supplying the anterior scalp (Fig. 29.10a).
4. The marked incision is injected with 1 % lidocaine with 1:100,000 epinephrine.
5. The incision is carried down sharply to the cranium from the temporal line on one side to the other side.
6. Lateral to the temporal line, the incision is carried down to the deep temporalis fascia, which is continuous with the periosteal layer. This allows the elevation of scalp in the same plane.
7. To minimize bleeding, Rainey clips are placed at the incision edges.
8. Elevation of the pericranium with the scalp flap has the advantage of preventing desiccation of the pericranial flap and also allows inclusion of the subaponeurotic tissue (loose areolar tissue) in the flap, making the flap more robust.
9. The scalp flap is then elevated anteriorly to the orbital rim. The supraorbital neurovascular pedicle may arise from a foramen or a notch. Should there be a foramen, the supraorbital and supratrochlear neurovascular pedicle may be freed via osteotomies using a 2–3 mm osteotome to prevent traction injury to the flap pedicle.
10. The pericranial flap is then raised by sharply dissecting in a subgaleal plane using tenotomy scissors. Care has to be taken as one approaches the superior orbital rim to avoid transecting through the penetrating branch of the supraorbital and supratrochlear arteries, which may arise 10 mm above the orbital rim.
11. Next, the high-speed drill is used to open a 1 × 15 mm osteotomy at the nasion through a separate horizontal incision, therefore communicating the coronal approach with the frontonasal area and the anterior skull base resection site (Fig. 29.10b).
12. The flap is then transposed through the nasion osteotomy into the nasal cavity.
13. An intranasal bolster is placed to support the flap (Fig. 29.10c, d).
14. The coronal incision is closed meticulously in a multilayered fashion.

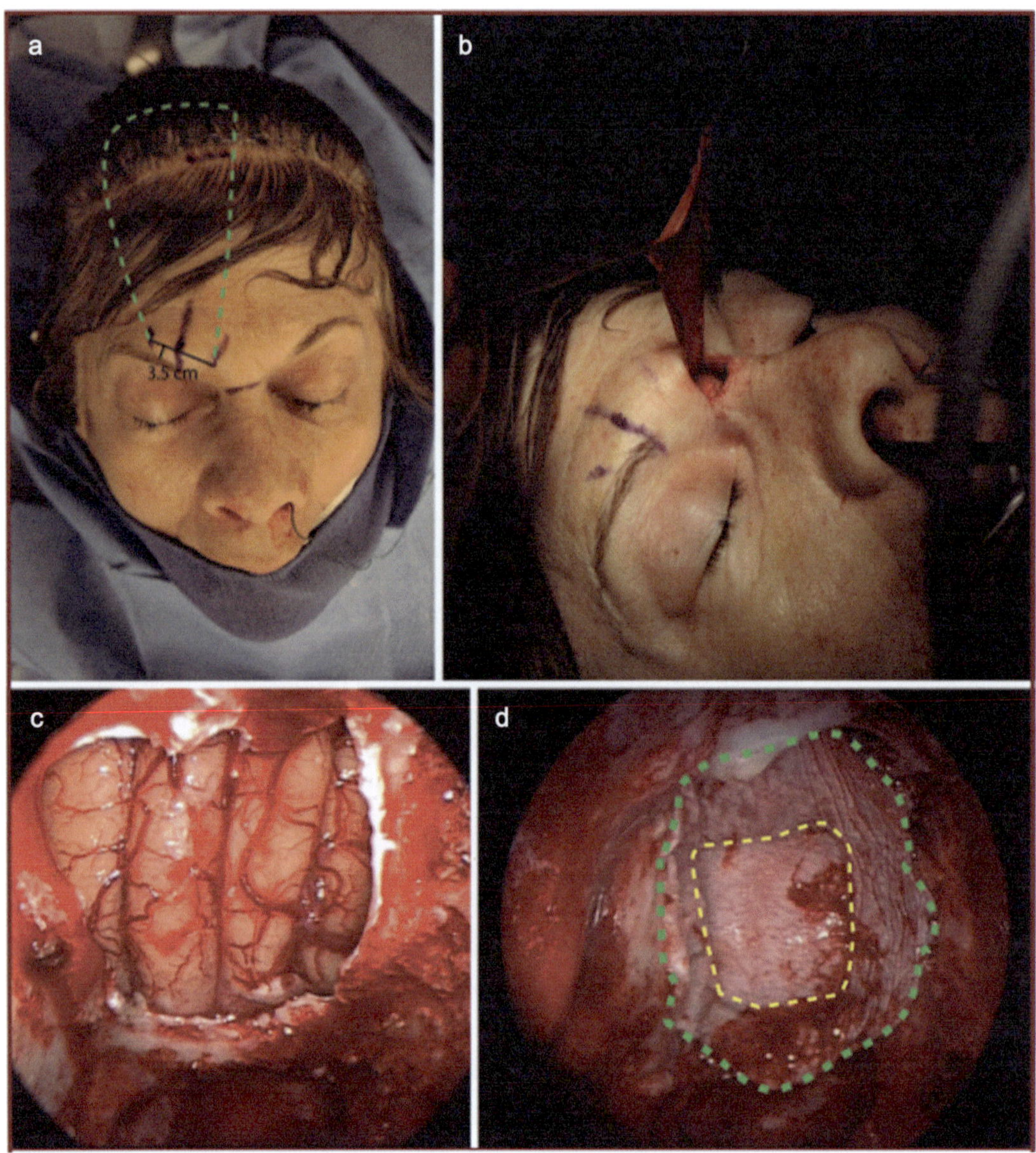

Fig. 29.10 (**a**) Preoperative incision planning for harvesting pericranial flap (*green dashed line*). The pericranial flap pedicle, located using a Doppler probe, is marked at the medial right brow (*three purple lines* represent the pedicle). (**b**) Rotated pericranial flap prior to passage into the nasal cavity. (**c**) Anterior cranial fossa defect after tumor resection. (**d**) Intranasal defect with pericranial flap onlay. *Yellow dashed line* anterior to cranial fossa defect, *Green dashed line* the pericranial flap onlay covering the defect (Reproduced with permission: Patel et al. [43]. Walters Kluwer Health)

Variations

1. If an extended resection mandates a longer flap, then step 3 may be modified such as to incise down to the loose areolar tissue and then dissect posteriorly prior to incising into the pericranium.
2. Note that the pericranium has bilateral neurovascular pedicles; however, a pericranial flap may be supported by only one vascular pedicle allowing the sacrifice of the other side. Variations include raising a wide flap that includes both pedicles, as is the preference

when a transcranial or subfrontal approach is performed; raising two separate flaps with their own respective pedicles; or raising a single side.

29.3.2.4 Temporoparietal Fascia Flap

Indications

The temporoparietal fascia flap is a regional vascularized pedicled flap comprising a strong fascial layer that connects the overlying fibrous septae of the subcutaneous tissue at the temporoparietal region of the scalp. This flap relies on very consistent vascular anatomy, has large dimensions, and is very pliable. Its use in skull base reconstruction after endonasal endoscopic resection requires a transpterygoid tunnel [44]. This allows the use of the transpterygoid temporoparietal fascia flap for the repair of skull base defects by transposing the flap from the temporal to the infratemporal fossa and then advancing it into the nasal cavity through an expanded pterygopalatine fossa.

The transpterygoid temporoparietal fascia flap will cover defects of the clivus and parasellar region [44]. However, its arc of rotation (90°) and tunneled pedicle through the pterygopalatine fossa limit the coverage of anterior skull base defects such as the planum sphenoidale and cribriform plate. A transpterygoid temporoparietal fascia flap is most useful to reconstruct large defects of the posterior and middle cranial base when intranasal vascularized flaps are not feasible or when the extent of the defect mandates the use of multiple flaps.

Contraindications

Careful consideration is necessary in any patient who has undergone a rhytidectomy, parotid surgery, and excision of scalp lesions, in any patient who suffered a zygoma fracture, in any patient with giant cell arteritis, and/or in any patient who has undergone a superficial temporal artery biopsy. This flap requires an external incision and, therefore, does have the potential to risk alopecia in the region of the scar. A transpterygoid temporoparietal fascia flap should also be avoided in a patient who has undergone irradiation of the scalp due to the risk of subsequent scalp necrosis [45].

Anatomy

The transpterygoid temporoparietal fascia flap is based on the anterior branch of the superficial temporal artery, a terminal branch of the external carotid artery, and the one or two veins that accompany it. This artery runs behind the temporomandibular joint, crosses the posterior aspect of the root of the zygoma, and ascends anterior to the tragus of the ear [41]. The superficial temporal artery divides into its terminal frontal and parietal branches approximately 3 cm above the zygomatic arch. The veins usually run superficial to the artery. It supplies the skin overlying the temporalis fascia, the fascia itself, and temporalis muscle [41].

The temporoparietal fascia (also known as the superficial temporal fascia) is 2–3 mm in thickness over the parietal region and extends in a fanlike manner from the preauricular region, comprising a surface area as large as 17 × 14 cm [44, 8]. The transpterygoid temporoparietal fascia flap has a long vascular pedicle and a robust blood supply.

The temporoparietal fascia is directly continuous with the galea superiorly and the superficial musculoaponeurotic system (SMAS) inferiorly [41]. Frontal and temporal branches of the facial nerve travel under (rarely within) the temporoparietal fascia and superficial to the superficial layer of the deep temporalis fascia (Fig. 29.11a). Topographically, the frontal branch runs along a line drawn from the attachment of the ear lobule (5 mm below the tragus) to a point approximately 1.5 cm superior to the lateral aspect of the ipsilateral eyebrow [46]. Therefore, care must be taken when elevating this flap to preserve the facial nerve branches as discussed below.

Technique [47, 1]

A. Creating a “window” for the transposition of the flap
   1. First, the nasal cavity is decongested and prepared as previously described.
   2. A standard endoscopic transpterygoid, transmaxillary approach is performed to create a window for the flap to be tunneled into the nasal cavity from the neck [47, 1].

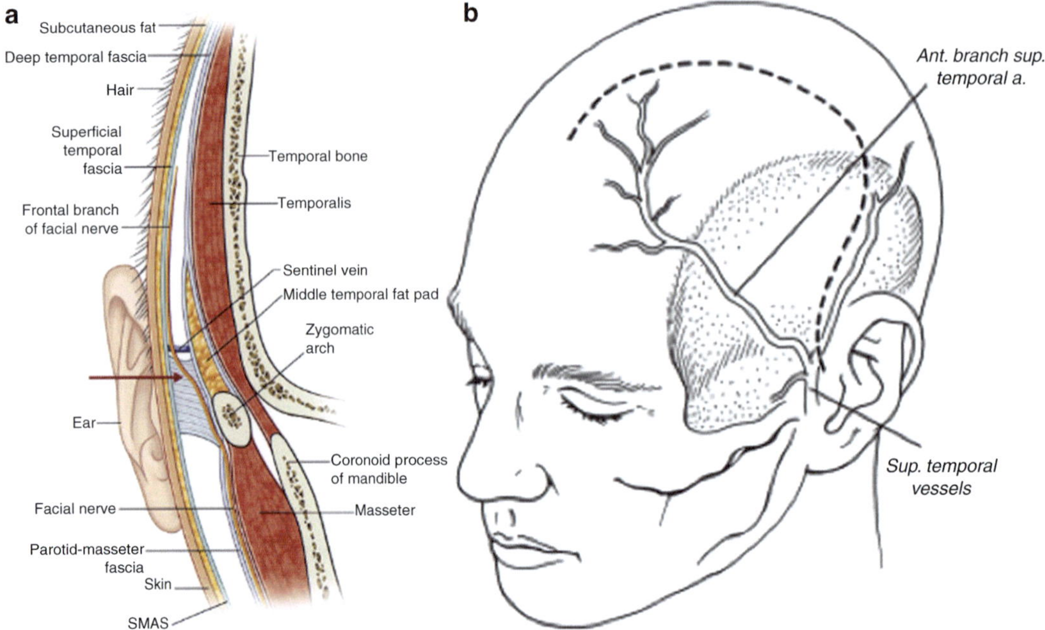

Fig. 29.11 (**a**) Schematic demonstrating the relationship of the frontal branch of the facial nerve to the temporoparietal fascia/superficial temporal fascia and superficial layer of the deep temporalis fascia (Reproduced with permission: Neligan et al. [67]). (**b**) Hemicoronal incision and blood supply for temporoparietal fascial flap (Reproduced with permission: Fortes et al. [8]. Wiley and Sons)

3. A transpterygoid temporoparietal fascia flap is preferably harvested ipsilateral to a transpterygoid endonasal approach, as this facilitates its transposition into the nasal cavity (contributes to the corridor).
4. Anterior and posterior ethmoidectomies and a large maxillary antrostomy facilitate the transpterygoid transposition.
5. The ipsilateral sphenopalatine artery is identified and ligated at the level of the sphenopalatine foramen. The posterior wall of the maxillary sinus is removed using Kerrison rongeurs to expose the pterygopalatine fossa.
6. Additional removal to include the lateral wall of the maxillary sinus expands the pterygomaxillary fissure, thus widening the communication with the infratemporal fossa.
7. Inferior displacement of the soft tissues of the pterygopalatine fossa exposes the anterior aspect of the pterygoid process. This requires the division of the vidian nerve and artery in order to allow the inferior displacement of the soft tissues; however, the sphenopalatine ganglion is preserved.
8. Care is taken not to injure the internal maxillary artery during this maneuver.
9. The most anterior aspect of the lateral pterygoid plate may be reduced with a high-speed drill to further enlarge the corridor for the transposition of the transpterygoid temporoparietal fascia flap.

B. Elevation of temporoparietal fascial flap
   1. A hemicoronal incision is carried down to the level of the hair follicles. The temporoparietal fascia is dissected from the subcutaneous tissue, thus leaving the transpterygoid temporoparietal fascia flap attached to the cranium (Fig. 29.11b).
   2. Once enough surface area is exposed, the fascia is incised at its lateral margins and is elevated from the cranium and the superficial layer of the deep temporal fascia down to its pedicle. This dissection must not extend anterior to an imaginary line between

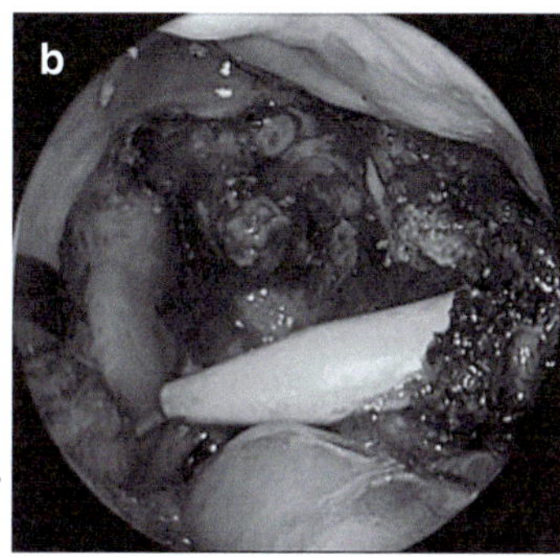

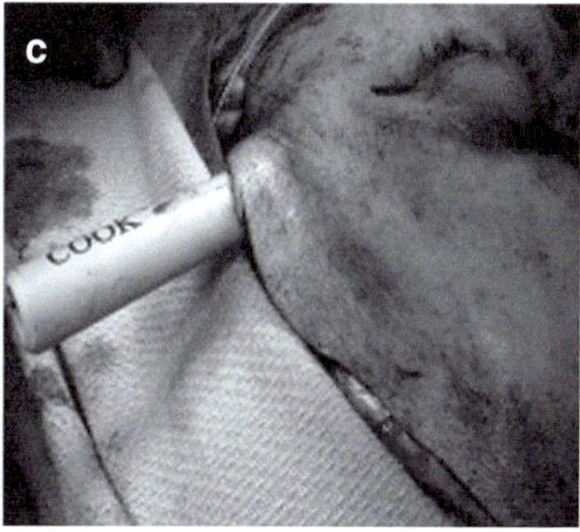

Fig. 29.12 Drawing (**a**) and intraoperative endoscopic (**b**) and external view (**c**) of guide wire and dilator being advanced into nasal cavity (Reproduced with permission: Fortes et al. [8]. Wiley and Sons)

the tragus and the lateral eyebrow or dissect anterior to the hairline in order to preserve the frontal branch of the facial nerve.

C. Creating an infratemporal/transpterygoid tunnel
   1. The superficial layer of the deep temporal fascia is incised vertically and is separated from the temporal muscle following a subfascial plane of dissection. This dissection is then carried inferiorly to elevate the periosteum from the medial surface of zygoma.
   2. This allows communication in the temporal, infratemporal, and pterygopalatine fossae. This tunnel may be expanded using percutaneous tracheostomy dilators.
   3. After an adequate tunnel is opened, the flap is tied to the external end of the guide wire. As the nasal end of the guide wire is pulled out through the nostril, it draws the flap through the tunnel into the nasal cavity (Fig. 29.12). Care must be taken to avoid rotation of the flap or pedicle, which may compromise the blood supply.
   4. This flap requires preservation of the venous outflow; thus, avoidance of excessive pressure over the pedicle is a critical consideration.
   5. Finally, the flap is placed and bolstered over the defect avoiding compression of the flap or pedicle, especially over each turn where they are most vulnerable.
   6. External incisions are closed with a single layer of 4-0 sutures after the insertion of a suction drain.

29.3.2.5 Occipital Galeopericranial Flap

Indications

The pedicle of this flap is approximately 8 cm long and provides a variable surface area of up to 44 cm^2 [48]. The occipital galeopericranial flap has not been applied clinically, thus remains as a theoretical possibility. Technically this flap can cover anterior skull base, posterior midline, and middle cranial fossa skull base defects. Unfortunately, the pedicle of this flap (especially its vein) is easily compressed, and it is, therefore, used only as a last resort.

29.3.2.6 Facial Artery Myomucosal/Buccinator Flap

Indications

This flap provides an area of up to 15.9 cm^2 of coverage and up to 16 cm in length [49]. This flap has been described as a possibility to reconstruct defects of the planum sphenoidale, sella turcica, frontal sinus, and fovea ethmoidalis [49]. However, due to the very distant location of the planum sphenoidale from the anterior maxillary tunnel required for this flap, we would recommend consideration of other flaps for lesions in this location. This flap may be a myomucosal flap (facial artery myomucosal (FAMM) flap) or a muscular flap (facial artery buccinator (FAB) flap).

Advantages of the FAMM/FAB flap include [49] the following:

- Reliability and low failure rate.
- Versatility due to its long pedicle and wide arc of rotation.

- Minimal donor site morbidity.
- Superior esthetics due to the absence of a visible scar.
- Robustness, as it may include mucosa and muscle.
- Can be harvested *after* the skull base resection; thus, it can be customized to the defect.
- It is harvested from site that is distant to the tumor, therefore outside any previously irradiated field.
- It withstands postoperative radiation therapy if required.
- Its length may be extended by harvesting the mandibular periosteum.

Disadvantages of the FAMM/FAB flap include the following:

- Possibility of flap migration due to gravitational pull of the vertically oriented pedicle
- Possible obstruction of the maxillary sinus
- Potential dental or facial paresthesia
- Potential epiphora
- Potential introduction of oral flora into a sterile field
- Risk of donor site fibrosis causing trismus

Contraindications

Careful consideration should be taken in any patient with previous intraoral neoplasms and trismus or in any patient who has undergone surgery in the region of the buccal mucosa.

Anatomy

This flap is based on the facial artery, a branch of the external carotid artery. As the facial artery ascends over the mandible, at the anterior border of the masseter muscle, it runs deep to the dilator muscles of the lips and superficial to the buccinator muscle [41]. It sends branches to the upper and lower lip and continues its ascent toward the medial aspect of the eye where it becomes the angular artery. The facial artery runs 1–1.6 cm from the oral commissure [50]. This flap derives its blood supply from reverse flow via the angular artery, which anastomoses with the infraorbital, dorsal nasal, and ophthalmic arteries, part of the internal carotid artery system [51]. Its venous supply is dependent on the venous buccal plexus, and therefore, the facial vein does not necessarily need to be harvested with the artery to ensure its survival. Due to the varied branching patterns of the facial artery, preoperative imaging (such as a CT angiogram or intraoperative Doppler) is recommended when planning to use this flap for skull base reconstruction.

Technique [51]

A. Flap elevation
   1. The flap may be a myomucosal flap (FAMM) or a myofascial flap (buccinators/FAB flap). Intraoral incisions are made accordingly including or excluding mucosa.
   2. Intraoral incisions are made in a “boot” or “L” shape in the buccal region (Fig. 29.13). For a myofascial flap (buccinator flap), a posteriorly based mucosal flap is elevated prior to step 4 (alternatively, it may be harvested via a longitudinal incision).
   3. An inferior incision is made first just superior to the level of the mandibular gingivobuccal sulcus. The incision is deepened through the buccinator muscle, and the facial artery is immediately identified superficial to the buccinator. The artery is ligated proximally to allow for increased length of the pedicle.
   4. An anterior incision is made about 1.5 cm from the oral commissure running parallel to the facial artery/angular artery axis.
   5. Next another parallel incision is made just anterior to the opening of the parotid duct.
   6. A horizontal superior incision is made to connect the previously made parallel incisions. The height of the superior incision determines the size of the flap and is made depending on the skull base defect.
   7. The flap is then elevated superficial to the facial artery.

B. Tunneling the flap
   1. The flap is transposed into the nasal cavity by creating a tunnel from the oral cavity into the nasal cavity. This can be done in a variety of ways, but the two most common routes are an anterior maxillotomy with a medial maxillectomy and via gingivobuccal incision to reach the lateral skull base.
   2. A separate incision is made in the maxillary gingivobuccal region.

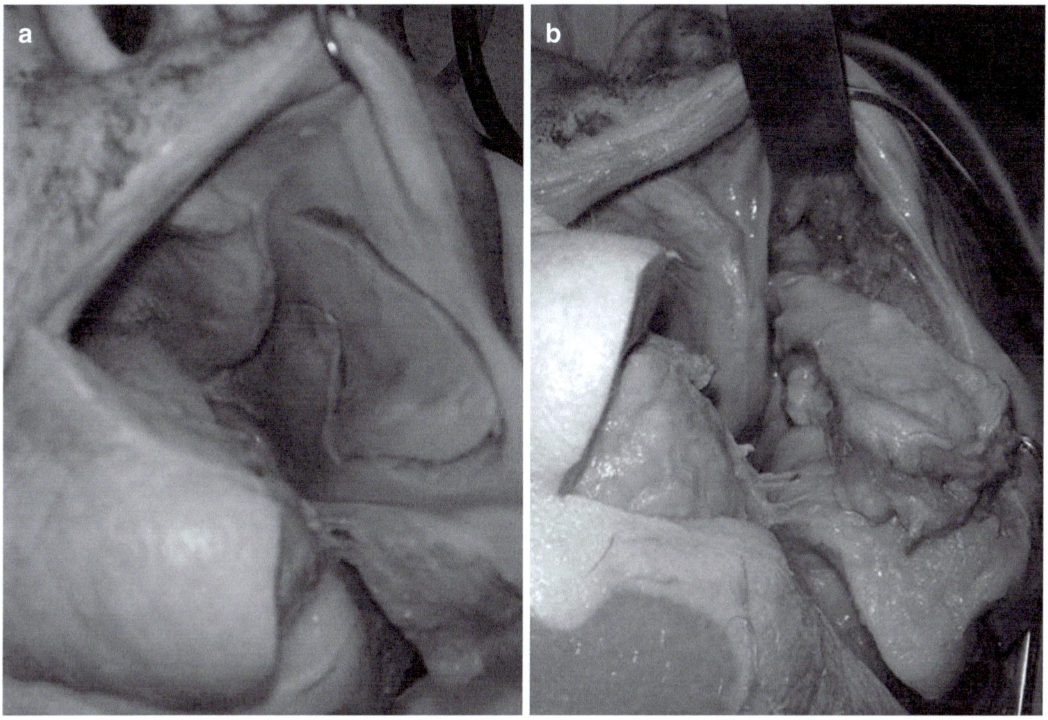

Fig. 29.13 Facial buccinator myomucosal flap. (**a**) Flap in situ in a fresh specimen. (**b**) Flap raised in a fresh specimen (Reproduced with permission: Rivera-Serrano et al. [51]. Wiley and Sons)

3. Transantral/transmaxillary osteotomies are then created and are limited superiorly by the infraorbital nerve. The inferior limit is level with the hard palate and maxillary floor.
4. An endoscopic medial maxillectomy is performed after preparation of the nose as described earlier.
5. The myofascial flap is then introduced into the nasal cavity via an anterior maxillary osteotomy and placed over the defect.
6. The buccal defect is closed primarily or may be allowed to heal by secondary intention. Alternatively, a split-thickness skin graft may be placed over the defect.

Postoperatively, we recommend the use of a Therabite (Atos Medical, Hörby, Sweden) device to avoid donor site fibrosis and trismus.

29.3.2.7 Oliver Pedicled Palatal Flap

The Oliver pedicled palatal flap provides up to 18.5 cm^2 surface area and requires a palatal defect of approximately 1.5 cm^2 for successful harvesting of the entire palatal mucosa and transposition into the nasal cavity [52]. The palatal flap was initially described for use in palatal lengthening during cleft palate repair [53].

Indications

The Oliver pedicled palatal flap can reach defects involving the planum, sella, and clivus down to the level of the foramen magnum [52]. It requires experience and skill to dissect and has the potential for significant donor site morbidity. This flap may be harvested after surgical resection and can therefore be specifically tailored to the size and shape of the defect.

Contraindications

Risks of this flap include the possibility of an oronasal fistula, which relegates this flap to one of last resort. A fistula may be overcome by preserving the mucosa of the nasal floor or using a posteriorly based nasal floor mucoperiosteal flap, acellular dermis to reconstruct the palatal defect, and a molded splint screwed into place for 2 weeks [54, 55, 53, 52]. Complete palatal

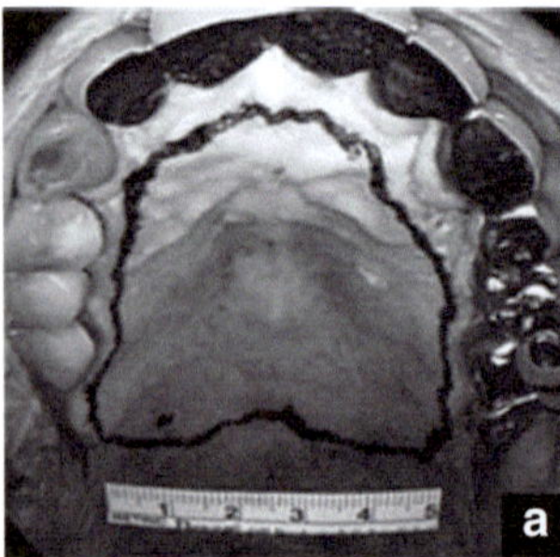
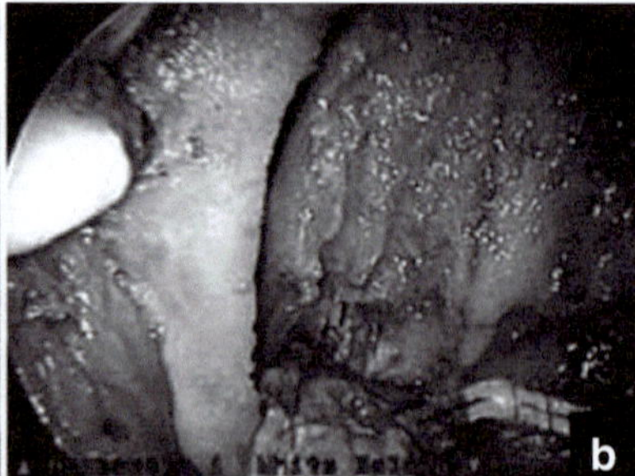
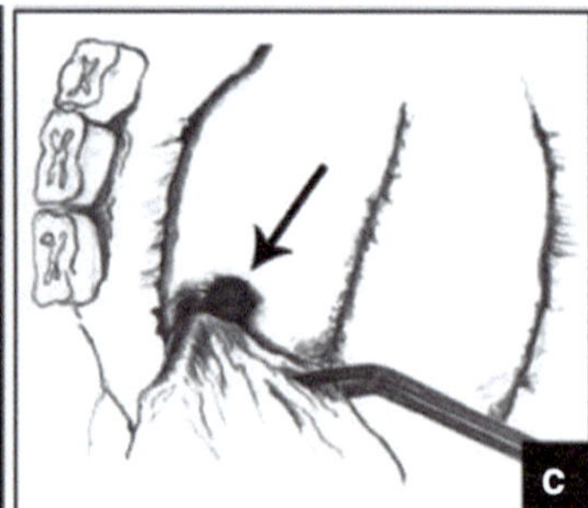

Fig. 29.14 Harvest and transposition of the palatal flap into the nasal cavity. (**a**) Outline of the palatal flap. (**b**, **c**) Palatal flap harvest (anatomic and illustration) with preservation of the greater palatine vasculature. Enlarged foramen (*arrow*) (Reproduced with permission: Oliver et al. [52]. John Wiley and Sons)

remucosalization occurs in 3–4 weeks [56]. Use of this flap theoretically risks the introduction of oral flora into the operative field. This risk may be reduced with the preoperative use of a chlorhexidine mouthwash and gargle [57].

Anatomy

The Oliver pedicled palatal flap is based on the greater palatine artery. The greater palatine artery is a branch of the internal maxillary artery and branches off within the pterygopalatine fossa [41]. The artery enters the greater palatine canal formed by a border between the crest of the palatine bone and the body of the maxilla [41]. It exits via the greater palatine foramen at the junction of the hard and soft palate and runs anteriorly along the hard palate to anastomose with the posterior septal branch of the sphenopalatine artery [41]. Due to a midline vascular network, the entire palatal mucosa may be harvested and based on a single greater palatine artery [58, 59]. This flap has a pedicle that is up to 3 cm long [52].

Technique [52]

Harvesting and transposition of the palatal flap requires a combined transoral and transnasal approach.

A. Transoral approach (Fig. 29.14)
   1. The greater palatine foramen is identified by palpation located just anterior to the junction of the hard and soft palate.
   2. An anterior incision is made about 2–5 mm from the teeth on the hard palate. Depending on the size of the defect, the incision may be extended to the contralateral hard palate to harvest a larger flap.
   3. The incisions are then extended posteriorly toward the junction of the hard and soft palate (Fig. 29.14a).
   4. A subperiosteal dissection is followed from anterior to posterior to elevate the palatal flap toward the greater palatine foramen.
   5. The greater palatine/descending palatine pedicle is identified at the foramen (Fig. 29.14b, c).
   6. The foramen is then drilled in a controlled fashion using a 2 mm coarse diamond high-speed drill to create a palatal defect up to 1.5 cm^2 through which the palatal flap can be delivered into the nasal cavity.

B. Endonasal approach
   1. The pterygopalatine fossa is identified in the standard fashion. An ipsilateral uncinectomy is performed to identify the natural maxillary ostium. The maxillary ostium is widened posteriorly toward the posterior wall of the maxillary sinus. Submucoperiosteal dissection in a medial direction results in identification of the crista ethmoidalis, sphenopalatine foramen, and the branches of the sphenopalatine artery. The pterygopalatine fossa is exposed removing the ascending process of the palatine bone.
   2. The mucosa of the lateral nasal wall and nasal floor is elevated after transecting the

inferior turbinate. The incision extends from the lateral wall through the nasal floor onto the septum.

3. An anterior to posterior submucoperiosteal elevation is performed along the septum and nasal floor to the ascending process of the palatine bone.
4. The anteromedial wall of the pterygopalatine fossa and the pterygopalatine canal is then drilled approximately around and inferiorly toward the previously enlarged greater palatine foramen, thus exposing and mobilizing the greater palatine/descending palatine neurovascular bundle.
5. The palatal flap is then transposed through the drilled tunnel from the oral cavity to the nasal cavity.
6. The palatal island flap is used to cover the skull base defect.
7. The oroantral defect is repaired using acellular dermis and by replacing the previously elevated submucoperiosteal flap.

Bolster

We prefer to place absorbable packing such as Nasopore (Polyganics, Groningen, the Netherlands) as the first layer adjacent to the repair/flap. Occasionally, apply absorbable hemostatic paste of thrombin-soaked gelatin granules (Floseal, Baxter International, Deerfield, IL, USA). We then place removable packing, such as Merocel sponges (Medtronic Inc, Minneapolis, USA), superficial to this and ensure the sponges are placed firmly against the repair sight. We have not found biologic glues to be of any added benefit; therefore, we do not use them.

Packing materials remain in situ for 5–7 days and are removed in the office under endoscopic visualization. Patients are encouraged to spray their nose with saline a minimum of three times daily while the packing remains in situ. Once the packing is removed, the patients commence saline irrigations a minimum of three times daily with a high-volume, low-flow device such as an irrigation bottle. In supporting our multilayered skull base reconstruction, we avoid the use of Foley catheters due to the fact that they do not provide even pressure throughout the skull base and nasal cavity and may cause pressure necrosis [60, 61].

29.4 Discussion

The ultimate goal of skull base reconstruction is to separate the cranial cavity from the sinonasal tract, thus preventing ascending infection [62]. Other aims include the elimination of dead space, promotion of wound healing, and preservation of neurovascular and ocular function [16]. In our hands, reconstruction of large skull base defects with free tissue grafts, either autologous or synthetic, is associated with a high incidence of postoperative CSF leaks [17]. Persistent CSF leaks in this scenario are commonly associated with failure to integrate or migration of part of the graft or flap. The latter was more frequent at the point of maximum pressure, the most dependent part, or its superior margin where the graft is most vulnerable to migration [63]. Vascularized flaps were developed to overcome the initial unacceptably high rates of postoperative CSF leaks associated with free tissue graft reconstruction after EEA. Adoption of the posterior pedicle nasoseptal flap leads to a dramatic drop of postoperative CSF leak to rates of less than 5 % [17, 12]. Based on our experience, we strongly advocate the use of vascularized flaps in patients who are at high risk for a postoperative CSF leak. This includes large skull base defects, patients with high intracranial pressure (>30 cm H_2O), patients with a wide opening of the arachnoid cisterns (e.g., meningiomas, craniopharyngiomas), and patients with significant meningo-/meningoencephaloceles and with extensive removal of dura (e.g., esthesioneuroblastomas). We also recommend the use of vascularized flaps when the internal carotid artery (ICA) or other major neurovascular structures are exposed and in patients who had undergone radiation therapy or in whom postoperative radiotherapy is planned.

Obviously, there are several options of vascularized flaps for the reconstruction of skull base defects, and a pertinent dilemma is which of the described 11 vascularized flaps is the best match for different clinical situations (Table 29.1). The posterior pedicle nasoseptal flap is our preferred choice in most situations, as it may be used to reconstruct defects located anywhere from posterior wall of frontal sinus to the lower clivus, and, as in all other intranasal flaps, it does not require to go to a separate site for harvesting. Skull base lesions associated with these defects include skull base meningiomas, craniopharyngiomas, encephaloceles, esthesioneuroblastomas, chordomas, and even large pituitary tumors with suprasellar or anterior extension. A posterior pedicle nasoseptal flap is also useful to cover exposed neurovascular structures such as the internal carotid artery [17, 12].

Donor site morbidity after harvesting the posterior pedicle nasoseptal flap, such as crusting, cacosmia, and anosmia, is often an issue in postoperative care, significantly impacting the quality of life in these patients. Therefore, harvesting of the posterior pedicle nasoseptal flap, for the reconstruction of skull base defects, is usually accompanied by the harvesting of a reverse rotation flap to cover the posterior pedicle nasoseptal flap donor site. This flap is very effective in expediting the nasoseptal remucosalization and thus improving the postoperative quality of life in patients after EEA. If this flap is not available, we use a free mucoperiosteal graft harvested from the middle turbinate.

It should be emphasized, however, that in patients with uncomplicated pituitary adenomas, Rathke's cleft cysts, or other sellar pathologies, a flap is rarely required. Free tissue grafts solve the great majority of CSF leaks associated with surgery of the sella [64, 65]. Nonetheless in our practice, a nasoseptal rescue flap technique plays an important role, preserving the pedicle of the posterior pedicle nasoseptal flap while avoiding its sinonasal morbidity [66].

In patients in whom the posterior pedicle nasoseptal flap is not feasible, we may use one of two lateral nasal wall flaps. The anteriorly based lateral nasal wall flap is ideal for the patients with defects resulting from a transcribiform or transplanum approach. Conversely, the posteriorly based lateral nasal wall flap is excellent for large skull base defects resulting from transcribiform, transplanum, transsellar, transclival, or middle cranial fossa approaches. When dealing with lesser defects of the fovea ethmoidalis, planum sphenoidale, and sella, the middle turbinate flap is an alternative, especially when the other intranasal flaps are not feasible. Endoscopic skull base surgeons should be aware that these techniques require greater experience and skills than the posterior pedicle nasoseptal flap.

When intranasal flaps are not feasible, we refer to extranasal or regional vascularized flaps. In our center, the two most commonly used regional vascularized flaps are the transpterygoid temporoparietal fascia flap and the transfrontal pericranial flap. The transpterygoid temporoparietal fascia flap is ideal for middle and posterior skull base defects, whereas the transfrontal pericranial flap is ideal for anterior skull base defects [13]. A transpterygoid temporoparietal fascia flap is ill suited for anterior skull base defects due to the length required to tunnel the flap through the pterygopalatine fossa. Similarly, the transfrontal pericranial flap is not recommended for posterior defects since it would require sacrifice of the ethmoid sinuses, septum, and possibly olfaction. However, the biggest disadvantage of extranasal flaps is the need for an external approach with potential additional morbidity (i.e., paresthesia of the forehead, paresis of the frontal branch of the facial nerve, alopecia, unsightly scar).

Postoperative management and instructions are equally important after any skull base repair. General principles of postoperative management following skull base surgery include the following:

- A perioperative, intravenous, fourth-generation cephalosporin or a customized antibiotic regimen targeting specific flora (with adequate CSF penetration) is used for 48 h. Oral broad-spectrum antibiotics then continue until the nasal packing is removed.
- A postoperative computed tomography scan is routinely performed within the first 24 h after surgery to rule out the presence of intracranial bleeding, parenchymal injury, or tension pneumocephalus. A contrasted magnetic resonance imaging (MRI) is also performed after oncologic surgery to ascertain the adequacy of

the resection. As a secondary gain, this MRI can also ascertain the adequacy of the reconstruction and the vascularity of the reconstructive flap.

- Nasal packing is removed 5–7 days postoperatively.
- The patient is advised and continually reminded to avoid nasal blowing, to sneeze and cough with an open mouth, and to avoid any activities that may increase intracranial pressure such as abdominal straining, leaning forward, lifting anything heavier than 15 lb, or using tight collars (e.g., turtle neck sweater, tie).
- Provide the patient with stool softeners to avoid constipation.
- Advise patients on how to perform nasal irrigations.
- Postoperative nasal irrigations and frequent outpatient debridements (for at least the first 4 weeks) are imperative to minimize crusting.

Conclusions

A myriad of intranasal pedicled flaps are available to reconstruct skull base defects resulting from EEAs, accidental trauma, or other pathologies. We advocate the use of the posterior pedicle nasoseptal flap for the reconstruction of extensive defects of anterior, middle, and posterior cranial base. Nevertheless, mastering of the skills of extranasal or regional vascularized flaps is fundamental as they may offer reconstructive alternatives, especially when the posterior pedicle nasoseptal flap is not a desirable or available option, when open approaches are needed, or when intranasal vascularized flaps are not available.

References

1. Kassam AB, Gardner P, Snyderman C, Mintz A, Carrau R (2005) Expanded endonasal approach: fully endoscopic, completely transnasal approach to the middle third of the clivus, petrous bone, middle cranial fossa, and infratemporal fossa. Neurosurg Focus 19(1):E6
2. Kassam AB, Snyderman C, Gardner P, Carrau R, Spiro R (2005) The expanded endonasal approach: a fully endoscopic transnasal approach and resection of the odontoid process: technical case report. Neurosurgery 1 Suppl:E213; discussion E213
3. Kassam A, Thomas AJ, Snyderman C, Carrau R, Gardner P, Mintz A, Kanaan H, Horowitz M, Pollack IF (2007) Fully endoscopic expanded endonasal approach treating skull base lesions in pediatric patients. J Neurosurg 106(2 Suppl):75–86. doi:10.3171/ped.2007.106.2.75
4. Briggs RJ, Wormald PJ (2004) Endoscopic transnasal intradural repair of anterior skull base cerebrospinal fluid fistulae. J Clin Neurosci 11(6):597–599. doi:10.1016/j.jocn.2003.09.011
5. Hegazy HM, Carrau RL, Snyderman CH, Kassam A, Zweig J (2000) Transnasal endoscopic repair of cerebrospinal fluid rhinorrhea: a meta-analysis. Laryngoscope 110(7):1166–1172. doi:10.1097/00005537-200007000-00019
6. Zweig JL, Carrau RL, Celin SE, Schaitkin BM, Pollice PA, Snyderman CH, Kassam A, Hegazy H (2000) Endoscopic repair of cerebrospinal fluid leaks to the sinonasal tract: predictors of success. Otolaryngol Head Neck Surg 123(3):195–201. doi:10.1067/mhn.2000.107452
7. Cavallo LM, Messina A, Cappabianca P, Esposito F, de Divitiis E, Gardner P, Tschabitscher M (2005) Endoscopic endonasal surgery of the midline skull base: anatomical study and clinical considerations. Neurosurg Focus 19(1):E2
8. Fortes FS, Carrau RL, Snyderman CH, Kassam A, Prevedello D, Vescan A, Mintz A, Gardner P (2007) Transpterygoid transposition of a temporoparietal fascia flap: a new method for skull base reconstruction after endoscopic expanded endonasal approaches. Laryngoscope 117(6):970–976. doi:10.1097/MLG.0b013e3180471482
9. Fortes FS, Carrau RL, Snyderman CH, Prevedello D, Vescan A, Mintz A, Gardner P, Kassam AB (2007) The posterior pedicle inferior turbinate flap: a new vascularized flap for skull base reconstruction. Laryngoscope 117(8):1329–1332. doi:10.1097/mlg.0b013e318062111f
10. Gardner PA, Kassam AB, Thomas A, Snyderman CH, Carrau RL, Mintz AH, Prevedello DM (2008) Endoscopic endonasal resection of anterior cranial base meningiomas. Neurosurgery 63(1):36–52. doi:10.1227/01.NEU.0000335069.30319.1E; discussion 52–54
11. Harvey RJ, Parmar P, Sacks R, Zanation AM (2012) Endoscopic skull base reconstruction of large dural defects: a systematic review of published evidence. Laryngoscope 122(2):452–459. doi:10.1002/lary.22475
12. Kassam AB, Thomas A, Carrau RL, Snyderman CH, Vescan A, Prevedello D, Mintz A, Gardner P (2008) Endoscopic reconstruction of the cranial base using a pedicled nasoseptal flap. Neurosurgery 63(1 Suppl 1):ONS44–ONS52. doi:10.1227/01.neu.0000335010.53122.75; discussion ONS52–53
13. Snyderman CH, Janecka IP, Sekhar LN, Sen CN, Eibling DE (1990) Anterior cranial base

reconstruction: role of galeal and pericranial flaps. Laryngoscope 100(6):607–614. doi:10.1288/00005537-199006000-00011
14. Patel MR, Taylor RJ, Hackman TG, Germanwala AV, Sasaki-Adams D, Ewend MG, Zanation AM (2014) Beyond the nasoseptal flap: outcomes and pearls with secondary flaps in endoscopic endonasal skull base reconstruction. Laryngoscope 124(4):846–852. doi:10.1002/lary.24319
15. Leng LZ, Brown S, Anand VK, Schwartz TH (2008) "Gasket-seal" watertight closure in minimal-access endoscopic cranial base surgery. Neurosurgery 62(5 Suppl 2):ONSE342–ONSE343. doi:10.1227/01.neu.0000326017.84315.1f; discussion ONSE343
16. Germani RM, Vivero R, Herzallah IR, Casiano RR (2007) Endoscopic reconstruction of large anterior skull base defects using acellular dermal allograft. Am J Rhinol 21(5):615–618. doi:10.2500/ajr.2007.21.3080
17. Hadad G, Bassagasteguy L, Carrau RL, Mataza JC, Kassam A, Snyderman CH, Mintz A (2006) A novel reconstructive technique after endoscopic expanded endonasal approaches: vascular pedicle nasoseptal flap. Laryngoscope 116(10):1882–1886. doi:10.1097/01.mlg.0000234933.37779.e4
18. Pinheiro-Neto CD, Prevedello DM, Carrau RL, Snyderman CH, Mintz A, Gardner P, Kassam A (2007) Improving the design of the pedicled nasoseptal flap for skull base reconstruction: a radioanatomic study. Laryngoscope 117(9):1560–1569. doi:10.1097/MLG.0b013e31806db514
19. Shah RN, Surowitz JB, Patel MR, Huang BY, Snyderman CH, Carrau RL, Kassam AB, Germanwala AV, Zanation AM (2009) Endoscopic pedicled nasoseptal flap reconstruction for pediatric skull base defects. Laryngoscope 119(6):1067–1075. doi:10.1002/lary.20216
20. Zhang X, Wang EW, Wei H, Shi J, Snyderman CH, Gardner PA, Fernandez-Miranda JC (2014) Anatomy of the posterior septal artery with surgical implications on the vascularized pedicled nasoseptal flap. Head Neck. doi:10.1002/hed.23775
21. Pinheiro-Neto CD, Ramos HF, Peris-Celda M, Fernandez-Miranda JC, Gardner PA, Snyderman CH, Sennes LU (2011) Study of the nasoseptal flap for endoscopic anterior cranial base reconstruction. Laryngoscope 121(12):2514–2520. doi:10.1002/lary.22353
22. Peris-Celda M, Pinheiro-Neto CD, Funaki T, Fernandez-Miranda JC, Gardner P, Snyderman C, Rhoton AL (2013) The extended nasoseptal flap for skull base reconstruction of the clival region: an anatomical and radiological study. J Neurol Surg B Skull Base 74(6):369–385. doi:10.1055/s-0033-1347368
23. Pinheiro-Neto C, Snyderman C (2013) Nasoseptal flap. In: Bleier B (ed) Comprehensive techniques in CSF leak repair and skull base reconstruction, vol 74, Advances in otorhinolaryngol. Karger, Basel, pp 42–55
24. Caicedo-Granados E, Carrau R, Snyderman CH, Prevedello D, Fernandez-Miranda J, Gardner P, Kassam A (2010) Reverse rotation flap for reconstruction of donor site after vascular pedicled nasoseptal flap in skull base surgery. Laryngoscope 120(8):1550–1552. doi:10.1002/lary.20975
25. Kasemsiri P, Carrau RL, Otto BA, Tang IP, Prevedello DM, Muto J, Caicedo E (2013) Reconstruction of the pedicled nasoseptal flap donor site with a contralateral reverse rotation flap: technical modifications and outcomes. Laryngoscope 123(11):2601–2604. doi:10.1002/lary.24088
26. Padgham N, Vaughan-Jones R (1991) Cadaver studies of the anatomy of arterial supply to the inferior turbinates. J R Soc Med 84(12):728–730
27. Hadar T, Ophir D, Yaniv E, Berger G (2005) Inferior turbinate arterial supply: histologic analysis and clinical implications. J Otolaryngol 34(1):46–50
28. Murakami CS, Kriet JD, Ierokomos AP (1999) Nasal reconstruction using the inferior turbinate mucosal flap. Arch Facial Plast Surg 1(2):97–100
29. Navarro J (2001) The nasal cavity and paranasal sinuses: surgical anatomy. Springer, Berlin
30. Harvey RJ, Sheahan PO, Schlosser RJ (2009) Inferior turbinate pedicle flap for endoscopic skull base defect repair. Am J Rhinol Allergy 23(5):522–526. doi:10.2500/ajra.2009.23.3354
31. Chiu T (2009) A study of the maxillary and sphenopalatine arteries in the pterygopalatine fossa and at the sphenopalatine foramen. Rhinology 47(3):264–270
32. Schwartzbauer HR, Shete M, Tami TA (2003) Endoscopic anatomy of the sphenopalatine and posterior nasal arteries: implications for the endoscopic management of epistaxis. Am J Rhinol 17(1):63–66
33. Patel MR, Stadler ME, Snyderman CH, Carrau RL, Kassam AB, Germanwala AV, Gardner P, Zanation AM (2010) How to choose? Endoscopic skull base reconstructive options and limitations. Skull Base 20(6):397–404. doi:10.1055/s-0030-1253573
34. Prevedello DM, Barges-Coll J, Fernandez-Miranda JC, Morera V, Jacobson D, Madhok R, dos Santos MC, Zanation A, Snyderman CH, Gardner P, Kassam AB, Carrau R (2009) Middle turbinate flap for skull base reconstruction: cadaveric feasibility study. Laryngoscope 119(11):2094–2098. doi:10.1002/lary.20226
35. Kim G, Hang A, Mitchell C, Zanation A (2013) Pedicled extranasal flaps in skull base reconstruction. In: Comprehensive techniques in CSF leak repair and skull base reconstruction, vol 74, Advances in otorhinolaryngol. Karger, Basel, pp 71–80
36. Hadad G, Rivera-Serrano CM, Bassagaisteguy LH, Carrau RL, Fernandez-Miranda J, Prevedello DM, Kassam AB (2011) Anterior pedicle lateral nasal wall flap: a novel technique for the reconstruction of anterior skull base defects. Laryngoscope 121(8):1606–1610. doi:10.1002/lary.21889
37. Rivera-Serrano CM, Bassagaisteguy LH, Hadad G, Carrau RL, Kelly D, Prevedello DM,

Fernandez-Miranda J, Kassam AB (2011) Posterior pedicle lateral nasal wall flap: new reconstructive technique for large defects of the skull base. Am J Rhinol Allergy 25(6):e212–e216. doi:10.2500/ajra.2011.25.3693
38. Price JC, Loury M, Carson B, Johns ME (1988) The pericranial flap for reconstruction of anterior skull base defects. Laryngoscope 98(11):1159–1164. doi:10.1288/00005537-198811000-00002
39. Smith JE, Ducic Y (2004) The versatile extended pericranial flap for closure of skull base defects. Otolaryngol Head Neck Surg 130(6):704–711. doi:10.1016/j.otohns.2004.01.004
40. Yoshioka N, Rhoton AL Jr (2005) Vascular anatomy of the anteriorly based pericranial flap. Neurosurgery 57(1 Suppl):11–16; discussion 11–16
41. McMinn R (2005) Last's anatomy: regional and applied, 9th edn. Churchill Livingstone, London
42. Ashwini LS, Mohandas Rao KG, Saran S, Somayaji SN (2012) Morphological and morphometric analysis of supraorbital foramen and supraorbital notch: a study on dry human skulls. Oman Med J 27(2):129–133. doi:10.5001/omj.2012.27
43. Patel MR, Shah RN, Snyderman CH, Carrau RL, Germanwala AV, Kassam AB, Zanation AM (2010) Pericranial flap for endoscopic anterior skull-base reconstruction: clinical outcomes and radioanatomic analysis of preoperative planning. Neurosurgery 66(3):506–512. doi:10.1227/01.NEU.0000365620.59677.FF; discussion 512
44. David SK, Cheney ML (1995) An anatomic study of the temporoparietal fascial flap. Arch Otolaryngol Head Neck Surg 121(10):1153–1156
45. Bhatki A, Pant H, Snyderman C, Carrau R, Kassam A, Prevedello D, Gardner P (2010) Reconstruction of the cranial base following endonasal skull base surgery: regional tissue flaps. Oper Tech Otolaryngol Head Neck Surg 21:83–90
46. Larrabee WJ, Makielski K (1993) Surgical anatomy of the face. Raven, New York
47. Cavallo LM, Messina A, Gardner P, Esposito F, Kassam AB, Cappabianca P, de Divitiis E, Tschabitscher M (2005) Extended endoscopic endonasal approach to the pterygopalatine fossa: anatomical study and clinical considerations. Neurosurg Focus 19(1):E5
48. Rivera-Serrano CM, Snyderman CH, Carrau RL, Durmaz A, Gardner PA (2011) Transparapharyngeal and transpterygoid transposition of a pedicled occipital galeopericranial flap: a new flap for skull base reconstruction. Laryngoscope 121(5):914–922. doi:10.1002/lary.21376
49. Xie L, Lavigne F, Rahal A, Moubayed SP, Ayad T (2013) Facial artery musculomucosal flap for reconstruction of skull base defects: a cadaveric study. Laryngoscope 123(8):1854–1861. doi:10.1002/lary.23939
50. Dupoirieux L, Plane L, Gard C, Penneau M (1999) Anatomical basis and results of the facial artery musculomucosal flap for oral reconstruction. Br J Oral Maxillofac Surg 37(1):25–28. doi:10.1054/bjom.1998.0301
51. Rivera-Serrano CM, Oliver CL, Sok J, Prevedello DM, Gardner P, Snyderman CH, Kassam AB, Carrau RL (2010) Pedicled facial buccinator (FAB) flap: a new flap for reconstruction of skull base defects. Laryngoscope 120(10):1922–1930. doi:10.1002/lary.21049
52. Oliver CL, Hackman TG, Carrau RL, Snyderman CH, Kassam AB, Prevedello DM, Gardner P (2008) Palatal flap modifications allow pedicled reconstruction of the skull base. Laryngoscope 118(12):2102–2106. doi:10.1097/MLG.0b013e318184e719
53. Millard D (1962) Wide and or short cleft palate. Plast Reconstr Surg 29:40–57
54. Hackman T, Chicoine MR, Uppaluri R (2009) Novel application of the palatal island flap for endoscopic skull base reconstruction. Laryngoscope 119(8):1463–1466. doi:10.1002/lary.20298
55. Kirschner RE, Cabiling DS, Slemp AE, Siddiqi F, LaRossa DD, Losee JE (2006) Repair of oronasal fistulae with acellular dermal matrices. Plast Reconstr Surg 118(6):1431–1440. doi:10.1097/01.prs.0000239612.35581.c3
56. Genden EM, Lee BB, Urken ML (2001) The palatal island flap for reconstruction of palatal and retromolar trigone defects revisited. Arch Otolaryngol Head Neck Surg 127(7):837–841
57. Balbuena L, Stambaugh KI, Ramirez SG, Yeager C (1998) Effects of topical oral antiseptic rinses on bacterial counts of saliva in healthy human subjects. Otolaryngol Head Neck Surg 118(5):625–629
58. Gullane PJ, Arena S (1985) Extended palatal island mucoperiosteal flap. Arch Otolaryngol 111(5):330–332
59. Maher WP (1977) Distribution of palatal and other arteries in cleft and non-cleft human palates. Cleft Palate J 14(1):1–12
60. Klinger M, Siegert R (1997) Microcirculation of the nasal mucosa during use of balloon tamponade. Laryngorhinootologie 76(3):127–130. doi:10.1055/s-2007-997400
61. Weber R, Keerl R, Hochapfel F, Draf W, Toffel PH (2001) Packing in endonasal surgery. Am J Otolaryngol 22(5):306–320. doi:10.1053/ajot.2001.26499
62. Seiler RW, Mariani L (2000) Sellar reconstruction with resorbable vicryl patches, gelatin foam, and fibrin glue in transsphenoidal surgery: a 10-year experience with 376 patients. J Neurosurg 93(5):762–765. doi:10.3171/jns.2000.93.5.0762
63. Zanation AM, Thorp BD, Parmar P, Harvey RJ (2011) Reconstructive options for endoscopic skull base surgery. Otolaryngol Clin North Am 44(5):1201–1222. doi:10.1016/j.otc.2011.06.016
64. Cappabianca P, Cavallo LM, Esposito F, Valente V, De Divitiis E (2002) Sellar repair in endoscopic endonasal transsphenoidal surgery: results of 170 cases. Neurosurgery 51(6):1365–1371; discussion 1371–1372

65. Cappabianca P, Cavallo LM, Valente V, Romano I, D'Enza AI, Esposito F, de Divitiis E (2004) Sellar repair with fibrin sealant and collagen fleece after endoscopic endonasal transsphenoidal surgery. Surg Neurol 62(3):227–233. doi:10.1016/j.surneu.2004.01.016; discussion 233
66. Rivera-Serrano CM, Snyderman CH, Gardner P, Prevedello D, Wheless S, Kassam AB, Carrau RL, Germanwala A, Zanation A (2011) Nasoseptal "rescue" flap: a novel modification of the nasoseptal flap technique for pituitary surgery. Laryngoscope 121(5):990–993. doi:10.1002/lary.21419
67. Neligan PC, Rodriguez ED, Losee JE (2012) Plastic surgery, vol 3, Craniofacial, head and neck surgery pediatric plastic surgery. Elsevier, Oxford

Index

A
Abdominal free fat, 340
Abducens nerve, 15, 284, 304
Abuhusain, H.J., 223–234
Acromegaly, 4, 53
ACTH pituitary adenomas, 12
Adamantinomatous craniopharyngiomas, 124
Adler, J.R., 275
Aggressive adjuvant radiotherapy, 301
Al-Mefty classification, 211
Al-Mefty, O., 237
Angileri, F.F., 155–161
Angiography, 39
Anterior clinoid process, 132
Anterior commissure, 126
Anterior communicating artery complex, 121
Anterior cranial fossa, 211
  anatomy of, 240
Anterior cranial fossa meningiomas
  attachement site, 212
  diaphragma sellae meningiomas, 211
  olfactory groove, 211
  operating microscope, 212
  planum sphenoidale, 211
  space-occupying lesions, 212
  tuberculum sellae, 211
  visual impairment, 212
Anterior pituitary insifufficency, 116
Anterior skull base (ASB)
  dorsal, 237
  meningiomas, 269
  ventral, 237
Apparent diffuse coefficient (ADC), 41
Arachnoid cysts, 179
  base of brain, located at, 201
  cranio-vertebral region, 205
  size reduction, 186
Arachnoid diverticulum, 173
Asymptomatic, incidentally discovered cysts, 179

B
Babinski, J., 62
Barbaro, N., 271
Barkhoudarian, G., 137–152
Barrande, G., 52
Barret, J.O., 61
Basilar plexus, 309
Bassagasteguy, L.H., 298, 336
Bath-plug technique, 335
Beadles, C., 61
Beta-catenin, 62
Biermasz, N.R., 52
Bilateral inferior petrosal sinus sampling (BIPSS), 4
Bilateral posterior pedicle nasoseptal flap, 338
Binostril approach, 306
Biologic glue, 340
Bi-pedicled flap, 342
Biroli, A., 89–96
Bitemporal hemianopia, 4
Bolster, 357
Boyce, R., 61
Brada, M., 52
Brain retraction, 289
Brainstem, 290
Breen, P., 52
Brell, M., 271
Bresson, D., 301–311
Bridging vein, 158
Briganti, F., 69–87
Broca's motor speech area, 126
Brunetti, A., 61–65
Brunori, A., 105–111
Buccinator flap
  anatomy
    dilator muscles, 354
    infraorbital, dorsal nasal and ophthalmic arteries, 354
  "boot" or "L" shape, 354
  flap tunneling, 354–355
  wide arc of rotation, 353
Buglione, M., 271

C
Caggiano, C., 289–298
Caicedo, E., 341
Califano, G., 211–213
Campbell, R.G., 333–359
Capone, C., 121–134

P. Cappabianca et al. (eds.), *Midline Skull Base Surgery*, DOI 10.1007/978-3-319-21533-4

Cappabianca, P., 3–7, 11–31, 61–65, 69–87, 121–134, 283–285, 289–298
Caranci, F., 11–31
Carbon ion radiotherapy
  nerve neuropathy, 327
  skull base chordomas, 327
Carcinomas, 36
Carella, R., 271
Carotid arteries, 290
Carotid canal unroofing, 308
Carotid cisterns, 145
Carotid-oculomotor windows, 141
Carrau-Hadad (C-H) flap, 347–348
  lacrimal bone, 347
  mucoperiosteum, 348
  nasolacrimal duct, 347
  posteriorly based lateral nasal wall flap, 347
Carrau, R.L., 6, 70, 216, 333–359
Cascone, D., 179–198
Castinetti, F., 54
Catapano, G., 237–251
Cavallo, L.M., 11–31, 69–87, 289–298
Cavernous segment, ICA, 304
Cavernous sinus (CS), 14, 35
Cerebral radionecrosis, 270
Cerebrospinal fluid (CSF), 183, 201, 215, 230, 245
  accumulations, 265
  egress, 145
  leak, 177, 333
  rhinorrhea, 147
Chiaramonte, C., 211–213
Chibbaro, S., 301–311, 313–320
Choana, 13
Choi, J.W., 180, 184
Cholesterol crystals, 89
Chondroid, 283
Chondromas, 292
Chondrosarcomas, 36, 292
  low-grade, 284
Chordoid meningiomas, 284
Chordomas, 36, 283, 301, 323
  carbon ion radiotherapy, 327
  conventional chordoma, 283
  extradural, 285
  fractionated radiotherapy, 323–324
  malignant chordomas, 284
  neuronavigation system, 285
  proton beam treatment, 285
  skull base, 285
  skull base tumor, 311
  stereotactic radiosurgery, 324–326
  surgery, 290
  transfacial, 285
  transoral, 285
Choroidal fissure, 157
Choudhri, O., 184
Chung, W.Y., 166
Cinalli, G., 179–198
Circle of Willis, 132
Circumferential devascularization, 217
Clival chordomas, 289
  anatomy, 293–295
  indications, 289–290
  radiology, 290–293
  surgical approach
    inferior third, 297
    middle third, 296–297
    reconstruction, 297–298
    superior third, 296
Clival recess, 304
Clivus, 283
  inferior third, 295
  middle third, 294–295
  upper third, 294
Clivus and craniocervical junction
  stability, 320
  ventral, 320
Colin, P., 52, 53
Colombo, F., 272, 273, 275
Combined endoscopic-microsurgical procedure, 103
Combined transcranial/endonasal procedure, 248
Combs, S.E., 164, 165, 271
Condra, K., 271
Conformal radiotherapy, 50
Connell, P., 270, 271
Conservative management, 204
Conti, A., 269–276
Contiguous CSF pathway, 179
Contrast enhancement, 38
Conventional external beam radiotherapy, 50
Conventionally fractionated radiotherapy
  cerebral radionecrosis, 270
  hypopituitarism, 270
  meningiomas, 270
  standard fractionation scheme, 270
Conventional radiotherapy
  craniopharyngiomas, 164
  external beam, 163
  irradiation and timing, 164
  progression-free survival, 163
Corpus callosum, 127
Corsten, M., 215–220
Cosmetic closure, 152
Cranial nerves, 218
  monitoring, 142, 306
Craniocervical junction (CCJ), 302
  disorders, 320
  lateral aspect, 310–311
Craniopharyngeal duct, 121
Craniopharyngioma cyst, 150
Craniopharyngiomas (CPs), 61, 89, 110, 121, 141
  adamantinomatous, 62, 90
  adjuvant therapies, 95–96
  classifications, 62–63
  cyst drainage, 65
  debulking, 159
  dissection, 159
  equipment, 91

fronto-temporal approach, 63
hypothalamic derangement, 64
indications, 90–91
intraventricular, 62
median midline location, 64
modern treatment targets, 65
neuroimaging, 64
origination, 62
papillary, 62
pathology, 90
postoperative management, 94–95
prechiasmatic, 62
radiology, 90
results, 95
retrochiasmatic, 62
subchiasmatic, 62
surgical approach, 91–94
symptoms, 90
third ventricle, 155
Craniotome, 130
Crista galli, 241
CSF. *See* Cerebrospinal fluid (CSF)
CT angiography, 39, 305
CT-cystography, 102
Cushing, H., 6, 63, 211, 212, 227, 237, 238
Cushing's disease, 4, 51, 53, 55
CyberKnife (CK), 165, 166
Cyst(s)
cisternostomy, 186, 192
communication, 179
of craniovertebral junction, 203–204
drainage, 65, 115, 175, 176
fenestration, 175
interpeduncular, 201
intrasellar, 201
marsupialization, 100
membrane, 176
recurrence, 115
retroclival, 203
shunting, 191
suprasellar, 201
Cystic craniopharyngiomas, 105
Cystosphenoidostomy, 105–109, 111
endoscopic transsphenoidal approach., 107
microsurgical, 107
Cysto-ventriculo-cisternostomy, 65, 105, 106, 111
Cystoventriculostomy, 100, 110, 192
Cyst-peritoneal shunt, 204

D

D'Amico, A., 283–285
Dandy's keyhole, 249
Dandy's point, 243
Dandy, W.E., 6, 212
3D CISS sequences, 303
de Angelis, M., 11–31, 89–96
de Divitiis, E., 110
de Divitiis, O., 121–134, 211–213
de Notaris, M., 237–251
Debulking, 81, 132
Debus, J., 271
Decq, P., 185
Del Basso De Caro, M., 3–7, 61–65, 283–285
Delitala, A., 105–111
3-D endoscopes, 91
Derome, P., 64, 69
Devin, J.K., 54
Di Lorenzo, P., 121–134
Di Martino, G., 179–198
Di Nuzzo, G., 237–251
Di Rocco, F., 180, 183, 184
Di Somma, A., 69–87
Diabetes insipidus (DI), 90, 95, 174
Diaphragma, 93
Diaphragma sellae, 13, 70, 242
Diaphragmatic defect, 177
DiBiase, S., 275
Differential diagnosis, 292
Diffusion-weighted imaging (DWI), 41, 122
Distal dural ring, 13
Donor site morbidity, 358
Dopamine-agonist drugs, 5
Dorello's canal, 294, 305
Dorsum sellae, 309
Dorward, N.L., 89–96
Double surgical corridor
extracapsular, 12
intracapsular, 12
Draf 3, 218
Dufour, H., 271
Dural attachment, 213
Durante, F., 211
Dynamic sequences, 5
Dysphagia, 317

E

Ecchordosis physaliphora, 284
Egyptian technique, 6
Eiselsberg, A., 6
Elefante, A., 121–134
El-Ghandour, N.M., 184
Elhammady, M.S., 184
Endonasal approach, 254
palatal island flap, 357
pterygopalatine canal, 357
pterygopalatine fossa, 356
submucoperiosteal elevation, 357
Endoscope, 6, 253
0-degree, 175
wide anatomic view, 12
Endoscopic-assisted techniques, 247–248
Endoscopic cyst decompression, 102
Endoscopic endonasal approach, 35, 64, 70, 116, 295
anatomy, 72–76
neuroradiology, 70–72
post-operative management, 84–87
reconstruction techniques, 82–84

Endoscopic endonasal odontoidectomy
  atlanto-axial dislocation, 313
  basilar impression, 313
  indication
    C1-C2 junction, 314
    dens, 314
    odontoid resection, 314
  surgical technique
    navigation, 314
    odontoid process, 315
    reconstruction, 316
  variations, technical
    anterior arch of C1, 316
    posterior fixation, 317
    subaxial instability, 317
Endoscopic fenestration, 204
Endoscopic third ventriculostomy (ETV), 195
Enseñat, J., 237–251
ENT steps, 307
Epaminonda, P., 52
Epidermoids, 122
Erdheim, J., 61
Esposito, F., 113–118, 173–177
Estrada, J., 51, 52
Ethmoido-pterygo-sphenoidal (EPS), 35
Etus, V., 184
Eustachian tube, 308, 310
Expanded endonasal approach (EEA), 215, 290, 302
  advantages, 317
  alternative way, 311
  anatomy, 216
  buccinators, 216
  lateral nasal wall, 216
  meningiomas, 217
  pedicled pericranial flaps, 216
  skull base, 215
  skull base reconstruction, 216
  temporoparietal flaps, 216
  tumor relative to cranial nerves, 217
  turbinate flaps, 216
Extended approaches, 7, 29–31
Extended, suprasellar area, 69
Extended transsphenoidal method, 89
"Extended" variation, 12
External beam radiotherapy (EBRT), 49, 269, 323
  toxicity of, 51
Extranasal flaps, 348
  frontal and temporal scalp, anatomy, 348
Extranasal/regional vascularized flaps, 359

F

Facial artery buccinator-FAB-flap, 353
Facial artery myomucosal (FAMM), 353
  migration, gravitational pull, 353
Facial nerve
  frontalis branch, 147
  frontalis muscle branch, 144
  frontotemporal branch, 255
  temporal branch, 226
Falciform ligament, 262
Falx cerebri, 249
  inferior sagittal sinuses, 241
  superior sagittal sinuses, 241
Far medial approach, 219
Fast imaging employing steady state acquisition (FIESTA), 40
Fat pad, 126
Fenestration, 133
FIESTA sequences, 303
Fish-hooks, 130
Fitzek, M.M., 167
Flaps, muscle
  latissimus dorsi, 336
  pectoralis major, 336
  sternocleidomastoid, 336
  temporalis, 336
  trapezius, 336
Flap tunneling, 354–355
Flickinger, J.C., 164
Flow artifact, 183
Fokas, E., 271
Foramen magnum, 219
Foraminoplasty, 100–101
Forbes, A., 271
Fornix, 126, 157
Fractionated radiotherapy (fXRT), 94, 323–324
Fractionated stereotactic radiotherapy (FSRT), 53, 55, 163, 270–271, 323
Frank, G., 35–47
Franzin, A., 54
Frazier, C.H., 238
Free abdominal fat, 335
Free microvascular flaps, 336
Friedman, W.A., 273
Frio, F., 69–87
Fritzek, M.M., 164
Froelich, S., 301–311
Frohlich, A., 62
Frontal branch, 126
Frontal fossa, SO approach, 146
Frontal sinus, 256
Frontal sinus pneumatization
  extent, 139
  size, 139
Frontal skullbase, 253
Frontobasal cortex, 259
Frontotemporal approach
  anatomy, 125–128
  indications, 121
  neuroradiology, 122–125
  surgical technique, 128–134
Fronto-zygomatic process, 125

G

Gaillard, S., 313–320
Galea aponeurotica, 125
Gamma knife (GK), 50, 272, 325
Gangemi, M., 99–103

Ganz, J., 274
Gasket seal closure technique, 335
Gerardi, R.M., 289–298
Germinomas, 122
GH receptor antagonists, 6
GH-secreting pituitary adenomas, 55
Giannetti, A.V., 192
Giant cystic craniopharyngioma, 103
Giordano, D., 6
Gittoes, N.J., 52
Gliomas, 52
Goldberg, I., 271
Goldsmith, B., 270, 271
Goumnerova, L., 186
Gowers, W., 212
Granata, F., 155–161
Granata, R., 237–251
Greater sphenoidal wing, 132
Grigsby, G.W., 52
Growth hormone (GH), 51, 53
Growth hormone secreting lesions, 11
Guiot, G., 64, 69
Guthrie, 213
Gutin, P.H., 110

H
Habrand, J.L., 164
Hadad-Bassagaisteguy 2 flap, 334, 345–346
  facial artery, 346
  middle turbinate, 346
  nasolacrimal duct, 346
  posterolateral nasal artery, 346
  sphenopalatine neurovascular bundle, 346
Hadad, G., 31, 298, 336
Hajek, M., 6
Half-moon shaped bone flap, 145
Halstead, A.E., 6, 63
Hamm, K., 271
Hardy, J., 6
Harrabi, S.B., 164
Hasegawa, T., 273
Hashizume, C., 164
Hemostasis, 320
Henzel, M., 271
Herman, P., 301–311
Hetelekidis, S., 164
Heuer, G.J., 6
High field MRI, 38
High-flow CSF leaks, 334
Hirsch, O., 6
Horsley, V., 6, 212
Hydrocephalus, 158
Hyperostosis, 238
Hyperostotic bone, 246
Hyperprolactinemia, 4
Hypofractionated radiosurgery, 276
Hypofractionated stereotactic radiotherapy (HSRT), 325
Hypoglossal canal, 311
Hypoglossal nerves, 290
Hyponatremia, 116
Hypopituitarism, 4, 53
Hypothalamic derangement, 64
Hypothalamic injuries, 65
Hypothalamus, 155, 157

I
Image-guided radiotherapy (IGRT), 270
Image-guided robotic radiosurgery system (Cyberknife), 55
Immunohistochemical reactions, 5
IMRT/proton beam therapy, 95
Indication, endocrine dysfunction, 5
Inferior hypophyseal artery, 14
Inferior turbinate flap
  dominant blood, 343
  inferior turbinate branch, 343
  ipsilateral sphenopalatine artery ligation, 343
  nasolacrimal duct, 343
  submucoperiosteal elevation, 343
Infrapetrous extension, 297
Infundibulum displacement, 148
Intensity-modulated radiation therapy (IMRT), 50, 272, 323
Interforniceal approach, 159
Interhemispheric arachnoid cysts
  aqueduct obstruction, 187
  corpus callosum, absence of, 191
  cyst-cisternostomy, 192
  cyst-ventriculostomy, 192
  lumboperitoneal shunt, 192
  Mori classification, 190
Interhemispheric fissure, 157, 158
Internal carotid artery (ICA), 46
Interpeduncular cysts, 201
Intracavernous ICA aneurism, 39
Intracavitary chemotherapy, 102
Intracavitary radiotherapy
  intracavitary RT, 166
  phosphorus-32, 166
  Yttrium-90, 166
Intracranial tumors, 65
Intracystic chemotherapy, 96
Intrasellar cysts, 201
Intraventricular craniopharyngiomas, 99
Invasive variant, 63
Ipsilateral frontal fossa, 141
Iwai, Y., 54
Iwata, H., 55, 166

J
Jagannathan, J., 54
Jalali, R., 271
Jezkova, J., 54
Jho, H.D., 6
Jugular foramen, 295

K
Kalani, M.Y.S., 223–234
Kanavel, A.B., 6
Kanesaka, N., 164
Karabagli, H., 183, 184
Kassam, A., 63, 70, 215–220, 296
Kaul, D., 271
Kelly, D.F., 137–152
Kennedy, R.F., 212
Key-hole approaches, 204
Keyhole paradigm, 228
K_i-67 labeling index, 211
Kilian, G., 6
Kim, J.O., 52
Kirollos, R.W., 186
Knosp, E., 19, 39
Kobayashi, T., 165, 166
Kocher, T., 6
Koechlin, N.O., 223–234
Kollovà, A., 273
Kondziolka, D., 272, 273, 275
Kong, D.S., 52
Krause, F., 238
Kreil, W., 273

L
Lamina terminalis, 121, 241
Lateral compartment, 45
Lateral optocarotid recess, 13
Lee, M., 166
Left middle turbinate, resection of, 307
Leksell, 96
Levy, M.L., 184
Lewis, D., 63
Liden, 96
Liliequist membrane, 294
Linac SRS, 50
Liscak, V., 54
Liu, X., 54
Liu, Y., 242
Lo, S., 271
Long-term complications, 327
Long-term effectiveness, radiation, 51
Losa, M., 54
Low-profile micro-instrumentation, 143
Luglietto, D., 11–31
Lumboperitoneal shunt, 192
Luu, Q.T., 164

M
MacEwen, W., 211
Macroadenomas, 3, 293
Maffei, L., 69–87
Magnetic resonance imaging (MRI), 16, 38, 49, 70, 122, 156, 212, 225, 238, 284
Maguire, P., 271
Maher, C.O., 186
Maire, J., 271
Maiuri, F., 201–206
Malar eminence, 128
Malik, I., 273
Mammillary body angle (MBA), 156
Mark, R.J., 164
Marruzzo, D., 105–111
Marsupialization, 100, 175
Mass effect, 4
Masson-Cote, L., 164
Mayfield-Kees pin headrest, 128
Mc Arthur, L., 238
McCollough, W.M., 52
McLaughlin, N., 173
Meckel's cave, 219
Medial compartment, CS, 44
Medial optocarotid recess, 13
Medial sphenoid wing meningiomas, 265
Median skull base, 333
Medical and surgical treatment, failure of, 5
Melloni, I., 105–111
Mendenhall, W., 271
Meningiomas, 36, 52, 293
Meningitis, 320
Merchant, T.E., 164
Metastasis, 36, 301
Metellus, P., 271, 274
Meyer, F.B., 173
Microadenomas, 3
Micro-Doppler, 47
Microsurgical approach, 204
Microsurgical removal, 102
Middle fossa
  CSF diversion procedure, 184
  cyst-cisternostomy, 183
  cyst disappearance, 183
  cyst-peritoneal shunt, 184
  endoscopic fenestration, 181
  flow artifact, 183
  "functional" symptoms, 180
  microsurgical fenestration, 181
  pulsation through fenestration, 183
  repeat endoscopy, 184
  SPECT evaluation, 181
  Sylvian fissure, 181
  Tulium LASER coagulation, 183
Middle turbinate flap
  middle turbinate mucoperiosteum, 344
  mucoperiosteum, 344
  sphenopalatine artery, 344
  sphenopalatine foramen, 345
Miles, J., 110
Milker-Zabel, S., 53, 271, 272
Mingione, V., 54
Minimally invasive, 320
Minimally invasive keyhole technique, 152
Mini pterional approach, 213
Mini-pterional approach
  anterior cranial fossa meningiomas, 223
    anatomy, 225–228
    indications, 223–224

neuroimaging, 224–225
sugical technique, 228–234
Minniti, G., 49–55, 163–167, 270, 271, 323–327
Miralbell, R., 271
Mirone, G., 179–198
Miyajima, M., 185
Monolateral ethmoidectomy, 46
Moon, S.H., 164
Mori classification, 190
Mori, K., 190
Motor oil, 62
Mott, F.W., 61
MR spectroscopy (MRS), 122
Mucin-secreting goblet cells, 113
Mucocutaneous junction, 339
Mucoperichondrium and mucoperiosteum, 338, 340
Mucoperiosteal graft, 358
Muller, H.L., 63
Multidisciplinary approach, 5
Multi-fraction SRS, 325
Multilayer technique, 297, 334
Multilobulated cystic craniopharyngioma, 151
Multiple cystic components, 145
Multiple techniques
inlay, 334
onlay, 334
Murphy, 126
Myriad, 217

N
N-acetylaspartate, 122
Nakamura, M., 237
Nasal cavity, endoscope
nasal septum, 13
nasal turbinates, 13
Nasal irrigations, 359
Nasal packing, 359
Nasopharyngeal malignancies, 293
Nasopharynx, 297, 310, 340
Nasoseptal flap (NSF), 216, 305
harvesting, 308
pedicle, 307
Navigation system, 306
Neuroendoscopic approach, 111
Neuroendoscopic management, 110
Neuroendoscopy
advantage, 179
procedure, 106
Neuroimaging, 16–22
Neurological function, preservation of, 302
Neuronavigation, 42, 143, 158
Neuro-navigation system, 314
Nicolato, A., 102, 273, 275
Niola, M., 289–298
Niranjan, A., 166
Noel, G., 271, 272
Non-strictly IVC, 100
Normal positioning, 74
Normo-fixed variant, 128
Notochordal tissue, 283
Nutting, C., 271

O
Occipital condyles, 285
Occipital galeopericranial flap, 353
Oculomotor nerve, 15
Ogunbameru, I., 137–152
Olfactory groove meningiomas, 218, 241, 260–261
Olfactory nerves, 132, 241
Oliver pedicled palatal flap, 355–357
endonasal approach, 356–357
palatine artery, 356
transoral approach, 356
Ommaya reservoirs, 102
One nostril/binostril approach, 306
Open transoral, 317
Optic canal invasion, 224
Optic cisterns, 145
Opticocarotid cisterns, 145
Optico-carotid windows, 141
Orbital apex, 132
Orbito-temporal periosteal fold (OTPF), 131
Orbitozygomatic craniotomy, 142
OsiriX software, 239
Otto, B.A., 333–359

P
Paek, S.H., 52
Palatine bone/maxilla, 339
Pan, L., 54
Pannullo, S.C., 273
Papillary type, 90
Paraclival segment, ICA, 305
Parasellar regions, 89
Park, K.J., 54
Pascual, J.M., 100
Pasquini, E., 35–47
Patil, C.G., 273
Patwa, H., 333–359
Paul, F.T., 6
Pedicled flaps, 334
buccinator flap, 353–355
Carrau-Hadad (C-H) flap, 347–348
Hadad-Bassagaisteguy 2 flap, 345–346
inferior turbinate flap, 342–344
middle turbinate flap, 344–345
occipital galeopericranial flap, 353
Oliver pedicled palatal flap, 355–357
posterior pedicle nasoseptal flap, 336–341
rescue flap, 342
reverse flap, 341–342
temporoparietal fascia flap, 351–353
transfrontal pericranial flap, 348–351
Pedicled nasoseptal flap, 72
Pedicle, harvesting of, 339
Peele, K., 271
Pemberton, L.S., 163, 164

Perfusion-weighted imaging (PWI), 122
Pericranium, 125
Periosteal suture, 260
Perneczky, A., 205, 213
Persistent CSF leaks, 357
Petroclival synchondrosis, 295
Petrous apex, 309
Physaliphorous cells, 284
Pirzkall, A., 271
Pitanguy, I., 126
Pituitary
  apoplexy, 5
  mobilized, 309
  stalk, 94, 132
Pituitary adenomas (PTA), 36
  non-functioning adenomas, 3
  secreting, 3
Pituitary surgery
  effective teamwork, 3
  skills, 3
Pituitary transposition/trans-dorsum sellae technique, 296
Planum sphenoidale, 12
Planum sphenoidal meningiomas, 241
Plasmocytoma, 293
Pneumatization, degree of, 13
Pollock, B., 54, 273
Pontoriero, A., 269–276
Posterior ascending segment, 304
Posterior clinoids, 309
Posterior intercavernous sinuses (PIS), 294
Posterior pedicle nasoseptal flap, 336–341, 358
Posterior septal artery, 338
Postero-superior compartment, 46
Post-fixed variant, 128
Post-operative CSF leak, 138, 176
Pouratian, N., 54
Pourel, N., 271
Prats-Galino, A., 237–251
Pre-fixed optic chiasm, 141
Pre-fixed variant, 128
Preoperative embolization, 238
Prevedello, D.M., 294, 333–359
Progression-free survival (PFS), 163
Prolactinomas, 12, 51, 54
Proton beam radiotherapy
  re-irradiation, 326
  skull base chordomas, 326
Proton MRS, 122
Proton radiotherapy, 166, 272
Protons, 55
Protuberances, 13
Proximal dural ring, 13
Proximal Sylvian fissure dissection, 146
Pseudoaneurysm, formation of, 335
Pseudo-intraventricular craniopharyngioma, 100
Pterion, 126, 226
Pterional approach, 121
Pterional craniotomy, 142
Pterional frontotemporal approach
  transcranial surgery, 205
Pterygoid plates, 43
Pterygoid process, 310
Pterygopalatine fossa, 338

Q

Quadrangular space, 219
Quadrigeminal cysts
  aqueduct distortion, 195
  cyst neuronavigation, 196
  endoscopic third ventriculostomy, 195
  endoscopy, 196
  increased ICP, 196
  VP shunts, 196

R

Radiation-induced complications, 269
Radiation toxicity, 50
Radical resection, 301
Radio-induced optic neuropathy, 275
Radiologic spacer, 335
Radiotherapeutic planning, 49
Radiotherapy, 49, 305
  long-term toxicity, 272
Rajan, B., 164
Ramos, A.S., 126
Raney clips, 129
Ransohoff, J., 237
Rathke's cleft cysts (RCCs), 113
  clinical symptoms, 115–118
  endoscopic endonasal "extended" approaches, 114
  extent of resection, 115–118
  intra-suprasellar, 114–115
  purely suprasellar, 115
  recurrence rate, 115–118
  standard endoscopic endonasal approach, 114
Rathke's pouch, 90
Recurrent craniopharyngioma, 339
Recurrent Heubner arteries, 127
Redo procedure, 307
Regine, W.F., 164
Regional vascularized flaps, 358
Relative cerebral blood volume (rCBV), 122
Reliable bony landmarks, 303
Reliable reconstruction, 334
Rescue flap
  CSF leak, 342
  mucocutaneous junction, 342
Retrochiasmal craniopharyngiomas, 138
Retroclival cysts, 203
Retrosigmoid approach
  transcranial surgery, 205–206
Reverse flap
  anterior ethmoid artery, 341
  artilaginous septum, 341
  intraoperative image guidance, 341
  nasal crusting, 341
  transmural sutures, 341
Rhoton, A.L., 293

Right middle turbinectomy, 338
Rigid endoscope, 142
Rizk, E., 187
Roche, P., 273
Ronson, B.B., 52
Roug, S., 53
Rovin, R., 215–220

S

Sagittal plane, types
    transclival, 333
    transfrontal, 333
    transodontoid, 333
    transplanum, 333
    transsellar, 333
Sajja, R., 271
Saleem, M.A., 165, 166
Samii, M., 63
Sandwich technique, 84, 298
Sarcomatous elements, 284
Scaringi, C., 49–55, 163–167, 323–327
Schloffer, H., 6, 63
Schroeder, H.W.S., 253–267
Schulz-Ertner, D., 164
Secondarily intraventricular craniopharyngioma, 100
Selch, M., 164, 271
Sella-clival junction, 296
Sellar regions, 89
Seneca, V., 237–251
Septal flap, 92
Sequestered fragments, 290
Sheehan, J.P., 54
Shi, X.E., 90
Simpson, D., 213, 224
Simpson Grade I, 242
Single fraction radiosurgery (SRS), 50, 53, 55, 94, 325
Skull base
    anatomy, 43, 255
    meningiomas, 239
    reconstruction, 357
Skull base lesions, defects
    chordomas, 358
    craniopharyngiomas, 358
    encephaloceles, 358
    esthesioneuroblastomas, 358
    pituitary tumors, suprasellar/anterior extension, 358
    skull base meningiomas, 358
Slater, J.D., 271
Solari, D., 11–31, 69–87, 289–298
Solda, F., 271
Solid craniopharyngioma, 151
Somatostatin analogues, 6
Somma, T., 121–134
Spacca, B., 183, 184
Spatulae, 129
Spaziante, R., 105–111, 177
Spennato, P., 179–198
Sphenoethmoid recess, 13
Sphenoid meningiomas
    classification of, 227–228
Sphenoid ostium, 339
Sphenoidotomy, 6
Sphenoid sinus, 290, 308
    pneumatization of, 294
Sphenoid wing meningiomas, 255
Spheno-occipital synchondrosis, 290
Sphenopalatine artery (SPA), 13, 338
    ligation, 310
    position of, 307
Sphenopalatine foramen (SPF), 304, 338
Squamopapillary craniopharyngioma, 72
Stagno, V., 11–31
Stalk-infundibulum axis, 70
"Standard" approach, 69
Standard endoscopic endonasal transsphenoidal
        approach, 11, 175
Standard frontolateral approach, 260
Standard transoral-transpalatal approach, 317
Starke, R.M., 54
Stereotactic irradiation, 50
Stereotactic radiosurgery (SRS), 163, 272–276, 323
    complications, 275
    CyberKnife, 273
    Gammaknife, 272
    hypofractionated treatments, 274
    perioptic meningiomas, 275
    radiation doses, 274
    radio-induced optic neuropathy, 275
    5-session scheme, 275
    tumor control, concept of, 275
Stereotactic radiotherapy (SRT), 6, 148, 152
Stereotactic techniques
    Cyberknife device, 165
    3D conformal, 165
    dose-dependent risk, radiation optic
        neuropathy, 165
    Gamma Knife, 165
    hypofractionated treatment, 166
    hypopituitarism development, 165
    linear accelerator (Linac SRS), 165
    recurrent craniopharyngiomas, 165
Stratified squamous epithelial cells, 113
Strictly IVC, 100
Stripp, D.C., 164
Subchiasmatic space, 16
Subfrontal approach, 237, 241
Subfrontal bilateral approach, 237
    arachnoid plane, 249
    bicoronal skin incision, 248
    Dandy's keyhole, 249
    falx cerebri, 249
    galea, 250
    hyperostotic bone, 250
    optic chiasm and hypothalamus, 249
    subgaleal plane, 248
    superior temporal line, 249
    vascularized pedicled graft, 251
    vascularized pericranium, 250
Subfrontal bilateral craniotomy, 238
Subfrontal/pterional approach, 185
Subfrontal route, 237

Subfrontal unilateral approach
  cerebrospinal fluid, release of, 245
  Dandy's point, 243
  devascularization, 246
  extradural/intradural route, 247
  galeaperiostal flap, 244
  hyperostotic bone, 246
  superficial temporal artery, 242
  venous drainage, 242
Suboccipital midline approach
  transcranial surgery, 206
Subtotal/partial resections, 99
Successful reconstruction, 334
"Sunburst" pattern, 238
Superficial musculo-aponeurotic system (SMAS), 351
Superficial temporal artery, 126, 226
Superior hypophyseal artery, 296
Superior temporal line, 129
Suprachiasmatic region, 16
Supracondylar/transjugular tubercle approach, 297
Supraorbital (SO) approach
  anatomical studies, 141–142
  complications, 147–148
  craniopharyngiomas, 137
  illustrative cases, 148–152
  indications, 138–139
  neuroradiology, 139–141
  recurrent craniopharyngioma, 152
  relative contraindication, 141
  surgical technique, 142–147
  transcranial surgery, 205
Supraorbital (SO) craniotomy, 149, 253
  anterior cranial fossa meningiomas
    anatomy, 255
    indications, 253–254
    neuroradiology, 254–255
    surgical technique, 255–260
  olfactory groove, 254
  planum sphenoidale, 254
  tuberculum sellae, 254
  vs. endonasal approach, 266–267
Supraorbital (SO) eyebrow craniotomy, 137
Supraorbital foramen, 129
Supraorbital "keyhole" craniotomy, 213
Supraorbital notch, 144
Supraorbital region, 146
Supraorbital *vs.* endonasal approach, 266–267
  anterior skullbase meningiomas, 266
  CSF leak rates, 267
  endonasal route, 267
  nasoseptal flap, 266
Suprasellar arachnoid cysts (SACs), 173, 174
  arachnoid diverticulum, 173
  diaphragma sellae, 173
  empty sella, 173
  endoscopic endonasal marsupialization, 177
  preoperative/postoperative assessment, 174
  surgical treatment, 175–177
Suprasellar cysts, 201
  chiasm and hypothalamic-pituitary axis, 185
  cyst-cisternostomy, 186
  subfrontal/pterional approach, 185
  ventriculocystostomy, 185
  wide fenestration, 185, 186
Suprasellar meningiomas
  classification of, 242
Suprasellar notch (SSN), 16, 74
Surgical approach, key factors, 138
Sylvian cerebral fissure, 126
Sylvian fissure, 181, 238
Syndrome of inappropriate secretion of anti-diuretic hormone (SIADH), 116

T

Tailored surgical working corridors, 217
Tang, I.P., 333–359
Tanji, M., 137–152
Tedeschi, E., 289–298
Temporalis muscle, 146
Temporal muscle dissection
  interfascial, 130
  subfascial, 130
  submuscular, 130
Temporo-parietal fascia, 125
Temporoparietal fascia flap
  anatomy
    superficial temporal artery, 351
    temporalis muscle, 351
  hemicoronal incision, 352
  infratemporal/transpterygoid tunnel, 353
  ipsilateral sphenopalatine artery, 352
  sphenopalatine ganglion preservation, 352
  transpterygoid, 351
  window, creating, 351
Teo, C., 223–234
Third ventricle, 90, 121
Thumb sign, 291
Tomasello, F., 155–161
Torres, R., 271, 274
Toxicity, 55
Transcallosal approach
  anatomy, 157
  indications, 155
  neuroradiology, 155–156
  surgical technique, 157–161
  transcranial surgery, 205
Transcondylar route, 297
Transcranial surgery, 6, 12
  endoscopic endonasal trans-sfenoidal approach, 204
  pterional frontotemporal approach, 205
  retrosigmoid approach, 205–206
  suboccipital midline approach, 206
  suboccipital retrosigmoid approach, 205
  supraorbital approach, 205
  third ventricle enlargement, 204

transcallosal approach, 205
ventricle-cyst-cisternostomy, 204
Transfrontal pericranial flap, 358
anterior pericranium, 348
Draf III frontal sinus resection, 349
frontalis layer, 349
superficial temporal artery, 349
supraorbital and supratrochlear neurovascular bundles, 348
transcranial or subfrontal approach, 351
Transmural sutures, 341
Transoral approach, 356
Transoral microscopic approach, 313
Transoral way, 317
Transplanum/transtuberculum approach, 218
Transpterygoid infrapetrous approach, 219
Transpterygoid temporoparietal fascia, 358
Transsphenoidal approach, 6, 11
Transsphenoidal route, 175
Transventricular neuroendoscopy, 100
Trigeminal nerve, ophthalmic division, 15
Trochlear nerve, 15
Tsang, R.W., 52
Tschabitscher, M., 11–31
Tuberculum sellae, 16, 116, 134
Tuberculum sellae meningiomas, 242, 262–265
Tumors(s)
calcifications, 156
cystic, 99
lateral extension, 310
lower clivus, 310
mixed, 99
parasellar, 137
progression, 51
sellar, 137
suprasellar, 137

U
Ulfarsson, E., 166
Ultrasonic aspirator, 128
Unilateral subfrontal approach, 237
Upper clivus, 309
Uy, N., 271

V
Variants
normo-fixed, 128
post-fixed, 128
pre-fixed, 128
Varlotto, J.M., 164
Vascular involvement, 224
Vascularized flaps, 357
Vascularized pedicled graft, 251
Vendrely, V., 271
Ventral corridors, 289
Ventriculocystostomy, 185, 196
Vernimmen, F., 271
Vertebrobasilar junction, 219
Vertebro-basilar junction (VBJ), 297
Vidian nerve, 296
Vik-Mo, E.O., 54
Villa, A., 3–7
Villavicencio, A., 273
Visual deficit, 5
Voges, J., 54
Vomer/nasal cartilage, 339

W
Weber, D., 271
Weiss, M.H., 64
Wenkel, E., 271, 272
WHO classification, 211
Wilson, P.J., 52, 54
Winkler, P.A., 121–134

X
Xu, Z., 166

Y
Yasargil, M.G., 62, 106, 129, 213, 228
Yomo, S., 166

Z
Zenker, F.A., 61
Zierhut, D., 52
Zona, G., 105–111
Zygomatic arch, 125

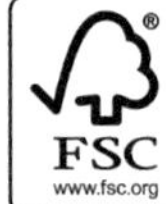

MIX
Papier aus verantwortungsvollen Quellen
Paper from responsible sources
FSC® C105338

If you have any concerns about our products,
you can contact us on
ProductSafety@springernature.com

In case Publisher is established outside the EU,
the EU authorized representative is:
Springer Nature Customer Service Center GmbH
Europaplatz 3, 69115 Heidelberg, Germany

Printed by Libri Plureos GmbH
in Hamburg, Germany